# Electronic Health Records

## Understanding and Using Computerized Medical Records

**Third Edition**

Richard Gartee

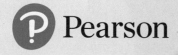 Pearson

330 Hudson Street, NY NY 10013

**Publisher:** Julie Levin Alexander
**Publisher's Assistant:** Sarah Henrich
**Director, Portfolio Management:** Marlene Pratt
**Program Manager:** Faye Gemmellaro
**Program Management, Team Lead:** Melissa Bashe
**Project Management, Team Lead:** Cindy Zonneveld
**Editorial Assistant:** Lauren Bonilla
**Developmental Editor:** Jill Rembetski
**Marketing Manager:** Brittany Hammond
**Senior Marketing Coordinator:** Alicia Wozniak

**Full-Service Project Management:** iEnergizer Aptara®, Ltd.
**Product Strategy Manager:** Amanda Killeen
**Senior Operations Specialist:** Mary Ann Gloriande
**Digital Program Manager:** Amy Peltier
**Digital Project Manager:** Brian Prybella
**Art Director:** Mary Siener
**Cover Image:** Shutterstock: everything possible
**Composition:** iEnergizer Aptara®, Ltd.
**Printing and Binding:** RR Donnelley/Kendallville
**Cover Printer:** Phoenix Color/Hagerstown

All trademarks used in this book are the property of their respective owners.

**Notice:** The authors and the publisher of this volume have taken care that the information and technical recommendations contained herein are based on research and expert consultation and are accurate and compatible with the standards generally accepted at the time of publication. Nevertheless, as new information becomes available, changes in clinical and technical practices become necessary. The reader is advised to carefully consult manufacturers' instructions and information material for all supplies and equipment before use, and to consult with a health care professional as necessary. This advice is especially important when using new supplies or equipment for clinical purposes. The authors and publisher disclaim all responsibility for any liability, loss, injury, or damage incurred as a consequence, directly or indirectly, of the use and application of any of the contents of this volume.

Credits and acknowledgments borrowed from other sources and reproduced, with permission, in this textbook appear on page.

**Library of Congress Cataloging-in-Publication Data**
Names: Gartee, Richard, author.
  Title: Electronic health records : understanding and using computerized
    medical records / Richard Gartee.
  Description: 3rd edition. | Boston : Pearson, 2016.
  Identifiers: LCCN 2016009987 | ISBN 9780134257501 | ISBN 0134257502
  Subjects: | MESH: Electronic Health Records | Forms and Records
  Control–methods
  Classification: LCC R864 | NLM WX 175 | DDC 610.285–dc23 LC record available at
    http://lccn.loc.gov/2016009987

1 16

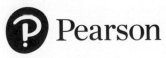

ISBN 10:    0-13-425750-2
ISBN 13: 978-0-13-425750-1

*For Hayley and RJ*

# Contents

Chapter 7

## Problem Lists, Lab Results, and Body Mass Index  254

## Chapter 11 — Privacy and Security of Health Records 443

# Preface

## Introduction

When the first edition of this textbook was published, it predicted that electronic health records would be the "next big thing" in healthcare. Surely that was an optimistic prediction considering at the time only forward thinking clinicians and early adopters of technology were using computers to document their patient encounters. A decade later, the majority of office-based physicians use certified EHR systems, and you would be hard pressed to find a hospital whose records are not computerized.

The upshot is that anyone who works in a healthcare setting needs to understand and be able to use electronic health records. For some healthcare students the proposition of having to learn to interact and care for a patient while documenting the encounter in a computer seems scary. Do not worry. This course will help you build, through practical experience, an understanding and a level of comfort with computerized medical records that can be applied directly in the clinical workplace.

This book was the first of its kind: A textbook focused on training users of an EHR through an innovative "learn by doing" approach. Since the first edition, over 120,000 doctors, nurses, medical assistants, physician assistants, and other healthcare students have made it the bestselling EHR textbook. This third edition continues the mission of providing the learner with a thorough understanding of the EHR that is continuously reinforced by actual EHR experiences.

Updated to reflect the latest rules, regulations, and innovations in EHR, this new edition has more hands-on exercises than previous editions. These exercises use real EHR software to transform theoretical EHR concepts into practical understanding.

Using the combination of textbook and software, you will ready yourself to join an educated clinical workforce that understands and is comfortable with computerized health records. It is my hope that practical application of this new edition will prepare you, the learner, for a bright future in healthcare.

## The Development and Organization of the Text

This book is organized to provide learners with a comprehensive understanding of the history, theory, and functional benefits of Electronic Health Records. Each chapter builds on the knowledge acquired in previous chapters.

**Chapter 1: History and Evolution of Electronic Health Records**   provides a foundation for student learning, introducing concepts and topics that are explained in depth in subsequent chapters. The chapter begins with a definition of Electronic Health Records and identifies the eight core EHR functions that became the basis for certified EHR systems. The chapter then discusses why EHRs are important, and the economic, social, and governmental forces that drove their adoption. Illustrated scenarios compare the workflow of a medical office using paper charts versus one using electronic charts, and the differences between inpatient and outpatient settings. Additional topics include how a medical practice is changed by adoption of an EHR, what constitutes meaningful use of an EHR, as well as patient registration and appointment scheduling.

**Chapter 2: Functional EHR Systems**   explains that the format EHR data is stored in determines the potential uses of EHR data to improve patient care and safety. Chapter 2 describes the various forms of EHR data and the value of using standardized codes for that data. Guided exercises provide the students with an opportunity to explore a component found in most EHR systems—Document Imaging. Major EHR nomenclatures are discussed. The student not only achieves knowledge of EHR nomenclatures and their history, but also their importance in enabling different healthcare systems to exchange data. Functional benefits of an EHR such as trending changes in patients' health, generating medical alerts and decision support such as the drug interaction checking feature of electronic prescription writing software also are covered.

**Chapter 3: Learning Medical Record Software**   introduces the Quippe Student Edition software, which will be used for the remainder of the book. In a series of brief hands-on exercises, the student becomes familiar with EHR concepts, learns to navigate the software, and creates several actual encounter notes. Students also learn how to produce a PDF of their work to print or download.

**Chapter 4: Increased Familiarity with EHR Software**   reinforces the student's computer skills with additional guided exercises. Critical thinking exercises provide step-by-step instructions, but do not provide screen figures for reference. These help students evaluate how well they can use the Student Edition software. A Testing Your Skill exercise at the end of most chapters challenges students to document a patient encounter from a case study.

**Chapter 5: Data Entry at the Point of Care**   stresses the importance of entering data at the time of the encounter, not after the fact. Students learn how to increase data entry speed by using EHR features of Lists, Forms, and pertinent negatives.

**Chapter 6: Understanding Electronic Orders**   continues to build EHR computer skills as students learn how to search the EHR nomenclature and prompt for diagnosis-based order protocols. Students are introduced to computerized order entry and electronic prescriptions that are now required in all certified EHR systems. The workflows of electronic laboratory and radiology order systems are illustrated. Electronic prescription writing illustrates the "closed loop safe medication administration" standard. Hands-on exercises are used for each feature.

**Chapter 7: Problem Lists, Lab Results, and Body Mass Index**   expands on concepts introduced in Chapters 1–6. Hands-on exercises allow students to understand and use patients' longitudinal records while documenting encounters. Students work with problem lists, create problem-oriented charts, and retrieve pending lab results. Students gain firsthand experience trending changes in patients' weight and learn to calculate Body Mass Index from vital signs measurements.

**Chapter 8: Flow Sheets, Annotated Drawings, and Graphs**   teaches the concept of flow sheets and provides students hands-on experiences using flow sheets for several types of patients. Additionally, students learn to annotate medical illustrations electronically to document observations in the EHR and to create graphs of patients' weight and body mass index for patient education.

**Chapter 9: Using the EHR to Improve Patient Health**   focuses on preventative care with hands-on exercises on pediatric wellness visits, immunizations, and preventative care screening. Students extend their understanding of trending by learning about pediatric growth charts. Preventive care screening is emphasized with hand-on exercises demonstrating clinical quality measures. The concept of Patient-Centered Medical Home also is introduced.

**Chapter 10: Decision Support and Patient Involvement**   includes a thorough discussion of the Internet's impact on healthcare, the practice of medicine online, telemedicine, and teleradiology. Hands-on exercises include using integrated decision support documents, online patient education material, and Internet medical research. Patient entry of symptoms and history using the Internet, and E-visits, are experienced by students first-hand. The chapter also covers what is necessary to secure remote provider access.

**Chapter 11: Privacy and Security of Health Records**   provides a thorough presentation of HIPAA privacy and security regulations that are of paramount concern in any medical setting. Critical thinking exercises help the learner put the material in context of their experiences. Chapter 11 also covers HIPAA transactions and code sets, preparing the students for Chapter 12, which ties EHR codes to billing codes.

**Chapter 12: EHR Coding and Reimbursement**   deals with the fact that providers get paid for the vast majority of their work by filing health insurance claims. Health plans require that the codes billed be supported by the encounter documentation. EHR systems help ensure that the documentation matches the code. Using the EHR, this chapter takes a unique approach that helps the student understand the relationship of the encounter note to the Evaluation and Management codes. Hands-on exercises use visual and tactile methods to simplify complicated billing rules and explain how key components determine the billing code.

# Learning Made Easy

## A Unique Approach to Learning Electronic Health Records

This textbook–software package introduces learners to the electronic health record (EHR) through practical applications and guided exercises. The textbook and Student Edition software combination provides a complete learning system. Chapters integrate the history, theory, and benefits of EHR with the opportunity to experience the EHR environment firsthand by completing guided exercises and critical thinking exercises using actual EHR software. Each chapter builds on the knowledge acquired in previous chapters.

## Applying Theory to Practice

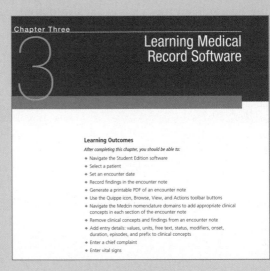

**Chapter Three**

# 3

## Learning Medical Record Software

### Learning Outcomes

*After completing this chapter, you should be able to:*

- Navigate the Student Edition software
- Select a patient
- Set an encounter date
- Record findings in the encounter note
- Generate a printable PDF of an encounter note
- Use the Quippe icon, Browse, View, and Actions toolbar buttons
- Navigate the Medcin nomenclature domains to add appropriate clinical concepts in each section of the encounter note
- Remove clinical concepts and findings from an encounter note
- Add entry details: values, units, free text, status, modifiers, onset, duration, episodes, and prefix to clinical concepts
- Enter a chief complaint
- Enter vital signs

▲ **LEARNING OUTCOMES** Each chapter begins with a list of learning outcomes that highlight the key concepts contained in that chapter.

▼ **KEY TERMS** Key terms are highlighted in a special color throughout chapters and their definitions are also provided in the Glossary for later reference.

**and Secondary Diagnoses**

pt of the primary diagnosis is also important. The primary diagnosis is the ny the patient came to the office or hospital. Other conditions that are during the visit are listed as secondary diagnoses (also called comorbidity). tal, secondary diagnoses are classified as POA, present on admission, or HAC, quired condition.

tions that exist concurrently with the primary diagnosis should be reviewed, or treated and documented in the exam note. Often this is facilitated by a st, which is a summary of ongoing or previous conditions. The problem list linician keep track of the patient's needs beyond the scope of the chief com-today's visit. You will see an example of a problem list in Chapter 7.

**Diagnoses**

iagnoses occur mainly in patients with ongoing or chronic conditions requir-r visits. It is correct and appropriate to continue to use diagnosis codes from for as long as the patient continues to have the illness or condition and that is clearly documented in the record. For example, a patient with diabetes poorly controlled might be seen regularly. With this disease, on some visits t will likely have other problems as well. Therefore, the diagnosis "Diabetes should be included in every visit note and on insurance claims for those visits.

**-Out Diagnosis**

osis for a patient may take more than one visit to be determined or confirmed, npatient billing guidelines do not allow for "possible," "probable," "sus-rule-out," or similar diagnoses. Although the prefix "possible" may be appro-necessary in the exam note, the insurance claim for an outpatient visit should

▼ **ACRONYMS** Acronyms and their meanings are provided in an easy-to-locate quick reference table.

| Acronyms Used in This Book | | | |
|---|---|---|---|
| ABG | Arterial Blood Gas | EDI | Electronic Data Interchange |
| ABN | Advance Beneficiary Notice | EFT | Electronic Funds Transfer |
| ABN | Abnormal | EHR | Electronic Health Record |
| ACA | Affordable Care Act | EMR | Electronic Medical Record |
| ACE | angiotensin-converting-enzyme | ENT | Ears, Nose, Throat |
| AHIMA | American Health Information Management Association | EPHI | Protected Health Information in Electronic form |
| AHRQ | Agency for Healthcare Research and Quality | EPs | Eligible Professionals |
| AMA | Against Medical Advice | ER | Emergency Department or Emergency Room |
| ARRA | American Recovery and Reinvestment Act | FDA | Food and Drug Administration |
| BID | Twice Daily | FEIN | Federal Employer Identification Number |
| BIPAP | Bilevel Positive Airway Pressure | GI | Gastrointestinal |
| BMI | Body Mass Index | H&P | History and Physical |
| BMP | Basic Metabolic Panel | HAC | Hospital Acquired Condition |
| CAT | Computerized Axial Tomography | HCAHPS | Hospital Consumer Assessment Healthcare Providers and Systems |
| CBC | Complete Blood Count | HCPCS | Healthcare Common Procedure Coding System |
| CC | Chief Complaint | | |
| CCC | Clinical Care Classification system | HDL-C | High-Density Lipoprotein (cholesterol test) |
| CCU | Critical Care Unit | HEENT | Head, Eyes, Ears, Nose, (Mouth), and Throat |
| CDC | Centers for Disease Control and Prevention | HepB | Hepatitis B (vaccine) |
| CDISC | Clinical Data Interchange Standards Consortium | HHS | U.S. Department of Health and Human Services |
| CDR | Clinical Data Repository | Hib | Haemophilus influenzae type B (vaccine) |
| CHF | Congestive Heart Failure | HIE | Health Information Exchange |
| CIR | Citywide Immunization Registry (New York City) | HIM | Health Information Management |
| | | HIMSS | Health Information Management Systems Society |
| CME | Continuing Medical Education | HIPAA | Health Insurance Portability and Accountability Act |
| CMS | Centers for Medicare and Medicaid Services | | |
| COB | Coordination of Benefits | HITECH | Health Information Technology for Economic and Clinical Health |
| CPOE | Computerized Provider Order Entry | | |
| CPR | Cardio-Pulmonary Resuscitation | HIV | Human Immunodeficiency Virus |
| CPRI | Computer-Based Patient Record Institute | HL7 | Health Level 7 |
| CPT-4 | Current Procedural Terminology, 4th Revision | HPI | History of Present Illness |
| CRNA | Certified Registered Nurse Anesthesiologist | ICD-9-CM | International Classification of Diseases, ninth revision, with clinical modifications |
| CT | Computed Tomography | ICD-10CM | International Classification of Diseases, tenth revision, with clinical modifications |
| CVP | Cerebral Vascular Pressure | | |
| DAW | Dispense As Written | IMH | Instant Medical History |
| DICOM | Digital Imaging and Communications in Medicine | IOM | Institute of Medicine |
| | | IPV | Inactivated Polio Virus (vaccine) |
| DTaP | Diphtheria, Tetanus, Pertussis (vaccine) | IT | Information Technology |
| DUR | Drug Utilization Review | JCAHO | The Joint Commission on Accreditation of Healthcare Organizations |
| DVT | Deep Vein Thrombosis | | |
| E&M | Evaluation and Management codes | LAN | Local Area Networks |
| ECG or EKG | Electrocardiogram | LIS | Laboratory Information System |

◄ **NOTES** Note boxes found within the chapters emphasize important points or provide additional information.

NOTE

In exercises that permit you to use the current date the patient's age may differ from the age shown in the textbook figures or given in the case study.

► **ALERTS** Alert boxes found within the chapters caution or remind learners about information related to using the software.

ALERT

Make certain you set the date and time correctly for this exercise.

◀ **REAL-LIFE STORY** Each chapter features a Real-Life Story told by a doctor, nurse, administrator, physician assistant, or patient about their experiences with EHR. These vignettes help learners connect chapter content to real life in the clinic.

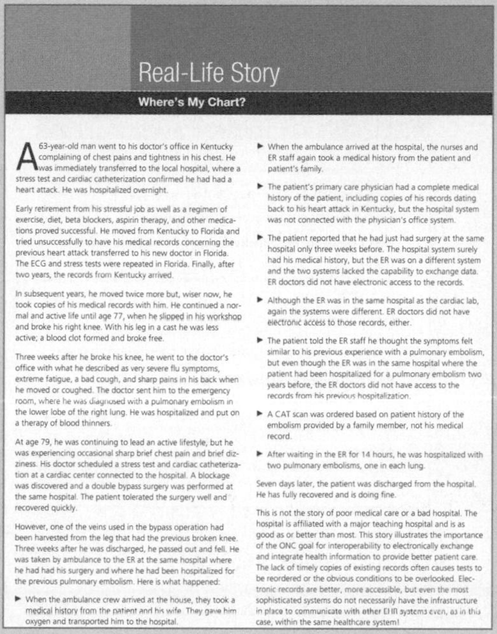

Real-Life Story

Where's My Chart?

A 63-year-old man went to his doctor's office in Kentucky complaining of chest pains and tightness in his chest. He was immediately transferred to the local hospital, where a stress test and cardiac catheterization confirmed he had had a heart attack. He was hospitalized overnight.

Early retirement from his stressful job as well as a regimen of exercise, diet, beta blockers, aspirin therapy, and other medications proved successful. He moved from Kentucky to Florida and tried unsuccessfully to have his medical records concerning the previous heart attack transferred to his new doctor in Florida. The ECG and stress tests were repeated in Florida. Finally, after two years, the records from Kentucky arrived.

In subsequent years, he moved twice more but, wiser now, he took copies of his medical records with him. He continued a normal and active life until age 77, when he slipped in his workshop and broke his right knee. With his leg in a cast he was less active; a blood clot formed and broke free.

Three weeks after he broke his knee, he went to the doctor's office with what he described as very severe flu symptoms, extreme fatigue, a bad cough, and sharp pains in his back when he moved or coughed. The doctor sent him to the emergency room, where he was diagnosed with a pulmonary embolism in the lower lobe of the right lung. He was hospitalized and put on a therapy of blood thinners.

At age 79, he was continuing to lead an active lifestyle, but he was experiencing occasional sharp brief chest pain and brief dizziness. His doctor scheduled a stress test and cardiac catheterization at a cardiac center connected to the hospital. A blockage was discovered and a double bypass surgery was performed at the same hospital. The patient tolerated the surgery well and recovered quickly.

However, one of the veins used in the bypass operation had been harvested from the leg that had the previous broken knee. Three weeks after he was discharged, he passed out and fell. He was taken by ambulance to the ER at the same hospital where he had had his surgery and where he had been hospitalized for the previous pulmonary embolism. Here is what happened:

- When the ambulance crew arrived at the house, they took a medical history from the patient and his wife. They gave him oxygen and transported him to the hospital.
- When the ambulance arrived at the hospital, the nurses and ER staff again took a medical history from the patient and patient's family.
- The patient's primary care physician had a complete medical history of the patient, including copies of his records dating back to his heart attack in Kentucky, but the hospital system was not connected with the physician's office system.
- The patient reported that he had just had surgery at the same hospital only three weeks before. The hospital system surely had his medical history, but the ER was on a different system and the two systems lacked the capability to exchange data. ER doctors did not have electronic access to the records.
- Although the ER was in the same hospital as the cardiac lab, again the systems were different. ER doctors did not have electronic access to those records, either.
- The patient told the ER staff he thought the symptoms felt similar to his previous experience with a pulmonary embolism, but even though the ER was in the same hospital where the patient had been hospitalized for a pulmonary embolism two years before, the ER doctors did not have access to the records from his previous hospitalization.
- A CAT scan was ordered based on patient history of the embolism provided by a family member, not his medical record.
- After waiting in the ER for 14 hours, he was hospitalized with two pulmonary embolisms, one in each lung.

Seven days later, the patient was discharged from the hospital. He has fully recovered and is doing fine.

This is not the story of poor medical care or a bad hospital. The hospital is affiliated with a major teaching hospital and is as good as or better than most. This story illustrates the importance of the ONC goal for interoperability to electronically exchange and integrate health information to provide better patient care. The lack of timely copies of existing records often causes tests to be reordered or the obvious conditions to be overlooked. Electronic records are better, more accessible, but even the most sophisticated systems do not necessarily have the infrastructure in place to communicate with other EHR systems even, as in this case, within the same healthcare system!

▶ **CHAPTER SUMMARY** Summaries at the end of each chapter synthesize key points for students and include a reference table of exercises that cover specific EHR skills.

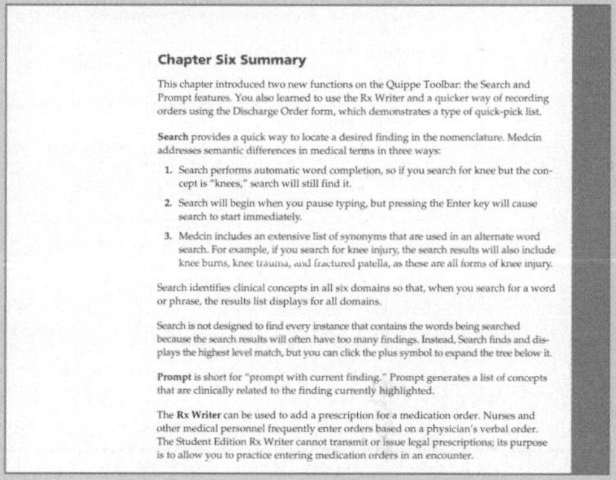

**Chapter Six Summary**

This chapter introduced two new functions on the Quippe Toolbar: the Search and Prompt features. You also learned to use the Rx Writer and a quicker way of recording orders using the Discharge Order form, which demonstrates a type of quick-pick list.

**Search** provides a quick way to locate a desired finding in the nomenclature. Medcin addresses semantic differences in medical terms in three ways:

1. Search performs automatic word completion, so if you search for knee but the concept is "knees," search will still find it.
2. Search will begin when you pause typing, but pressing the Enter key will cause search to start immediately.
3. Medcin includes an extensive list of synonyms that are used in an alternate word search. For example, if you search for knee injury, the search results will also include knee burns, knee trauma, and fractured patella, as these are all forms of knee injury.

Search identifies clinical concepts in all six domains so that, when you search for a word or phrase, the results list displays for all domains.

Search is not designed to find every instance that contains the words being searched because the search results will often have too many findings. Instead, Search finds and displays the highest level match, but you can click the plus symbol to expand the tree below it.

**Prompt** is short for "prompt with current finding." Prompt generates a list of concepts that are clinically related to the finding currently highlighted.

The **Rx Writer** can be used to add a prescription for a medication order. Nurses and other medical personnel frequently enter orders based on a physician's verbal order. The Student Edition Rx Writer cannot transmit or issue legal prescriptions; its purpose is to allow you to practice entering medication orders in an encounter.

## Practice Opportunities

◀ **GUIDED EXERCISES** Guided hands-on exercises using a step-by-step approach allow the students to learn by doing. The companion Student Edition software provides a computer experience using real EHR software actually found in medical facilities.

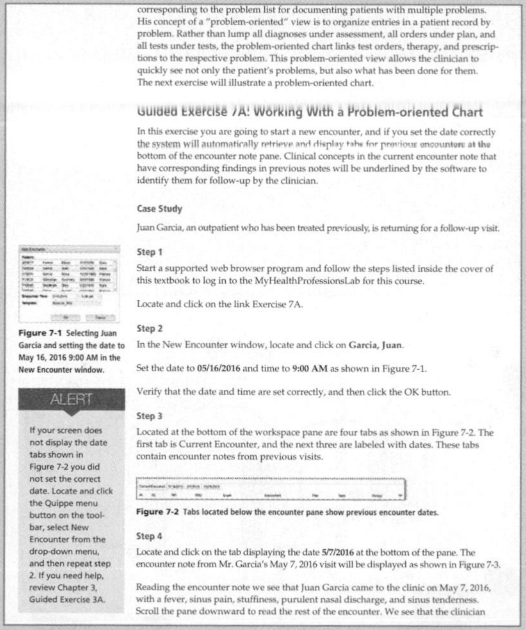

corresponding to the problem list for documenting patients with multiple problems. His concept of a "problem-oriented" view is to organize entries in a patient record by problem. Rather than lump all diagnoses under assessment, all orders under plan, and all tests under tests, the problem-oriented chart links test orders, therapy, and prescriptions to the respective problem. This problem-oriented view allows the clinician to quickly see not only the patient's problems, but also what has been done for them. The next exercise will illustrate a problem-oriented chart.

**Guided Exercise 7A: Working With a Problem-oriented Chart**

In this exercise you are going to start a new encounter, and if you set the date correctly the system will automatically retrieve and display tabs for previous encounters at the bottom of the encounter note pane. Clinical concepts in the current encounter note that have corresponding findings in previous notes will be underlined by the software to identify them for follow-up by the clinician.

**Case Study**

Juan Garcia, an outpatient who has been treated previously, is returning for a follow-up visit.

**Step 1**

Start a supported web browser program and follow the steps listed inside the cover of this textbook to log in to the MyHealthProfessionsLab for this course.

Locate and click on the link Exercise 7A.

**Figure 7-1** Selecting Juan Garcia and setting the date to May 16, 2016 9:00 AM in the New Encounter window.

**Step 2**

In the New Encounter window, locate and click on **Garcia, Juan**.

Set the date to **05/16/2016** and time to **9:00 AM** as shown in Figure 7-1.

Verify that the date and time are set correctly, and then click the OK button.

ALERT

If your screen does not display the date tabs shown in Figure 7-2 you did not set the correct date. Locate and click the Quippe menu button on the toolbar, select New Encounter from the drop-down menu, and then repeat step 2. If you need help, review Chapter 3, Guided Exercise 3A.

**Step 3**

Located at the bottom of the workspace pane are four tabs as shown in Figure 7-2. The first tab is Current Encounter, and the next three are labeled with dates. These tabs contain encounter notes from previous visits.

**Figure 7-2** Tabs located below the encounter pane show previous encounter dates.

**Step 4**

Locate and click on the tab displaying the date **5/7/2016** at the bottom of the pane. The encounter note from Mr. Garcia's May 7, 2016 visit will be displayed as shown in Figure 7-3.

Reading the encounter note we see that Juan Garcia came to the clinic on May 7, 2016, with a fever, sinus pain, stuffiness, purulent nasal discharge, and sinus tenderness. Scroll the pane downward to read the rest of the encounter. We see that the clinician

▼ **CRITICAL THINKING EXERCISES** Hands-on critical thinking exercises challenge learners to extend what they have learned through their completion of the guided exercises by applying their knowledge in a new way.

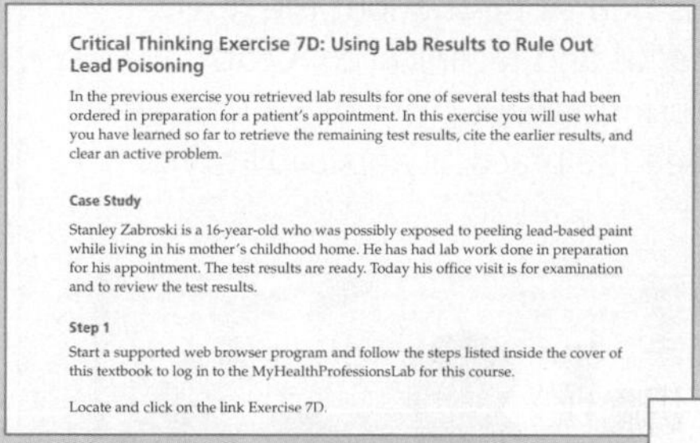

**Critical Thinking Exercise 7D: Using Lab Results to Rule Out Lead Poisoning**

In the previous exercise you retrieved lab results for one of several tests that had been ordered in preparation for a patient's appointment. In this exercise you will use what you have learned so far to retrieve the remaining test results, cite the earlier results, and clear an active problem.

**Case Study**

Stanley Zabroski is a 16-year-old who was possibly exposed to peeling lead-based paint while living in his mother's childhood home. He has had lab work done in preparation for his appointment. The test results are ready. Today his office visit is for examination and to review the test results.

**Step 1**

Start a supported web browser program and follow the steps listed inside the cover of this textbook to log in to the MyHealthProfessionsLab for this course.

Locate and click on the link Exercise 7D.

▶ **TESTING YOUR SKILL EXERCISES** Hands-on skill exercises challenge students to extrapolate information from a case study and apply their learned experience to document a patient visit.

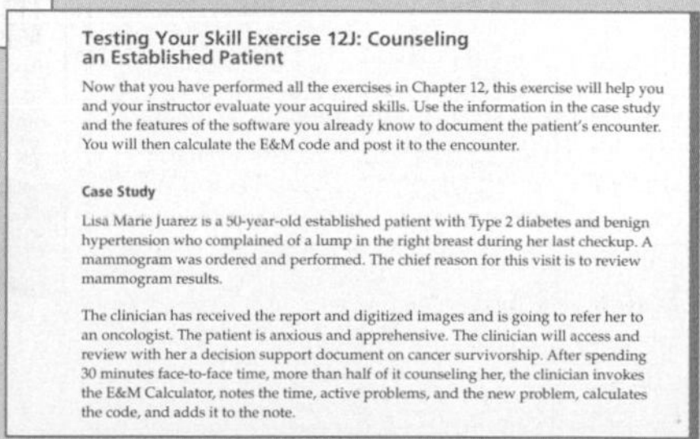

**Testing Your Skill Exercise 12J: Counseling an Established Patient**

Now that you have performed all the exercises in Chapter 12, this exercise will help you and your instructor evaluate your acquired skills. Use the information in the case study and the features of the software you already know to document the patient's encounter. You will then calculate the E&M code and post it to the encounter.

**Case Study**

Lisa Marie Juarez is a 50-year-old established patient with Type 2 diabetes and benign hypertension who complained of a lump in the right breast during her last checkup. A mammogram was ordered and performed. The chief reason for this visit is to review mammogram results.

The clinician has received the report and digitized images and is going to refer her to an oncologist. The patient is anxious and apprehensive. The clinician will access and review with her a decision support document on cancer survivorship. After spending 30 minutes face-to-face time, more than half of it counseling her, the clinician invokes the E&M Calculator, notes the time, active problems, and the new problem, calculates the code, and adds it to the note.

**▼ TESTING YOUR KNOWLEDGE** Online multiple-choice questions at the end of each chapter allow learners to test their knowledge and think critically.

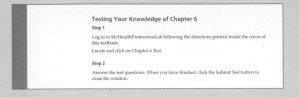

**► COMPREHENSIVE EVALUATION** Learners will test their mastery of the material through two comprehensive evaluations found at the midpoint and end of the text. Each evaluation includes a written exam and hands-on critical thinking exercises.

### Comprehensive Evaluation of Chapters 1–6

This comprehensive evaluation will enable you and your instructor to determine your understanding of the material covered so far. Complete both the online test and the two exercises provided below. Depending on the time provided, it may be necessary to do this in two separate sessions. Your instructor will advise you. Do not begin the Part III exercise if there will not be enough class time to complete it.

**Part I–Testing Your Knowledge of Chapters 1–6**

**Step 1**

Log in to MyHealthProfessionsLab following the directions printed inside the cover of this textbook.

Locate and click on Comprehensive Evaluation Test 1.

**Step 2**

Answer the test questions. When you have finished, click the Submit Test button.

**Part II–Guided Exercise CE1: Document Image Retrieval**

Use the document image simulation program to retrieve scanned documents and locate the answers to five questions from information contained in them.

**Case Study**

Raj Patel is an 80-year-old male who arrives in the emergency department accompanied by his daughter. His daughter informs the triage nurse that Mr. Patel was previously an inpatient at this hospital.

---

## Visualizing the Electronic Health Record

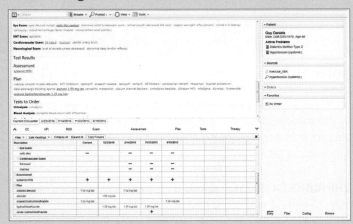

**► SCREEN CAPTURES** Easy-to-follow, step-by-step screen captures of the computer screens from the Student Edition software illustrate the steps of the exercise. They serve as a ready reference to help learners orient themselves and assess their progress as they master content.

**▼ FIGURES AND TABLES** Numerous figures throughout the text help learners visualize workflow scenarios and technical concepts. Photographs of healthcare providers using various types of EHR systems and medical devices make it easy to see the practical applicability in a medical office.

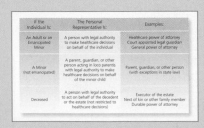

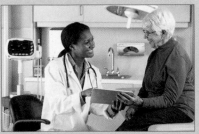

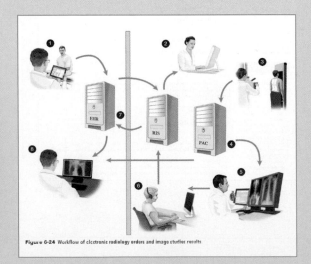

Figure 6-24 Workflow of electronic radiology orders and image studies results.

# The Student Edition Software

- The Quippe® software used for this course is the latest version of the same clinical documentation tool found in commercial EHR software, and contains the entire Medcin nomenclature used in professional EHR systems. Because leading EHR systems for medical offices use the Medcin nomenclature as the technology underlying commercial EHR systems, students in most cases may apply skills they acquire in this course directly to an EHR application in their office. Those systems may not be identical to the student software, but they will seem very familiar to someone who has completed this course.
- The web-based Student Edition software is accessed through Pearson's MyHealthProfessionsLab. The Student Edition software does not need to be downloaded or installed. Its web-based architecture makes it independent of the type of computer or operating system, so long as a compatible web browser is used. This is ideal for distance learning students or those who wish to work outside the classroom.
- Hands-on exercises are short and have been designed to be completed in a normal class time.
- The web-based software allows all students to work simultaneously and yet keeps each student's work separate.
- Most exercises are scored automatically at the end of the exercise so students can see in the LMS how they have done without delay.
- Encounter notes created during the exercises can be output to a PDF file, which may be downloaded or printed for the student's record or to turn in.
- Free Adobe Reader software may be used to print the PDF to any compatible printer.

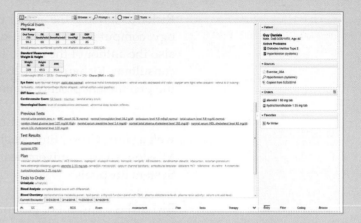

# Software Requirements

To complete the exercises in this book, you will need Internet access. You will also need to purchase an access code card and register for the MyHealthProfessionsLab for this course. Instructions are provided on the inside cover of this book.

You must use a compatible web browser. Because browsers change over time, you will find the current list of compatible browsers on the MyHealthProfessionsLab site.

Although a device may have Internet capability, some device screens may be too small to easily navigate the software, in which case a computer or a tablet with a larger screen should be used.

Ideally, use a mouse with at least two buttons that respectively perform the right- and left-click functions.

### Software License Notice

The Quippe Student Edition software is licensed only for educational purposes, to allow the student to perform exercises in the textbook.

By using this program, a healthcare provider agrees that this product is not intended to suggest or replace any medical decisions or actions with respect to the patient's medical care and that the sole and exclusive responsibility for determining the accuracy, completeness, or appropriateness of any diagnostic, clinical, billing, or other medical information provided by the program and any underlying clinical database resides solely with the healthcare provider. Licensor assumes no responsibility for how such materials are used and disclaims all warranties, whether expressed or implied, including any warranty as to the quality, accuracy, or suitability of this information and product for any particular purpose.

# About the Author

Richard Gartee is the author of seven college textbooks on health information technology, computerized medical systems, managed care, and electronic health records. He is also the author of the novel, *Lancelot's Grail*. Before becoming a full-time author and consultant, Richard spent 20 years in the design, development, and implementation of the preeminent practice management and electronic health records systems.

Richard also served as a liaison to other companies in the medical computer industry as well as Blue Cross/Blue Shield, a U.S. Department of Commerce International Trade Mission, various universities, and EHR design consultant for the Aravind Eye Care System hospitals.

Richard is a current or past member of many of the professional organizations and national standards groups recommended in this book:

◆ American Health Information Management Association (AHIMA)

◆ Healthcare Information Management Systems Society (HIMSS)

◆ American National Standards Institute (ANSI) X12n Committee for Development of Electronic Claims Standards

◆ Health Level Seven (HL7) Committee for Development of Claims Attachment Standards

◆ Workgroup for Electronic Data Interchange (WEDI) Task Force for Development of Electronic Remittance Guidelines

◆ A faculty member/speaker at the Medical Records Institute international Electronic Health Records Conference (TEPR) for 12 years

# Acknowledgments

This book was made possible by the contribution of many individuals and several of the most prominent commercial EHR vendors, whom I personally would like to thank and acknowledge here.

I first would like to thank Peter S. Goltra, David Lareau, Dan Gainer, Karen Chapman, and Roy Soltoff of Medicomp Systems, Inc. for allowing us to use Quippe software for the Student Edition.

Peter S. Goltra is the father of the Medcin nomenclature. He is the founder of Medicomp Systems, which he established in 1978 to develop advanced documentation and diagnostic tools for use by physicians at the point of care. His honors include an award from the American Medical Informatics Association for contributions to the field of medical informatics.

David Lareau is chief executive officer of Medicomp Systems, Inc. Before joining Medicomp in 1995, Mr. Lareau founded and served as CEO of a medical software and billing company and served as controller of one of the nation's largest distribution companies. In addition to his CEO duties, David has responsibility for operations and product management, including customer relations and marketing. David is the leading proponent of the Medcin nomenclature, having personally presented it to thousands of physicians, key EHR developers, and decision makers during his tenure.

Dan Gainer is Chief Technology Officer of Medicomp. Gainer joined Medicomp in 2005 as a Senior Software Engineer and led the charge to move the company to web-based capabilities. Gainer was instrumental in Medicomp's development and launch of Quippe and continues to lead the development team to expand Quippe products and offerings.

Dan has more than 23 years' experience in software development in a number of industries including healthcare, accounting, education, and financial services. Before joining Medicomp, Gainer co-founded a company that provides accounting software for small businesses that contract with the federal government.

Karen Chapman is senior product manager at Medicomp Systems, Inc. Prior to joining Medicomp Systems, Karen spearheaded the training and implementation efforts for the Department of Defense's EHR, which includes the Medicomp MEDCIN Engine, developing training curriculum, implementation best practices, and conducting multiple training courses. Karen joined Medicomp in 2013, where she now focuses on all aspects of Quippe including overall direction, new features, testing, release, and customer support and training.

Roy Soltoff is senior developer at Medicomp Systems. Mr. Soltoff has been involved in software development, starting with AT&T in 1964. He joined the Medicomp development staff in 1992 and has been responsible for significant advances in clinical user interface design.

The medical content and EHR theory of the textbook were greatly enhanced by my acquaintance with Allen R. Wenner, MD, a physician, teacher, author, speaker, and expert on information technology, and with John Bachman, MD, professor of family medicine at Mayo Clinic, Rochester, Minnesota. I would also like to thank Kimberly Freese Beal, MD, and Sharyl Beal, RN, MSN, for their advice on several of the exercises, and Jim O'Connor, MD, for his advice on asthma codes.

My special thanks go to the many individuals who shared firsthand experiences in real-life stories and allowed them to be used in this book. Their unique perspectives help the student understand the relationship of the conceptual to the practical. I would like to thank Richard A. Gartee, Michelle White (whose story was written by Julie DeSantis), Allen R. Wenner, MD, Sharyl Beal, RN, MSN, Michael Lukowski, MD, Marney Thompson, RN, Henry Palmer, MD, Primetime Medical (who contributed the real-life story of Mr. John Gould), Alison Connelly, P.A., Tanya Townsend, CIO, Karen L. Smith, MD, and Philip C. Yount, MD.

I am also indebted to Greenway Health, LLC and Primetime Medical Software & Instant Medical History for allowing their copyrighted work to be reprinted herein.

Also thanks to Michael Lukowski, MD for allowing me to reproduce his GYN form.

I would also like to acknowledge the help of all my editors who assisted me with this work.

# Reviewers

I would like to thank the academic reviewers, who took time to review and comment on this book.

**Reviewers for the 3rd Edition**

**Natasha Bratton**
Program Coordinator
Centura College
North Charleston, SC

**Marion Bucci, M.Ed., RMA**
Faculty - Healthcare Professions
Montgomery County Community College
Blue Bell, PA

**Angela Chisley, AHI, RMA, CMAA, EHR Trainer**
Adjunct Professor
University of the District of Columbia; College of Southern Maryland
Washington, DC

**Pamela Christianson, MS, CMA (AAMA), CPhT (PTCB)**
Program Director - Medical Assisting/ Pharmacy Technician
Great Falls College - Montana State University
Great Falls, MT

**Abbie Clavio, MD, RMA, CBCS**
Professor/Instructor
Technical Career Institute College of Technology; Metropolitan College of New York
New York, NY

**Kathryn Hansen, BS, CPC, CPMA, REEGT**
Adjunct Faculty
Medtech College; Bluegrass Community and Technical College
Lexington, KY

**Gloria Madison, MS, RHIA, CHDA, CHTS-IM**
Program Director - Health Information Technology
Moraine Park Technical College
West Bend, WI

**Sharone Roberts, CEHRS, NCICS, CCS**
Program Manager
Harris School of Business
Cherry Hill, NJ

**Staci Waldrep, MS, RHIT**
Program Director - Health Information Technology
Lamar Institute of Technology
Beaumont, TX

**Barb Westrick, AAS, CMA, CPC**
Program Chair - Medical Assisting and Medical Insurance Billing/Office Administration
Ross Medical Education Center
Brighton, MI

## Quippe Advisory Board and Medcin Consulting Editors

Finally, I would like to recognize the work of the doctors who consulted on the development of the Medcin nomenclature and serve on the Quippe Advisory board. These clinicians did not review the exercises in this book, but they did review the medical accuracy of the Medcin nomenclature that underlies this entire work. Therefore, I would like to acknowledge their work in the development and evolution of the knowledge base on which the Quippe Student Edition is based.

**Jay Anders, MD**
Chief Medical Officer
Medicomp Systems, Inc.
Washington, DC

**Robert G. Barone, MD**
Clinical Instructor
University of Medicine and Dentistry of New Jersey
Newark, NJ

**J. Gregory Cairncross, MD**
Department Head of Clinical Neurological Sciences
Alberta Health Services
Calgary, Alberta, Canada

**Edmund M. Herrold, MD, PhD**
Director of Clinical Cardiology and Professor of Medicine
The State University of New York, Downstate Medical College
Associate Professor in the Department of Medicine
Division of Cardiology and Department of Cardiothoracic Surgery
Cornell University Medical College
New York, NY

**Paul F. Miskovitz, MD**
Clinical Associate Professor of Medicine in Gastroenterology and Hepatology
Cornell University Medical College
Attending Physician
New York Presbyterian Hospital
New York, NY

# History and Evolution of Electronic Health Records

## Learning Outcomes

*After completing this chapter, you should be able to:*

◆ Define electronic health records

◆ Understand the core functions of an electronic health record as defined by the Institute of Medicine

◆ Discuss social forces that are driving the adoption of electronic health records

◆ Describe federal government strategies to promote electronic health record adoption

◆ Explain why patient visits should be documented at the point of care

◆ Explain why electronic health records are important

◆ Describe the flow of medical information into the chart

◆ Compare the workflow of an office using paper charts with an office using an electronic health record

◆ Contrast inpatient and outpatient charts

◆ Discuss patient registration and appointment scheduling

## History of Electronic Health Records

The idea of computerizing patients' medical records has been around for years, but only in the past decade has it become widely adopted. Prior to the electronic health record (EHR), a patient's medical records consisted of handwritten notes, typed reports, and test results stored in a paper file system. Today paper medical records are used in fewer healthcare facilities. The transition to electronic health records is well underway.

## Institute of Medicine (IOM)

Beginning in 1991, the IOM (a division of the National Academies of Sciences, Engineering, and Medicine) sponsored studies and created reports that led the way toward the concepts we have in place today for electronic health records. Originally, the IOM called them *computer-based patient records*.[1] During their evolution, EHRs have had many other names, including *electronic medical records, computerized medical records, longitudinal patient records*, and *electronic charts*. All of these names referred to something intended to replace the paper chart. In 2003, the IOM chose the name *electronic health records*, or EHR, because "health" means "a state of well-being," and the goal of computerizing medical records is to improve the delivery of safe, quality care focused on patients' health.

The IOM report[2] put forth a set of eight core functions that an EHR should be capable of performing. The influence this report had on the development of EHR cannot be overstated. The eight core functions listed here became determining factors in the evolution of EHR, and the ability to perform these functions is the criteria by which EHRs are judged.

The eight core functions are as follows:

**Health information and data** This function provides a defined data set that includes such items as medical and nursing diagnoses, a medication list, allergies, demographics, clinical narratives, and laboratory test results. Further, it provides improved access to information needed by care providers when they need it.

**Result management** Computerized results can be accessed more easily (than paper reports) by the provider at the time and place they are needed.

◆ Reduced lag time allows for quicker recognition and treatment of medical problems.

◆ The automated display of previous test results makes it possible to reduce redundant and additional testing.

◆ Having electronic results can allow for better interpretation and for easier detection of abnormalities, thereby ensuring appropriate follow-up.

◆ Access to electronic consults and patient consents can establish critical links and improve care coordination among multiple providers, as well as between provider and patient.

**Order management** Computerized provider order entry (CPOE) systems can improve workflow processes by eliminating lost orders and ambiguities caused by illegible handwriting, generating related orders automatically, monitoring for duplicate orders, and reducing the time required to fill orders.

◆ CPOE systems for medications reduce the number of errors in medication dose and frequency, drug allergies, and drug–drug interactions.

◆ The use of CPOE, in conjunction with an EHR, also improves clinician productivity.

**Decision support** Computerized decision support systems include prevention, prescribing of drugs, diagnosis and management, and detection of adverse events and disease outbreaks.

◆ Computer reminders and prompts improve preventive practices in areas such as vaccinations, breast cancer screening, colorectal screening, and cardiovascular risk reduction.

---

[1] R. S. Dick and E. B. Steen, *The Computer-based Patient Record: An Essential Technology for Health Care* (Washington, DC: Institute of Medicine, National Academy Press, 1991, revised 1997, 2000).
[2] Ibid.

**Electronic communication and connectivity** Electronic communication among care partners can enhance patient safety and quality of care, especially for patients who have multiple providers in multiple settings that must coordinate care plans.

◆ Electronic connectivity is essential in creating and populating EHR systems with data from laboratory, pharmacy, radiology, and other providers.

◆ Secure e-mail and web messaging have been shown to be effective in facilitating communication both among providers and with patients, thus allowing for greater continuity of care and more timely interventions.

◆ Automatic alerts to providers regarding abnormal laboratory results reduce the time until an appropriate treatment is ordered.

◆ Electronic communication is fundamental to the creation of an integrated health record, both within a setting and across settings and institutions.

**Patient support** Computer-based patient education has been found to be successful in improving control of chronic illnesses, such as diabetes, in primary care.

◆ Examples of home monitoring by patients using electronic devices include self-testing by patients with asthma (spirometry), glucose monitors for patients with diabetes, and Holter monitors for patients with heart conditions. Data from monitoring devices can be merged into the EHR, as shown in Figure 1-1.

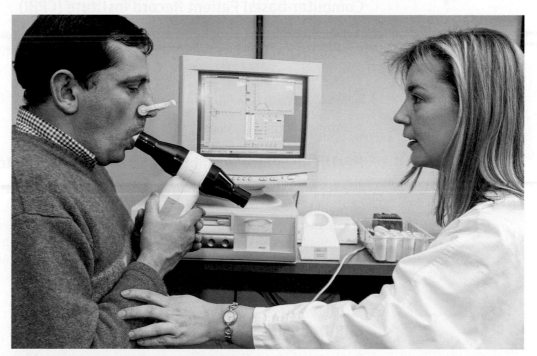

Courtesy of Javier Larrea/age fotostock/Getty Images

**Figure 1-1** Data from the digital spirometer transfers to the EHR.

**Administrative processes and reporting** Electronic scheduling systems increase the efficiency of healthcare organizations and provide better, timelier service to patients.

◆ Communication and content standards are important in the billing and claims management area.

◆ Electronic authorization and prior approvals can eliminate delays and confusion; immediate validation of insurance eligibility results in more timely payments and less paperwork.

- EHR data can be analyzed to identify patients who are potentially eligible for clinical trials, as well as candidates for chronic disease management programs.

- Reporting tools support drug recalls.

**Reporting and population health** Public- and private-sector reporting requirements at the federal, state, and local levels for patient safety and quality, as well as for public health, are more easily met with computerized data because it

- eliminates the labor-intensive and time-consuming abstraction of data from paper records and the errors that often occur in a manual process.

- facilitates the reporting of key quality indicators used for the internal quality improvement efforts of many healthcare organizations.

- improves public health surveillance and timely reporting of adverse reactions and disease outbreaks.

Later in this chapter, we will discuss initiatives by the U.S. government to encourage the development of healthcare information technology. The IOM definitions of core functions influenced and were adapted into the strategic framework developed by the government. Subsequent chapters will refer back to these eight core functions as you learn to use the EHR functionality that evolved to meet them.

## Computer-based Patient Record Institute (CPRI)

Another early contributor to the thinking on EHR systems was the **Computer-based Patient Record Institute (CPRI)**, which identified three key criteria for an EHR:

- Capture data at the point of care

- Integrate data from multiple sources

- Provide decision support

## Health Insurance Portability and Accountability Act (HIPAA)

The **Health Insurance Portability and Accountability Act (HIPAA)**, which will be covered in Chapter 11, did not define an EHR, but perhaps the HIPAA Security Rule broadened the definition. The Security Rule established protection for *all* personally identifiable health information stored in electronic format. Thus, everything about a patient stored in a healthcare provider's system is protected and treated as part of the patient's EHR. HIPAA also standardized transaction formats for several Administrative Processes identified in the IOM report.

## EHR Defined

In *Electronic Health Records: Changing the Vision*, authors Murphy, Waters, Hanken, and Pfeiffer define the EHR to include "any information relating to the past, present or future physical/mental health, or condition of an individual which resides in electronic system(s) used to capture, transmit, receive, store, retrieve, link and manipulate multimedia data for the primary purpose of providing healthcare and health-related services."[3]

The core functions defined by the IOM and CPRI suggest that the EHR is not just what data is stored, but what can be done with it. In the broadest sense, *Electronic Health Records are the portions of a patient's medical records that are stored in a computer system as*

---

[3]Gretchen Murphy, Kathleen Waters, Mary A. Hanken, and Maureen Pfeiffer, eds., *Electronic Health Records: Changing the Vision* (Philadelphia: W. B. Saunders Company, 1999), 5.

*well as the functional benefits derived from having an electronic health record.* EHRs focus on and promote the total health of the patient.

## Social Forces Driving EHR Adoption

Visionary leaders in medical informatics had been making the case for the EHR for a long time. However, the combination of several important reports caught the public's attention and set in motion economic and political forces that drove the transformation of our medical records systems.

### Health Safety

The IOM published a report that stated the following: "Healthcare in the United States is not as safe as it should be—and can be. At least 44,000 people, and perhaps as many as 98,000 people, die in hospitals each year as a result of medical errors that could have been prevented, according to estimates from two major studies.

"Beyond their cost in human lives, preventable medical errors exact other significant tolls. They have been estimated to result in total costs (including the expense of additional care necessitated by the errors, lost income and household productivity, and disability) of between $17 billion and $29 billion per year in hospitals nationwide. Errors also are costly in terms of loss of trust in the healthcare system by patients and diminished satisfaction by both patients and health professionals.

"A variety of factors have contributed to the nation's epidemic of medical errors. One oft-cited problem arises from the decentralized and fragmented nature of the healthcare delivery system—or 'non-system,' to some observers. When patients see multiple providers in different settings, none of whom has access to complete information, it becomes easier for things to go wrong."[4]

Over a decade later, the IOM reported[5] medical errors still occurring routinely, citing a study of 10 North Carolina hospitals over a 5-year period that found approximately 18 percent of patients were harmed by medical care, with 63 percent of those cases being judged as preventable. These findings were reinforced by a nationwide study revealing that one in seven Medicare patients suffered harm from hospital care, with an additional one in seven suffering temporary harm from care-related problems that were detected in time and corrected; 44 percent of these errors were found to be preventable.

In the report conclusion, the IOM committee recommended ten actions to achieve the best care at lower costs. Five of them involving EHR were:

◆ Improve the digital infrastructure capacity to capture clinical, care delivery process, and financial data,

◆ Streamline and revise research regulations to improve care, promote the capture of clinical data, and generate knowledge.

◆ Accelerate integration of the best clinical knowledge into care decisions through clinical decision support.

---

[4]Linda T. Kohn, Janet M. Corrigan, and Molla S. Donaldson, eds., *To Err Is Human: Building a Safer Health System* (Washington, DC: Committee on Quality of Healthcare in America, Institute of Medicine, 1999).
[5]Mark Smith, Robert Saunders, Leigh Stuckhardt, and J. Michael McGinnis, eds., *Best Care at Lower Cost: The Path to Continuously Learning Health Care in America* (Washington, DC: Committee on the Learning Health Care System in America, The National Academies Press, 2012).

- ◆ Offer patient-centered care involving patients and families in decisions regarding health and health care, tailored to fit their preferences.
- ◆ Improve continuity of care by coordination and communication within and across organizations.

## Health Costs

The 1999 IOM report got the attention of the press and public. It also got the attention of 150 of the nation's largest employers who sponsored employee health insurance programs and had become frustrated by the increasing costs of health insurance benefits for which they had little or no say about the quality of care. Following the release of the IOM report, these employers formed the Leapfrog group.

A study by the Center for Information Technology Leadership found more than 130,000 life-threatening situations caused by adverse drug reactions alone. The study suggested that $44 billion could be saved annually by installing computerized physician order entry systems in ambulatory settings.

Leapfrog created a strategy that tied purchase of group health insurance benefits to quality care standards. It also promoted computerized provider order entry (CPOE) as a means of reducing errors.

## Changing Society

Changes in the way we live have also made paper medical records outdated. In an increasingly mobile society, patients relocate and change doctors more frequently, thus needing to transfer their medical records from previous doctors to new ones. Additionally, many patients no longer have a single general practitioner who provides their total care. Increased specialization and the development of new methods of diagnostic and preventive medicine require the ability to share exam records among different specialists and testing facilities.

The Internet, one of the strongest forces for social change in the past two decades, has also affected healthcare. Consumers became accustomed to being able to access very sensitive information securely over the web. They ask, "If I can bank online securely; if I can trade stocks and see my brokerage account; if I can check in for my airline flight and print my boarding passes; why can't I see my lab test result online?"

The World Wide Web also gave patients unprecedented access to medical information and research. There are literally millions of health-related pieces of information on the web. Patients are arriving at their doctors' offices armed with questions and sometimes answers. Medical information previously unavailable to the average consumer is now as easy to access as searching Google™ or WebMD®.

In response medical offices created interactive web sites (portals) to allow patients to view their records, make appointments, or request prescription renewals. In a number of states it is even possible for patients and doctors to conduct medical visits via the Internet. These are called E-visits and will be discussed further in Chapter 10.

The increased capabilities of smart phones and other mobile devices to track and store heart rate and other personal fitness data as well as to link to devices that measure respiration rate, blood pressure, and blood glucose levels provide a wealth of self-generated patient health data. The challenge is how to integrate that data into the provider's decision-making process.

## Group Discussion Topic: EHR News

1. The topic of EHR is frequently in the news. Describe something you have read or seen on the web or television about EHR.

## Forces Driving EHR Evolution

The response to the IOM report on the rate of preventable medical errors was swift and positive, within both the government and private sectors. Almost immediately, President Bill Clinton's administration issued an executive order instructing government agencies that conduct or oversee healthcare programs to implement proven techniques for reducing medical errors and creating a task force to find new strategies for reducing errors. Congress appropriated $50 million to the Agency for Healthcare Research and Quality (AHRQ) to support a variety of efforts targeted at reducing medical errors.

President George W. Bush followed through by establishing the **Office of the National Coordinator for Health Information Technology (ONC)**, under the U.S. Department of Health and Human Services (HHS), to "develop, maintain, and direct the implementation of a strategic plan to guide the nationwide implementation of interoperable health information technology in both the public and private healthcare sectors that will reduce medical errors, improve quality, and produce greater value for healthcare expenditures."[6]

President Barack Obama identified the EHR as a priority for his administration and signed into law the **Health Information Technology for Economic and Clinical Health (HITECH) Act**, which promoted the widespread adoption of EHR.[7] Note that the HITECH Act is contained within the American Recovery and Reinvestment Act (ARRA); therefore, you may see it referred to by the ARRA designation as well.

## Office of National Coordinator for Health Information Technology

David J. Brailer, M.D., Ph.D., the first National Coordinator, acted quickly. Ten weeks after his appointment, the ONC delivered a framework for strategic action outlining 4 goals and 12 strategies for national adoption of health information technology.[8] The document outlined a vision for consumer-centric and information-rich healthcare derived from the widespread adoption of health information technology and set a 10-year time frame for that to happen.

## Strategic Framework

The framework as first published listed four major goals and a corresponding set of strategies. These were:

1. Inform Clinical Practice
2. Interconnect Clinicians
3. Personalize Care
4. Improve Population Health

---

[6]President George W. Bush, Executive Order #13335, April 27, 2004.
[7]H.R. 1 American Recovery and Reinvestment Act of 2009, Title XIII Health Information Technology for Economic and Clinical Health, February 17, 2009.
[8]*The Decade of Health Information Technology: Delivering Consumer-centric and Information-rich Healthcare* (Washington, DC: U.S. Department of Health and Human Services, July 21, 2004).

## Federal Health IT Strategic Plan

In June of 2008, the ONC published an update to the strategic framework called the *Federal Health IT Strategic Plan*.[9] (IT is an acronym for information technology.) The plan had two goals, patient-focused healthcare and population health, with four objectives under each goal. The themes of privacy and security, interoperability, IT adoption, and collaborative governance recur across the goals, but they apply in very different ways to healthcare and population health.

Achievement of the eight objectives was tied to measurable outcomes, describing 43 strategies that needed to be done to achieve the objectives. Each strategy was associated with a milestone against which progress could be assessed. The plan included a set of illustrative actions to implement each strategy.

## The HITECH Act

In 2009 the federal government passed the HITECH Act,[10] which showed that it firmly believed in the benefits of using EHR. The act encouraged widespread adoption of EHR by authorizing the Centers for Medicare & Medicaid Services (CMS) to make incentive payments to doctors and hospitals that use a certified EHR. These incentives were intended to drive adoption of EHR in order to reach the goal of every American having a secure EHR. To achieve this vision of a transformed healthcare system that health information technology can facilitate, this Act included three critical short-term prerequisites:

◆ Clinicians and hospitals must acquire and implement certified EHR in a way that fully integrates these tools into the care delivery process.

◆ Technical, legal, and financial supports must be in place to enable information to flow securely to wherever it is needed to support healthcare and population health.

◆ A skilled workforce must be able to facilitate the implementation and support of EHR, exchange of health information among healthcare providers and public health authorities, and the redesign of workflows within the healthcare settings.

Providers who implemented and proved meaningful use of a certified EHR prior to 2015 were eligible for incentives. This meant a practice adopting an EHR was actually paid more than a practice continuing to use paper charts.

After 2015, Medicare began to administer financial penalties for physicians and hospitals that do not use an EHR. These involve reducing the provider's payments by 1 percent per year for up to five years.

## Strategic Plan Updates

The HITECH Act requires the ONC, in consultation with other appropriate federal agencies, to update the Federal Health IT Strategic Plan at regular intervals. The HITECH Act requires that the update include specific objectives, milestones, and metrics with respect to the following:

1. The electronic exchange and use of health information and the enterprise integration of such information.

2. The use of an EHR for each person in the United States.

---

[9]*Federal Health IT Strategic Plan (ONC): 2008–2012* (Washington, DC: U.S. Department of Health and Human Services, Office of National Coordinator, June 3, 2008, pp. iii–iv).
[10]H.R. 1 American Recovery and Reinvestment Act of 2009, Title XIII Health Information Technology for Economic and Clinical Health, February 17, 2009.

3. The incorporation of privacy and security protections for electronic exchange of an individual's individually identifiable health information.

4. Establishing security methods to ensure appropriate authorization and electronic authentication of health information and specifying technologies or methodologies for rendering health information unusable, unreadable, or indecipherable.

5. Specifying a framework for coordination and flow of recommendations and policies under this subtitle among the Secretary, the National Coordinator, the HIT Policy Committee, the HIT Standards Committee, and other health information exchanges and other relevant entities.

6. Methods to foster the public understanding of health information technology.

7. Strategies to enhance the use of health information technology in improving the quality of healthcare, reducing medical errors, reducing health disparities, improving public health, increasing prevention and coordination with community resources, and improving the continuity of care among healthcare settings.

8. Specific plans for ensuring that populations with unique needs, such as children, are appropriately addressed in the technology design, as appropriate, which may include technology that automates enrollment and retention for eligible individuals.

In compliance with the HITECH act, the ONC issued Strategic Plan updates to cover the period 2011–2015, and a subsequent update for the period 2015–2020.

The 2015–2020 plan "focuses on advancing health information technology innovation and use for a variety of purposes; however, the use of health IT is not in itself an end goal. The work described in this Plan aims to modernize the U.S. health IT infrastructure so that individuals, their providers, and communities can use it to help achieve health and wellness goals."[11] The 2015–2020 plan framework has four goals and 13 objectives:

### Goal 1: Advance Person-Centered and Self-Managed Health

◆ Objective A: Empower individual, family, and caregiver health management and engagement

◆ Objective B: Foster individual, provider, and community partnerships

### Goal 2: Transform Health Care Delivery and Community Health

◆ Objective A: Improve health care quality, access, and experience through safe, timely, effective, efficient, equitable, and person-centered care

◆ Objective B: Support the delivery of high-value health care

◆ Objective C: Protect and promote public health and healthy, resilient communities

### Goal 3: Foster Research, Scientific Knowledge, and Innovation

◆ Objective A: Increase access to and usability of high-quality electronic health information and services

◆ Objective B: Accelerate the development and commercialization of innovative technologies and solutions

◆ Objective C: Invest, disseminate, and translate research on how health IT can improve health and care delivery

---

[11]*The ONC-Coordinated Federal Health IT Strategic Plan: 2015–2020* (Washington, DC: Office of National Coordinator for Health Information Technology, 2015).

**Goal 4: Enhance Nation's Health IT Infrastructure**

◆ Objective A: Finalize and implement the Nationwide Interoperability Roadmap

◆ Objective B: Protect the privacy and security of health information

◆ Objective C: Identify, prioritize, and advance technical standards to support secure and interoperable health information and health IT

◆ Objective D: Increase user and market confidence in the safety and safe use of health IT products, systems, and services

◆ Objective E: Advance a national communications infrastructure that supports health, safety, and care delivery

## Meaningful Use of a Certified EHR

The HITECH act specifies the following three components of Meaningful Use:

1. Use of certified EHR in a meaningful manner

2. Use of certified EHR technology for electronic exchange of health information to improve quality of healthcare

3. Use of certified EHR technology to submit clinical quality measures (CQM) and other such measures selected by the Secretary of Health and Human Services

The key terms here are *certified EHR* and *meaningful use*. What is a certified EHR, and how is meaningful use determined?

## Certified EHR

Under the CMS EHR incentive programs, eligible health care providers must adopt and meaningfully use a "certified EHR" that has been certified by an ONC Authorized Certification Body (ONC-ACB). To synchronize the two regulations, the ONC published the Health Information Technology: Initial Set of Standards, Implementation Specifications, and Certification Criteria for Electronic Health Record Technology Final Rule[12] on the same date as the CMS Final Rule. The following year HHS established through ONC a permanent certification program for health information technology.[13] The purpose of the certification program was to reduce the financial risk for the provider by ensuring that if they used an EHR certified by the ONC-ACB it would be capable of meeting the meaningful use performance requirements.

The ONC certification criteria represent the minimum capabilities an EHR needed to include and have properly implemented in order to achieve certification. The criteria do not preclude developers from including additional capabilities that are not required for the purposes of certification.

## Meaningful Use and Clinical Quality Measures

CMS officially published the Electronic Health Record Incentive Program Final Rule July 28, 2010, which finalized the incentive program and defined the criteria for determining "meaningful use."[14]

Requirements for meaningful use incentive payments were implemented over a multi-year period, in three stages. Stage 1, spanning the years 2011 and 2013, set the baseline

---

[12]U.S. Department of Health and Human Services, 45 CFR Part 170; Final Rule, July 28, 2010.

[13]U.S. Department of Health and Human Services, 45 CFR Part 170; Establishment of the Permanent Certification for Health Information Technology, Final Rule, January 7, 2011.

[14]U.S. Department of Health and Human Services, 42 CFR Parts 412, 413, 422, and 495; Final Rule July 28, 2010.

for electronic data capture and information sharing. Stage 2 began in 2014 and retained the core requirements and menu structure for meaningful use objectives established in Stage 1. Although some Stage 1 objectives were either combined or eliminated, most of the Stage 1 objectives became core objectives under the Stage 2 criteria. Stage 3, in 2016, strengthened the core objective "to protect patient health information" through the implementation of appropriate technical, administrative, and physical safeguards.

The meaningful use requirements for hospital and eligible professionals (EPs) differ. The table in Figure 1-2 combines the Meaningful Use Objectives for Eligible Professionals from Stages 1, 2, and 3. The table cell color helps associate the meaningful use objectives to the goals of the strategic plans (discussed above) listed in the first row of the table.

**Figure 1-2** Table of Meaningful Use Objectives for Eligible Professionals.

## Eligible Professionals Meaningful Use Objectives

| Improve Quality, Safety, Efficiency | Engage Patients & Families | Improve Care Coordination | Improve Public & Population Health | Ensure Privacy & Security of PHI |
|---|---|---|---|---|
| EPs Core Objectives (all must be met*) | | | Menu of Additional Objectives (EPs choose from list) | |
| Use computerized provider order entry (CPOE) for medication, laboratory and radiology orders | | | Record electronic notes in patient records | |
| Generate and transmit permissible prescriptions electronically | | | Imaging results accessible | |
| Record demographic information | | | Record patient family health history | |
| Record and chart changes in vital signs | | | Identify and report cancer cases to a state cancer registry | |
| Record smoking status for patients 13 years old or older | | | Identify and report specific cases to another specialized registry | |
| Use clinical decision support to improve performance on high-priority health conditions | | | Submit electronic syndromic surveillance data to public health agencies | |
| Provide patients the ability to view online, download, and transmit their health information | | | | |
| Provide clinical summaries for patients for each office visit | | | | |
| Protect electronic health information created or maintained by the Certified EHR Technology through implementation of appropriate technical, administrative, and physical safeguards | | | | |
| Incorporate clinical lab-test results into Certified EHR Technology | | | | |
| Generate lists of patients by specific conditions to use for quality improvement, reduction of disparities, research, or outreach | | | | |
| Use clinically relevant information to identify patients who should receive reminders for preventive/follow-up care | | | | |
| Use certified EHR technology to identify patient-specific education resources. | | | | |
| Perform medication reconciliation | | | | |
| Provide summary of care record for each transition of care or referral | | | | |
| Submit electronic data to immunization registries | | | | |
| Use secure electronic messaging to communicate with patients on relevant health information | | | | |
| *Exclusions are provided for objectives outside of the normal scope of a provider's clinical practice. | | | | |

A key core requirement is to report **Clinical Quality Measures** (CQM). CMS uses **clinical quality measures** in a variety of quality initiatives that include quality improvement and public reporting. ONC certified that electronic health record (EHR) technologies are capable of accurately calculating the electronic clinical quality measure results. Four federal agencies—the Agency for Healthcare Research and Quality (AHRQ), CMS, the National Library of Medicine (NLM), and ONC—define the CQM components comprised of definitions, measure logic, data elements, and value sets.

The purpose of clinical quality measures is to help meet the strategic goals of improving patient health. An example of this is the requirement to record patients' tobacco use status and counsel patients on tobacco cessation methods. Chapter 9 will cover recording clinical quality measures in the EHR.

## EHR Adoption After HITECH

At the beginning of the 21st century, adoption of electronic health records among physicians was moving slowly. In the past decade, EHR adoption among hospitals and physicians has grown substantially, especially since the passage of the HITECH act.

"From 2010 (the earliest year that trend data are available) to 2013, physician adoption of EHRs able to support various Stage 2 meaningful use objectives increased significantly,"[15] as shown in Figure 1-3.

**Figure 1-3** Percentage of office-based physicians in the United States with EHR systems, 2001–2013.

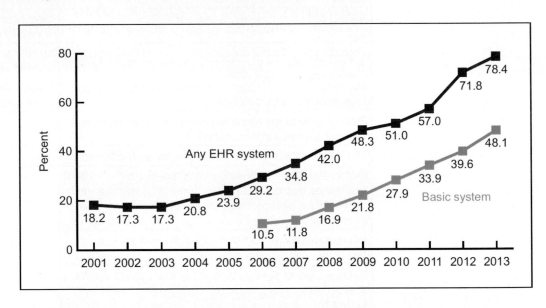

"In 2013, 59 percent of hospitals and 48 percent of physicians had at least a basic EHR system, respective increases of 47 percentage points and 26 percentage points since 2009, the year the HITECH Act was signed into law. Moreover, there is widespread participation among eligible hospitals and professionals in the CMS EHR Incentive Programs. As of June 2014, 75 percent (403,000+) of the nation's eligible professionals and 92 percent (4,500+) of eligible hospitals and CAHs had received incentive payments."[16]

---

[15]Hsiao C.-J., and Hing E. Use and characteristics of electronic health record systems among office-based physician practices: United States, 2001–2013. NCHS data brief, no. 143. Hyattsville, MD: National Center for Health Statistics. 2014. http://www.cdc.gov/nchs/data/databriefs/db143.htm
[16]2014 Report to Congress on Health IT Adoption and HIE, The Office of the National Coordinator for Health Information Technology (ONC) Office of the Secretary, U.S. Department of Health and Human Services, Washington, DC, 2014.

**Figure 1-4** Office-based physicians with a certified electronic health record system, by physician specialty: United States, 2013–2014

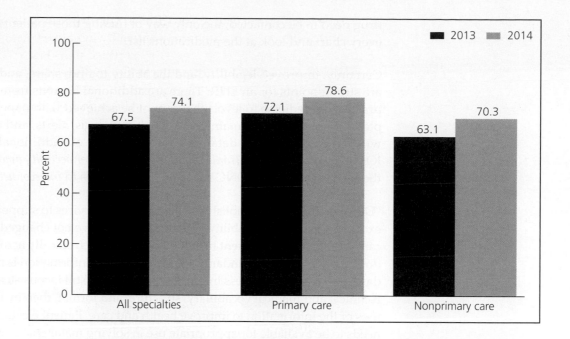

Adoption of certified EHR systems by office-based physicians increased from 2013 to 2014. In 2014, 74.1% of office-based physicians had a certified EHR system, up from 67.5% in 2013 (as shown in Figure 1-4). The HITECH Act of 2009 gave eligible physicians monetary incentives to adopt a certified EHR system and may be one of the reasons for the continued rise in physician adoption of these systems.

The percentage of physicians with a certified EHR system ranged from 58.8% in Alaska to 88.6% in Minnesota.[17]

## Why Interoperability Is Important

An ONC report to Congress states: "(EHR) progress has laid a strong base for health IT adoption and created a growing demand for its interoperability that not only supports the care continuum, but also supports health generally."[18]

Historically, a patient's medical records consisted of handwritten notes, typed reports, and test results stored in a paper file system. A separate file folder was created and stored at each location where the patient was examined or treated. X-ray films and other radiology records typically were stored separately from the chart, even when they were created at the same medical office.

These are some of the drawbacks to paper records: Handwritten records often are abbreviated, cryptic, or illegible. When information is to be used by another medical practice, the charts must be copied and faxed or mailed to the other office. Even in one practice with multiple locations, the chart must be transported from one office to another when a patient is seen at a different location than usual. Paper records are not easily searchable. For example, if a practice is notified that all patients on a particular

[17]Jamoom EW, Yang N, Hing E. Adoption of certified electronic health record systems and electronic information sharing in physician offices: United States, 2013 and 2014. NCHS data brief, no 236. Hyattsville, MD: National Center for Health Statistics. 2016. http://www.cdc.gov/nchs/data/databriefs/db236.htm

[18]2014 Report to Congress on Health IT Adoption and HIE, The Office of the National Coordinator for Health Information Technology (ONC) Office of the Secretary, U.S. Department of Health and Human Services, Washington, DC, 2014.

drug need to be contacted, the only way of finding those patients is literally to open every chart and look at the medications list.

Certainly, improved legibility, and the ability to find, share, and search patient records are strong points for an EHR. There are additional benefits from an EHR that take the practice of medicine to levels that cannot be achieved with paper records. Four examples of these are health maintenance, trend analysis, alerts, and decision support. These will be covered in more detail in Chapter 2. There are additional criteria, however. The IOM report calls for *electronic communication and connectivity among care partners*, and the second goal of the ONC strategic framework is to *interconnect clinicians*.

"Despite progress in establishing standards and services to support health information exchange and interoperability, practice patterns have not changed to the point that health care providers share patient health information electronically across organizational, vendor, and geographic boundaries. Electronic health information is not yet sufficiently standardized to allow seamless interoperability, as it is still inconsistently expressed through technical and medical vocabulary, structure, and format, thereby limiting the potential uses of the information to improve health and care. Patient electronic health information needs to be available for appropriate use in solving major challenges, such as providing more effective care and informing and accelerating scientific research."[19]

In Chapter 2 we will discuss the structured data EHR as well as standardized codified medical vocabulary the ONC report says is necessary to support the exchange of healthcare data between provider systems and which supports improved patient and population health.

The need for EHR and better connectivity between EHR systems is demonstrated in the Real-Life Story: Where's My Chart?

## Group Discussion Topic: When the Chart Is Lacking

After reading the Real-Life Story: "Where's My Chart?" discuss the following:

1. What are the dangers to the patient of a provider who does not have access to paper charts?

2. What is the likelihood of the second incident of the pulmonary embolism being overlooked?

3. How would the patient care have been improved if the various EHR systems had been able to exchange patient records electronically?

## Documenting at the Point of Care

Another item noted in the ONC report was the need for practice patterns to change. A goal of using an EHR system is to improve the accuracy and completeness of the patient record. One way to achieve this is to record the information in the EHR at the time it is happening. This is called **point-of-care documentation**. In a physician's office, this means completing the encounter note before the patient ever leaves the office. In an inpatient setting, this means that nurses enter vital signs and nursing notes at bedside, not at the end of their shift.

---

[19]2014 Report to Congress on Health IT Adoption and HIE, The Office of the National Coordinator for Health Information Technology (ONC) Office of the Secretary, U.S. Department of Health and Human Services, Washington, DC, 2014.

# Real-Life Story

A 63-year-old man went to his doctor's office in Kentucky complaining of chest pains and tightness in his chest. He was immediately transferred to the local hospital, where a stress test and cardiac catheterization confirmed he had had a heart attack. He was hospitalized overnight.

Early retirement from his stressful job as well as a regimen of exercise, diet, beta blockers, aspirin therapy, and other medications proved successful. He moved from Kentucky to Florida and tried unsuccessfully to have his medical records concerning the previous heart attack transferred to his new doctor in Florida. The ECG and stress tests were repeated in Florida. Finally, after two years, the records from Kentucky arrived.

In subsequent years, he moved twice more but, wiser now, he took copies of his medical records with him. He continued a normal and active life until age 77, when he slipped in his workshop and broke his right knee. With his leg in a cast he was less active; a blood clot formed and broke free.

Three weeks after he broke his knee, he went to the doctor's office with what he described as very severe flu symptoms, extreme fatigue, a bad cough, and sharp pains in his back when he moved or coughed. The doctor sent him to the emergency room, where he was diagnosed with a pulmonary embolism in the lower lobe of the right lung. He was hospitalized and put on a therapy of blood thinners.

At age 79, he was continuing to lead an active lifestyle, but he was experiencing occasional sharp brief chest pain and brief dizziness. His doctor scheduled a stress test and cardiac catheterization at a cardiac center connected to the hospital. A blockage was discovered and a double bypass surgery was performed at the same hospital. The patient tolerated the surgery well and recovered quickly.

However, one of the veins used in the bypass operation had been harvested from the leg that had the previous broken knee. Three weeks after he was discharged, he passed out and fell. He was taken by ambulance to the ER at the same hospital where he had had his surgery and where he had been hospitalized for the previous pulmonary embolism. Here is what happened:

▶ When the ambulance crew arrived at the house, they took a medical history from the patient and his wife. They gave him oxygen and transported him to the hospital.

▶ When the ambulance arrived at the hospital, the nurses and ER staff again took a medical history from the patient and patient's family.

▶ The patient's primary care physician had a complete medical history of the patient, including copies of his records dating back to his heart attack in Kentucky, but the hospital system was not connected with the physician's office system.

▶ The patient reported that he had just had surgery at the same hospital only three weeks before. The hospital system surely had his medical history, but the ER was on a different system and the two systems lacked the capability to exchange data. ER doctors did not have electronic access to the records.

▶ Although the ER was in the same hospital as the cardiac lab, again the systems were different. ER doctors did not have electronic access to those records, either.

▶ The patient told the ER staff he thought the symptoms felt similar to his previous experience with a pulmonary embolism, but even though the ER was in the same hospital where the patient had been hospitalized for a pulmonary embolism two years before, the ER doctors did not have access to the records from his previous hospitalization.

▶ A CAT scan was ordered based on patient history of the embolism provided by a family member, not his medical record.

▶ After waiting in the ER for 14 hours, he was hospitalized with two pulmonary embolisms, one in each lung.

Seven days later, the patient was discharged from the hospital. He has fully recovered and is doing fine.

This is not the story of poor medical care or a bad hospital. The hospital is affiliated with a major teaching hospital and is as good as or better than most. This story illustrates the importance of the ONC goal for interoperability to electronically exchange and integrate health information to provide better patient care. The lack of timely copies of existing records often causes tests to be reordered or the obvious conditions to be overlooked. Electronic records are better, more accessible, but even the most sophisticated systems do not necessarily have the infrastructure in place to communicate with other EHR systems even, as in this case, within the same healthcare system!

Using a point-of-care EHR, when the visit is complete, the note is complete. The clinician can then provide not only patient education materials for patients to take home, but also can actually print a copy of the finished note. Giving patients a copy of the notes from that day's visit is one of the core Meaningful Use Objectives required of eligible professionals by CMS. Providing a summary of the visit helps patients remember the key elements of their treatment plan. They also will have a clearer understanding of their condition as well as information on any tests that may have been ordered or performed.

Leading physician experts on EHR, Allen R. Wenner, an MD in Columbia, South Carolina, and John W. Bachman, an MD and professor of Family Medicine at the Mayo Medical School in Rochester, Minnesota, wrote concerning outpatient practices: "Documenting an encounter at the point of care is the most efficient method of practicing medicine because the physician completes the medical record at the time of a patient's visit. Dictation time is saved and the need for personal dictation aides is eliminated. Thus, point-of-care documentation is less expensive than traditional dictation with its associated high cost of transcription. In addition, the physician can sign the note immediately.

Patient care is improved because the patient can leave with a complete copy of the medical record, a step that stimulates compliance. The delivery process is improved with point-of-care documentation because referrals can be accomplished with full information available at the time that the referral is needed. For these benefits to occur, the clinical workflow changes to improve efficiency, increase data accuracy, and lower the overall cost of healthcare delivery."[20]

John Bachman has formulated what he refers to as Bachman's Rule and Bachman's Law. These are defined as follows:

Bachman's Rule: "A patient who has a copy of a note is impressed by the fact that all the information they provided and were given is included for them to review. It also is useful in that it has immunizations prevention information and instructions. Outcome studies have shown it to be helpful in compliance and improvement of health; crossing the Quality Chasm."

Bachman's Law: "A clinician who gives a patient a copy of their note has all their work complete. Consequently there is no dictation, rework, signing, or any activity of maintaining the administrative workflow. This saves a great deal of money and means the workflow systems are extremely efficient."

Underscoring Bachman and Wenner are the CMS regulations for meaningful use,[21] which require eligible professionals to provide clinical summaries to patients each office visit.

The availability of information from the EHR during the patient visit is an invaluable tool in counseling and patient education. The clinician has access to graphs, medical images, test results, and anatomical drawings, all of which are useful in explaining something related to the patient's condition or in illustrating an upcoming procedure. Using a Tablet, the clinician in Figure 1-5 is able to document the encounter while with the patient.

---

[20]Allen R. Wenner and John W. Bachman,"Transforming the Physician Practice: Interviewing Patients with a Computer,"Chap. 26 in *Healthcare Information Management Systems: Cases, Strategies, and Solutions*, 3rd ed., ed. Marion J. Ball, Charlotte A. Weaver, and Joan M. Kiel (New York: Springer Science+Business Media, Inc., 2004), 297–319. Copyright © 2004 Springer Science+Business Media, Inc., New York.
[21]U.S. Department of Health and Human Services, 42 CFR Parts 412, 413, 422, and 495; Final Rule July 28, 2010.

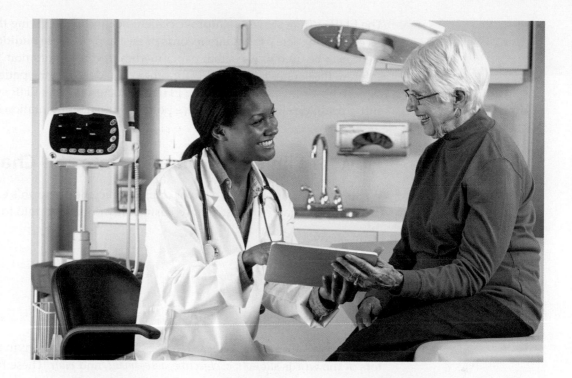

**Figure 1-5** A clinician documents the visit while with the patient.

As stated earlier, adopting an EHR may change the way doctors work. Experience has shown that patients react favorably to the use of a computer during the exam, especially when they are part of the process, able to see the screen, and able to participate in the review of their information. However, Wenner and Bachman describe three types of patient–physician relationships:[22]

1. The doctor is paternalistic, telling the patient what to do.

2. The doctor gives the patient information and the patient decides what to do.

3. Patients and doctors share information to determine the best plan for given conditions.

Figure 1-6, provided by Dr. Wenner, lists the stages of change resulting from adoption of an EHR. Wenner and Bachman believe patients will help the physician when they are given some degree of control, as reflected in points 2 and 3.

**Figure 1-6** Stages of change in EHR adoption.

| | Stages of Change in EHR Technology Adoption | | |
|---|---|---|---|
| Stage | Technology Adoption | Medical Records | Medical Practice |
| Stage I | Do it the old way | The paper chart used and viewed as an historical document by physicians | Health care providers are the center of healthcare |
| Stage II | Adopt technology but continue to do it the old way | Transcribing dictation onto paper, using the EHR for data storage only managed by staff | Providers continue to dominate medical decisions and maintain all healthcare data |
| Stage III | Change the workflow to leverage the technology Paperless medical office | Use EHR at the point-of-care with providers and patients participating to allow real-time continuity of care | Patients and providers will share decision making as healthcare information is available to both |

[22]Ibid.

The EHR system strives to improve patient healthcare by giving the provider and patient access to complete, up-to-date records of past and present conditions; it also enables the records to be used in ways that paper medical records could not. The sooner the data is entered, the sooner it is available for other providers and the patient. Chapters 2–12 will explore how data is entered in the EHR and focus on ways EHR systems speed up data entry, enabling clinicians to achieve point-of-care documentation in real time.

## Flow of Clinical Information into the Chart

Whether medical records are paper or electronic, the clinician's exam notes are usually documented in a defined structure, historically organized into four components:

◆ Subjective

◆ Objective

◆ Assessment

◆ Plan

Charts in this format are referred to as *SOAP notes*; the acronym represents the first letters of the words *subjective, objective, assessment*, and *plan*. These four basic components are frequently subdivided into additional sections. For example, history and symptoms are two sections under subjective. Another example is the problem-oriented format, which subdivides the assessment component by diagnosis (problem) and groups treatment plans under each problem. Still, the overarching structure may be thought of as following the SOAP format.

To better understand the functional benefits of EHR, let us compare the workflow in a medical office using paper charts with a medical office using an EHR system.

### Workflow of an Office Using Paper Charts

Follow the arrows in Figure 1-7 as you read the following description of a workflow in a primary care medical practice using paper charts.

**1** An established patient phones the medical office and schedules an appointment.

**2** The night before the appointment, the patient charts are pulled from the medical record filing system and organized for the next day's patients.

**3** On the day of the appointment, the patient arrives at the office and is asked to confirm that insurance and demographic information on file is correct.

The patient is given a clipboard with a blank medical history form and asked to complete it. The form asks the reason for today's visit and asks the patient to report any previous history, any changes to medications, new allergies, and so on.

**4** The patient is moved to an exam room and is asked to wait.

**Subjective**—The patient is asked to describe in his or her own words what the problem is, what the symptoms are, and what he or she is experiencing.

A nurse or medical assistant measures the patient's height and weight, takes vital signs, reviews the form the patient completed, and may ask for more detail about the reason for the visit, which usually is called the *chief complaint*. The vital signs and chief complaint are written on a form that is placed at the front of the chart along with the updated patient form.

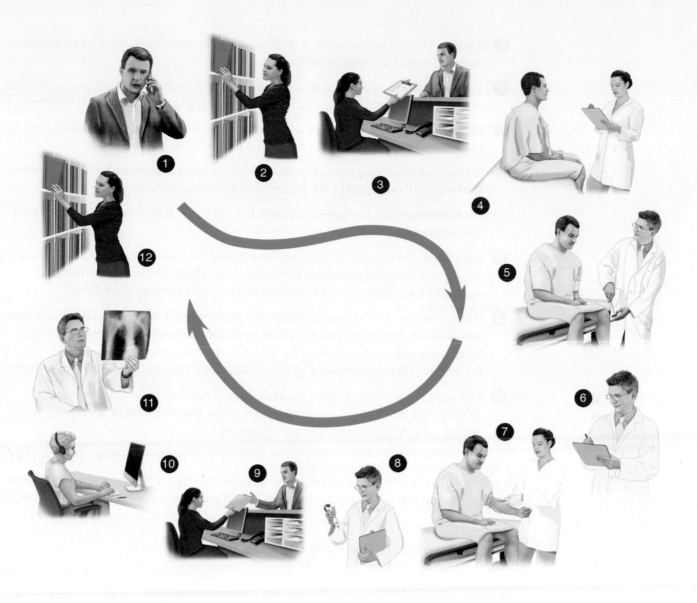

**Figure 1-7** Workflow in a medical office using paper charts.

**⑤** The clinician (doctor or other licensed healthcare provider) enters the exam room and discusses the reason for the visit and reviews the symptoms.

> **Objective**—The clinician performs a physical exam and makes observations about what he or she finds.

> **Assessment**—Applying his or her training to the subjective and objective findings, the clinician arrives at a decision of what might be the cause of the patient's condition, or what further tests might be necessary.

> **Plan of Treatment**—The clinician prescribes a treatment, medication, or orders further tests. Perhaps a follow-up visit at a later date is recommended. A note will be made in the chart of each element of the plan.

**⑥** If medications have been ordered, a handwritten prescription will be given to the patient or phoned to the pharmacy. A note of the prescription will be written in the patient's chart.

> The doctor marks one or more billing codes and one or more diagnosis codes on the chart and leaves the exam room.

**7** If lab work has been ordered, a medical assistant will obtain the necessary specimen and send the order to the lab.

**8** The clinician creates the exam note from memory, either handwriting in the chart or dictating the subjective, objective, assessment, plan, and treatment information.

**9** When the patient is dressed, the patient will be escorted to the check-out area. The patient may be given education material or medication instructions.

If x-rays or other diagnostic tests have been ordered at another facility, the office staff may call on behalf of the patient and schedule the tests.

If a follow-up visit has been indicated, the patient will be scheduled for the next appointment.

**10** If dictated, the encounter notes are later transcribed and returned to the clinician to review before being permanently stored in the chart. The completed chart is reviewed by a billing coder to determine the codes for medical billing.

**11** If lab, x-ray, or other diagnostic tests have been ordered, the results and reports are subsequently sent to the practice either by fax or on paper a number of days later. When received, they are filed in the patient's chart and the chart is sent to the clinician for review. They are reviewed by the clinician, and then re-filed in the paper chart.

**12** The paper chart is filed again. Note that the chart may have to be pulled and re-filed each time a new document, such as the transcription or lab report, was added, which required the clinician's review.

One obvious downside to paper charts is accessibility. If the patient chart is needed for a follow-up visit or by another provider, it is possible that it has not been returned to the file room while it is pending dictation or while the provider is reviewing test results.

## Workflow of an Office Fully Using an EHR

Follow the arrows in Figure 1-8 as you read the following description of a workflow of a patient visit to an office that fully uses the electronic capabilities that are available in EHR systems today, including patient participation in the process and the capabilities of the Internet.

**1** An established patient phones the doctor's office and schedules an appointment.

**Internet alternative:** Patients are increasingly able to request an appointment and receive a confirmation via the Internet by visiting the practice portal.

**2** The night before the appointment, the medical office computer electronically verifies insurance eligibility for patients scheduled the next day.

**3** On the day of the appointment, the patient arrives at the office and is asked to confirm that the demographic information on file is still correct.

**4** A receptionist, nurse, or medical assistant asks the patient to complete a medical history and reason for today's visit using a computer in a private area of the waiting room. The patient completes a computer-guided questionnaire concerning his symptoms and medical history.

**Internet alternative:** Some medical practices' portals enable patients to complete the history and symptom questionnaire via the Internet before coming to the office.

**5** When the patient has completed the questionnaire, the system alerts the nurse or medical assistant that the patient is ready to move to an exam room.

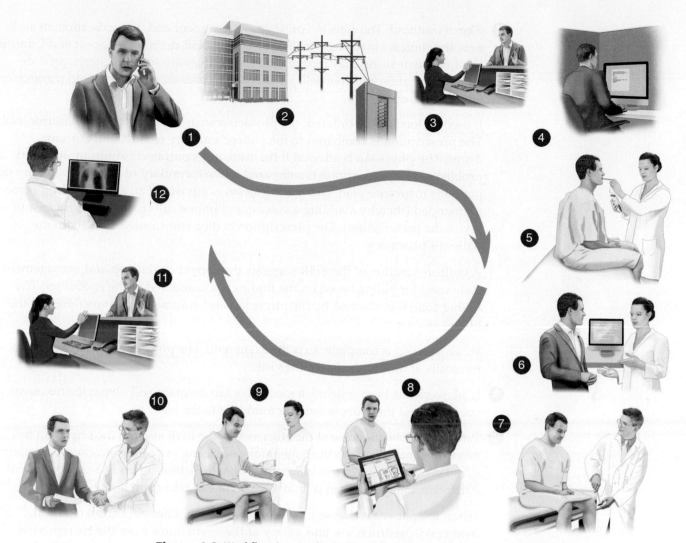

**Figure 1-8** Workflow in a medical office fully using an EHR.

The nurse or medical assistant measures the patient's height and weight and records it in the EHR. Using a digital device, vital signs for blood pressure, temperature, and pulse are recorded and wirelessly transferred into the EHR.

**6** *Subjective:* The nurse or medical assistant reviews with the patient the patient-entered symptoms and history. Where necessary, the nurse or medical assistant edits the record to add clarification or refinement.

The clinician enters the exam room and discusses the reason for the visit and reviews with the patient the information already in the chart.

**7** *Objective:* The clinician performs the physical exam. The clinician typically makes a mental provisional diagnosis. This is used to select a list or template of findings to quickly record the physical exam in the EHR.

The EHR presents a list of problems the patient reported in past visits that have not been resolved. The clinician reviews each, examining additional body systems as necessary, and marks the improvement, worsening, or resolution of each problem.

**Assessment:** Applying his or her training to the subjective and objective findings, the clinician arrives at a decision of one or more diagnoses and decides if further tests might be warranted.

**⑧** *Plan of treatment:* The clinician prescribes a treatment and/or medication; in addition, the clinician may order further tests. The EHR decisions support and Clinical Quality care features may recommend preventive care screening tests, provide patient education and counseling materials, or present evidence-based research on the patient's condition.

If medication is to be ordered, the physician writes the prescription electronically. The prescription is compared to the patient's allergy records and current drugs. The physician is advised if there are any contraindications or potential problems. The prescription is compared to the formulary of drugs covered by the patient's insurance plan, and the physician is advised if an alternate drug is recommended (thereby avoiding a subsequent phone call from the pharmacist to revise the prescription). The prescription is then transmitted directly to the patient's pharmacy.

A built-in function of the EHR suggests the correct evaluation and management code used for billing based on the findings documented in the encounter. The billing code is confirmed by the physician and automatically transferred to the billing system.

When the visit is complete, so is the exam note. The physician signs the note electronically at the conclusion of the visit.

**⑨** If lab work has been ordered, a medical or lab assistant will obtain the necessary specimen and the order is sent electronically to the lab.

**⑩** *Patient education:* Because of the efficiency of the EHR system, the physician has more personal time with the patient for counseling or patient education. In many systems the provider can display and annotate pictures of body areas for patient education, and print them so that the patient can take them home.

When the patient is dressed, he or she is given patient education material, medication instructions, and a copy of the exam notes from the current visit. Allowing the patient to take away a written record of the visit meets CMS requirements and enables better compliance with the doctor's plan of care and recommended treatments.

**Internet alternative:** The patient may also have access to his health records through the practice's secure Internet portal.

**⑪** The patient is escorted to the checkout area.

If x-rays or other diagnostic tests have been ordered at another facility, the office staff may call on behalf of the patient and schedule the tests.

If a follow-up visit has been indicated, the patient will be scheduled for the next appointment.

**⑫** If lab tests were ordered, the results are sent to the doctor electronically, are reviewed on screen, and automatically merged into the EHR.

If radiology or other diagnostic reports are sent to the practice electronically as text reports, they are imported into the EHR and can be reviewed by the physician.

Accessibility is not a problem in the EHR system because there is no chart to re-file. Multiple providers can access the patient's chart, even simultaneously; for example, a physician could review the previous lab results before entering the exam room, even if the nurse was currently entering vital signs in the chart.

## Group Discussion About Workflow

Having compared the two workflow scenarios, we see the immediate advantages of the EHR for the patient and clinician. Think about the workflow of the office that used paper charts (refer to Figure 1-7 if necessary.) Answer the following questions about the first workflow:

1. What was the medical assistant, nurse, or clinician doing at the time of the patient interaction?

2. Could they have recorded this data in a computer?

3. Could they have saved time later?

4. Could the data be entered by someone other than the person seeing the patient?

   The patient completed a form concerning any previous history, any changes to medications, new allergies, and so on.

5. Could the patient have used a computer, or could the form have been designed to be read by a computer?

6. Could the patient have completed the information before the visit?

   The nurse or medical assistant recorded various health measurements (vital signs) in the exam room.

7. Could the nurse or medical assistant have recorded the chief complaint or the vital signs in a computer instead of on a paper chart?

8. Were any of the instruments used capable of transferring their measurements to a computer system?

   During the physical exam, the clinician made observations and an assessment. This was later dictated from memory, subsequently transcribed by a typist, and finally reviewed and signed by the physician.

9. Is the time it would take to record the observations and assessment in the exam comparable to the time it takes to dictate and review the transcribed notes later?

   The clinician prescribed medications and ordered tests.

10. Would the time spent entering the prescriptions on a computer justify the benefits of electronic prescribing?

11. Are results available electronically from laboratories that the medical practice uses?

12. Would ordering a test electronically improve the matching of results to orders when the tests were completed?

## Inpatient Charts versus Outpatient Charts

The previous figures illustrated the differences between two medical offices, one using a paper chart and another using an EHR. The differences between a hospital using a paper chart and a hospital fully using electronic records are even more significant. However, there are also differences in the type of chart each facility uses and overall workflow process. In this section we are going to compare both.

Although some patients are admitted to the hospital through the emergency department or by transfer from another facility, most patient admissions begin in the

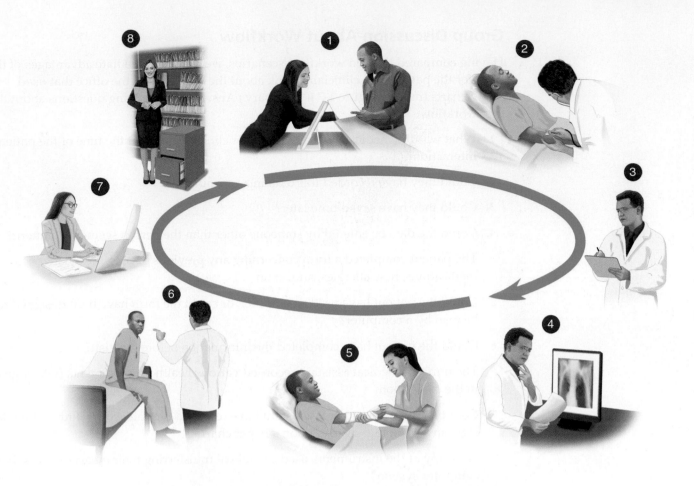

**Figure 1-9** Flow of an inpatient from admission through discharge.

registration department. As depicted in Figure 1-9, the steps involved in an inpatient admission and discharge include the following:

❶ When the patient arrives, patient demographic and insurance information is collected or updated, and an account is set up for the patient stay. Even if the patient has been an inpatient previously, a new account is created (although previous patients will use their existing medical record number).

❷ An admitting and/or attending doctor is assigned to the patient. In some facilities this is a hospitalist, a physician who works full-time in the hospital. A physician is required to perform a complete history and physical on an inpatient within 24 hours of the admission. In an outpatient facility, no such time limit is imposed on when or what type of physical is performed.

❸ The doctor orders tests, medications, and procedures.

❹ The doctor reviews the results of tests and diagnostic procedures when they are ready.

❺ Nurses provide most of the patient care, administer medications, take samples for tests, measure vital signs, perform nursing assessments and nursing interventions, and enter nursing notes into the chart.

❻ When a patient leaves an inpatient facility, there is also a formal discharge process. Normally, the physician performs a final examination of the patient and writes a discharge order. Discharge does not necessarily mean the patient goes home. Patients may be discharged to a skilled nursing facility or a rehabilitation facility for further care. Patients who leave without a doctor's order are discharged AMA (against medical advice).

**7** Following discharge, the Health Information Management (HIM) department examines the patient's chart to determine if it has any missing or unsigned documents (called chart deficiencies). Once the chart is complete, it is given to a professional coder to determine the proper billing codes.

**8** In a facility using paper charts, the last step is to file the chart.

There are also several significant differences in the content and purpose of a patient chart used in an acute care facility and that used by a medical office: the amount of information gathered about each patient and the number of individuals who will need access to it. Figure 1-10 highlights some of the differences between inpatient and outpatient charts.

**Figure 1-10** Contents typical of acute care versus ambulatory patient charts.

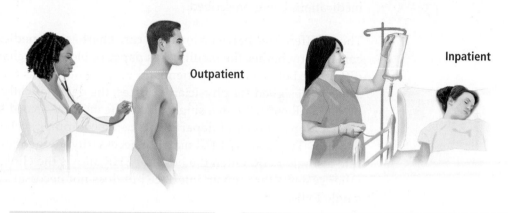

Outpatient

Inpatient

| Outpatient | Inpatient |
|---|---|
| Most physician offices have a single chart for the patient. Notes for each visit, test results, and any other reports are added to the chart. | A hospital chart for an episode of care includes all data for a specific stay. Previous hospitalizations are unique episodes of care linked by the patient's medical record number. |
| The quantity of data in an outpatient chart is relatively low by comparison. | The quantity of data in an inpatient chart is likely to be much larger. Vital signs are taken and nurses' notes are added numerous times per day; dietitians, respiratory therapists, and other providers add to the chart; there are typically many more orders for labs, medications, and so on. |
| The central element in the chart is the physician's exam note. | Physician exams tend to be brief; the main focus of the chart is the physician orders and nurse's notes indicating the patient's response. |

In an ambulatory setting such as a physician's office, the patient visits the physician's office a number of times over a period of months or years. Although items produced outside each visit, such as lab results and consult reports, are also integrated into the patient's chart, the most important element of the outpatient chart is the doctor's notes about each visit. The clinician reviews previous notes on each subsequent visit, using them to follow up on past ailments and to measure the patient's progress in managing chronic problems.

The medical chart is primarily used by the clinician, nurse, and medical assistant, but is also used briefly by the administrative staff to prepare billings following each visit. The focus of the chart is the longitudinal care of the patient. As such, it usually contains all records of the patient's visits and any reports or results received from other providers.

The inpatient chart, however, focuses on the treatment of a specific ailment or condition for which the patient was hospitalized. Data are gathered more frequently during the inpatient's stay, resulting in a substantially large amount of information gathered during a short period of time. In most hospitals, a new episode chart or medical record is started for each hospital stay. Although records from previous hospitalizations are available for reference, they are not incorporated into the current episode chart, except as described in the admitting physician's history and physical notes.

Because a large number of caregivers are involved with the patient's stay in an acute care facility, there are a larger number of individuals with a legitimate need to access a patient's record than in an ambulatory care setting. These caregivers include not only nurses and physicians, but also other specialists that may consult on the case; radiologists, respiratory therapists, dietitians, and in many hospitals, even the hospital pharmacists have access to records when consulting with the ordering physicians about the medications being prescribed.

These differences between an acute care chart and a medical office chart are consistent whether the facility uses paper or electronic charts. However, another difference between the inpatient and outpatient EHR is the system itself. In most systems designed for physician's offices, the data typically is received and stored by the EHR software in a single electronic medical record system. Most hospitals have a large number of departments using computer systems from many different vendors. The hospital EHR may not necessarily merge the data from these systems into a single EHR. Often the hospital EHR allows the clinician to view data in these other systems through an interface but does not necessarily store the data in a single EHR.

## Patient Registration and Appointment Scheduling

Although the subject of this book is Electronic Health Records, the first three elements in the preceding workflow diagrams involve software modules other than the EHR. These are the patient administration (or registration) module and the appointment schedule. If you have worked in a medical office, or previously taken a course in practice management, these functions may be familiar to you. While you will not be adding patients or scheduling appointments in this book, brief tutorials on these two functions may be helpful in understanding the overall workflow of a medical practice. Additionally, the registration and scheduling processes are fundamental. Nothing about the patient's care can be documented in the computer until the patient is set up, and except for emergency departments or walk-in clinics, the schedule is essential to ensuring the provider has sufficient time with each patient.

### Patient Administration

Health information systems for both inpatient and outpatient facilities have a patient registration component used to add new patients to the system as well as to add or edit information about existing patients.

The patient registration process records demographic information about the patient as well as account and insurance information that will be necessary to obtain payment for the services rendered. Additional data may also be gathered to help the practice better serve the patient or meet certain reporting requirements. Some examples of additional data include the patient's ethnicity, preferred language, emergency contact information, and HIPAA privacy preferences.

In addition to adding patient demographic information, it is necessary to set up account and guarantor information, and, if the patient has health insurance, the policy information as well.

The module used to add and edit patient information will vary in appearance between different health information systems, but all registration systems gather the same essential data. In some medical offices a new patient may be partially registered to facilitate appointment scheduling, and the registration completed when the patient arrives for the appointment. Some practices also allow a new patient to register via a web portal. The concept of a web portal will be covered further in Chapter 10.

## Tutorial Exercise 1A: Overview of a Patient Administration Module

In this tutorial you will observe how patient information is added and edited in a medical office practice management system. The Patient Administration demonstrated in the tutorial is from Greenway Health's SuccessEHS, an integrated EHR and practice management solution. Figure 1-11 shows an example of a paper form that is used to gather the patient and insurance information for the registration clerk.

Here are terms used in the tutorial with which you may not be familiar:

♦ **Patient account:** Each patient must have an account. The account is used to post charges and payments and to conduct billing and reporting. The account number is not necessarily the same as the patient ID or patient chart number.

♦ **Guarantor:** The person responsible for paying amounts not covered by insurance is called the guarantor of the account. In many cases, the guarantor is the patient. In other cases, the guarantor may be a parent or spouse. When the patient is not the guarantor, the name, address, and phone numbers of the guarantor must be recorded so they can be used for account billing later.

♦ **Health plan or payer:** A health plan may be a for-profit or not-for-profit insurance company, an employer self-insurance fund, or a government program such as Medicare. Health plans are sometimes also referred to as payers. Generally, the billing address and other information necessary to file claims are in a master file. The registration clerk usually just has to select the plan from a list, and the address fields are automatically completed.

♦ **Policy number or member number:** A unique ID is assigned by a health plan to each policy or by a government program to each participant. HMO plans sometimes call this the member number; other plans may call it the insurance ID. Some plans assign a unique member number to each dependent as well. Keeping accurate records of these IDs is vital to getting paid by the health plan.

♦ **Group number:** In many cases health insurance is obtained through an employer who has negotiated special rates and coverage. In such cases, the insurance card may include a group number. This number is used to further identify the policy and the benefits to which the patient is entitled.

♦ **Policy holder:** The primary person who is named on the health insurance card is referred to as the *subscriber, insured party, enrollee, member, or policy holder*.

♦ **Beneficiary:** The beneficiary is a person who is entitled to receive benefits from the plan. Plan coverage is not limited to the policy holder and frequently includes spouses and children. In some systems these are called *dependents*.

◆ **Assignment of benefits:** Nearly all medical claims are filed by the provider, not the patient. The patient, during registration, signs a document authorizing the plan to pay the doctor directly. This is called assignment of benefits. The patient also authorizes the provider to submit information to the insurance plan for claims, eligibility and other business purposes.

### Case Study

John and Shirlee Colby are bringing their new baby, John, Jr., for his first visit to the pediatrician. Before being seen by the doctor, the new patient must be added to the system. The parents have completed the paper form shown in Figure 1-11.

### Step 1

You will need access to the Internet for this exercise. Start a supported web browser program and follow the steps listed inside the cover of this textbook to log in to the MyHealthProfessionsLab for this course.

### Step 2

Locate and click on the link **Exercise 1A**. This will open a video window.

Watch the video demonstrating the process of adding demographic information for a new patient.

### Step 3

Answer the onscreen questions at the end of the tutorial.

When you are finished click the Submit Quiz button to complete Exercise 1A.

After completing the tutorial, think about how many of the patient data fields will be used by the EHR system. In addition to the patient's name and medical record number used for the chart, the date of birth will be used to calculate the patient's age at each encounter. Gender will determine gender specific components of the examination, recommended tests, and clinical quality measures. The patient's pharmacy data will allow for electronic transmission of prescriptions. Race and ethnicity are used to prompt clinicians to screen for health conditions found in certain population groups.

## Patient and Provider Scheduling

Scheduling is central to a successful, smooth-running medical practice. With the exception of walk-in urgent care centers, most ambulatory care is delivered in scheduled patient appointments. The appointment schedule provides the framework for balanced and judicious scheduling of the provider's time. Enough time must be allotted for quality patient care, but the provider's time must not be wasted.

A typical patient encounter has several stages. The first part of the appointment consists of a medical assistant or nurse discussing the reason for the visit, past medical history, and measuring vital signs; the doctor comes in later. Where is the doctor during the first part of the appointment? With another patient, of course. From a scheduling perspective the two patients have overlapping appointments. This is called double booking.

However, patients are treated for many different reasons, and the time required of the doctor is not the same for all visits. Therefore, the type of appointment becomes a factor

# PATIENT REGISTRATION FORM

## PLEASE PRINT AND COMPLETE ALL ENTRIES

| PATIENT NAME (FIRST - MIDDLE INITIAL - LAST) **John T Colby, Jr.** | ADDRESS **2407 Grandview Avenue** | | |
|---|---|---|---|
| CITY, STATE **Mason, KY 41054-0001** | ZIP **41054** | HOME PHONE | CELL PHONE **859-555-5169** |

| DATE OF BIRTH **04/21/2015** | PATIENT SSN 555-55-5555 | GENDER ☒ Male ☐ Female | MARITAL STATUS ☒ Single ☐ Married ☐ Other_____ |
|---|---|---|---|

| NICKNAME | RACE – ETHINICITY **White** | PREFERRED LANGUAGE **English** | EMPLOYMENT STATUS ☐ Fulltime ☐ Part-time ☒ Not Employed ☐ Retired ☐ Student |
|---|---|---|---|

| PATIENT EMPLOYER NAME | PATIENT EMPLOYER ADDRESS (STREET ADDRESS - CITY - STATE - ZIP) | WORK PHONE |
|---|---|---|

## GUARANTOR/RESPONSIBLE PARTY INFORMATION — PATIENT RELATIONSHIP TO GUARANTOR: ☐ Self ☐ Spouse ☒ Child ☐ Other

| NAME (FIRST - MIDDLE INITIAL - LAST) **John T Colby** | ADDRESS (if different from patient) **Same** | | |
|---|---|---|---|
| HOME PHONE **859-555-5169** | WORK PHONE | SSN **000-00-2285** | BIRTH DATE **2/24/70** | EMPLOYER **Home Depot** |

## INSURANCE INFORMATION

| PRIMARY INSURANCE PLAN NAME **Cigna** | PLAN ADDRESS (STREET - CITY - STATE - ZIP) **PO Box 182223, Mason, KY 40154** | | PLAN PHONE |
|---|---|---|---|
| POLICY NUMBER **HX0002285** | POLICY HOLDER NAME **John T Colby** | DATE OF BIRTH **2/24/70** | GENDER ☒ Male ☐ Female |
| GROUP NUMBER/ NAME **None** | HOLDER ADDRESS (STREET - CITY - STATE - ZIP) **Same as patient** | PATIENT RELATIONSHIP TO HOLDER: ☐ Self ☐ Spouse ☒ Child ☐ Other | |
| SECONDARY INSURANCE PLAN NAME | PLAN ADDRESS (STREET CITY STATE ZIP) | | PLAN PHONE |
| POLICY NUMBER | POLICY HOLDER NAME | DATE OF BIRTH | GENDER ☐ Male ☐ Female |
| GROUP NUMBER/NAME | HOLDER ADDRESS (STREET - CITY - STATE - ZIP) | PATIENT RELATIONSHIP TO HOLDER: ☐ Self ☐ Spouse ☐ Child ☐ Other | |

## OTHER INFORMATION

| PRIMARY DOCTOR **Dr. Lora Jordan** | REFFERING DOCTOR **None** | |
|---|---|---|
| IN CASE OF EMERGENCY CONTACT **Shirlee Colby** | RELATIONSHIP **Mother** | PHONE NUMBER **859-555-0947** |
| PREFERRED METHOD OF CONTACT (Check all that apply). ☒ Home Phone ☐ Cell Phone ☒ Mail ☐ Email ☒ OK to leave message | EMAIL ADDRESS | I WOULD LIKE A CODE TO ACCESS THE WELL CARE ONLINE PORTAL ☐ Yes ☐ No |

## ASSIGNMENT AND CONSENT FOR RELEASE OF INFORMATION

I hereby authorize my insurance benefits be paid directly to the physician/provider. I also authorize the physician/provider to release any information required in the processing of this claim and all future claims. I agree to be financially responsible for non-covered services. If my account is sent to a collection agency, I agree to pay all collection and attorney fees.

I acknowledge that I have been offered a copy of Well Clinic's HIPAA Privacy Policy and I understand that:

- Well Care Clinic and its employees are permitted to share/disclose my health information for purposes of my Treatment, obtaining Payment and for Operation of the clinic (hereafter TPO.)

- I may make a request in writing at any time to inspect and/or obtain a copy of my health information maintained at this facility as provided in the Federal Privacy Rule 45 CFR (164.524).

- If I wish to do so I may also designate a Personal Representative to act in my behalf in all matters regarding my Protected PHI information.

- My records are protected and cannot be disclosed to a third party without my written Authorization except for TPO or when required by applicable federal and state laws governing the use and disclosure of protected health information.

- I may authorize the release of my information to Third Party by signing an Authorization request. A separate Authorization must be signed for each third party. Well Care Clinic is not responsible if the Recipient i authorize re-discloses my health information.

| SIGNATURE OF PATIENT OR LEGAL REPRESENTATIVE **John T. Colby** | DATE **2-10-2015** | RELATIONSHIP IF SIGNED BY LEGAL REPRESENTATIVE: **Father** |
|---|---|---|

**Figure 1-11** Example of paper patient information form used for patient registration.

in determining if appointments can overlap. How much of a resource's time is required for each type of appointment can be expressed as a percentage or "**percent effort**."

For example, appointment type A is 30 minutes long and requires 15 minutes of the doctor's time, or 50 percent effort. Appointment type B is 30 minutes long, but requires 20 minutes of the doctor's time, or 66 percent effort. Scheduling two overlapping type A appointments will not cause a problem. But scheduling appointments of types A and B at the same time would be a problem because the sum of the percent effort would require 116 percent of the provider's time. This is called overbooking.

As long as the cumulative percent for multiple appointments in the same time period doesn't exceed 100 percent the provider will be able to give sufficient time to each patient. The ideal schedule keeps the provider busy but not overcommitted. When a doctor is consistently overbooked, the doctor's schedule gets backed up, and the patients are kept waiting.

Another consideration is that not all providers work at the same pace, or perform exams in the same way. Therefore the percent effort can vary by provider even for the same type of appointment. Computerized scheduling systems assist the office in maintaining optimal schedules for all.

Not all appointments are with patients. Doctors have meetings, vacations, and personal appointments of their own. These are recorded in the schedule as *nonpatient* appointments. These have the effect of blocking the designated time and help make the scheduling person aware of times when the doctor is unavailable for patient appointments.

A typical scheduling module allows the user to view, schedule, and search for both patient and nonpatient appointments. It is also used to reschedule or cancel appointments and generate scheduling reports. It can also be used to check patients in or mark that a patient has arrived.

## Tutorial Exercise 1B: Overview of a Scheduling Module

In this exercise you will learn about the Scheduling module and how to add patient appointments. The Appointment Scheduling module demonstrated in this tutorial organizes schedules in Appointment books. When the user opens an appointment book, they see the schedule for a particular resource such as a doctor. As you will see in the tutorial, however, appointment books can be opened in such a way that multiple schedules can be viewed side by side in columns.

### Case Study

An appointment clerk in a multidoctor practice adds, cancels, and reschedules patient appointments and blocks time on the doctors' schedules for a meeting.

### Step 1

You will need access to the Internet for this exercise. Start a supported web browser program and follow the steps listed inside the cover of this textbook to log in to the MyHealthProfessionsLab for this course.

### Step 2

Locate and click on the link **Exercise 1B**. This will open a video window.

Watch the video demonstrating the process of scheduling patient appointments.

**Step 3**

Answer the onscreen questions at the end of the tutorial.

When you are finished, click the Submit Quiz button.

Now that you have seen patient registration, an appointment book, and how appointment schedules are managed, we will concentrate on EHR functions for the remaining chapters.

## Chapter One Summary

*Electronic Health Records are the portions of a patient's medical records that are stored in a computer system as well as the functional benefits derived from having an electronic health record.*

The IOM set forth eight core functions that an EHR should be capable of performing:

◆ **Health information and data**  Provide improved access to information needed by care providers, using a defined data set that includes medical and nursing diagnoses, a medication list, allergies, demographics, clinical narratives, laboratory test results, and more.

◆ **Result management**  Electronic results for better interpretation, and quicker recognition and treatment of medical problems; reduces redundant testing and improves care coordination among multiple providers.

◆ **Order management**  CPOE systems improve workflow, eliminate lost orders and ambiguities caused by illegible handwriting, monitor for duplicate orders, and reduce the time required to fill orders.

◆ **Decision support**  Includes prevention, prescribing of drugs, diagnosis and management, and detection of adverse events and disease outbreaks.

◆ Computer reminders and prompts improve preventive practices in areas such as vaccinations, breast cancer screening, colorectal screening, and cardiovascular risk reduction.

◆ **Electronic communication and connectivity**  Among care partners, enhances patient safety and quality of care, especially for patients who have multiple providers.

◆ **Patient support**  For example, patient education and home monitoring by patients using electronic devices.

◆ **Administrative processes and reporting**  Increases the efficiency of healthcare organizations and provides better, timelier service to patients.

◆ **Reporting and population health**  Facilitates the reporting of key quality indicators and timely reporting of adverse reactions and disease outbreaks.

The CPRI identified three key criteria for an EHR:

◆ Capture data at the point of care

◆ Integrate data from multiple sources

◆ Provide decision support

The ONC created a strategic framework for achieving widespread adoption of EHR within 10 years.

The HITECH Act provides CMS incentives for providers to use a certified EHR.

ONC seeks to reduce the risk of EHR investment by establishing Authorized Testing and Certification Bodies to certify EHR systems.

A patient encounter document is organized into four components:

◆ Subjective

◆ Objective

◆ Assessment

◆ Plan

EHR systems strive to improve patient healthcare by giving the provider and patient access to complete, up-to-date records of past and present conditions.

Documenting at the point of care means the providers (clinicians, nurses, and medical assistants) record findings at the time of the encounter, not after they have left the patient.

Implementing an EHR requires changes in the way providers work, including the type of clinician–patient interaction the clinicians hope to achieve.

Before the patient encounter can be documented in an EHR, the patient must first be added to the system and in most practices scheduled. During patient registration the system automatically assigns a patient number. Patients are also assigned to an account. The account is used for charge and payment posting, and for billing.

The demographic portion of registration is divided into two sections, patient information and guarantor information. The guarantor is the person responsible for paying the account. The guarantor may be the patient, a spouse, a parent, or even an employer.

When the patient is not the guarantor, the name, address, and phone number of the guarantor must be recorded so they can be used for account billing later. The employer field on the demographic tab records the guarantor's employer. When the patient is not the guarantor, the patient's employer is recorded on the Additional Data tab.

Insurance information is recorded on the insurance tab and is used to submit claims, preauthorization, and determining eligibility.

The health plan, sometimes called the payer, is a third party who pays all or a portion of the patient's medical bill. Health plans include profit and not-for-profit insurance companies, government programs, and employer self-insurance funds.

Patients can have multiple insurance plans. The rank field is used to indicate which should be billed: primary, secondary, and so on.

The beneficiary is a person entitled to receive benefits from the plan. Some plans call beneficiaries members.

Health plans assign a unique ID to each policy and sometimes each member of a policy.

Employers or other groups negotiate special rates and coverage. A Group Name or Group Number assigned by the plan helps assure the patient receives these special rates.

The person who holds the policy or coverage is called the policy holder. In some cases (such as worker's compensation) the policy holder may be a nonperson such as a corporation or business. Other terms used for policy holder include subscriber, insured party, enrollee, or member.

An assignment of benefits authorizes the health plan to pay the doctor directly. The patient also authorizes the provider to submit information to the insurance plan for claims, eligibility, and other business purposes. These authorizations may be part of the registration form or a separate document.

Scheduling is essential to keeping most ambulatory care practices running smoothly. Balanced and judicious scheduling of the provider's time must allow enough time for quality patient care without wasting the provider's time between patients. Since the provider is with the patient for only a portion of the typical patient encounter, offices often overlap the appointments of multiple patients. This is called double booking.

The amount of the provider's time required for each type of appointment can be expressed as a percentage. The tutorial called this the percent effort. Different appointment types have different percent effort. Double booked appointments can be scheduled unless the cumulative percent effort in a slot exceeds 100 percent. If this occurs, the user is warned. If the user overrides the warning, the slot is considered overbooked. An override code is required to overbook a time slot.

## Testing Your Knowledge of Chapter 1

### Step 1

Log in to MyHealthProfessionsLab following the directions printed inside the cover of this textbook.

Locate and click on Chapter 1 Test.

### Step 2

Answer the test questions. When you have finished, click the Submit Test button to close the window.

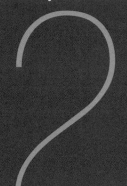

# Functional EHR Systems

## Learning Outcomes

*After completing this chapter, you should be able to:*

- ◆ Compare different formats of EHR data
- ◆ Describe the importance of codified EHR
- ◆ Have an understanding of prominent EHR code sets such as SNOMED-CT, Medcin, LOINC, and CCC
- ◆ Explain different methods of capturing and recording EHR data
- ◆ Catalog and retrieve documents and images from a digital image system
- ◆ Discuss the exchange of data between EHR and other systems
- ◆ Discuss the benefits of patient-entered data
- ◆ Describe the functional benefits from a codified EHR
- ◆ Compare different formats of lab result data
- ◆ Discuss alert systems and drug utilization review
- ◆ Describe two important components of health maintenance
- ◆ Provide examples of EHR decision support

## Format of Data Determines Potential Benefits

The ability to easily find, share, and search patient records makes an EHR superior to a paper record system. Remember, however, that Chapter 1 defined the EHR as the portions of the patient's medical record stored in the computer system *as well as the functional benefits derived from them.*

The IOM defined eight core functions that an EHR should be capable of performing. Four of the *functional benefits* identified by the IOM are health maintenance, trend analysis, alerts, and decision support. The form in which the data is stored determines to what extent the computer can use the content of the EHR to provide additional functions that improve the quality of care.

CMS states on their website: "In order to capture and share patient data efficiently, providers need an EHR that stores data in a structured format. Structured data allows patient information to be easily retrieved and transferred, and it allows the provider to use the EHR in ways that can aid patient care."[1] This chapter will examine the forms in which EHR data is stored, explore how functional benefits are derived from it, and see how data may be entered.

## EHR Data Formats

The various ways in which medical records data are stored in the database may be broadly categorized into three forms:

### Digital images

This form of EHR data can be retrieved and displayed by the computer, but a human is required to interpret the meaning of the content. This category may be subcategorized into:

**Diagnostic images** such as digital x-rays, CAT scans, digital pathology, and even annotated drawings

**Scanned documents** such as paper forms, old medical records, letters, or even sound files of dictated notes

### Text files

The second type of data includes word processing files of transcribed exam notes and also text reports. It is principally obtained in the EHR by importing text files from outside sources. Here is an example of text data: "The patient injured his knee on March 31, 2016, but it was improved as of April 28, 2016."

### Discrete data

This third form of stored information in an EHR is the easiest for the computer to use. It can be instantly searched, retrieved, and combined or reported in different ways. Discrete data in an EHR may be subcategorized into:

**Fielded data** in which each piece of information is stored separately in an assigned position in a computer record called a *field*. The meaning of the information is inferred from its position in the record. For example, a record of fielded data might look like this:

"knee injury","20160331","improved","20160428"

The data in this record are stored in four fields (in this example surrounded by quotation marks). The computer would look for the name of the problem in the first field, the date of onset in the second field, the status of the problem in the third field, and the date of the last exam in the fourth field.

**Coded data** is fielded data that also contains codes in addition to or in place of descriptive text. Codes eliminate ambiguities about the clinician's meaning, improve data specificity, and act as a universal language between disparate computer systems.

---

[1] www.cms.gov/regulations-and-guidance/legislation/ehrincentiveprograms/certification.html, on September 24, 2015.

A codified EHR record of the same knee problem might look like this:

"8442", "knee injury","20160331","improved","20160428"

The first field holds a code number identifying a specific type of injury.

### Limitations of Certain Types of Data

An EHR offers improved accessibility to patient records over a paper chart. That is certainly a functional benefit of any EHR regardless of the format of its data. However, to achieve its full functional benefits, the computer must be able to quickly and accurately identify the information contained within the records.

**Digital image** data can be retrieved and displayed by the computer, but a human is required to interpret the meaning of the content. Although this is beneficial for sharing diagnostic images, if the bulk of the EHR is simply scanned paper documents, only one or two of the IOM criteria defined in Chapter 1 are satisfied.

**Text data** are useful for healthcare providers and ancillary staff to read and can be searched by the computer for research purposes. However, text data is seldom used for generating alerts, trend analysis, decision support, or other real-time EHR functions because the search capability is slow and the results often ambiguous.

**Fielded data** is the most common way to store information in computers and EHR systems. It is fast and efficient and uses very little storage space. However, unless the fielded data is also codified, the meaning of the data can be ambiguous.

Within medicine, many different terms are used to describe the same symptom, condition, or observation. Additionally, clinicians often use short abbreviations to document their observations in a patient chart. This makes it difficult for a computer to compare notes from one physician to another. For example, providers at two different clinics might record a knee injury problem differently:

Dr. 1: "twisted his knee"

Dr. 2: "knee sprain"

A search of medical records with "knee injury" in the problem field might not find the records created by either clinician.

**Coded data** is when a code is stored in the medical record in addition to the text description—the record is then considered codified. The EHR system can instantly find and match the desired information by code regardless of the clinician's choice of words. Continuing with the previous example, if the records of both Dr. 1 and Dr. 2 contained the code 8442, then the computer would recognize the knee injury. A codified EHR is more useful than a text-based record for precisely identifying the clinician's finding or treatment.

EHR data stored in a fielded, codified form adds significant value, but if the codes are not standard it will be difficult to exchange medical record data between different EHR systems or facilities. Remember, the exchange of data is one of the eight core functions defined by the IOM. Using a national standard code set instead of proprietary codes to codify the data will better enable the exchange of medical records among systems, improve the accuracy of the content, and open the door to the other functional benefits derived from having an electronic health record.

## Standard EHR Coding Systems

EHR coding systems are called nomenclatures. EHR nomenclatures differ from other code sets and classification systems in that they are designed to codify the details and nuance of the patient–clinician encounter. EHR nomenclatures are different from code sets used for billing and reimbursement in this respect. For example, a procedure code used for billing an office visit does not describe what the clinician observed during the visit, just the type of visit and complexity of the exam. EHR nomenclatures need to have a lot more codes to describe the details of the exam; for this reason, they are said to be more *granular*. Two prominent nomenclatures for EHR records are SNOMED-CT® and Medcin®. Another prominent coding system, LOINC®, is used for lab results.

Unfortunately, many hospital systems use none of these standard systems, having instead developed internal coding schemes applicable only to their facilities. These work within the organization but create problems when trying to integrate other software or exchange data with other facilities. To create an EHR that is able to receive, create, and compare medical information from numerous sources, it is necessary to adopt a coding system that is used by other providers—in other words, a national standard.

## Prominent EHR Code Sets

EHR nomenclatures have hundreds of thousands of codes to represent not only procedures and diseases but also the symptoms, observations, history, medications, and myriad other details. The level of **granularity** determines how fine a level of detail is represented by a code in the nomenclature.

However, too much granularity can make a code set difficult to use at the point of care. The point of care is when both the clinician and patient are present. Extremely granular code sets, called *reference terminologies*, are impractical for a clinician to use in an exam. Designed for data analysis, these code sets often are applied to the medical records after the fact for a specific research project.

To balance the need for granularity with the practical requirements of point-of-care documentation, EHR nomenclatures define **clinical concepts** or **findings**, which are codified observations, medically meaningful to the clinician. Some systems of clinical vocabulary are just "data dictionaries" that are used to standardize medical terms.

For example, a data dictionary will have the terms *eye, arm, leg, chest, nostril, left, right, red, yellow, radiating, discharge,* and *pain.* These terms could be combined in many ways, some of them meaningless. EHR nomenclatures precorrelate those terms into relevant *clinical concepts* which become easier to record as *findings*.

Precorrelating clinical concepts means to use one code that represents the combination of several individual terms in a manner that is clinically relevant. For example using one code to record the finding "chest pain radiating to the left arm" combines five clinical terms into a meaningful symptom.

Linked or indexed concepts in an EHR nomenclature enable clinicians to quickly locate related symptoms, elements of the physical exam, assessments, and treatments when documenting the visit.

The following sections will provide a brief history and purpose of several of the most prominent coding standards you are likely to encounter or use in an EHR.

**SNOMED-CT**    SNOMED stands for Systematized Nomenclature of Medicine; CT stands for Clinical Terms. **SNOMED-CT** is a comprehensive clinical terminology, originally created by the College of American Pathologists, but now owned, maintained, and distributed by the International Health Terminology Standards Development

Organisation, a not-for-profit association in Denmark. SNOMED-CT is one of a suite of designated standards for use in U.S. Federal Government systems for the electronic exchange of clinical health information.

**SNOMED-CT Structure**    The SNOMED-CT Core terminology contains over 400,000 healthcare *concepts*, organized into the following 18 hierarchical categories:

- Body structure
- Clinical finding
- Environments or geographical location
- Event
- Linkage concept
- Observable entity
- Organism
- Pharmaceutical/biological product
- Physical force
- Physical object
- Procedure
- Qualifier value
- Record artifact
- Situation with explicit context
- Social context
- Special concept
- Staging and scales
- Substance

Semantic relationships between concepts in the SNOMED-CT nomenclature are of two types: *Is-A* relationships and *Attribute* relationships.

**Is-A** relationships connect concepts within a single hierarchy. For example, the disease concept Bronchial Pneumonia *Is-A* Pneumonia (also a disease concept).

**Attribute** relationships connect concepts from two different hierarchies. For example, the disease concept Bronchial Pneumonia has the associated *Attribute* Inflammation (which is from a different hierarchy, morphology).

**Medcin**    Medcin is a medical nomenclature and knowledge base developed by Medicomp Systems, Inc., in collaboration with physicians on staff at Cornell, Harvard, Johns Hopkins, and other major medical centers. Medcin is the nomenclature standard used in U.S. Department of Defense medical facilities worldwide, and in software of many prominent U.S. EHR companies.

The purpose of the Medcin nomenclature and the intent of the design differentiate it from other coding standards. SNOMED-CT and other reference coding systems were designed to classify or index medical information for research or other purposes and later expanded for use by practicing physicians. Medcin was designed for point-of-care use by the clinician. Medcin is not just a list of medical terms, but rather a list of precorrelated clinical concepts that are medically meaningful to the clinician at the point of care.

**Medcin Structure** The Medcin nomenclature consists of more than 340,000 clinical concepts or "findings" divided into six domains:

◆ Symptoms

◆ History

◆ Physical examination

◆ Tests

◆ Diagnoses, syndromes, and conditions

◆ Therapy

Medcin differs from other EHR coding systems in that the nomenclature is not just a codified list of terms. The Medcin nomenclature is contained in a "knowledge base" with a diagnostic index of more than 68 million links between clinically related concepts. This "knowledge" enables an EHR system based on Medcin to quickly find other clinical concepts that are likely to be needed; this in turn reduces the time it takes to create exam notes.

This difference means a physician selects fewer individual codes to complete the patient exam note. For example, SNOMED-CT has a code for "arm" and a code for "pain," Medcin has the clinical concept "arm pain." Medcin often has additional clinical concepts that infer important nuances; for example, the clinical concept "arm tenderness" might more accurately describe the patient's symptom than arm pain.

SNOMED-CT was historically developed as a reference terminology. It provides very granular coding that normalizes data for research and reporting. Its structure provides millions of semantic links based on a term, word, or concept. Figure 2-1 shows the SNOMED-CT finding Asthma with its various Is-A relationships.

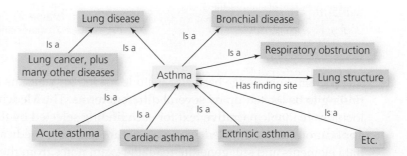

**Figure 2-1** SNOMED-CT links for the term "Asthma."

Figure 2-1 and Figure 2-2 compare the structure of SNOMED-CT and Medcin using the finding for asthma. As you can see from the comparison, the Medcin knowledge base relates asthma to 279 total direct links (only 70 are shown in Figure 2-2). Each of these has relevancy to point-of-care use for an asthma patient. SNOMED-CT links include obvious links to asthma but not directly to the symptoms, tests, or therapy. Links in Figure 2-1 also connect to lungs and other lung diseases not related to asthma. Such associations are sometimes useful when coding records for research but can make it difficult for the clinician to use such a system while seeing the patient.

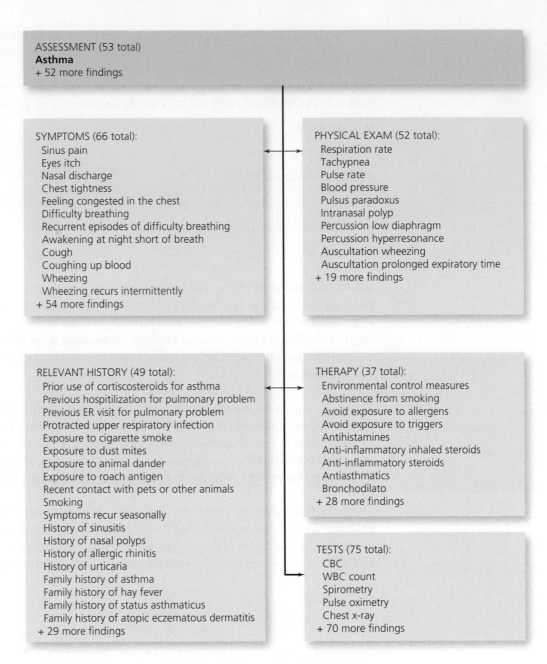

**Figure 2-2** Medcin links for the term "Asthma."

ASSESSMENT (53 total)
**Asthma**
+ 52 more findings

SYMPTOMS (66 total):
  Sinus pain
  Eyes itch
  Nasal discharge
  Chest tightness
  Feeling congested in the chest
  Difficulty breathing
  Recurrent episodes of difficulty breathing
  Awakening at night short of breath
  Cough
  Coughing up blood
  Wheezing
  Wheezing recurs intermittently
+ 54 more findings

PHYSICAL EXAM (52 total):
  Respiration rate
  Tachypnea
  Pulse rate
  Blood pressure
  Pulsus paradoxus
  Intranasal polyp
  Percussion low diaphragm
  Percussion hyperresonance
  Auscultation wheezing
  Auscultation prolonged expiratory time
+ 19 more findings

RELEVANT HISTORY (49 total):
  Prior use of cortiscosteroids for asthma
  Previous hospitilization for pulmonary problem
  Previous ER visit for pulmonary problem
  Protracted upper respiratory infection
  Exposure to cigarette smoke
  Exposure to dust mites
  Exposure to animal dander
  Exposure to roach antigen
  Recent contact with pets or other animals
  Smoking
  Symptoms recur seasonally
  History of sinusitis
  History of nasal polyps
  History of allergic rhinitis
  History of urticaria
  Family history of asthma
  Family history of hay fever
  Family history of status asthmaticus
  Family history of atopic eczematous dermatitis
+ 29 more findings

THERAPY (37 total):
  Environmental control measures
  Abstinence from smoking
  Avoid exposure to allergens
  Avoid exposure to triggers
  Antihistamines
  Anti-inflammatory inhaled steroids
  Anti-inflammatory steroids
  Antiasthmatics
  Bronchodilato
+ 28 more findings

TESTS (75 total):
  CBC
  WBC count
  Spirometry
  Pulse oximetry
  Chest x-ray
+ 70 more findings

The Medcin knowledge base also includes 600,000 synonyms for findings, allowing a finding to be looked up by several different terms. The Medcin knowledge base includes readable narrative text for each finding selected by the clinician. EHR applications using the Medcin nomenclature can store medical information as coded data elements and still generate readable exam notes from the same data.

An EHR system based on Medcin enables the clinician to select fewer individual codes and to quickly locate other clinical concepts that are likely to be needed. This difference from SNOMED-CT means it takes less time for a clinician to create patient exam notes and makes it possible to complete the exam note at the time of the encounter.

Many experts feel that for point-of-care documentation medical nomenclatures such as Medcin are the key to successful adoption of an EHR by clinicians. Because Medcin is used in many commercial EHR systems, it has been selected as the EHR nomenclature for the student exercises in this textbook. You will learn more about Medcin in subsequent chapters.

**LOINC** LOINC stands for Logical Observation Identifiers Names and Codes. LOINC was created and is maintained by the Regenstrief Institute, which is closely affiliated with the Indiana University School of Medicine. While not a full medical nomenclature, LOINC standardizes codes for laboratory test orders and results, such as blood hemoglobin and serum potassium, and also clinical observations, such as vital signs or ECG.

LOINC is important because when laboratories and other diagnostic services report test results using their own internal proprietary codes it makes it difficult for the receiving EHR to compare results from multiple lab facilities—like comparing apples and oranges. LOINC provides a universal coding system for mapping laboratory tests and results to a common terminology in the EHR. This then makes it possible for a computer program to find and report comparable test values regardless of where the test was processed.

The LOINC terminology is divided into three portions: laboratory, clinical (nonlaboratory), and HIPAA. The largest number of codes is in the laboratory section. The second largest section of LOINC is the clinical section, which includes codes for vital signs, ECG, ultrasound, cardiac echogram, and many other clinical observations.

A third section of LOINC has been created to categorize codes for a HIPAA claims attachment transaction. Claims attachments are used to submit additional supporting information with an insurance claim.

The wide acceptance of LOINC is attributable in part to its adoption by HL7 (discussed later in this chapter). HL7 uses LOINC codes in its clinical messages

**Clinical Care Classification System (CCC)** Twelve standards for coded nursing languages are recognized by the American Nurses Association today for use in the assessment, diagnosis, intervention, and outcome of nursing care. Using a commonly understood codified structure enables nurses to create and communicate a patient plan of care that is evidence based, facilitates documentation of the practice of nursing in the EHR, and permits data sharing to improve patient care outcomes. This chapter does not include a comprehensive explanation of all 12 coding structures, but will briefly discuss one of them, the Clinical Care Classification (CCC) System, which codifies the discrete elements of nursing practice.

Developed by Virginia Saba at Georgetown University, the CCC System was accepted by the Department of Health and Human Services in 2007 as the first national nursing terminology and is an American Nurses Association–recognized, comprehensive, coded nursing terminology standard.

The CCC System consists of a unique four-level framework and coding structure for capturing the essence of patient care in all healthcare settings. The CCC System is used to document a nursing plan of care following the six steps of the nursing process model.

The CCC system provides standardized coding concepts for nursing diagnoses, outcomes, nursing interventions, and actions in two interrelated terminologies based on ICD-10. CCC defines 21 Care Components that provide a framework to interrelate the 176 CCC Nursing Diagnoses and 201 core Nursing Actions/Interventions (804 nursing concepts). The complete CCC system has been integrated into the Medcin nomenclature used for this course, and CCC codes have been added to the SNOMED-CT and LOINC code sets as well.

**RxNorm** RxNorm provides normalized names and codes for drugs, and links drugs to codified vocabularies commonly used in pharmacy management and drug interaction software including NDF-RT. (NDF-RT is a terminology from the Veterans Health Administration used to code clinical drug properties, including mechanism of action, physiologic effect, and therapeutic category.) RxNorm codes are incorporated into Medcin and SNOMED-CT.

**UMLS**   UMLS stands for Unified Medical Language System®. It is maintained by the National Library of Medicine (NLM). Because students may find mention of UMLS elsewhere, it is mentioned here. However, UMLS is not itself a medical terminology, but rather a resource of software tools and data created from many medical nomenclatures, including those described in this chapter. UMLS is described as a "meta-thesaurus." It can be used to retrieve and integrate biomedical information and provide cross-references among selected vocabularies.

## How EHR Code Sets Differ From Code Sets Used for Billing

Code sets that have been created or adapted for reimbursement are not suitable for codifying clinical records. They are too general—simply reporting what service was rendered or a condition that was diagnosed. They lack sufficient granularity to document what was reported by the patient and observed by the clinician that led to the diagnosis and procedure. However, since this is a discussion of coding systems we will briefly mention two standard code sets whose use is required by HIPAA. These are not EHR nomenclatures, but are required for billing and will be explained more fully in Chapter 12.

If you have worked in a medical facility or taken a course on practice management, you may have already heard of the next two code sets.

**ICD-10CM**   ICD stands for International Classification of Diseases, which is a system of standardized codes developed collaboratively between the World Health Organization (WHO) and ten international centers. The coding system as it is today evolved from the International List of Causes of Death, which was used by physicians, medical examiners, and coroners to facilitate standardized mortality studies. In 1948, WHO expanded and renamed the system to make it useful for codifying patient medical conditions as well.

The numeral 10 represents the 10th revision of the coding system. The preceding versions were revised about every 10 years from 1900–1979. After the ninth revision was published, however, the United States National Center for Health Statistics modified the system to add clinical information codes. The code set was distinguished by the letters "CM" for Clinical Modification. When, in 1989, the U.S. Congress made ICD-9CM mandatory on Part B Medicare claims, the code set became firmly linked to billing. Because of this, although WHO continued to evolve the ICD codes, the U.S. healthcare system could not easily adopt the new revision. Finally, in 2015, U.S. providers were required to transition from ICD-9CM to ICD-10CM for health insurance claims.

ICD-10CM differs from EHR nomenclatures in that it primarily codes the assessment portion of the encounter. An unrelated code set with a similar name, ICD-10PCS, is used to classify procedures performed in an inpatient facility for billing.

**CPT-4®**   CPT stands for Current Procedural Terminology. The numeral 4 represents the fourth edition of the coding system. CPT-4 codes are standardized codes for reporting medical services, procedures, and treatments performed for patients in ambulatory settings. A different code set (ICD-10PCS) is used for inpatient procedures.

CPT was created in 1968 by the American Medical Society to provide a uniform code set that accurately identified medical, surgical, and diagnostic services. In 1983, CPT-4 codes became standard for private insurance, Medicare, and Medicaid claims when it was adopted by the government as part of the Healthcare Common Procedure Coding System (HCPCS).

CPT-4 differs from EHR nomenclatures in that a CPT-4 only identifies the event of a patient encounter, performed test, or procedure. The code set lacks granularity to describe the signs, symptoms, or clinical concepts of the patient encounter or service. Conversely, findings in the symptoms, history, physical exam, and plan domains are used to determine the CPT-4 code for an encounter, as we shall see in Chapter 12.

**Code Usage** A big difference between EHR nomenclatures and billing code sets is the users' awareness of the codes themselves. EHR nomenclature codes are typically invisible to the user. Daily clinical users may not even be aware of which nomenclature underlies the EHR they are using. EHR users are able to locate desired clinical concepts by description and never need to know the underlying code number. EHR nomenclatures tie assessments codes directly to the ICD-10CM code for the provider. Medcin-based EHRs can also analyze the findings in the note and suggest the appropriate CPT-4 codes. Still, providers and/or their staff must know the ICD-10CM and CPT-4 codes to assign the appropriate codes to bill for the encounter.

## Exchanging Data with Other Standard Code Sets

The Medcin knowledge base contains cross-references to map Medcin to SNOMED-CT, ICD-10-CM, CPT-4, LOINC, CCC, and RxNorm drug codes. This allows the EHR to exchange information with billing, laboratory, pharmacy, and other systems that use one of the standardized code sets we have discussed. The following examples illustrate how the Medcin codes[2] for three findings map to other standard vocabularies:

| *test to measure:* Hemoglobin Level | |
|---|---|
| **Vocabulary** | **Code** |
| Medcin | 12004 |
| CPT-4 | 85018 |
| LOINC | 718-7 |
| SNOMED-CT | 271026005 |

| *finding:* Allergy to penicillin | |
|---|---|
| **Vocabulary** | **Code** |
| Medcin | 4927 |
| ICD-10CM | Z88.0 |
| SNOMED-CT | 91936005 |

| *nursing diagnosis finding:* Cardiac output alteration | |
|---|---|
| **Vocabulary** | **Code** |
| Medcin | 314435 |
| CCC | C05.0 |
| LOINC | 28149-3 |
| SNOMED-CT | 129900004 |

---

[2]Code mapping © 2016 - Medicomp Systems Inc - All rights reserved. Used with permission.

# Capturing and Recording EHR Data

The value of having an EHR is evident, but how does the data get into the EHR? Thus far we have discussed three forms of EHR data. In subsequent chapters we will explore how healthcare providers (clinicians, nurses, and medical assistants) create codified EHR. But before we move on, let us briefly examine how digital image data and text file data are added to the EHR and used. We will also discuss additional sources of EHR data that can be imported directly into the system.

## Importing Digital Images

As discussed previously, digital image data may be subcategorized into diagnostic images and scanned document images. Even with the implementation of a codified EHR, there will always be some paper documents. Obviously there are all the old paper charts of established patients, but there is also a continuing influx of patient-related paper medical documents from outside sources.

Most healthcare organizations choose to bring incoming paper documents such as referral forms into the EHR as scanned images. Although document images do not offer all the benefits of a codified medical record, they do provide widespread accessibility and a means to include source documents for a complete electronic chart.

Most document image systems have a computer program to associate various ID fields and keywords with scanned images. This is called *cataloging the image*. Catalog data adds the capability to search for the electronic document images in multiple ways.

## Guided Exercise 2A: Exploring a Document Imaging System

In this exercise you will experience how an imaging system works.

### Case Study

Memorial Hospital has begun to archive older paper and film records into the EHR document image system. In this exercise you are going to retrieve and view some records from 2012.

### Step 1

You will need access to the Internet for this exercise. Start a supported web browser program and follow the steps listed inside the cover of this textbook to log in to the MyHealthProfessionsLab for this course.

### Step 2

Locate and click on the link **Exercise 2A**.

A screen similar to Figure 2-3 will be displayed.

#### The Document/Image System Window
As you proceed through the following steps, you will be introduced to names, functions, and components of the Document/Image System window. This program simulates many of the features typically found in an EHR document/image management system.

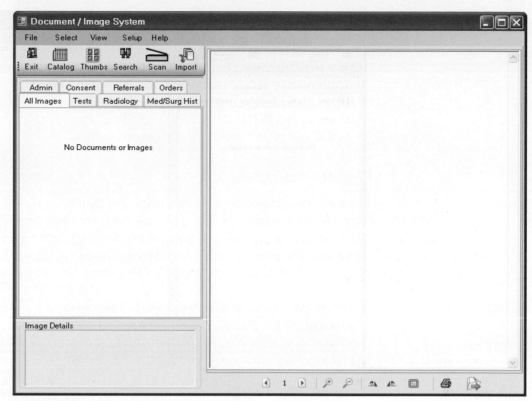

**Figure 2-3** Document/Image System window.

**The Menu Bar** At the top of the screen, the words "File," "Select," "View," "Setup," and "Help" are the menus of functions typically found in document image software. We call this the *Menu bar*. When you position the mouse over one of these words and click the mouse once, a list of functions will drop down below the word.

Once a menu list appears, clicking one of the items will invoke that function. Clicking the mouse anywhere except on the list will close the list. Certain items on the menu are displayed in gray text. These items are not available until a patient or document has been selected. The Setup and Help options are not available in this simulation.

### Step 3

Position the mouse pointer over the word "Select" in the Menu bar at the top of the screen and click the mouse button once. A list of the Select menu functions will appear (see Figure 2-4).

### Step 4

Move the mouse pointer vertically down the list over the word "Patient" and click the mouse to invoke the Patient Selection window shown in Figure 2-5.

### Step 5

Find the patient named Raj Patel in the Patient Selection window. Position the mouse pointer over the patient name and double-click the mouse. (*Double-click* means to click the mouse button twice, very rapidly.)

Once a patient is selected, the patient's name, age, and sex are displayed in the title at the top of the window.

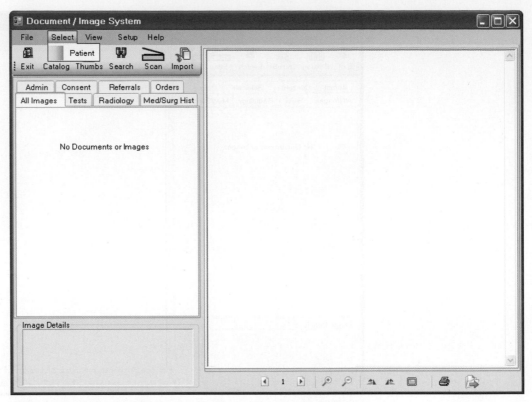

**Figure 2-4** Document/Image System after clicking the Select menu.

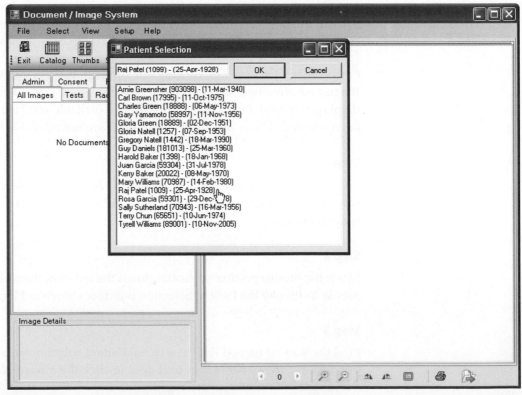

**Figure 2-5** Selecting Raj Patel from the Patient Selection window.

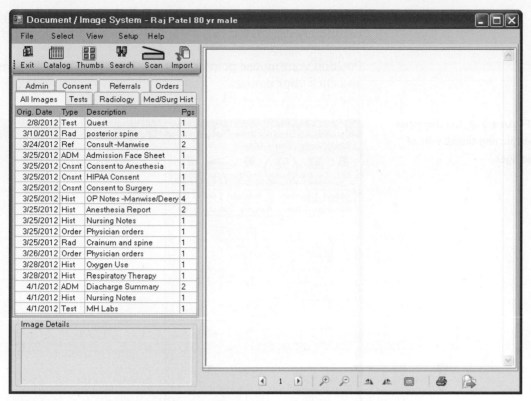

**Figure 2-6** Left pane displays catalog list of documents and images for Raj Patel.

Compare your screen to Figure 2-6 as you read the following information:

### The Toolbar

Also located at the top of your screen is a row of icon buttons called a *Toolbar*. The purpose of the Toolbar is to allow quick access to commonly used functions. Most Windows programs feature a Toolbar, so you may already be familiar with the concept.

### The Catalog Pane

The middle portion of the screen is divided into two window panes. The left pane (just below the Toolbar) is where a list of cataloged documents display once a patient is selected. At the top of the catalog pane are eight tabs. These look like tabs on file folders. The tabs are used to limit the list to images by category, making it easier to find a specific type of image quickly. The initial tab is All Images, listed in date order.

### Step 6

Locate the Toolbar in the Document/Image System window. The first icon, labeled "Exit," will close the simulation program and return you to the MyHealthProfessionsLab page. Do not click it yet.

The next two buttons are used to change display of items in the Catalog pane from a list to thumbnails. Thumbnails are small versions of the document or image.

Position your mouse pointer over the Thumbs icon on the Toolbar (circled in Figure 2-7) and click your mouse.

**Figure 2-7** Catalog pane displaying thumbnails of images.

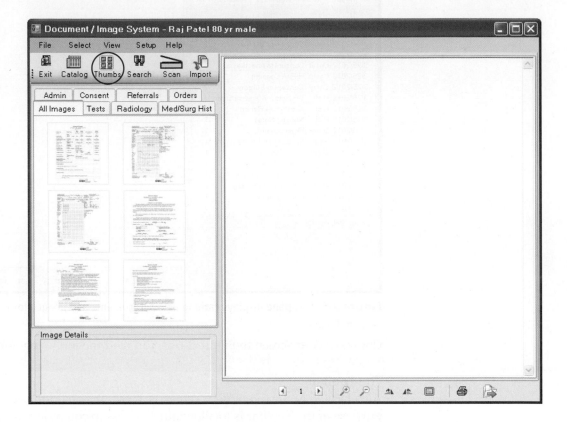

Compare your screen to Figure 2-7.

Now position your mouse pointer over the Catalog icon on the Toolbar and click your mouse. Your screen should again resemble Figure 2-6.

### Step 7

Locate the Med/Srg Hist tab above the Catalog pane. Position your mouse pointer over it and click your mouse. The list should now be shorter as it is limited to items cataloged in the category of Medical/Surgical History.

### Step 8

Locate the catalog item Anesthesia Report and click on it. Compare your screen to Figure 2-8 as you read the following information.

### The Image Viewer Pane

The right pane of the window will dynamically display the corresponding image for a catalog entry that is clicked.

### Item Details

Just below the Catalog pane is a gray panel that displays information about a selected catalog item such as the user who scanned the document, relevant dates, and a longer description of the item.

**Figure 2-8** Catalog on Med/Srg tab, Anesthesia Report, displayed in the Image Viewer pane.

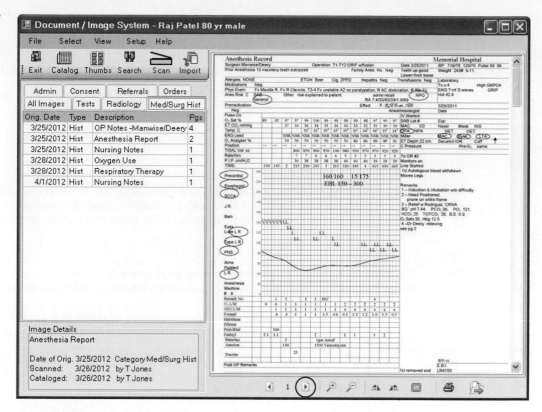

## Image Tools

Just below the Image Viewer pane is a row of icon buttons used to change the displayed image. These include the ability to page through multipage documents, and enlarge or reduce the displayed image.

### Step 9

Locate the image tools buttons just below the viewer pane. The first three icons become active whenever a multipage document is selected. The Anesthesia Report has two pages. Locate and click on the Next page button (circled in red in Figure 2-6). The button displays the next page of a multipage document. The numeral between the two buttons is the page number currently displayed. You screen should now display the second page of the report and the Image Tool should display the numeral two.

The Previous page button is the first icon in the image tools. Locate it and click on it. The image tool area should now display the numeral one, and the image viewer should again display the first page of the report.

The next two icons resemble magnifying glasses. One includes a plus sign—this is the Zoom In tool; it enlarges the text in the viewer. The other magnifying glass has a minus sign—this is the Zoom Out tool; it reduces the enlarged view to show more of the page in the viewer.

Locate and click on the Zoom In icon to see how it works.

### Step 10

Locate and click the Exit button in the Document Image program toolbar. Answer the questions presented. When you have finished, click the Submit Quiz button.

## Cataloging Digital Images

The process of scanning documents or importing scanned images into an image system includes not only capturing the image but tying it to the correct patient and entering

Memorial Hospital
876 Memory Ln, Anywhere, ID 83776
(208) 378-5555
CONSENT TO USE AND DISCLOSE HEALTH INFORMATION
for Treatment, Payment, or Healthcare operations

I understand that as part of my healthcare, Memorial Hospital originates and maintains health records describing my health history, symptoms, examination and test results, diagnoses, treatment, and any plans for future care or treatment. I understand that this information serves as:

- a basis for planning my care and treatment
- a means of communication among the many health professionals who contribute to my care
- a source of information for applying my diagnosis and surgical information to my bill
- a means by which a third-party payer can verify that services billed were actually provided
- and a tool for routine healthcare operations such as assessing quality and reviewing the competence of healthcare professionals

I understand and have been provided with a *Notice of Privacy Practices* that provides a more complete description of information uses and disclosures. I understand that I have the right to review the notice prior to signing this consent. I understand that Memorial Hospital reserves the right to change their notice and practices and prior to implementation will mail a copy of any revised notice to the address I've provided. I understand that I have the right to object to the use of my health information for directory purposes. I understand that I have the right to request restrictions as to how my health information may be used or disclosed to carry out treatment, payment, or healthcare operations and that Memorial Hospital is not required to agree to the restrictions requested. I understand that I may revoke this consent in writing, except to the extent that the hospital and its employees have already take action in reliance thereon.

I request the following restrictions to the use or disclosure of my health information:

Signature of Patient or Legal Representative Witness

Date Notice Effective Date or Version

__X__ Accepted _____ Denied

Signature: ____**Raj Patel**_____      Date: ____**3-24-2016**_____

Patient:   Patel, Raj
Med Rec #:   837155

**Figure 2-9** HIPAA Consent Form with barcode.

data into the computer about the document such as the date, provider, type of image, and so on. This is called *cataloging the image*. Figure 2-10, shown later, is an example of an image catalog system.

Document images are scanned and cataloged into the EHR by many different people, including nurses, medical assistants, and personnel in the patient registration and Health Information Management departments. During scanning and cataloging, quality control is most important. Once a document has been scanned and cataloged, the original may be shipped to a remote storage facility or shredded. In either case, the original document may no longer be available for comparison. Although the scanned document image is stored safely on the computer, if it has been incorrectly cataloged it may not be easy to locate.

For the most part, the catalog data is entered by hand, but in some instances the image cataloging can be automated. Here are some examples of automated image cataloging:

Paper forms can include a barcode to identify catalog data; the scanning software interprets the barcode and automatically creates the catalog record. For example, Figure 2-9 shows a HIPAA authorization form that was printed for patient signature. The form includes a barcode identifying the patient, date, and document type, allowing automatic cataloging of the signed copy when it is scanned by the Document/Image System.

Another type of technology uses Optical Character Recognition (OCR) software to recognize text characters in images. Some document imaging systems can be programmed to find and use the text contained in the scanned document to populate the fields in the catalog records. Typically, only a few types of documents are processed this way, as each document type requires custom programming. Nonetheless, when an organization images thousands of the same type of document, it can be worth it. For example, your bank keeps an image of the front and back of each check it processes. Because the account number and check number are in a consistent place at the bottom of the check, the bank's computers can automatically catalog each image to the correct account as it is scanned.

## Guided Exercise 2B: Importing and Cataloging Images

In this exercise you will learn how to catalog images in a document imaging system. You will need access to the Internet for this exercise.

### Case Study

As Memorial Hospital continues to archive older paper and film records into the EHR document image system, you will catalog a scanned report and two diagnostic images from 2012.

### Step 1

If you are still logged in from the previous exercise, proceed to Step 2; otherwise, start your web browser program and follow the steps listed inside the cover of this text to log in to MyHealthProfessionsLab.

### Step 2

Locate and click on the link **Exercise 2B**. A new window will open with the Document/Image System simulation program previously shown in Figure 2-3.

### Step 3

Position your mouse pointer over the word "Select" in the Menu bar at the top of the screen and click the mouse button once.

Move the mouse pointer vertically down the list over the word "Patient" and click the mouse to invoke the Patient Selection window shown in Figure 2-10.

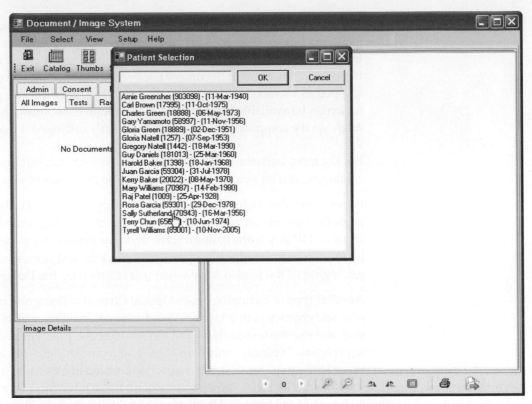

**Figure 2-10** Selecting Sally Sutherland from the Patient Selection window.

### Step 4

Find the patient named **Sally Sutherland** in the Patient Selection window. Position the mouse pointer over the patient name and double-click the mouse.

Once a patient is selected, the patient's name, age, and sex are displayed in the title at the top of the window. The Catalog pane displays the message "No Documents or Images" because Sally has no documents or images in the catalog.

### Step 5

Because you may not have a scanner connected to your computer, you are going to import a file that has already been scanned but not yet cataloged.

Locate and click on the Toolbar Import button.

The Open Media File window, displaying available files, will open. Compare your screen to Figure 2-11.

### Step 6

Locate and click on the thumbnail image of the **radiologist report document** (suth70943rpt.tif)

Locate and click on the Open button.

Compare your screen to Figure 2-12.

**Figure 2-11** Open Media window displays after clicking the Import icon.

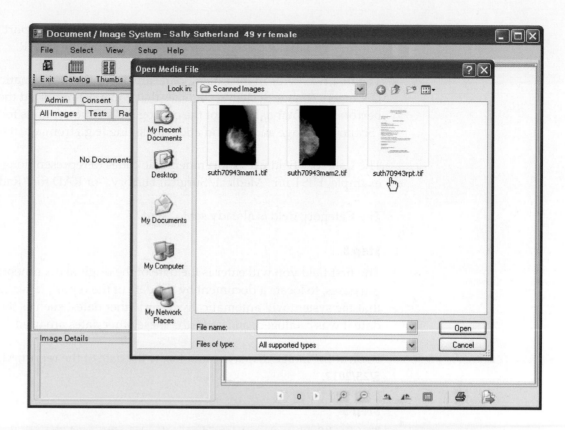

**Figure 2-12** Data entry fields in Catalog pane; Image Viewer displays the imported Radiology report.

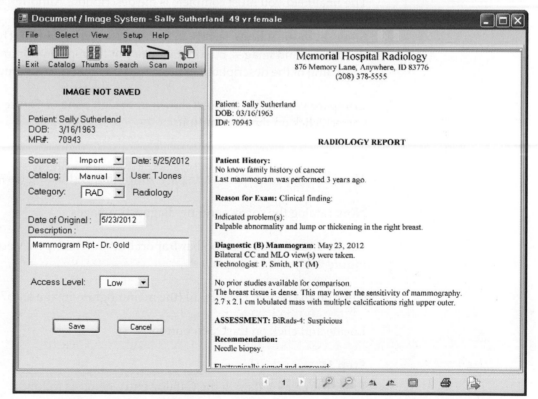

## Step 7

The imported file displays in the Image Viewer pane, and data entry fields replace the catalog list. The fields shown in Figure 2-12 are the minimum for most Document/Image systems. The actual fields in a catalog record will differ by software vendor or medical facility.

The image you have imported should be the radiologist's report. The Catalog pane reminds you that it has not been saved into the patient's EHR.

The first two fields in the catalog pane are determined automatically because the Document/Image System recognizes that you have imported the file and that you are performing a manual entry of the catalog data. Other options for these fields are "Scanned" image and "Automatic" cataloging (e.g., from a barcode).

The Category field uses short mnemonic codes to represent longer category names, for example, HIST for "Medical/Surgical History," or RAD for "Radiology."

The Category field is already set to "RAD."

### Step 8

The first field you will enter is the date of the original document; this is for reference purposes, to locate a document by the date of the report, letter, surgery, and so on. Note that the system will automatically record other dates, such as the date of the scan, the date it was cataloged, and so forth. These other dates are used for audit purposes.

Look at the image displayed and locate the date of the report, May 23, 2012. Enter **5/23/2012.**

### Step 9

The final field you must complete is the description. Although the field can hold a lengthy description, only the first portion of it is displayed in the catalog list, which is used by others at the healthcare facility to find the document/image. Therefore, when cataloging documents and images, be sure that you put the most important information at the beginning of the description. In this case, you will type **Mammogram Rpt - Dr. Gold.**

Compare your fields to those shown in the left pane of Figure 2-12. If everything is correct, click on the Save button.

### Step 10

The Catalog pane will now display your cataloged listing (as shown in Figure 2-13).

Now catalog the corresponding diagnostic images.

Locate and click on the Toolbar Import button. The Open Media window (shown in Figure 2-11) will be displayed.

Click on the **center** Thumbnail (the mammogram image suth70943mam2.tif).

Locate and click on the Open button.

### Step 11

Enter the catalog data in the Catalog entry fields as follows:

Date: **5/23/2012**

Description: **Mammogram right breast w/ abnormality**

Click the Save button.

The Catalog pane will now display two listings (as shown in Figure 2-14).

**Figure 2-13** Cataloged mammogram report.

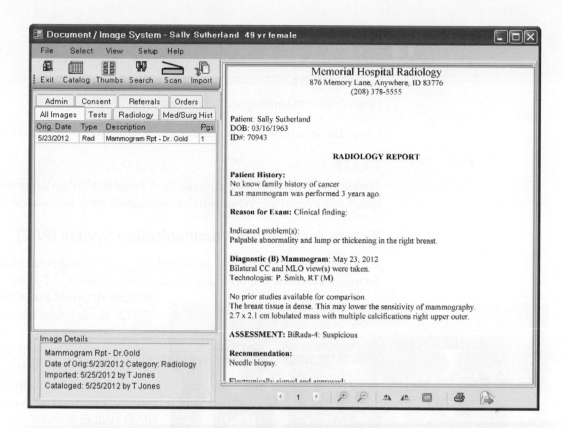

**Figure 2-14** Cataloged mammogram image.

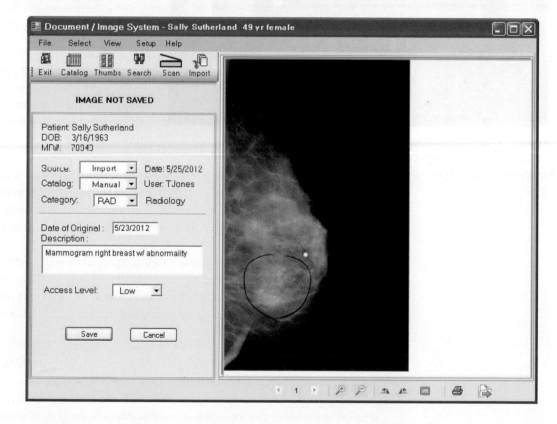

### Step 12

Catalog the other mammogram image by clicking the Toolbar Import button. When the Open Media window appears, click on the **left** Thumbnail (the mammogram image suth70943mam1.tif).

Locate and click on the Open button.

Enter the catalog data in the Catalog entry fields as follows:

Date: **5/23/2012**

Description: **Mammogram left breast**

Click the Save button. The Catalog pane will now display three listings.

**Step 13**

Locate and click the Exit button in the Document Image program toolbar. Answer the questions presented. When you have finished, click the Submit Quiz button.

## Picture Archival and Communication System (PAC)

In the previous exercise you imported diagnostic images (mammograms) into the EHR. At many facilities, digital images such as x-rays and CAT scans reside on a separate

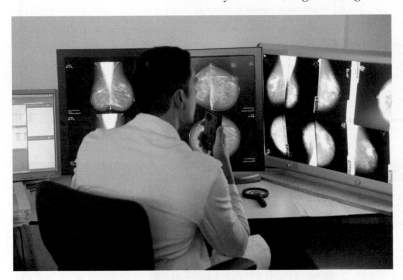

Courtesy of Javier Larrea/age fotostock/Getty Images

**Figure 2-15** Radiologist dictates report while interpreting radiology study on a PAC system.

Picture Archival and Communication System (PAC). These images can be associated with the radiology report in the EHR and appear to be part of the EHR record, even though they are on a separate system. In those facilities, the diagnostic image is not actually imported into the EHR, but rather linked to the patient EHR record. A PAC system is shown in Figure 2-15.

## Importing Text to the EHR

The second form of data we discussed is text data; that is, data that consists of words, sentences, and paragraphs, but is not fielded data. Frequently this type of data comes from word processing files that result from transcribed dictation. A good example of this is the radiologist's report. A radiologist is a specialist who interprets diagnostic images. Radiologists often dictate their impressions of a study. Their dictation is later typed by a medical transcriptionist. The word processing file containing the radiology report can be imported directly into the EHR, eliminating the steps of printing and scanning.

Similarly, a healthcare facility implementing an EHR will eventually need to bring old paper charts into the Document/Image system. If the facility has retained word processing files of transcribed dictation, importing them as EHR text records instead of scanning the printed pages from the paper chart increases the amount of the EHR that is text data and reduces the number of pages to be scanned.

Although imported text data are not codified like those created when clinicians enter actual data, they may be preferable to a scanned image for two reasons. First, the text records are searchable by computer. Second, text data can be dynamically reformatted for display on smaller devices such as mobile phones; images of scanned documents cannot.

For example, a text document viewed on a small device such as a mobile phone might display in a font suitable for that device. If the same document were a scanned image, it might be too small to read, thus requiring the clinician to zoom the image and making it cumbersome to read.

## Importing Coded EHR Data

As we have already learned, the very best form of EHR data is fielded, codified data. In addition to the coded data that will be created by the clinician using an EHR, many other sources of codified data can be imported. Importing coded data produces a better EHR and eliminates the need to re-key data or scan reports into the chart.

For example, electronic lab order and results systems can be interfaced to send the orders and merge test results directly into the patient's chart. The numerical data that makes up many lab results lends itself to trend analysis, graphs, and comparison with other tests. The ability to review and present results in this manner allows providers to see the immediate, tangible benefits of using an EHR and improves patient care.

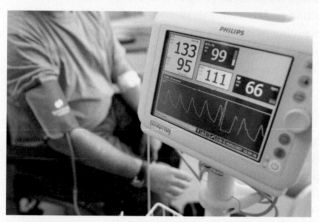

Other sources of EHR data available for import into the EHR include vital signs when they are measured with modern electronic devices (as shown in Figure 2-16). Similarly, glucose monitors and Holter monitors are devices that gather and store data about the patient. Most of these medical devices have the ability to transfer the data they have collected to a computer.

When clinicians use the EHR to write prescriptions, the orders are also automatically recorded in the EHR as part of the workflow. This keeps a record of the patient's past prescriptions and makes renewing prescriptions much faster for the provider.

**Courtesy of Frederik Astier/Science Source**

**Figure 2-16** Taking a patient's vital signs with an electronic device.

## Patient-Entered Data

Numerous studies have shown that patient data also can become a significant contributor to the EHR, for some of the following reasons:

◆ Only the patient has the information about what symptoms were present at the outset of the illness.

◆ Only the patient knows the outcome of medical treatment of those symptoms.

◆ The patient is also the source of past medical, family, and social history.

◆ Patient-entered data is a more accurate reflection of a patient's complaints.

◆ Patients who can review their histories are better prepared for the visit.

According to Dr. Allen Wenner, up to 67 percent of the nurse or clinician's time with the patient is spent entering the patient's symptoms into the visit documentation. A computer program developed by Dr. Wenner, allows patients to enter their history and symptom information on a computer in the waiting room or via the Internet prior to the visit. Patients do not have access to the EHR, but use a separate program that is linked to the EHR. The patient-entered data is reviewed by the doctor or nurse during the exam and before being merged into the EHR. You will have an opportunity to explore this concept yourself in Chapter 10.

## Provider-Entered Data

Finally, the surest source of reliable coded EHR data is that entered by the providers (doctor, nurse, and medical assistant) during the patient encounter using a standardized nomenclature. That process will be the subject of subsequent chapters in this text.

# Health Information Exchange

**Health information exchange (HIE)** is the electronic transmission of healthcare-related data among facilities, health information organizations, and government agencies, according to national standards for interoperability, security, and confidentiality. HIE allows doctors, nurses, pharmacists, other healthcare providers, and patients to appropriately access and securely share a patient's vital medical information electronically—improving the speed, quality, safety, and cost of patient care.

HIE is an important part of the health information technology infrastructure under development in the United States, and of the associated National Health Information Network. For HIE to successfully exchange data requires not only standardized code sets, but also that the sending and receiving systems both use the same standard protocols defining how the transmitted records are formatted and organized. In this section we discuss several standards organizations and methods of accomplishing HIE.

## HL7

**Health Level 7 (HL7)** is a nonprofit organization and the leading messaging standard used by healthcare computer systems to exchange information. The organization comprises healthcare providers, institutions, government representatives, and software developers. HL7 uses a consensus process to arrive at specifications acceptable to everyone involved. The HL7 specifications are updated regularly and released as new versions.

Hospitals and other large healthcare organizations often have many different computer systems created by unrelated vendors. These systems generate various portions of the patient's medical data. HL7 is used to translate and interface that data into the main EHR system. As a part of this course, it is not necessary to delve into the specific structure or flow of HL7 messages, but it is helpful to understand its advantages and limitations.

HL7 specifications are independent of any application or vendor; therefore, applications that can send and receive HL7 messages can potentially exchange information. That is its advantage and importance to an EHR system.

HL7 has been successful because it is very flexible both in its structure as well as its support for multiple coding standards. Nonetheless, when a message is received the codes and terms used by the other system may not match those used by the EHR. That is its disadvantage.

To overcome this problem, segments of the HL7 message that contain coded data also contain an identifier indicating which coding standard is being used. A special computer program called an *HL7 translator* is used to match the codes in the message with the codes in the EHR. The translator also can reconcile differences between HL7 versions from multiple systems.

## DICOM

**DICOM** stands for Digital Imaging and Communications in Medicine. It is the standard used for medical images, such as digital x-rays, CT scans, MRIs, and ultrasounds. Other uses include the images from angiography, endoscopy, laparoscopy, medical photography, and microscopy. It was created by the National Electrical Manufacturers Association and is the most widely used format for storing and sending diagnostic images.

DICOM is the standard for communication between diagnostic imaging equipment and the image processing software. The standard also defines the specification for a file that contains the actual digital image. A DICOM file includes a header that contains information about the image, dimensions, type of scan, image compression, and so on, as well as patient information such as ID number or name. DICOM-compatible software is required to view the image.

## CDISC

CDISC, which stands for Clinical Data Interchange Standards Consortium is a global, open, multidisciplinary, nonprofit organization that has established standards to support the acquisition, exchange, submission, and archiving of clinical research data and metadata. CDISC originated as a special interest group of the Drug Information Association but became its own entity and formed an alliance with HL7.

The CDISC mission is to develop and support global, platform-independent data standards that enable information system interoperability to improve medical research and related areas of healthcare. CDISC standards are vendor-neutral and platform-independent. CDISC is mentioned here because you may encounter CDISC if you work at a healthcare facility that participates in clinical trials.

## Biomedical Devices

Biomedical devices can output important and useful medical information that can be received and stored as data in the patient's EHR. However, the type of data and method of communicating between the device and EHR often are proprietary to the particular device. Therefore HL7 often is used to exchange demographic information between the device and the EHR system.

Still, the advantage of having the data in the EHR is so strong as to warrant the additional interfaces. Many of the patient monitoring, point-of-care testing, and biomedical devices in hospitals have the capability of exporting data to the EHR. Examples include instruments for measuring vital signs and cardiac and arterial blood gas monitors. Today, many of these devices have wired or wireless telemetry to transmit their information to nurses and into the EHR.

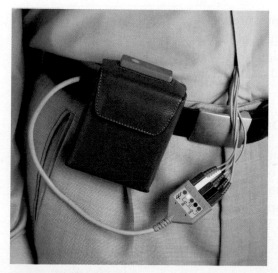

A similar capability is available in systems used in medical offices and for patient home monitoring such as the spirometer shown in Chapter 1, Figure 1-1. Other examples include electrocardiograms, ultrasounds, and the vital signs device shown earlier.

## Telemonitors

Many patients with chronic conditions are monitored at home using devices such as blood pressure monitors, glucose meters, and Holter monitors. Some of these devices store the readings and transfer the data to the doctor's system either by using a modem and phone line or by downloading from the device during a patient encounter. For blood pressure monitoring, if the device does not store the readings, the patient may keep a log, which is then entered into the patient's medical record at the doctor's office.

**Figure 2-17** Patient wearing a Holter monitor device.

One example of a telemonitor is the Holter monitor, a device the patient wears for 24 to 72 hours to measure and record information about the patient's heart. The data is then transferred either remotely or in person to the doctor's computer, where it is reviewed. Figure 2-17 shows a patient wearing a Holter monitor.

**By Julie DeSantis**

Hinsdale Hematology Oncology Associates, Ltd. (HHOA), of Hinsdale, Illinois, switched from traditional paper records to the advanced technology of wireless, mobile electronic medical records from IMPAC Medical Systems. At HHOA, the result of implementing an EHR is improved patient and clinician satisfaction, an increased patient load, and an elevated level of process efficiency that has paid for itself within 2 years of implementation.

Michele White, practice administrator at HHOA, said that patient confidence improved with the use of advanced technology, such as handheld devices and wireless laptop systems. "Our patients have noticed that our medical documentation is complete, up-to-date, and right at hand," she said. The patients have more confidence in our doctors, and have received more face-to-face interaction time during their visits, she said. "We have a high standard of care that we did not want to compromise, and with tablet PCs, wireless laptops, and the handheld devices—we have everything we need to access lab reports, scheduling, and more."

HHOA provides services to 80–100 patients a day—an increase in patient load since installing IMPAC. With 12 busy exam rooms and only 6 physicians, they use IMPAC's online transcription and report management system to quickly and accurately document

patient encounters and manage them online. In addition, HHOA uses a structured noting system for patient documentation within the EHR. All incoming lab results also are downloaded into the system via interface, and available from any laptop at the practice, ensuring the patient record is complete, up-to-date, and easily accessible to physicians and staff. "From an administrative and economic perspective, our mobile access to EHRs has meant that we did not need to purchase additional antivirus software and miscellaneous upgrades. We've saved a lot of money, while increasing efficiency, security, and reliability," White said.

For six years, HHOA used remote connection software in the physicians' homes to access the office. However, they have found remote access to the EHR from IMPAC to be faster, more reliable, and readily accessible from anywhere. There are six physicians on staff at HHOA, all with different technical knowledge, but "they are all comfortable with IMPAC's EHR," White explained. "They can get any reports they need and print right through the system when they are off-site."

---

[3]©2005 IMPAC Medical Systems, Inc. (edited by author). Used with permission.

---

When a patient is seen in a doctor's office, measurements of vital signs, a glucose test, or even an ECG reflect only the patient's condition at that particular time. The advantage of telemonitoring is that it allows the provider to study these values measured many times over the course of the patient's normal daily activity.

## Functional Benefits from Codified Records

The IOM report cited in Chapter 1 defined an EHR as more than simply storing medical records on a computer. IOM included a list of functional benefits the EHR should provide. Because coded EHR data is unambiguous, the computer can use it for trend analysis, alerts, health maintenance, decision support, orders and results, administrative processes, and population health reporting. We will now explore four of the functional benefits that can be derived from using a codified EHR.

### Trend Analysis

In healthcare, laboratory tests are used to measure the level of certain components present in specimens taken from the patient. When the same test is performed over a period of time, changes in the results can indicate a *trend* in the patient's health.

To spot a trend with a paper chart, the clinician must page through the reports and mentally remember the values to compare them. When a health record is electronic, it is easier to compare data from different dates, tests, or events. When the data is fielded and coded, it is possible to generate graphs and reports that support trend analysis.

To experience the differences in forms of data, we will compare a patient's lab results that have been stored in each of the three data formats we discussed earlier in this chapter.

## Critical Thinking Exercise 2C: Retrieving a Scanned Lab Report

In this exercise you will use what you have learned in Guided Exercise 2A to locate information from a recent lab report for a patient.

### Case Study

Patient Raj Patel is being seen. In this exercise you are going to retrieve and view some of his records from 2012.

### Step 1

You will need access to the Internet for this exercise. Start a supported web browser program and follow the steps listed inside the cover of this textbook to log in to the MyHealthProfessionsLab for this course.

### Step 2

Locate and click on the link **Exercise 2C**.

When the Document/Image System program is displayed in your browser, locate and click Select in the Menu bar at the top of the screen and click Patient on the drop-down menu.

When the list of patients is displayed, select patient **Raj Patel** by clicking on his name.

### Step 3

On **February 8, 2012**, the facility received the results of a lab test performed by **Quest** laboratories. The lab report was scanned and cataloged in Raj Patel's chart.

Locate the catalog entry for this lab report and click on it to display the report.

### Step 4

When the report is displayed in the Image Viewer, locate the results for the test component Triglycerides and note the value.

You may need to use the Zoom In button to read the value accurately.

### Step 5

Enter the value from the report in the text box and click the Submit Quiz button to complete Exercise 2C.

**Lab Report as Digital Image**   The previous exercise demonstrates the drawback of data in the format of a digital image. While cataloging scanned reports into the EHR has the advantage of making the results easier to locate and retrieve than a paper chart, it requires a human to identify and read the data values. Although the lab data are present in the image, there is no way to extract the values or compare them across repeated tests.

**Lab Report as Text Data**  If a lab results report was received as a text file, it might resemble Figure 2-18. The file could be imported into the EHR, but because the data is not fielded or codified, a computer might have difficulty accurately parsing the data in the report. Nonetheless a computer could easily search text records and locate those that contained the word *cholesterol*. This could be useful to quickly locate records of previous tests containing the same word.

**Figure 2-18** Text-based lab results.

```
Raj Patel: M: 3/5/1936:

Doctor's Laboratory
3/10/2016 11:30 AM

Tests
Blood Chemistry:                        Value        Normal Range
Total plasma cholesterol level          215 mg/dl      140 - 200
Plasma HDL cholesterol level            40 mg/dl        30 - 70
Plasma LDL cholesterol level            98 mg/dl        80 - 130
Total cholesterol/HDL ratio             5.4             4 - 6

Hematology:                             Value        Normal Range
INR                                     2.1            25 - 40
```

**Coded Lab Data**  If the test result data are fielded and coded, the computer can find matching results in the data and generate a cumulative summary report or a graph, making it easier to compare test results from different times and dates.

The cumulative summary report shown in Figure 2-19 has three sections of results: blood gases, whole blood chemistries, and general chemistry. Within each section are the results from tests performed five different times; the date and time are printed above each column of data.

The report is read from left to right; each row contains the name of the test component followed by result values for each of the five times. The two columns on the right are informational; they contain the range of values considered normal for each particular test and the unit of measure.

A simple graphing tool can turn numeric data in the EHR into a powerful visual aid that would be impractical to create from a paper chart. Figure 2-20 provides an example of how data from multiple lab tests can be quickly extracted and graphed for the clinician. The test result values of the patient's total cholesterol over a three-month period of time are trended with the green line. The reference ranges of normal high (200) and low (140) values are shown in the graph as red and blue lines, respectively.

The computer is able to generate this graph because the data is fielded and the different tests and components have unique codes. From all the possible tests a patient might have had, the computer can quickly find those coded as "total cholesterol." Using a graph, the clinician can easily see the trend of this patient's total cholesterol levels.

Trend analysis is not limited to lab test results. Graphs of patient weight loss or gain are used as patient education tools. Effects of medication can be measured by comparing changes in dosage to changes in blood pressure measurements. Flow sheets (shown later in Chapter 8) are another type of trend analysis tool.

```
****************************************** Blood Gases ******************************************

DATE:          [-------------------- 03/26/2016 --------------------]  03/25/2016
TIME:          2132         1920         1720         1506         1615        NORMAL       UNITS

pH-Arterial     7.30 L       7.36         7.38         7.47 H       7.48 H      7.35-7.45
PCO2-Arterial   47.4 H       41.1         38.3         34.8 L       33.0 L      35-45        mm Hg
PO2-Arterial    90.2        189.0 H      187.0 H      188.0 H      227.0 H      90-105       mm Hg
HCO3-Arterial   22.8         22.8         22.0         24.9         24.4        21-27        mEq/L
Base Excess-A                                          1.7          1.6         0-3          mEq/L
Base Deficit-A  3.2 H        1.9          2.3                                   0-3          mEq/L
O2 Sat Dir-A    96.0         99.3 H       99.5 H       99.6 H       99.9 H      95-99        % Saturation
O2 Content-A    15.9         15.3         14.6 L       10.3 L       14.4 L      15-17        vol %
Hemoglobin-BG   12.0         10.8         10.3         7.2          10.1                     g/dL
CarboxyHb-A     1.1 H        1.0 H        1.2 H        0.9          1.6 H       0.0-0.9      % Saturation
MetHb-A         0.9          0.4          0.7          0.4          0.8         0.0-0.9      % Saturation
FIO2                         .55          .56          0.54         .65                      %


************************************ Whole Blood Chemistries ************************************

DATE:          [--------------------03/26/2016----------------------]  03/25/2016
TIME:   2209    2132         1920         1720         1506         1615        NORMAL       UNITS

Sodium-WB                    142          142          142          139         135-145      mEq/L
Potassium-WB    3.5          3.3          3.0 L        2.9 L        2.7 L       3.3-4.6      mEq/L
Calcium Ionized      1.21    1.05         0.99 L       1.07         1.08        1.05-1.30    mmol/L
Lactic Acid-WB       1.3     0.8          1.1          0.8          0.5         0.3-1.5      mmol/L
Glucose-WB           197 H   156 H        165 H        118 H        90          65-99        mg/dL
Hematocrit-WB        37      34 L         32 L         22 L         31 L        36-46        %


*********************************** General Chemistry ***********************************

DATE:   04/01/2016 [---- 03/30/2016 ----] [---------- 03/29/16 ----------]  03/28/2016
TIME:   *0620    0653    0327    1835    0915    0532    2048    NORMAL       UNITS

Sodium           140                                     143             136-145      mmol/L
Potassium        2.7 L    3.0 L           2.9 L   3.0 L   2.7 L           3.3-5.1      mmol/L
Chloride         101                                     100             98-107       mmol/L
Carbon Dioxide   32 H                                    36 H            22-30        mmol/L
Urea Nitrogen    10                                      7               6-20         mg/dL
Creatinine       0.54                                    0.60            0.40-0.90    mg/dL
Glucose          115 H                                   96              65-99        mg/dL
Calcium          0.4                                     8.0             8.0-10.6     mg/dL
Magnesium        1.9                                     2.3     1.8     1.5-2.8      mg/dL
Phosphorus Inorg 2.3 L                                   2.8     1.8 L   2.7-4.5      mg/dL
CK Total                   165                                   273 H   30-170       U/L

------------------------------------------------------------------------------------------------
    H=Abnormal High          L=Abnormal Low          H*=Critical High          L*=Critical Low
    Date Printed: 04/01/2016          Admit Date: 03/25/2016          Discharge Date: 04/01/2016
                             INPATIENT MEDICAL RECORDS COPY                     Page: 1
```

**Figure 2-19** Cumulative summary lab report.

## Alerts

One of the important reasons for the widespread adoption of EHR is the potential to reduce medical errors. Paper charts and even electronic charts that are principally scanned images depend on the clinician noticing a risk factor about the patient. However, when an EHR consists primarily of fielded and codified data using standard nomenclature, rules can be set up that allow the computer to do the monitoring.

Alert is the term used in an EHR for a message or reminder that is automatically generated by the system. Alerts are based on programmed rules that cause the EHR to notify the provider when two or more conditions are met. For example, an electronic

**Figure 2-20** Graph of total cholesterol from codified lab results.

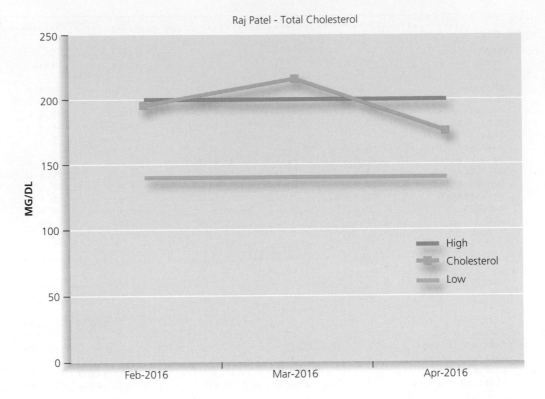

prescription system generates an alert when two drugs known to have adverse interactions are prescribed for the same patient.

Alerts can be programmed for just about anything in the EHR. However, the most prevalent alert systems are those implemented with electronic prescription systems. Interactions between multiple prescription drugs, allergic reactions to certain classes of drugs, and patient health conditions that contraindicate certain drugs can all contribute to suffering, additional illness, and in extreme cases even death.

When using paper-based medical charts, physicians had to consult the patient medication list, allergy list, and the *Physicians' Desk Reference* (for interactions) before writing a prescription. An EHR can present this information concurrently or even automatically check patient allergy and medication data for conflicts and warn the clinician before the prescription is written. As a further precaution, the pharmacy checks for drug conflicts and provides the patient with warning materials about the drug. Figure 2-21 shows a clinical warning alert generated by the SuccessEHS system. Let's take a closer look at how this process works.

**Drug Utilization Review**   When the clinician writing an electronic prescription selects a drug and enters the Sig[4] information, the EHR system scans the patient chart for allergy information, past and current diagnoses, and a list of current medications. This information is then passed to a **drug utilization review (DUR)** program that compares the prescription to a database of most known drugs. The database includes prescription drugs as well as over-the-counter drugs, and even nutritional herb and vitamin supplements. The DUR program performs the following functions:

◆ It checks the drug about to be prescribed against the patient medication list to determine if there is a conflict with any drug the patient is already taking. Certain drugs remain in the body for a period of time after the patient has stopped taking them. This latency period is factored in as well.

---

[4]The term Sig, from the Latin *signa*, refers to the instructions for labeling a prescription.

**Figure 2-21** Electronic prescription DUR alert.

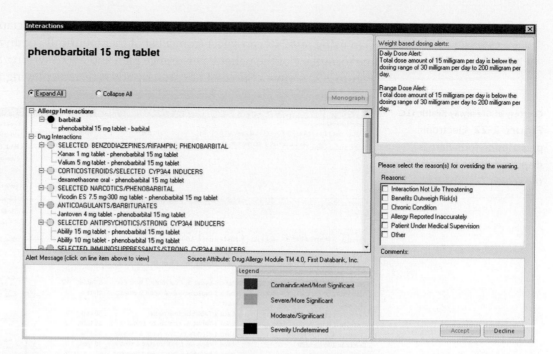

◆ It checks ingredients that make up the drug against the ingredients of current medications to see if they conflict or would hinder the effectiveness of the drug.

◆ Drugs are checked for duplicate therapy, which occurs when a patient is taking a different drug of the same class that would have the effect of an overdose.

◆ Allergy records are checked for food and drug allergies that would be aggravated by the new drug.

◆ It checks the patient's diagnosis history because some drugs cannot be given to patients with certain medical conditions.

◆ A patient education alert is created when the drug might be affected by certain foods or alcohol interactions.

◆ It checks the Sig, if it has been entered at the time of the DUR, to see if it matches recommended guidelines for the drug. Too much, too little, too many days, or too many refills could cause overdosing, underdosing (causing it to be ineffective), or abuse.

If the DUR software finds any of these conditions, the clinician is given an alert message explaining the conflict. The clinician can then alter the prescription or select a new drug, having never issued the incorrect one.

**Formulary Alerts**   Another type of alert found in many EHR prescription systems warns the clinician if the drug about to be prescribed is not covered by a patient's pharmacy benefit insurance.

Insurance plans provide **drug formularies** indicating preferred, nonpreferred, and non-covered drugs. Preferred brands have the lowest patient copay. Nonpreferred brands will require the patient to pay a larger portion of the prescription cost. Noncovered brands will require the patient to pay the entire cost. This is important because if a patient's insurance will not pay for it, the patient may choose not to fill the prescription or to take less than the amount prescribed.

If the clinician prescribes a drug that is not on the list, then when the patient tries to have the prescription filled, the pharmacy will call and ask the ordering clinician to change it.

This causes inconvenience to the patient and wastes the clinician's time. Instead, a clinician using an EHR can select from a list of therapeutically equivalent drugs that are on the formulary of the patient's insurance plan and avoid writing an incorrect prescription. Figure 2-22 shows a SuccessEHS prescription screen displaying formulary information.

Courtesy of Greenway Health, LLC.

**Figure 2-22** Electronic prescription formulary is displayed at the bottom of the screen.

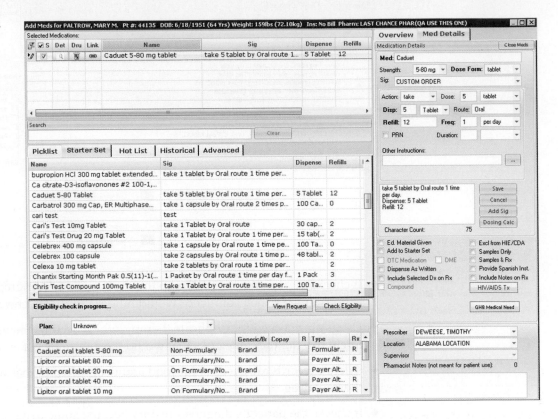

**Other Types of Alerts**  Electronic lab order systems can provide alerts as well. For example, certain tests are not covered by Medicare. CMS requires that patients sign a waiver indicating that they were notified that a test would not be covered. The waiver is called an **Advance Beneficiary Notice (ABN)**. The form is shown in Figure 2-23. When certain tests are ordered, the clinician is alerted if an ABN is required.

Another example is an alert that monitors changes in values of certain blood tests and pages a doctor whenever the value is outside a certain range.

Alerts can be generated by nonactions as well. Task list systems can notify an administrator when medical items are not handled in a timely fashion. CPOE systems can generate alerts when results for a pending test order have not been received within the time frame normally required for that type of test.

Once an EHR system contains codified data, an alert system is just a matter of programming a rule to watch for a certain event or detect a finding with a value above or below the desired limit.

## Health Maintenance

One of the best ways to maintain good health is to prevent disease, or if it occurs, to detect it early enough to be easily treated. This is one of the eight IOM core functions of an EHR and has become the basis of Clinical Quality Measures, which you will learn more about in Chapter 9. Two important components of health maintenance are preventive care screening and immunizations.

**A. Notifier:**

**B. Patient Name:**                                     **C. Identification Number:**

# Advance Beneficiary Notice of Noncoverage (ABN)

<u>NOTE:</u> If Medicare doesn't pay for **D.** _____ below, you may have to pay.
Medicare does not pay for everything, even some care that you or your health care provider have good reason to think you need. We expect Medicare may not pay for the **D.** _____ below.

| D. | E. Reason Medicare May Not Pay: | F. Estimated Cost |
|---|---|---|
|  |  |  |
|  |  |  |

## WHAT YOU NEED TO DO NOW:
- Read this notice, so you can make an informed decision about your care.
- Ask us any questions that you may have after you finish reading.
- Choose an option below about whether to receive the **D.** _____ listed above.
  **Note:** If you choose Option 1 or 2, we may help you to use any other insurance that you might have, but Medicare cannot require us to do this.

| **G. OPTIONS:    Check only one box.  We cannot choose a box for you.** |
|---|
| ☐ **OPTION 1.** I want the **D.** _____ listed above.  You may ask to be paid now, but I also want Medicare billed for an official decision on payment, which is sent to me on a Medicare Summary Notice (MSN).  I understand that if Medicare doesn't pay, I am responsible for payment, but **I can appeal to Medicare** by following the directions on the MSN.  If Medicare does pay, you will refund any payments I made to you, less co-pays or deductibles. |
| ☐ **OPTION 2.** I want the **D.** _____ listed above, but do not bill Medicare. You may ask to be paid now as I am responsible for payment. **I cannot appeal if Medicare is not billed**. |
| ☐ **OPTION 3.** I don't want the **D.** _____ listed above. I understand with this choice I am **not** responsible for payment, and **I cannot appeal to see if Medicare would pay.** |

**H. Additional Information:**


**This notice gives our opinion, not an official Medicare decision.** If you have other questions on this notice or Medicare billing, call **1-800-MEDICARE** (1-800-633-4227/**TTY:** 1-877-486-2048).
Signing below means that you have received and understand this notice. You also receive a copy.

| I. Signature: | J. Date: |
|---|---|
|  |  |

According to the Paperwork Reduction Act of 1995, no persons are required to respond to a collection of information unless it displays a valid OMB control number. The valid OMB control number for this information collection is 0938-0566. The time required to complete this information collection is estimated to average 7 minutes per response, including the time to review instructions, search existing data resources, gather the data needed, and complete and review the information collection. If you have comments concerning the accuracy of the time estimate or suggestions for improving this form, please write to: CMS, 7500 Security Boulevard, Attn: PRA Reports Clearance Officer, Baltimore, Maryland 21244-1850.

Form CMS-R-131 (03/11)                                    Form Approved OMB No. 0938-0566

**Figure 2-23** Sample advance beneficiary notice form.

**Preventive Care**   The simplest example of health maintenance is a card or letter reminding the patient that it is time for a checkup. In a paper-based office, creating this reminder is a manual process. However, when a medical practice has electronic records, preventive screening can become more dynamic and sophisticated.

Health maintenance systems, also known as preventive care systems, can go beyond simple reminders for an annual checkup. When an EHR has codified data, it can be electronically compared to the recommendations of the U.S. Preventive Services Task Force (described further in Chapter 9).

Using a sophisticated set of rules, the EHR software compares the list of tests recommended for patients of a certain age and sex to previous test results stored in the EHR. It also calculates the time since the test was last performed and compares that to the recommended interval for repeat testing. A guideline unique to the patient is generated and displayed on the clinician's computer. Using this information, the clinician can order tests, discuss important healthcare options, and recommend lifestyle changes to the patient at the point of care. Figure 2-24 shows a SuccessEHS screen used for ordering, tracking, and monitoring recommended preventive care measures for a patient.

**Courtesy of Greeenway Health, LLC.**

**Figure 2-24** Screen displaying the status of a patient's preventive care events.

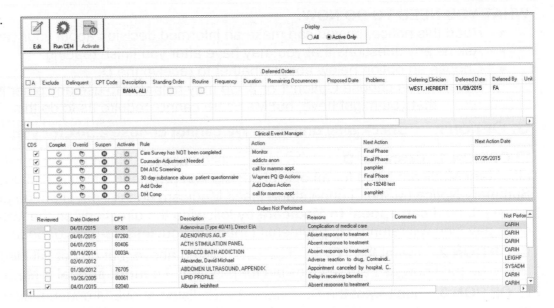

It would be difficult to create standardized rules for the preventive care system if the tests were not coded using a standardized coding system. Preventive care screening guidelines are not limited to lab tests; other examples include mammograms, hearing and vision screening, and certain elements of the physical examination.

**Immunizations**   The other important component of preventive care is immunizations. Immunization slows down or stops disease outbreaks. Vaccines prevent disease in the people who receive them and protect those who come into contact with unvaccinated individuals.

Immunizations must be acquired over time. Vaccines cannot be given all at once. Several require repeated applications over a period of time, and some, such as the measles vaccine, cannot be given to children under the age of one year. Therefore, the Centers for Disease Control and Prevention (CDC) and state health departments have designed a schedule to immunize children and adolescents from birth through 18 years of age. The CDC also publishes a recommended immunization schedule for adults. Adult immunizations are different from those given to a child.

Using the codified data in an EHR, computers can compare a patient's immunization history with the CDC-recommended vaccines and intervals and identify which immunizations the patient needs. EHR systems can also scan the data and generate letters to send to patients who have not been in recently but may need to renew their immunizations.

## Decision Support

Physicians are trained to analyze information from a patient's history, physical exams, and test results for a medical decision. They are also accustomed to researching the medical literature when faced with an unusual case. However, the quantity of information available to clinicians regarding conditions, disease management, protocols, case studies, and treatments far exceeds their available time to read it.

*Decision support* refers to the ability of EHR systems to store or quickly locate materials relevant to the findings of the current case. These might include defined protocols, results of case studies, or standard care guidelines prepared by specialists, medical societies, or government organizations.

Decision support is not about artificial intelligence replacing a physician with a computer; it is instead about providing help just when the clinician needs it. There are many examples of decision support systems, but let us look at four:

♦ **Prescriptions:** Decision support can include the drug formularies mentioned earlier. Formularies can be used to look up drugs by name or therapeutic class. Electronic prescription systems provide decision support to the clinician by comparing alternative brands that are therapeutically equivalent. They can also provide information on costs, indications for use, treatment recommendations, dosage, guidelines, and prescribing information.

♦ **Medical references:** Decision support systems can provide quick access to medical references directly from the EHR. This can make access to evidence-based guidelines or medical literature as easy as clicking on a link in the chart.

♦ **Protocols:** Protocols are one form of decision support that can ultimately speed up documentation of the patient exam and improve patient care. Protocols are standard plans of therapy established for different conditions. With a decision support system, when a doctor has diagnosed a patient with a particular condition, the appropriate protocol appears on the EHR screen and all therapies are ordered with a click of the mouse.

♦ **Medication dosing:** Many medications have serious side effects, some of which must be monitored by regular blood tests. When both the medications and lab results are stored in the EHR as codified data, it is possible for decision support software to compare changes in medication dosing with changes in the patient's test results. This assists the clinician in adjusting the patient's medication levels to obtain the maximum benefit to the patient.

## Meeting the IOM Definition of an EHR

Each of the functional benefits we have discussed—trend analysis, alerts, health maintenance, and decision support—are products of EHR systems that store medical records as codified, fielded data. It is only when these functional benefits are added to the clinical practice that the EHR approaches the vision of the IOM and meets the CMS "meaningful use" criteria discussed in Chapter 1.

# Chapter Two Summary

The IOM definition of an EHR went beyond a computer that just stores the patient's medical record to include *the functional benefits* derived from having an electronic health record. In this chapter we explored how the format that the data are stored in determines to what extent the data can be used to achieve that extended functionality.

The forms of EHR data are broadly categorized into three types:

1. Digital image data (provides increased accessibility)

2. Text-based data (provides accessibility and text search capability; can be displayed on different devices)

3. Discrete data, fielded and ideally codified (provides all of the above plus the capability to be used for alerts, health maintenance, and data exchange)

Increased benefits of an EHR can be realized when the information is stored as codified data. In addition, codified EHR data that adheres to a national standard enables the exchange and comparison of medical information from other facilities.

A code set designed specifically to record medical observations is referred to as a *clinical nomenclature*. Using an EHR nomenclature provides consistency in patient records and improves communication between different medical specialties.

EHR nomenclatures differ from other coding standards in several ways:

◆ EHR nomenclatures precorrelate individual terms into clinically relevant findings or codified observations that are medically meaningful to the clinician.

◆ Findings are often linked to other findings, which helps the clinician quickly locate associated information and shortens the time required to document the exam.

◆ EHR nomenclatures differ from billing codes in that EHR nomenclatures have many more codes used to describe the detail of the exam such as the symptoms, history, observations, and plan. Billing codes tend to represent simply that the service was rendered.

◆ Reference terminologies designed for research may codify each medical term, but these terms can combine in ways that are not clinically relevant; therefore, these nomenclatures are not easy to use at the point of care.

◆ EHR nomenclatures often include cross-references to other standard code sets. Coding systems not intended for EHR do not typically contain a map to other coding systems.

Several of the most prominent coding standards you are likely to encounter or use in an EHR were discussed in this chapter.

◆ SNOMED-CT is a robust clinical terminology originally developed by the College of American Pathologists and now maintained by an international organization.

◆ Medcin is a medical nomenclature and knowledge base used in many commercial EHR systems as well as the Department of Defense CHCS II system. Medcin differs from other EHR coding systems in that Medcin was designed for point-of-care use by the clinician, so that each finding represents a meaningful clinical observation or term. The Medcin findings are linked in a knowledge base. This enables a clinician to quickly find other clinical findings that are likely to be needed. This difference means a physician selects fewer individual codes to complete the patient exam note.

- LOINC stands for Logical Observation Identifier Names and Codes. LOINC is an important clinical terminology for laboratory test orders and results. LOINC has become one of the standard code sets designated by the U.S. government for the electronic exchange of clinical health information.

- RxNorm is a code set normalizing the names of drugs and linking other drug vocabularies.

- CCC stands for Clinical Classification Codes, a system of codes for nursing that is incorporated into other EHR nomenclatures, such as SNOMED-CT, Medcin, and LOINC.

EHR data may be captured in many ways:

- Scanning paper records

- Importing diagnostic images in digital format

- Importing text or word processing files

- Receiving data electronically from other systems using

  - HL7

  - DICOM

  - CDISK

- Biomedical devices

- Telemonitoring devices

- Patients may enter their own history and symptoms

- Providers record the EHR at the point of care

When EHR data is coded, it can be used for:

- Trend analysis, the comparison of multiple values or findings over a period of time

- Alerts, computer-prompted warnings such as a potential drug interaction or a lab result seriously above or below the expected range

- Health maintenance, which creates reminders of health screening, immunizations, and other preventive measures

- Decision support, systems to quickly locate materials relevant to the findings of the current case such as defined protocols, standard care guidelines, or medical research

## Testing Your Knowledge of Chapter 2

### Step 1

Log in to MyHealthProfessionsLab following the directions printed inside the cover of this text book.

Locate and click on Chapter 2 Test.

### Step 2

Answer the test questions. When you have finished, click the Submit Test button.

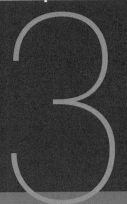

# Learning Medical Record Software

## Learning Outcomes

*After completing this chapter, you should be able to:*

- ◆ Navigate the Student Edition software
- ◆ Select a patient
- ◆ Set an encounter date
- ◆ Record findings in the encounter note
- ◆ Generate a printable PDF of an encounter note
- ◆ Use the Quippe icon, Browse, View, and Actions toolbar buttons
- ◆ Navigate the Medcin nomenclature domains to add appropriate clinical concepts in each section of the encounter note
- ◆ Remove clinical concepts and findings from an encounter note
- ◆ Add entry details: values, units, free text, status, modifiers, onset, duration, episodes, and prefix to clinical concepts
- ◆ Enter a chief complaint
- ◆ Enter vital signs

## Introducing the Quippe® Student Edition Software

In this chapter you will learn to document a patient encounter using Medcin, one of the standard EHR nomenclatures discussed in Chapter 2. Special Quippe Student Edition software has been created for you to use with this course. **Quippe** is a clinical documentation tool that many commercial software vendors use as the basis of their EHR applications to incorporate the Medcin knowledge base and utilize the rich intelligence and functionality of Medcin to enhance the clinical documentation and patient care experience. The evolution of EHR software design has resolved to a few methods of user input that seem to work best in medical offices. Quippe's customizable templates enable the

Student Edition software to represent the most commonly used interfaces, allowing you to become familiar with multiple styles of EHR systems.

Because the Student Edition is designed for the classroom, it will be different in some aspects from EHR systems you will encounter when working in a medical office or hospital. However, the concepts, skills, and familiarity with EHR systems you will acquire by practicing with the Student Edition software will transfer directly into the workplace.

The Student Edition software allows you to select clinical concepts for symptoms, history, physical examination, tests, diagnoses, and therapy to produce medical documents typical of the clinical notes created in a medical office that uses an EHR. At the conclusion of each exercise, you will check your work and submit it for a grade. The Student Edition software also allows you to create a printable PDF of your work. Some instructors may ask you to print or email the PDF. If a PDF is desired, it must be created **before** submitting the exercise for a grade.

## About the Exercises in This Book

The purpose of the exercises is to teach EHR concepts by providing hands-on experience. Completing the exercises in this and subsequent chapters of the book using real EHR software will give you practical experience in creating electronic health records. Each set of exercises is designed to illustrate one or more EHR concepts and will result in a documented encounter note. Once you have mastered the basics, you will learn in subsequent chapters how to increase data entry speed through the use of forms, lists, and flow sheets. These capabilities are useful to document a patient visit during the encounter. Later, you also will learn how information from previous exams can be used during patient encounters.

Brief case studies precede most exercises. These describe the patients and the reasons they have come to the medical facility. In a medical office or outpatient clinic, patients are also seen by licensed healthcare professionals who are not physicians. This textbook frequently uses the term *clinician* or *provider* to represent equally a nurse practitioner, physician assistant, or doctor.

Although the clinical notes produced by the textbook exercises are medically accurate, routine elements of a complete patient assessment that should normally be documented are frequently omitted from the exercise. This is done solely to facilitate completion of exercises in the allotted class time. Note that some exercises ask you to document items that would normally be entered by a physician, physician assistant, or nurse practitioner. The reason for including these components in the exercises is to demonstrate all aspects of the EHR.

It is important to remember that you cannot save a partially completed exercise and resume later where you left off. Exercises have been carefully designed to be completed in the allotted class time. When you finish one exercise, do not begin the next unless there will be sufficient time to complete it.

## Creating Your First Patient Encounter Note

When a doctor, nurse, or other healthcare provider examines a patient in a facility or at home, it is commonly referred to as an encounter. Similarly, an outpatient visit to a provider in a medical office or clinic is also called an *encounter*. Clinical notes documenting the encounter are variously referred to as *exam notes, provider notes*, or *encounter notes*. Whatever term is used, the encounter note is a record of the findings of an examination that occurred on a specific date and time. Although a portion of the data may be recorded by the medical assistant, another portion by the nurse, and yet another by a doctor, one completed encounter note should encompass the entire visit. However, when the patient returns for another visit, a new encounter is created.

## Guided Exercise 3A: Understanding the Software

This is the first of several exercises in this chapter designed to help you become familiar with the Student Edition software, the Medcin nomenclature, and the screen navigation controls.

### Case Study

Guy Daniels is a 46-year-old male patient who complains of headaches and admits he is under a lot of pressure at work. He is an existing patient with a history of hypertension and Type 2 diabetes.

### Step 1

You will need access to the Internet for this exercise. Start a supported web browser program and follow the steps listed inside the cover of this textbook to log in to the MyHealthProfessionsLab for this course.

### Step 2

Locate and click on the link **Exercise 3A**.

This will open the Quippe software window, in the center of which will be displayed the New Encounter window shown in Figure 3-1.

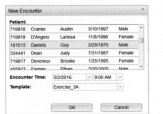

**Figure 3-1** Selecting Guy Daniels from the patient list in the New Encounter window.

### Step 3

The New Encounter window displays a list of patients, alphabetically by last name, and a field for setting the Encounter date and time. On the right edge of the patient list is a scroll bar.

You are probably familiar with the concept of scrolling a window. Position the mouse pointer on the scroll bar and hold the mouse button down while you drag the mouse in a downward motion. This action will scroll the list. Continue scrolling the list until you can see the patient name **Daniels, Guy**.

Position the mouse pointer on the patient named **Daniels, Guy** as shown in Figure 3-1 and single-click the mouse button. This will select Guy Daniels as the patient for this encounter.

### Step 4

In any type of medical facility it is important to accurately record the date and time of the encounter. In this step, you will learn how to set the date and time of the encounter.

#### Setting the Date to May 2, 2016

When you create a new encounter, the month, day, year, and time will default to current date and time settings in your own computer. The date and time are displayed in two fields just below the list of patients in Figure 3-1.

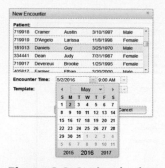

**Figure 3-2** Setting the date with the New Encounter window calendar.

One purpose of this exercise is to teach you how to set the date and time in the New Encounter window. Because it is unlikely that you are doing this exercise on May 2, 2016, you will need to manually set the date and time as instructed in this exercise.

There are two ways of doing this. You can click in the date field and type over the date using the format MM/DD/YYYY. Note: the typed date must include the slashes.

The alternative method is to select the date from a pop-up calendar, which is invoked by single-clicking on the small down-arrow next to the date field. The calendar window shown in Figure 3-2 will be displayed.

To navigate to the correct month you can click the small arrow buttons pointing left and right located at the top of the calendar window. Clicking the button with the right arrow advances the calendar one month for each click of the mouse. Clicking the button with the left arrow takes the calendar backward one month for each click. If you click on the name of the month, a drop-down list of months will appear, from which you can select the desired month.

If the month of May is not already displayed, use the navigation buttons at the top of the calendar or the month drop-down list to select **May**.

Tabs at the bottom of the calendar display the previous year, current year, and following year. Clicking the tab displaying the following year advances the calendar one year for each click of the mouse. Clicking the tab displaying the earliest year takes the calendar backward one year for each click. The year on the center tab is the year that will be used when the date is set.

If the year 2016 is not displayed on the center tab, click on whichever year tabs are necessary to display **2016** on the center tab.

Verify that the month is May and the year is 2016, and then locate and click on day **2.** Selecting the day of the month closes the calendar pop-up and sets the date.

### Setting the Encounter Time

In this exercise it will not be necessary for you to set a specific time. Therefore, the following explanation is for informational purposes only.

The time of the encounter is set in the field to the right of the date. For example, in Figure 3-2 the time of the encounter is 9:00 AM. Your time will likely be different. Clicking the down-arrow in the time field will invoke a drop-down list of times at fifteen-minute intervals. Clicking a time on the list will select it. Alternatively, time can also be set by typing directly into the time field using the HH:MM format and including either AM or PM.

Although it is not necessary to set a specific time in this exercise, you may optionally set the time using either method described above, if so desired.

NOTE

Setting the encounter date is only required in exercises containing a step for setting a specific date such as this one. The majority of exercises will function with any date. When using a current date, the patient's age displayed in your software may differ from the patient's age in the textbook figures and case studies.

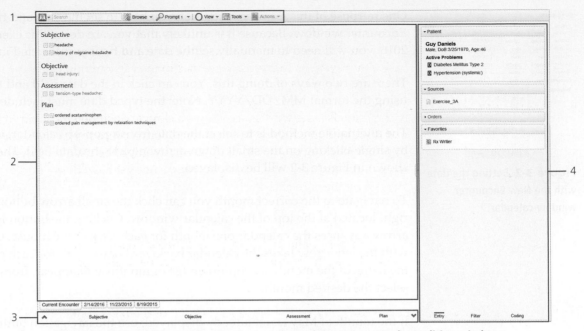

**Figure 3-3** Red boxes outline the four sections of the Quippe Student Edition window.

### Step 5

Verify that the patient **Daniels, Guy** is selected and that the date field displays **5/2/2016**. Locate the OK button at the bottom of the New Encounter window shown in Figure 3-1, and click it.

Your screen should resemble Figure 3-3 (without the red boxes, which were added to the figure for the following discussion).

### Navigating the Screen

This section will explain how the screen is organized and discuss some of the features you will use throughout the course.

The Quippe window contains four functional areas: the toolbar, the **workspace**, the **content pane**, and the **navigation bar**. Refer to Figure 3-3 and locate each of the sections indicated by the numerals 1–4.

**Section 1: The Toolbar** At the top of the window is a row of icon buttons called a *Toolbar*. The purpose of the Toolbar is to allow quick access to the application menu and commonly used functions. Toolbar functions will be explained in more detail later in this and other chapters, as you learn to use them.

**Section 2: The Workspace Pane** The middle portion of the screen (shown in Figure 3-3 with the numeral 2) is the area where clinical documentation takes place. This is the portion of the screen that holds content merged from various sources, where clinical concepts are recorded as findings, and additional details are added to recorded findings. The type of information displayed in the workspace is subject to the View button.

**Section 3: The Navigation Bar** is the narrow strip located below the workspace containing links to jump to section headings in the workspace. This will be used in a later exercise.

**Section 4: The Content Pane** is located along the right side of the application window. The content pane displays information about the patient, and the resources used in the workspace such as the exercise name, and any forms or lists added to the template during the exercise. (Forms and lists are topics of subsequent chapters.) The content pane may also list frequently used orders and other items the clinician might want to quickly add to an encounter note. The content pane can also be used to identify codes from other systems that cross-reference to the Medcin nomenclature such as ICD-10 and SNOMED codes.

In this exercise, the workspace shows a clinical document structured in the SOAP format discussed in Chapter 2. The medical terms preceded by Y/N check boxes are Medcin clinical concepts, which potentially might be used for this encounter. The gray color of the text indicates concepts that do not yet have normal or abnormal results entered by the clinician.

### Step 6

The workspace pane also allows the clinician to review notes from previous visits. Notice that at the bottom of the workspace pane are five tabs: Current Encounter and four with dates.

Locate and click on the tab at the bottom of the pane containing the date **2/14/2016**

A note from February 14, 2016, containing Mr. Daniels' lab results will be displayed. Compare your screen to Figure 3-4.

**Figure 3-4** Guy Daniels' previous encounter note.

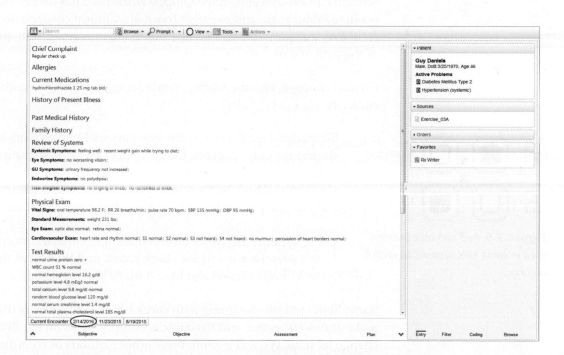

### Step 7

After you have reviewed the previous note, to return to the current encounter, click on the tab at the bottom of the workspace labeled Current Encounter.

On the current encounter you will have noticed that there are headings in a larger size typeface: Subjective, Objective, Assessment, and Plan. These are the sections of a SOAP note. The clinical concepts in the workspace are organized under them.

At the very bottom of the screen, below the workspace tabs, is the Navigation bar. This bar allows the clinician to quickly jump to various sections of the current encounter.

Although this encounter doesn't have many sections and clinical concepts, in subsequent exercises we will see that structured documentation often has more sections and significantly more clinical concepts. In longer documentation, the ability to quickly jump to a section without scrolling can save the clinician time.

Locate and click on each of the links in the navigation bar, in turn: Subjective, Objective, Assessment, and Plan. Notice as each section becomes outlined in a box. If the current encounter contained more data than would fit in the window, the window would have automatically scrolled to the section clicked.

To unselect the Navigation sections, position your mouse pointer over any white space in the current encounter that is not a heading or a clinical concept and click.

### Recording Clinical Findings

The main purpose of EHR software such as systems based on Medcin is to document clinical notes in a codified electronic medical record. This is done by recording a finding from the Medcin nomenclature list as normal or abnormal. The finding and accompanying text are automatically recorded in the encounter note displayed in the workspace pane. (The portion of the screen is indicated by the numeral 2 in Figure 3-3.)

Medcin clinical concepts in the Quippe workspace have three basic states: unentered, positive (abnormal), and negative (normal). Clinical concepts from a template, list, or form may appear in the workspace, but in the unentered state they will not become part of the patient's record.

Clinical concepts become *findings* when set to positive or negative by the documenting clinician.

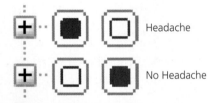

Headache

No Headache

**Figure 3-5** Red and blue buttons used in some EHR systems to record findings.

Slight differences exist in the way various EHR systems show a recorded finding during the entry process. Many Medcin-based systems use red and blue buttons adjacent to a finding, such as those shown in Figure 3-5. In an unselected state the center of both buttons is empty. Clicking a red button fills the button red to indicate the patient had a headache. Blue would indicate no headache.

Other systems use check boxes adjacent to clinical concepts to indicate Yes or No. In this exercise we will use check boxes, and the text of the finding will turn red if the Y box is clicked and blue if the N box is clicked.

Some EHR systems use forms with check boxes, while others dispense with check boxes and buttons altogether and the clinician simply clicks on the finding description to change its state. We will explore these other methods of recording clinical concepts in subsequent exercises.

Y N headache

**Figure 3-6** Y and N check boxes used in this exercise to record findings.

### Step 8

Locate the clinical concept headache, in the Subjective section. Position your mouse pointer on the rightmost box, containing the letter **Y**, and click it. The clinical concept will become a finding and turn red, as shown in Figure 3-6, indicating the patient reports having a headache.

Red indicates a positive or abnormal finding. The finding is abnormal because it is not normal to have a headache, and the finding is positive because the patient positively reported a headache.

### Step 9

Now position your mouse pointer on the box adjacent to headache, containing the letter N, and click it. The finding will now turn blue, indicating no headache.

Click the box containing the letter N again, and the finding will return to its neutral state as an unentered clinical concept.

### Step 10

The patient reported a headache, so again locate and click on the **Y** box for headache. The finding should turn red.

### Step 11

The patient denies any history of migraines, so locate and click the **N** box adjacent to **history of migraine headache**. The finding should turn blue.

Blue indicates a normal or negative finding. The finding is normal because it is normal not to have migraines, and the finding is negative because the patient said he didn't have them.

### Step 12

The clinician performs a physical examination of Mr. Daniels' head to determine if his headaches are caused by an injury. Proceed to the Objective section. Locate and click on the **N** box adjacent to **head injury**. The finding should turn blue.

### Step 13

After speaking with the patient, the clinician concludes Mr. Daniels is suffering from tension headaches. Proceed to the Assessment section. Locate and click on the **Y** box for **tension-type headache**. The finding should turn red.

### Step 14

The clinician orders **acetaminophen** and **learning relaxation techniques**. Proceed to the Plan section. Locate and click on the **Y** boxes for both clinical concepts. The findings should turn red.

### Printing Encounters and Submitting Your Work

Once all the clinical concepts in this exercise have been recorded as findings, compare your screen to Figure 3-7. If anything is incorrect, apply the procedures you learned in Step 9 to unset a finding, and then make the correction.

> **NOTE**
>
> The Student Edition software prints encounter notes by creating a PDF, or Portable Document Format, file, which you can print or download to your computer. You will need the free Adobe Reader or another compatible program to open this file.

### Step 15

You may wish to print your completed encounter notes, either to have a copy for yourself or because your instructor requires you to turn them in. This step will teach you how to create a PDF.

**Figure 3-7** Completed
encounter for Guy Daniels.

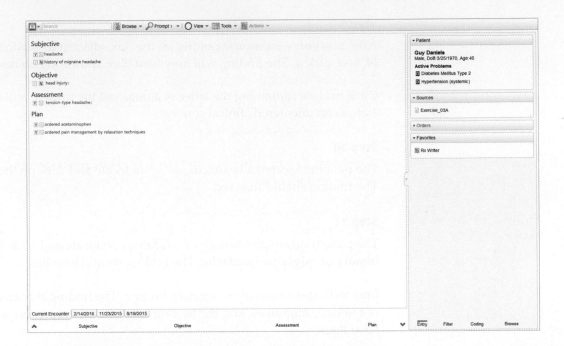

**Figure 3-8** Quippe
application menu.

Locate the toolbar above the workspace, and click on the blue Quippe icon button. This will drop down the Quippe application menu shown in Figure 3-8.

On the Quippe menu, locate and click the option Create PDF. A new tab or window containing a PDF will open in your browser, as shown in Figure 3-9. Use your browser's print or download function to perform either task.

In the next step you will learn how to submit your work to your instructor. If you wish to print or download the PDF, you must do so **before** clicking Submit for Grade, as that function ends your exercise session.

Compare your PDF to Figure 3-9. If there are any differences, review the previous steps in this exercise to find and correct your error. If everything is correct, proceed to step 16.

**Figure 3-9** PDF of Guy
Daniels' encounter note.

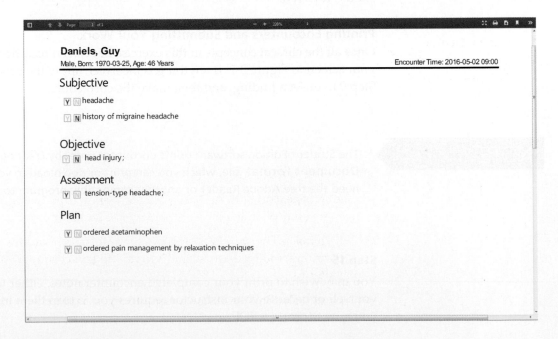

**Step 16**

The final step in every exercise will be to submit your completed work for a grade.

Locate the blue Quippe icon button on the toolbar and click it. This will drop down the Quippe application menu shown in Figure 3-8.

Click on the option Submit for Grade.

**Important: If you close, exit, or refresh your browser before clicking Submit for Grade, you will lose all work done in a session.**

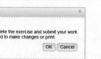

**Figure 3-10** Submit for Grade confirmation window.

The confirmation window shown in Figure 3-10 will display. If are satisfied everything is correct, click on the OK button. If you would like to change something in the exercise, click Cancel and continue working. However, after you have made your corrections remember to click on Submit for Grade to get credit for the exercise.

## Understanding the Toolbar

The Toolbar, located at the top of the window, above the workspace, consists of a row of icon buttons. The purpose of the Toolbar is to allow quick access to commonly used functions. In the previous exercise you clicked the first toolbar button, the Quippe icon, to invoke the Application menu, and you have already used two of the options on that menu.

With the exception of the Search box, in which you first type a term to search, the other toolbar buttons invoke a drop-down menu or list when you click on them. Once a list appears, moving the mouse pointer vertically over the list will highlight each item. In the Student Edition, highlight refers to a colored rectangle that appears over an item. Clicking on the highlighted item will invoke that function. Clicking the mouse anywhere in the application other than in the list will close the list.

For illustration purposes, Figure 3-11 collectively shows the drop-down lists from all the toolbar buttons. Note that in the application only one drop-down list appears at a time, and it is always positioned directly below the corresponding button.

**Figure 3-11** Student Edition toolbar showing drop-down menus for each button.

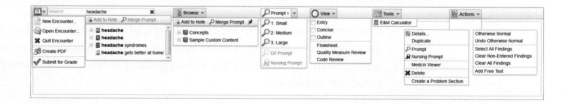

The Toolbar buttons are (from left to right):

◆ The Quippe icon button – when clicked displays the Quippe application menu, which you used in Exercise 3A (shown in Figure 3-8).

◆ Search box – The search box allows users to search various content, including the Medcin knowledge base for individual Medcin concepts(described further in Chapter 6).

◆ Browse – The Browse button is used to access and navigate the clinical concepts in the Medcin nomenclature as well as a directory of Forms and Lists (tools that may be used to add multiple clinical concepts into the workspace at once). Forms and Lists will be covered in Chapter 5.

◆ Prompt button – Executes an intelligent prompt on data entered in the current encounter (described further in Chapter 6).

◆ View – Changes the workspace display; entry view includes entered and unentered clinical concepts, concise view displays only recorded findings, and outline view headings of sections that contain recorded findings. Flowsheet, Clinical Measures Review, and Code Review are covered in Chapters 8–10.

◆ Tools – Accesses the E&M Calculator, which analyzes the encounter note and suggests the correct CPT-4 code for insurance billing (described further in Chapter 12).

◆ Actions – The Actions button only becomes active when an item in the workspace is selected. The functions on the Actions menu affect only the selected item, and options on the Actions drop-down menu vary by the type of item selected. The Actions drop-down menu shown in Figure 3-11 below the left side of the button is invoked when the selected item is a finding. The Actions drop-down menu below the right side of the button is invoked when the selected item is a section heading. Note: the Actions menu can also be invoked by right-clicking on a clinical concept or finding in the encounter note.

## Navigating Medcin Content

In the old days doctors simply handwrote a few notes about a patient's visit in a chart. Eventually, medical schools began to teach a disciplined approach to documenting patient visits. Clinicians learned to organize their notes in a structured format referred to by the acronym *SOAP*, as discussed in Chapter 1. However, the four broad headings—subjective, objective, assessment, and plan—encompass many different types of clinical concepts.

For example, subjective is the information the patient reports. It includes not only symptoms reported by the patient, but also history of the present illness, past medical history, family history, daily habits, and medications the patient is currently taking. Rather that lump all of these clinical concepts under a single heading, the format for structuring encounter notes evolved into a new standard, which better identified the information with additional headings.

In a similar manner, the Medcin nomenclature is organized into a hierarchy of six domains that correspond to six broad sections of a standard encounter note and are arranged in the order of a typical outpatient exam. The six domains fit into the SOAP structure as follows:

| | | |
|---|---|---|
| **Subjective** | S | Symptoms |
| | H | History |
| **Objective** | P | Physical Examination |
| | T | Tests (performed) |
| **Assessment** | D | Diagnoses, syndromes, and conditions |
| **Plan** | R | Therapy (plan, instructions, and ordered tests), medication, and treatment |

CMS initiatives led clinicians to adopt a structured note format with a more expansive set of headings, which better identified and grouped information in the encounter note.

To accommodate the CMS structure, clinical concepts in the Medcin knowledge base contain information as to which section of a structured note the finding would normally appear in. When Medcin clinical concepts are added to an encounter note, Quippe will automatically place them in the default section.

To help you become familiar with the Medcin nomenclature and with the additional CMS headings, the next exercise will start with a blank SOAP note, to which you will add Medcin clinical concepts. As you do so, the new headings will appear, but the main purpose of the exercise is to learn to navigate the Medcin nomenclature, locate clinical concepts, and add them to the workspace, so you can document the patient's visit.

The Quippe Student Edition software used for these exercises is not a simulation program, but actual EHR software containing the entire Medcin nomenclature, which consists of more than 340,000 clinical concepts with 68 million relationships.

Even after dividing the nomenclature into six broad domains, the nomenclature list is still too extensive to navigate easily. To help clinicians navigate such a robust nomenclature, each category is further subdivided by body systems, types of history, types of treatments, and more.

## Guided Exercise 3B: Adding Clinical Concepts to the Workspace

This exercise will use additional toolbar buttons, with emphasis on understanding how the Medcin nomenclature is organized, how to locate clinical concepts, and how to add them to the workspace.

### Case Study

When a person consumes excessive quantities of caffeinated beverages on a regular basis, a dependency can develop. If the person suddenly quits all caffeine, physical symptoms such as strong headaches can occur.

Briana Allen is a college student working part-time as a barista in a coffee shop. She was formerly a heavy coffee drinker who recently stopped all coffee. Today she visits her doctor's office complaining of headaches for the last five days.

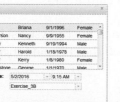

**Figure 3-12** Selecting Briana Allen from the patient list in the New Encounter window.

### Step 1

Start a supported web browser program and follow the steps listed inside the cover of this textbook to log in to the MyHealthProfessionsLab for this course.

Locate and click on the link **Exercise 3B**. This will open the Quippe software window with the New Encounter window shown in Figure 3-12 displayed in the center.

Notice that while the New Encounter window is displayed all the toolbar buttons are grayed out, indicating that they are not accessible. A toolbar button is grayed out when its particular function is not applicable to the currently selected clinical concept, or to the state of the encounter note, or when a pop-up window such as New Encounter is present.

### Step 2

In this step you will temporarily cancel the New Encounter window to allow access to the Quippe application menu while we discuss its options. Normally, you should never cancel the New Encounter window, because until a patient is selected you cannot record clinical concepts in the workspace pane.

Locate and click the Cancel button. This will close the New Encounter window.

Locate and click the Quippe icon button on the toolbar to access the Quippe application menu shown in Figure 3-8. In addition to the options used in the previous exercise are the following:

◆ New Encounter – restarts the encounter for the current exercise. This option is normally used only if you have made errors in the exercise and wish to start from scratch. Creating a new encounter will eliminate anything you did for this exercise. If any clinical concepts have been recorded, a dialogue box will ask you to confirm your intention to restart the exercise.

◆ Open Encounter – opens a patient's previous encounter.

◆ Quit Encounter – quits the exercise without saving any of your work, closes Quippe, and returns you to MyHealthProfessionsLab. This option is used **only** when there isn't sufficient class time to complete an exercise and submit it for a grade. If any clinical concepts have been recorded, a dialogue box will ask you to confirm your intention to quit the exercise.

On the Quippe application menu shown in Figure 3-8, locate and click the New Encounter option. This will invoke the New Encounter pop-up window you previously canceled.

### Step 3

In the New Encounter window locate and click on the patient name **Allen, Briana.**

You do not have to set a specific encounter date for this exercise; use the current date and time. Locate and click the OK button.

This will start a new encounter with a blank SOAP note in the workspace.

### Step 4

Locate and click on the toolbar Browse button. A drop-down menu containing the Concepts and Sample Custom Content book icons will be displayed.

Locate the icon that resembles a stickpin in the upper right corner of the Browse list and click on it. This will allow the list to remain open as you scroll and select clinical concepts in the next steps. The stickpin icon is circled in red in Figure 3-13.

Note: the stickpin icon will change to a red X. The X icon button in the Browse list is used when you no longer need to navigate the list and wish to turn off the stickpin function.

### Step 5

In the Browse drop-down list, locate and click the plus symbol next to the Concepts book icon. This will open the Medcin nomenclature list as shown in Figure 3-14.

### Step 6

Each of the six domains is preceded by a small plus symbol adjacent to a colored block letter. Locate and click on the small plus symbol next to Symptoms.

The list will expand to show symptom groups organized in order of body systems, listed head-to-toe.

Locate and click on the small plus symbol next to head symptoms. The list of concepts will expand to show symptoms related to various parts of the head.

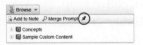

**Figure 3-13** Drop-down list invoked by the Browse button (with stickpin icon circled).

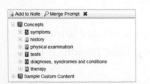

**Figure 3-14** Expanded Concepts list displays the six domains of the Medcin nomenclature.

**NOTE**

In exercises that permit you to use the current date the patient's age may differ from the age shown in the textbook figures or given in the case study.

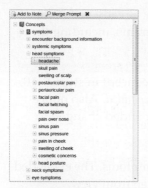

**Figure 3-15** Expanded list of clinical concepts for head symptoms with headache highlighted.

Compare your list with Figure 3-15. The list should have expanded to reveal many additional head clinical concepts. Notice that "head symptoms" is indented, and clinical concepts under that are further indented.

Notice also that some of the head symptoms have small plus symbols as well—for example, "headache" and "postauricular pain." These plus symbols indicate that even more specific clinical concepts are available for those items. Conversely, clinical concepts such as "skull pain" and "swelling of scalp" do not have small plus symbols. This means that there are not more specific clinical concepts available for those items.

### Step 7

Locate the clinical concept **headache** in the list of head symptoms and click on the word headache (not the plus symbol next to it). This will highlight headache, as shown in Figure 3-15. In the Student Edition, highlight refers to a colored rectangle that appears over or around an item.

Locate the Add to Note button at the top of the browse list, and click it. This will add the clinical concept to the SOAP note for us to use later. At this step we are not recording findings in the encounter note, merely adding clinical concepts to the workspace.

### Step 8

Remember, the small plus symbol indicates there are more specific clinical concepts hidden from view that are related to the clinical concept displayed.

Locate and click the small plus symbol next to the clinical concept headache. The list expands further.

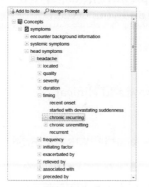

**Figure 3-16** Expanded list of clinical concepts for headache with chronic recurring highlighted.

Locate the word "timing," indented under headache, and click on the small plus symbol next to it. The list expands further, revealing various timing attributes of headache symptoms.

### Step 9

Locate the clinical concept **chronic/recurring** in the expanded list under timing, and click on the words "chronic/recurring" (not the plus symbol next to the clinical concept). This will highlight the clinical concept, as shown in Figure 3-16.

With the clinical concept highlighted, locate and click the Add to Note button at the top of the browse list.

### Step 10

Notice that even the detailed clinical concepts chronic/recurring and chronic/unremitting have small plus symbols, indicating that still further detailed clinical concepts are available.

Locate and click the small plus symbol next to the clinical concept chronic recurring to expand the list further, as shown in Figure 3-17.

Locate and click on the words "episodes recently worse" to highlight the clinical concept, and then click the Add to Note button at the top of the browse list.

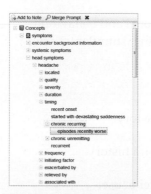

**Figure 3-17** Tree shows chronic recurring expanded and the concept "episodes recently worse" highlighted.

### Step 11

This type of list structure is called a *tree* because each indention of the list represents smaller branches of the clinical concept above it. Look again at Figure 3-17; notice how each new level is indented further than the one above it. You may already be familiar with this concept because it is used in many other computer programs, including the Windows operating system.

Each time you clicked on the small plus symbol next to a clinical concept in steps 6–10, the list grew. The term we use for this is to say that the tree has *expanded*. Also notice that the small plus symbols next to clinical concepts that were expanded changed to small minus signs.

Locate and click the minus sign next to the clinical concept head symptoms. The expanded list of various types of head symptom clinical concepts will be hidden from view.

When you clicked on the small minus symbol for head symptoms, the expanded clinical concepts indented under "head symptoms" were reduced back to just that one. The term we use for this is to say that the view of the tree has been *collapsed*. These are the terms that will be used when working with Medcin lists for the remainder of this book.

Locate and click the plus symbol next to the clinical concept head symptoms, and the list expands to the full extent it was in Figure 3-17.

### Step 12

Locate and click the minus sign next to the domain heading Symptoms. The expanded list of symptom clinical concepts will again be hidden from view and your screen should again resemble Figure 3-14.

### Step 13

Applying what you have learned in the previous steps, we will now add clinical concepts from other Medcin domains into the workspace pane.

Locate and click the plus symbol next to the domain History to expand it. A list of three types of history is displayed.

◆ Past medical history contains clinical concepts for recording conditions, injuries, medications, surgeries, and other health factors in the patient's medical history.

◆ Family medical history contains clinical concepts for documenting diseases, health factors, and longevity of close family members, especially factors that may indicate hereditary predisposition.

◆ Social history contains clinical concepts for documenting personal and behavioral factors that influence health; for example, diet, exercise, smoking, stimulants, drug and alcohol use, and others.

### Step 14

Locate and click the plus symbol next to the subheading Social history.

Locate and click the plus symbol next to the subheading Behavioral history.

Locate and click the plus symbol next to the clinical concept Caffeine use.

Locate and click the plus symbol next to the clinical concept daily coffee consumption.

Compare your expanded tree to Figure 3-18.

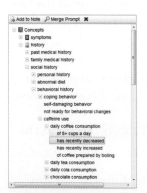

**Figure 3-18** Expanded social, behavioral history, caffeine use, and coffee consumption with two concepts highlighted.

## Step 15

Click on the words "of 8+ cups a day" to highlight the clinical concept, and then click the Add to Note button.

Click on the words "has recently decreased" to highlight the clinical concept, and then click the Add to Note button.

Locate and click the minus sign next to the domain heading History to hide the History tree.

## Step 16

Locate and click the plus symbol next to the domain heading Physical examination to expand it. The Physical examination section of the nomenclature will be displayed. Notice that the list is organized by body systems, essentially in the order you would perform a head-to-toe exam.

The physical examination category contains clinical concepts used to record the observations and results of the clinician's physical examination of the patient as well as measurements and vital signs recorded during the course of the encounter. The primary source of the Objective section of SOAP is the physical examination clinical concepts.

In the expanded tree of physical examination, locate and click on the small plus symbol next to head exam to expand the tree further.

Locate and click on the word "injury" in the expanded list to highlight it, and then click the Add to Note button. Compare your screen to Figure 3-19.

## Step 17

The clinical concepts added to the workspace thus far have been relatively easy to locate near the top of the tree. The final two sections of the encounter note (Assessment and Plan) will provide opportunities to scroll and expand the trees more extensively.

Locate and click the plus symbol next to the domain heading Diagnoses, syndromes and conditions to expand it.

Scroll the list downward until you see "neurologic disorders." Note: if you scroll the expanded tree to the bottom of the list, neurologic disorders is located about midway in the list (shown highlighted in Figure 3-20). Click on the small plus symbol next to neurologic disorders to expand the tree.

## Step 18

Scroll the list further downward until neurologic disorders is positioned at the top of the drop-down list as shown in Figure 3-21. This will enable you to more easily locate the next two clinical concepts to be expanded.

Locate headache syndromes (just below neurologic disorders) and click on the small plus symbol next to it.

Locate benign (in the expanded tree of headache syndromes) and click on the small plus symbol next to it.

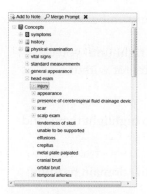

**Figure 3-19** Expanded Physical Examination tree for head exam; shows the injury concept highlighted.

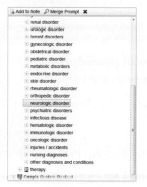

**Figure 3-20** Expanded diagnoses domain with Neurologic Disorder highlighted.

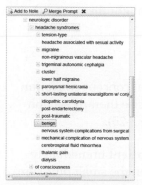

**Figure 3-21** Neurologic disorder scrolled to the top, headache syndromes expanded, benign highlighted.

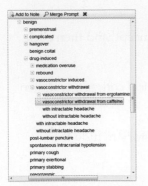

**Figure 3-22** Benign scrolled to the top, drug-induced and vasoconstrictor withdrawal expanded, vasoconstrictor withdrawal from caffeine highlighted.

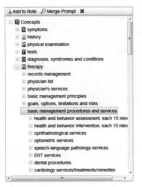

**Figure 3-23** Therapy domain expanded, basic management procedures and services highlighted and expanded.

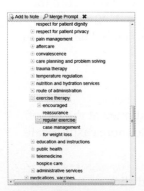

**Figure 3-24** Exercise therapy expanded to show the concept regular exercise highlighted.

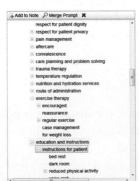

**Figure 3-25** Education and instructions expanded, instructions for patient highlighted.

### Step 19

As in the previous step, it will be easier for you to locate the next two concepts if you first scroll the list downward until benign is positioned at the top as shown in Figure 3-22.

Locate drug-induced and then click on the small plus symbol next to it.

Locate vasoconstrictor withdrawal and then click on the small plus symbol next to it.

Slide the horizontal scroll bar at the bottom of the list toward the right until you can read the full descriptions of the clinical concepts under vasoconstrictor withdrawal, as shown in Figure 3-22.

Click on the words "vasoconstrictor withdrawal from caffeine" to highlight them, and then click the Add to Note button.

Scroll to the top of the list and click the small minus sign next to the domain heading Diagnoses, syndromes, and conditions to collapse the tree.

### Step 20

Clinical concepts used in the Plan section of the encounter note are located in the Therapy domain. You will now add several items from this domain to the workspace.

Click the small plus symbol next to the domain heading Therapy.

Locate and click on the small plus symbol next to **basic management procedures and services** as shown in Figure 3-23. (Note that there is another concept in the list named basic management principles. Do not choose it by mistake.)

### Step 21

Scroll downward to locate the clinical concept **exercise therapy**. (It is located almost at the end of the indented section of basic management procedures and services, just above the concept "education and instructions." If you pass the concept "medicines, vaccines," you have scrolled too far.)

Click the small plus symbol to expand **exercise therapy** as shown in Figure 3-24.

Click on the words "regular exercise" to highlight them, and then click the Add to Note button.

### Step 22

Click the small plus symbol next to the clinical concept **education and instructions** (located just below the exercise therapy section used in the previous step, as shown in Figure 3-25).

Locate the clinical concept **instructions for patient** immediately below education and instructions, and click on the small plus symbol next to it.

### Step 23

Scroll the expanded tree downward until you locate **abstinence from alcohol.** (The concept is located quite far down the expanded

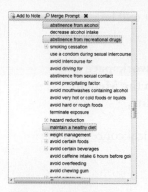

**Figure 3-26** Scroll abstinence from alcohol to the top to select three concepts.

section of instructions for patient.) Once you locate it, it will be easier to complete the remaining items in this step if you continue scrolling until abstinence from alcohol is positioned at the top of the list as shown in Figure 3-26.

Click on the words "abstinence from alcohol" to highlight the concept, and then click the Add to Note button.

Locate and click on the words "abstinence from recreational drugs" to highlight the concept, and then click the Add to Note button.

Locate and click on the words "maintain a healthy diet" (to highlight the concept), and then click the Add to Note button.

### Removing Clinical Concepts and Findings

### Step 24

Close the Browse drop-down list by clicking the toolbar Browse button.

Notice that additional section headings have appeared in the encounter note wherever clinical concepts were added.

Locate and click on the clinical concept abstinence from recreational drugs in the Plan section of the workspace. The concept will be enclosed in a rectangle. In Figure 3-27 the rectangle is yellow. The color could be different on your computer. This rectangle identifies the finding or section of the encounter pane that is *highlighted* or has focus.

**Figure 3-27** Finding highlighted. Delete function located on the Actions button drop-down menu.

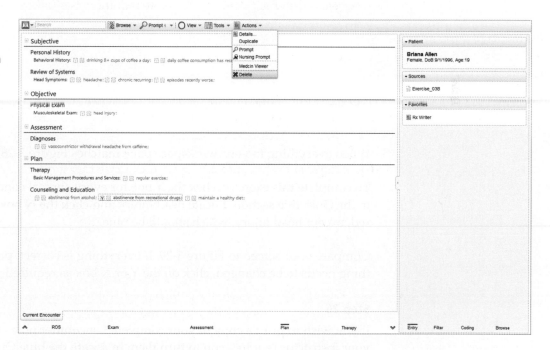

Locate and click the toolbar Actions button. The drop-down menu shown in Figure 3-27 will appear.

The Actions button is only available when a clinical concept, finding, or heading in the workspace has been selected, and actions taken affect only the item(s) within the highlight rectangle.

Locate and click the Actions menu option **Delete** and the concept will be removed from the encounter note.

> Note that this procedure only removes the finding from the workspace and current encounter. Clinical concepts will not be deleted from the Medcin nomenclature or previous patient encounters by this procedure.

The Actions menu can also be invoked by right-clicking on a clinical concept in the workspace.

## Step 25

Compare your screen to Figure 3-28. If any clinical concepts are missing or different from those in the figure, review steps 4–23 to identify and correct your error. If you have added an incorrect clinical concept, use the procedure in Step 24 to remove it.

**Figure 3-28** All clinical concepts added to the workspace from the Browse list.

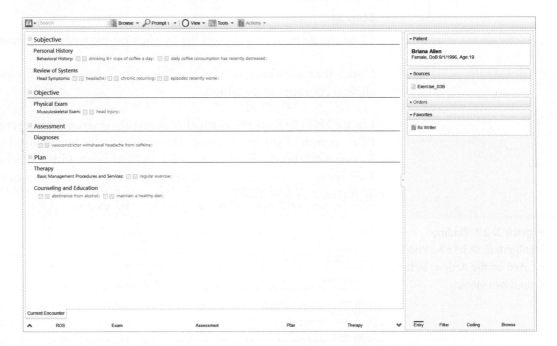

When everything in your workspace pane matches Figure 3-28 you can proceed.

To complete this exercise, click the **Y** box for every clinical concept **except head injury** in the Objective section. Locate head injury and click the **N** box. All findings should be red, except head injury, which should be blue.

Compare your screen to Figure 3-29. If everything is correct, proceed to Step 26. If anything needs to be changed, click on the Y or N box as required.

## Step 26

If you wish to print a copy of your completed encounter notes for yourself or because your instructor requires you to turn them in, locate the blue Quippe icon button on the toolbar and click it. This will drop down the Quippe application menu shown in Figure 3-8. Click the Create PDF option on the menu, and then download or print the resulting PDF. Do this before clicking Submit for Grade in Step 27.

## Step 27

The final step in every exercise is to submit your completed work for a grade.

**Figure 3-29** Completed encounter with recorded findings.

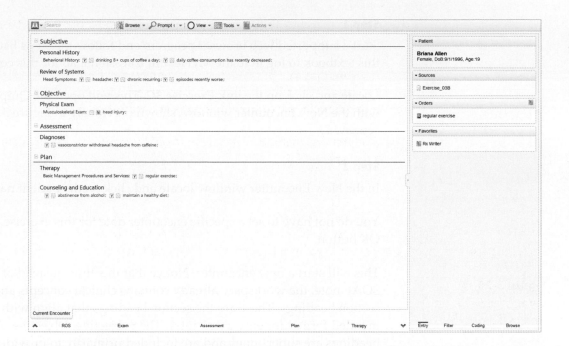

Locate the blue Quippe icon button on the toolbar and click it. This will drop down the Quippe application menu previously shown in Figure 3-8.

Locate and click on the menu option Submit for Grade. This will complete Exercise 3B.

**Important: If you close, exit, or refresh your browser before completing Submit for Grade, you will lose all work done in this session.**

## Using a More Specific Finding

In the previous exercise, you recorded a patient's symptom of chronic/recurring headaches by selecting three different clinical concepts from the list. There is nothing wrong with doing it that way if the natural flow of the exam progresses in that manner. For example, the patient reports having headaches. The clinician asks if they are recurring, and the patient says "yes." The clinician adds the clinical concept, but the patient also mentions that the headaches are getting worse. The clinician then adds the finding "worse."

However, if you have all of the information before adding the clinical concepts, you can simply select the most specific concept and Medcin will add the surrounding text. In this exercise, you will record all three pieces of information about the patient's symptom by clicking only two findings.

### Guided Exercise 3C: Patient with Caffeine Withdrawal Headache

This exercise will allow you to apply what you have learned in previous exercises to add clinical concepts and document a patient encounter. It will also show you the purpose of the View button on the toolbar.

#### Case Study

This exercise will use the same patient as the previous exercise: Briana Allen, a formerly heavy coffee drinker who recently stopped all coffee and has been experiencing withdrawal headaches.

### Step 1

Start a supported web browser program and follow the steps listed inside the cover of this textbook to log in to the MyHealthProfessionsLab for this course.

Locate and click on the link **Exercise 3C**. This will open the Quippe software window with the New Encounter window, shown previously in Figure 3-12, displayed in the center.

### Step 2

In the New Encounter window locate and click on the patient name **Allen, Briana.**

You do not have to set a specific encounter date for this exercise. Locate and click the OK button.

This will start a new encounter. Notice that this time, instead of starting with a blank SOAP note, the workspace already contains clinical concepts and significantly more section headings. These are the section headings that align with the CMS recommended format for encounter notes. The Subjective, Objective, Assessment, and Plan headings are superfluous and are included primarily to provide continuity from previous exercises.

### Step 3

The patient reports symptoms of chronic recurring headaches, the concept for which is not currently in your encounter note. Apply what you learned in the previous exercise to add clinical concepts to your workspace.

Locate and click on the toolbar Browse button. A drop-down menu containing the Concepts and Sample Custom Content book icons will be displayed.

Locate the icon that resembles a stickpin in the upper right corner of the Browse list and click on it. The stickpin icon is circled in red in Figure 3-13.

In the Browse drop-down list, locate and click the plus symbol next to the Concepts book icon. This will open the Medcin nomenclature list as shown in Figure 3-14.

### Step 4

Locate and click on the small plus symbol next to the domain Symptoms.

Locate and click on the small plus symbol next to head symptoms. The list of concepts will expand to show symptoms related to various parts of the head (as previously shown in Figure 3-15).

### Step 5

One positive effect of a nomenclature with a hierarchical structure such as Medcin is that when you add a clinical concept, it automatically inherits the parent concepts above it in the tree. For example, in the previous exercise you did not add head symptoms to the note, but when you added headache, it automatically inherited its position as a head symptom. This can be a time saver for the clinician because when adding clinical concepts it is only necessary to add the more specific concept.

This time instead of adding headache to the note, we will add chronic/recurring, as that is the type of headache Briana is reporting.

Locate the clinical concept **headache** in the list of head symptoms and click on the plus symbol next to it.

Locate **timing** in the expanded list under headache and click on the plus symbol next to it.

### Step 6

Locate the clinical concept **chronic/recurring** in the expanded list under timing, and click on the words "chronic/recurring" (not the plus symbol next to the clinical concept). This will highlight the clinical concept, as shown previously in Figure 3-16.

With the clinical concept highlighted, locate and click the Add to Note button at the top of the browse list.

### Step 7

Locate and click the small plus symbol next to the clinical concept chronic/recurring to expand the list further.

Locate and click on the words "episodes recently worse" to highlight the clinical concept, as shown previously in Figure 3-17, and then click the Add to Note button at the top of the browse list.

Click the Browse button on the toolbar to close the concepts list.

### Step 8

Compare your screen to Figure 3-30. Locate the Review of Systems section and notice that the clinical concept chronic/recurring includes the word headaches. This was added to the workspace as part of chronic/recurring without having to select and add headache, because it is the parent concept in the hierarchy.

**Figure 3-30** Clinical concepts chronic recurring headaches and episodes recently worse added to the workspace.

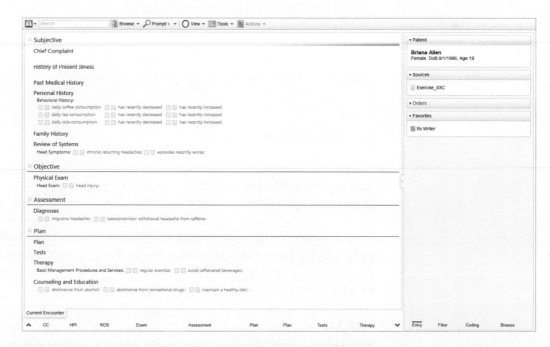

### Step 9

Locate the Personal History section and click on the **Y** check boxes next to **Daily coffee consumption** and **has recently decreased**. Both findings will turn red.

You will recall from an earlier exercise that Quippe findings have three states: gray (neutral), indicating an unentered clinical concept; red, indicating a positive or abnormal finding; and blue, indicating a normal or negative finding.

Notice the workspace contains many clinical concepts that are gray (neutral). Although these display in your workspace, they are not yet recorded in the encounter note.

### Step 10

As you learn to enter encounter notes of greater complexity we will use templates, lists, and forms that will provide significant numbers of clinical concepts to choose from. From time to time, you may wish to quickly view the note with only the entered findings. The toolbar View button contains options to change what is displayed in the workspace.

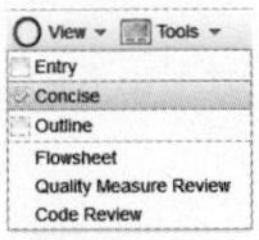

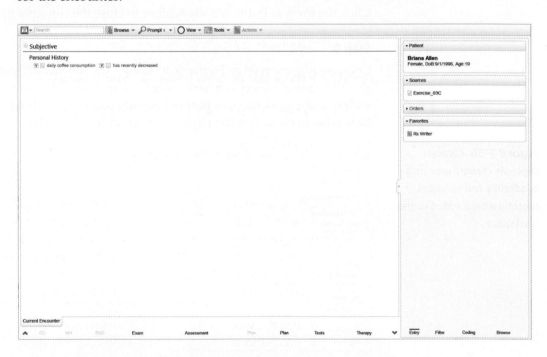

**Figure 3-31** Toolbar View button menu with Concise highlighted.

Locate and click the toolbar View button. A drop-down menu will appear.

Locate and click on the View menu option **Concise** as shown in Figure 3-31.

### Step 11

Compare your screen to Figure 3-32. Notice that only recorded findings are displayed. If the encounter note was printed or saved at this point, these would be the only data for the encounter.

**Figure 3-32** Concise view of encounter showing two recorded findings.

To return to the entry view, click the View button on the toolbar and select the menu option Entry from the drop-down menu. Your screen should again resemble Figure 3-30. You can toggle between Entry and Concise views anytime you wish to see exactly which data are recorded in the encounter.

### Step 12

Just because clinical concepts appear in a template does not mean they should all be recorded. Often numerous clinical concepts are included in a template, list, or form to minimize the need to add clinical concepts with the Browse button while documenting the encounter.

In this exercise, the template lists additional types of caffeinated beverages, but since the patient does not report using those, leave them unentered and proceed to the Review of Systems section.

Locate and click on the **Y** check boxes next to **chronic/recurring headaches** and **episodes recently worse**. Both findings will turn red.

### Step 13

As you have done in the previous exercise, locate the Physical Exam section and click the **N** check box next to **head injury**. The finding will turn blue.

### Step 14

Locate the Diagnoses section.

Locate and click the **Y** check box next to **vasoconstrictor withdrawal headache from caffeine**. The finding will turn red. Again, only the finding relevant to the patient's encounter is to be checked. The other diagnosis is left unentered.

### Step 15

Locate the Therapy section and click the **Y** check boxes next to **regular exercises** and **avoid caffeinated beverages**. Both findings will turn red.

### Step 16

Locate the Counseling and Education section.

Click the **Y** check box next to **abstinence from alcohol**.

Click the **Y** check box next to **abstinence from recreational drugs**.

Both findings will turn red.

### Step 17

One thing you may have discovered already is that if you accidentally clicked on a clinical concept it had the same effect as clicking the Y check box. As we discussed early in this chapter, various EHR systems use different methods to record a finding. Some use buttons, some use check boxes, and some systems support clinicians who want to merely see findings in an uncluttered note. In later chapters you will work with templates that do not use check boxes, so it is important to understand this concept now.

Locate and click the words "**maintain a healthy diet**" instead of either check box. The finding turns red, and the Y check box is automatically set.

Click again on the words "maintain a healthy diet." The finding turns blue, and the N check box is automatically set.

Click on the words "maintain a healthy diet" a third time. The finding is set to an unentered state, the clinical concept turns gray (neutral), and neither the Y nor the N check box is set.

Since the clinician does want the patient to maintain a healthy diet, set the finding in a positive state by clicking the clinical concept one more time. Make certain the finding maintain a healthy diet is red and the Y check box is set before proceeding to step 18.

### Step 18

Locate and click the toolbar View button. A drop-down menu will appear.

Locate and click on the View menu option **Concise** as shown previously in Figure 3-31.

Compare your screen to Figure 3-33. If everything is correct, proceed to step 19. If there are any differences, click the View button on the toolbar, select the Entry option on the drop-down menu, and then correct your work according to the preceding steps.

**Figure 3-33** Concise view of completed encounter with correctly recorded findings.

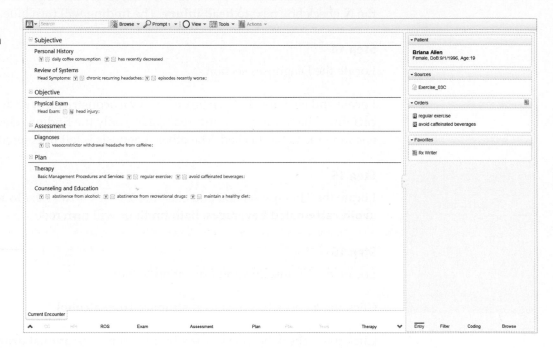

### Step 19

If you wish to print a copy of your completed encounter notes for yourself or because your instructor requires you to turn them in, locate and click the blue Quippe icon button on the toolbar. Select the option Create PDF on the drop-down menu and then download or print the resulting PDF. Do this before clicking Submit for Grade in Step 20.

### Step 20

The final step in every exercise is to submit your completed work for a grade.

Locate and click the blue Quippe icon button on the toolbar to display the drop-down menu shown previously in Figure 3-8.

Locate and click on the menu option Submit for Grade. This will complete Exercise 3C.

## Adding Details to the Findings

In addition to the medical terminology and surrounding narrative text that clicking a finding automatically records, it is sometimes necessary or desirable for the clinician to add details to a finding for further clarification or to alter the meaning of a finding. The added details appear in the encounter note and in some cases change the section of the note to which the finding belongs.

For example, migraine headache is a diagnosis. If prefixed with "Family history of," it is no longer an assessment, but is instead a history item that belongs in the Family history section. If the same clinical concept is given the prefix "History of," then the finding is about the patient and belongs in the Past Medical History section.

Details are added to a finding in Quippe via a pop-up window that is invoked by either clicking the Actions button on the toolbar or right-clicking on a finding. The window contains nine fields, which are used to add information or alter the meaning of the currently selected finding. The fields in the pop-up window are prefix, modifier, status, value, unit, note, onset, duration, and episodes. In subsequent exercises we will discuss and use each of the fields.

All of the fields in the Details pop-up window apply to a single finding, the one currently selected. Also, use caution if you select findings to add details by clicking with the left-mouse button. As you learned in Step 17 of the previous exercise, left-clicking on a finding can toggle its state—positive, negative, or unentered. After adding details, always verify the finding is in the positive or negative state required by the exercise.

## Guided Exercise 3D: Using the Details Pop-up Window

This exercise will use the same patient as the previous exercise, Briana Allen. In this exercise the patient provides additional information about her caffeine consumption and resulting headaches. You will learn to use the Details pop-up window to add information to Briana Allen's encounter.

### Case Study

While working as a barista, Briana Allen found herself consuming ten cups of coffee a day. When she completely stopped drinking coffee, she began experiencing withdrawal headaches, which have recurred for the last five days.

### Step 1

Start a supported web browser program and follow the steps listed inside the cover of this textbook to log in to the MyHealthProfessionsLab for this course.

Locate and click on the link **Exercise 3D**. This will open the Quippe software window with the New Encounter window, shown previously in Figure 3-12, displayed in the center.

### Step 2

In the New Encounter window locate and click on the patient name **Allen, Briana.**

You do not have to set a specific encounter date for this exercise; use the current date and time. Locate and click the OK button.

Notice that this time the workspace template contains only the CMS-recommended section headings. Use of the superfluous Subjective, Objective, Assessment, and Plan headings will be discontinued for this and most subsequent exercises.

### Step 3

The patient reports she was previously drinking ten cups of coffee a day, but doesn't anymore because she stopped drinking coffee entirely.

Locate and click on the clinical concept **daily coffee consumption**. The finding will turn red.

Locate and click the Actions button on the toolbar. The Actions menu shown previously in Figure 3-27 will drop-down.

Locate and click Details on the drop-down menu. The pop-up window shown in Figure 3-34 will be displayed.

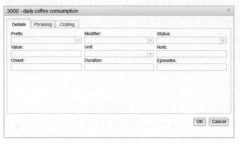

**Figure 3-34** Pop-up window for adding details to the finding daily coffee consumption.

### Value and Unit

### Step 4

At the top of the Details window will be the currently selected finding. Develop a habit of checking the name of the clinical concept displayed there to verify you are adding details to the intended finding.

The first two fields we are going to discuss are Value and Unit.

The Value field can be used to enter a numeric value about any finding. For example, the patient's weight would be entered in the value field of the weight finding, or the numeric result of a Hematocrit (a simple blood test performed in the doctor's office) would be entered in the value field Hematocrit finding.

The Unit field is related to the Value field in that it describes the unit of measure for the value. In the previous example, the unit for weight would be pounds or kilograms, and the unit for the hematocrit volume of red blood cells would be percent.

Medcin has built-in default units associated with certain clinical concepts. These appear in a drop-down list on the unit field. For example, weight has a drop-down list containing kilograms, pounds, or stones (British). In this exercise, coffee consumption is measured in cups. So the value will be the number the patient consumed and the unit would be "cups per day."

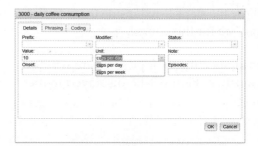

**Figure 3-35** Setting the value 10 and the unit cups per day in the Detail pop-up window.

Locate and click in the Value field. Type the number **10**.

Click in the Unit field and begin to type **cups per day**. A drop-down list will appear, giving you the choice of cups per day or cups per week, as shown in Figure 3-35. Select "cups per day" by clicking on it, or continue typing the entire phrase.

When you have both the Value and the Units set correctly, click the OK button to close the pop-up and add the information to the finding. The finding on your screen should now read "daily coffee consumption 10 cups per day."

### Free Text

### Step 5

In some cases the information to be added is merely something the patient said, or the clinician observed, and is not necessarily a concept in standard nomenclatures. The term for this type of EHR data is "free text," meaning that the text is not codified and might contain anything. Ideally, the less free text used in the EHR, the better. Still, there are many times when free text is appropriate—for example, adding a nuance to a

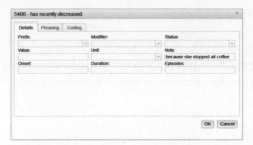

**Figure 3-36** Adding free-text note "because she stopped all coffee" to the finding.

finding that extends its meaning or entering text that more accurately portrays the patient's own words. In this step you will learn how to add free text into the note.

Locate and click on the clinical concept **has recently decreased**. The finding will turn red.

Click the Actions button on the toolbar and select the Detail option from the drop-down menu. The pop-up window shown in Figure 3-36 will be displayed.

Locate and click in the Note field and type the following: **because she stopped all coffee** (do not add punctuation, as Quippe will do this).

Verify that you have spelled everything correctly, and then click the OK button to close the pop-up and add the information to the finding. The finding on your screen should now read "daily coffee consumption has recently decreased because she stopped all coffee."

Note that each of the six Medcin domains has a special finding code named Free-text that can be used to enter larger blocks of text into an encounter note. One example of its use is to enter a narrative of a surgical procedure.

**Onset and Episodes**

**Step 6**

Locate and click on the clinical concept **chronic recurring headaches**. The finding will turn red.

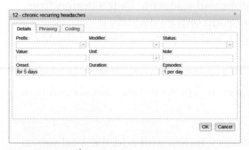

**Figure 3-37** Adding Onset and Episodes detail to the chronic recurring headaches finding.

Click the Actions button on the toolbar and select the Detail option from the drop-down menu. The pop-up window shown in Figure 3-34 will be displayed.

Locate and click in the Onset field, and then type **for 5 days**.

Locate and click in the Episode field, and then type **1 per day**.

Compare your screen to Figure 3-37 and, if everything is correct, click the OK button to close the Details window and add the onset and episode information to your finding. The finding on your screen should now read "chronic recurring headaches 1 per day for 5 days."

**Status and Duration**

**Step 7**

Locate and click on the clinical concept **episodes recently worse**. The finding will turn red.

Click the Actions button on the toolbar and select the Detail option from the drop-down menu. The Details pop-up window will be displayed.

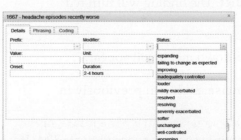

**Figure 3-38** Select **inadequately controlled** Status from the drop-down list; in Duration type 2-4 hours.

Locate and click the Status field. A drop-down list will appear as shown in Figure 3-38. Locate **inadequately controlled** in the list and click on it. The status field should now read "inadequately controlled."

Locate and click in the Duration field, and then type **2-4 hours**.

Verify that Status and Duration have been set correctly, then click the OK button to close the Details window and add the onset and episode information to your finding. The finding on your screen should now read "episodes recently worse 2-4 hours – inadequately controlled."

### Step 8

As you have done in the previous exercise, locate the Physical Exam section and click the **N** check box next to **head injury**. The finding will turn blue.

### Step 9

Locate the Assessment section.

Locate and click the **Y** check box next to **vasoconstrictor withdrawal headache from caffeine**. The finding will turn red.

### Step 10

Locate the Therapy section and click the **Y** check boxes next to **regular exercises** and **avoid caffeinated beverages**. Both findings will turn red.

### Modifier

### Step 11

Locate and click on the clinical concept **abstinence from alcohol** in the Counseling and Education section. The finding will turn red.

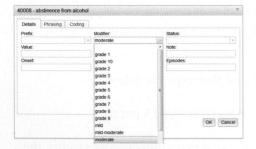

**Figure 3-39** Select moderate from the drop-down list for the Modifier field.

Click the Actions button on the toolbar and select the Detail option from the drop-down menu. The Details pop-up will be displayed.

Locate and click the Modifier field. A drop-down list will appear. The modifier list is longer than the others. Locate **moderate** in the list (shown highlighted in Figure 3-39) and click on it. The modifier field should now read "moderate."

Click the OK button to close the Details window and add the modifier to your finding. The finding on your screen should now read "moderate abstinence from alcohol."

### Step 12

Click the **Y** check box next to **maintain healthy diet**. The finding will turn red.

### Step 13

Locate and click the toolbar View button. A drop-down menu will appear.

Locate and click on the View menu option **Concise** as shown previously in Figure 3-31.

Compare your screen to Figure 3-40. If everything is correct, proceed to step 14. If there are any differences, click the View button on the toolbar, select the Entry option on the drop-down menu, and then correct your work according to the preceding steps.

> **NOTE**
>
> Modifier, Prefix, and other drop-down lists contain a blank in the first row. The blank is used to clear a field previously set by a drop-down list.

**Figure 3-40** Concise view of the completed encounter with correctly recorded findings and details.

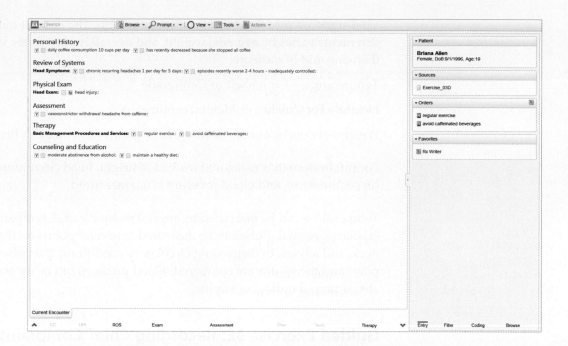

### Step 14

If wish to print a copy of your completed encounter notes for yourself or because your instructor requires you to turn them in, locate and click the blue Quippe icon button on the toolbar. Select the option Create PDF on the drop-down menu and then download or print the resulting PDF. Do this before clicking Submit for Grade in Step 15.

### Step 15

The final step in every exercise is to submit your completed work for a grade.

Locate and click the blue Quippe icon button on the toolbar to display the drop-down menu, and then select the menu option Submit for Grade. This will complete Exercise 3D.

## Chief Complaint and Vital Signs

There are two standard components of the encounter note, recorded by almost every type of practitioner, which we have omitted thus far. Typically, these are among the first things recorded in the encounter note. The exercises up to this point have not dealt with them because they focused on learning to navigate the software. Now that you are familiar with adding clinical concepts, recording and removing findings, and adding details to findings, it is an appropriate time to learn about Chief Complaint and Vital Signs.

The Chief Complaint is a description of the patient's reason for the visit, often paraphrasing the patient's words. Chief Complaint is a required element of the CMS recommended format, usually positioned at the head of the encounter note.

Vital Signs are measurements of the physical body functions (and size) expressed in numeric values. In the truest sense, only heart rate (pulse), respiration rate, and temperature are defined as actual vital signs, but nearly all practices also measure blood pressure, height, and weight. Many practitioners also measure the saturation of oxygen in the blood, and sometimes the waist circumference.

Vital signs are measured differently for children. The normal range for vital signs measurements varies by age, sex, weight, and overall health. Three vital signs have more than one unit of measure:

Temperature – Fahrenheit or Centigrade

Height – Feet/inches or Meters/centimeters

Weight – Pounds/ounces or Kilograms/grams (and Stone in Britain)

For infants length is measured instead of height, head circumference is also measured (in centimeters), and blood pressure is not measured.

Temperature can be measured by several methods: oral, tympanic, under the arm (axillary), or anal. Pulse can be measured at several points on the body, including wrist, neck, and ankles. In diagnosing circulatory conditions, the pulse is measured at each point and the results are compared. Blood pressure can be measured at left or right arm, also sitting, standing, or supine.

## Guided Exercise 3E: Recording Chief Complaint and Vital Signs

This exercise will add two remaining sections found in standard encounters to the relatively simplistic encounter note we have been developing for Briana Allen thus far. In this exercise you will learn to document the Chief Complaint, record vital signs, and then apply what you have learned in previous exercises to record other findings and complete the exercise.

### Case Study

This exercise will use the same patient as recent exercises, Briana Allen, who presents complaining of headaches lasting more than five days since she stopped drinking all coffee.

### Step 1

Start a supported web browser program and follow the steps listed inside the cover of this textbook to log in to the MyHealthProfessionsLab for this course.

Locate and click on the link **Exercise 3E**. This will open the Quippe software window with the New Encounter window displayed in the center.

As you have done in previous exercises, locate and click on the patient name **Allen, Briana**, and then click the OK button.

You do not have to set a specific encounter date for this exercise; use the current date and time.

### Step 2

When the encounter note is displayed, notice the Chief Complaint section heading at the top of the workspace. Although the Medcin nomenclature contains a clinical concept for Chief Complaint, it would waste the clinician's time to have to add it for every encounter. Therefore it is built into most encounter templates because it is part of the CMS recommended standard.

Click in the blank space located just below the Chief Complaint heading. This will open a free-text note field outlined in a colored box where you will type the following text:

**Headaches for more than 5 days**

The portion of the workspace containing the Chief Complaint note field is shown in Figure 3-41.

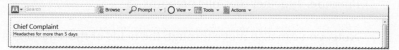

**Figure 3-41** Abridged image of the workspace showing the Chief Complaint field open.

When you have finished typing, you can click anywhere else in the workspace to close the field. If you need to modify or edit the Chief Complaint at any time, simply click on the field again to reopen it.

### Step 3

Locate the Personal History section and click on the **Y** check boxes next to **drinking 8+ cups of coffee per day** and **daily coffee consumption has recently decreased**. Both findings will turn red.

### Step 4

Locate and click on the clinical concept **chronic recurring headaches**. The finding will turn red.

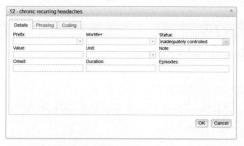

**Figure 3-42** Detail window with Status set to inadequately controlled.

Click the Actions button on the toolbar and select the Detail option from the drop-down menu. The Details pop-up window will be displayed.

Locate and click the Status field. A drop-down list will appear. Locate **inadequately controlled** in the list and click on it. The status field should now read "inadequately controlled."

Compare your screen to Figure 3-42 and, if everything is correct, click the OK button to close the Details window and add the status to your finding. The finding on your screen should now read: "chronic recurring headaches – inadequately controlled."

### Step 5

Locate and click the **Y** check box next to **episodes recently worse**. The finding will turn red.

### Step 6

Locate the Vital Signs table in the Physical Exam section. Enter Briana's vital signs into the corresponding fields, as follows:

Click in the field below the label "Oral Temp" and type her temperature: **98.6**

Click in the next field, below the label "PR." This is the patient's pulse, measured in beats per minute. Type her Pulse Rate: **78**

Click in the next field, below the label "RR." This is the respiration rate, measured in breaths per minute. Type her Respiration Rate: **24**

The next two fields are for recording blood pressure, which is often written as two numbers separated by a slash mark such as 120/78. The first number is called *systolic pressure*, and the second is called *diastolic pressure*. In the EHR, enter the numbers in separate fields, omitting the slash mark.

Click in the field, below the label "SBP." This acronym stands for Systolic Blood Pressure. Type her systolic pressure: **120**

Click in the next field, below the label "DBP." This acronym stands for Diastolic Blood Pressure. Type her diastolic pressure: **78**

Note: you can also move through the fields of the Vital Signs table by pressing the tab key on your keyboard.

> ### Systolic and Diastolic Blood Pressure
>
> The heart beats by contracting the heart muscle, which pushes blood through all the arteries in the body. The force of this action creates pressure on the walls of the arteries. The measurement of this pressure is called the *systolic pressure*. *Diastolic pressure* is the measure of pressure in the arteries between beats, when the heart relaxes and its chambers fill with blood.

### Step 7

Locate the Weight & Height table in the Physical Exam section. Briana weighs 100 pounds and is 5' 4" (64 inches) tall. Enter Briana's weight and height into the corresponding fields, as follows:

Click in the field below the label "Weight" and type **100**

Click (or tab to) the next field below the label "Height" and type **64**

### Step 8

As you have done in the previous exercise, locate the Physical Exam section and click the **N** check box next to **head injury**. The finding will turn blue.

### Step 9

Locate the Diagnoses section.

Locate and click the **Y** check box next to **vasoconstrictor withdrawal headache from caffeine**. The finding will turn red.

### Step 10

Locate the Therapy section and click the **Y** check boxes next to **regular exercises** and **avoid caffeinated beverages**. Both findings will turn red.

### Step 11

Locate the Counseling and Education section.

Click the **Y** check box next to **abstinence from alcohol**.

Click the **Y** check box next to **maintain a healthy diet**.

Both findings will turn red.

### Step 12

Compare your screen to Figure 3-43, being sure to verify that you have entered the numeric values for the vital signs, weight, and height correctly.

**Figure 3-43** Completed encounter note for Briana Allen showing the Vital Signs section with data.

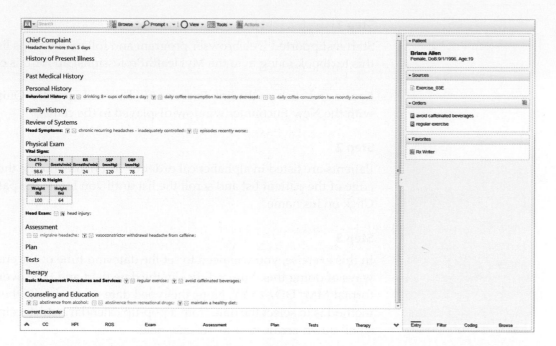

If everything is correct, proceed to step 13. If there are any differences, review steps 2–11 and correct your error.

### Step 13

If you wish to print a copy of your completed encounter notes for yourself or because your instructor requires you to turn them in, locate and click the blue Quippe icon button on the toolbar. Select the option Create PDF on the drop-down menu and then download or print the resulting PDF. Do this before clicking Submit for Grade in Step 14.

### Step 14

The final step in every exercise is to click the blue Quippe icon button on the toolbar, and then select the menu option Submit for Grade. This will complete Exercise 3E.

## Critical Thinking Exercise 3F: A Patient Suffering Withdrawal Headaches

This exercise will help you evaluate how well you can use the Student Edition software to create an encounter note. The exercise provides step-by-step instructions, but does not provide screen figures for reference. Previous exercises in this chapter covered features used in this exercise. If you have difficulty at any step during this exercise, refer to the Summary section at the end of the chapter where a table lists various tasks and the corresponding exercise/step where that feature was explained.

### Case Study

College student Ryan Poole has been trying to keep up with his busy schedule by using caffeine stimulants. When his friend Briana told him to stop drinking so much coffee, he switched to cola and started taking pep pills. He presents with a complaint of recurring headaches.

### Step 1

Start a supported web browser program and follow the steps listed inside the cover of this textbook to log in to the MyHealthProfessionsLab for this course.

Locate and click on the link **Exercise 3F**. This will open the Quippe software window with the New Encounter window displayed in the center.

### Step 2

Patients are listed in alphabetical order by last name. Locate the scroll bar on the right edge of the patient list and scroll the list until you locate the patient named **Poole, Ryan**. Click on his name.

### Step 3

In this exercise, you will need to set the date and time of the encounter. There are two ways of doing this. You can click in the date field and type over the date using the format MM/DD/YYYY. Note: the typed date must include the slashes. The alternative method is to select the date from a pop-up calendar, which is invoked by clicking on the small down-arrow next to the date field.

Locate the date field, and use either method to set the date to **May 3, 2016.**

### Step 4

In this exercise it will be necessary for you to set a specific time of the encounter. There are two methods for doing this. You can click the down-arrow in the time field to invoke a drop-down list of times at fifteen-minute intervals, then scroll the list to locate and click on the appropriate time to select it. Alternatively, time can also be set by typing directly into the time field using the HH:MM format and including either AM or PM.

Locate the time field, and use either method to set the time to **10:00 AM.**

### Step 5

Verify Ryan Poole is the selected patient, the date field displays 5/3/16, and the time field displays 10:00 AM. Locate and click the OK button.

When the encounter template is displayed in the workspace, locate and click in the blank space located just below the Chief Complaint heading. This will open a free-text note field outlined in a colored box where you will type the following text: **Headaches all week**.

### Step 6

The clinician asks the patient if he is currently taking any medications (he is).

Locate the clinical concept **taking medications** in the Current Medications section and click the **Y** check box next to it.

The patient reports that he has been taking aspirin for headaches, using caffeine pep pills, and drinking six colas a day to replace the eight to ten cups of coffee he was formerly drinking.

Add clinical concepts to Current Medications by clicking the Browse button on the toolbar. Click the red stickpin icon in the upper right corner of the drop-down list, and then click the small plus symbol next to Concepts.

**Step 7**

The concept list may automatically open to "taking medications." If it does not, use the following instructions to navigate the concept trees:

Locate and click the small plus symbol next to the History domain.

Locate and click the small plus symbol next to **past medical history**.

Locate **reported medication history** about halfway down the list, and click the small plus symbol next to it.

Locate **taking medications** and click the small plus symbol next to it.

Scroll the list downward until taking medications is positioned at the top. This will make it easier to locate the necessary clinical concepts to add in step 8.

**Step 8**

Locate the clinical concept **for headaches** about halfway down the indented list, and click on the words "for headaches" to highlight them. With the clinical concept highlighted, locate and click the Add to Note button at the top of the browse list.

**Step 9**

Further down the list, locate the clinical concept **aspirin** and click on the word "aspirin" (not the plus symbol next to it). With aspirin highlighted, locate and click the Add to Note button at the top of the browse list.

A few items below aspirin, locate the clinical concept **pep pills** and click on the words. With pep pills highlighted, locate and click the Add to Note button at the top of the browse list.

Click the Browse button on the toolbar to close the drop-down list.

Adding the above clinical concepts may have automatically set them as positive findings. If any of the added findings—pep pills, aspirin, or for headaches—are not red, click the **Y** check box next to them.

**Step 10**

The patient states he is allergic to pollen, but not allergic to any drugs.

Locate the Allergies section, and click the **Y** check boxes next to **allergies** and **allergies to pollen**. Both findings will turn red.

Locate and click the **N** check box next to **drugs**. The finding will turn blue.

**Step 11**

The patient states he has never had migraine headaches, but his mother used to have them.

Locate the Past Medical History section and click the **N** check box next to **history of migraines**. The finding will turn blue.

Proceed to the Family History section and click the **Y** check box next to **family history of migraines**. The finding will turn red.

**Step 12**

Locate the Behavioral History section, and click on the clinical concept **daily coffee consumption**. The finding will turn red.

Locate and click the Actions button on the toolbar, and then click Details in the drop-down menu. The Details entry pop-up window displays with the currently selected finding at the top. Verify that you are adding details to the intended finding.

Click in the Value field and type **8-10**

Click in the Unit field and begin typing **cups per day**. A drop-down list will appear. As soon as it appears, you can select cups per day.

Confirm you have both the Value and the Units set correctly, and then click the OK button to close the pop-up and add the information to the finding. The finding on your screen should now read "daily coffee consumption 8-10 cups per day."

Locate the clinical concept next to it, **has recently decreased**, and click the **Y** check box. The finding will turn red.

**Step 13**

You will recall the patient switched to cola when he gave up coffee.

Locate and click on the clinical concept **daily cola consumption**. The finding will turn red.

Locate and click the Actions button on the toolbar, and then click Details in the drop-down menu. The Details entry pop-up window displays with the currently selected finding at the top.

Click in the Value field and type the number **6.**

Click in the Unit field and begin typing **cans per day**. A drop-down list will appear. As soon as it appears, you can select cans per day.

Confirm you have both the Value and the Units set correctly, and then click the OK button to close the pop-up and add the information to the finding. The finding on your screen should now read "daily cola consumption 6 cans per day."

Since his cola consumption has *increased*, locate the clinical concept **has recently increased** in the row for cola, and click the **Y** check box. The finding will turn red.

**Step 14**

The patient denies using alcohol, recreational drugs, or smoking.

Locate and click the **N** check box for each of the following findings: **alcohol use**, **drug use**, and **smoking**. All three findings will turn blue.

**Step 15**

Locate the Review of Systems section and click on the clinical concept **chronic recurring headaches**. The finding will turn red.

Locate and click the Actions button on the toolbar, and then click Details in the drop-down menu, which will open the Details entry pop-up window.

Click in the Onset field and type **for 1 week**

Confirm you have typed the onset information correctly, and then click the OK button to close the pop-up and add the information to the finding. The finding on your screen should now read "chronic recurring headaches for 1 week."

### Step 16

Locate and click on the clinical concept **episodes recently worse**. The finding will turn red.

Locate and click the Actions button on the toolbar, and then click Details in the drop-down menu, which will open the Details entry pop-up window.

Locate and click the Status field. A drop-down list will appear. Locate **inadequately controlled** in the list and click on it. The status field should now read "inadequately controlled."

Locate and click in the Duration field, and then type **lasting 2-4 hours**.

Confirm you have both the Duration field and the Status set correctly, and then click the OK button to close the pop-up and add the information to the finding. The finding on your screen should now read "episodes recently worse lasting 2-4 hours – inadequately controlled."

### Step 17

Locate the Vital Signs table in the Physical Exam section. Enter Ryan's vital signs into the corresponding fields, as follows:

Click in the field below the label "Oral Temp." His temperature is **98.6**.

Click in the next field, below the label "PR." His pulse is **85**.

Click in the next field, below the label "RR." His respiration rate is **25**.

His blood pressure is 130/90. Click in the field, below the label "SBP." His systolic pressure is **130**.

Click in the next field, below the label "DBP." His diastolic pressure is **90**.

### Step 18

Ryan is 5′ 9″ (entered as 69 inches) and weighs 150 pounds. Enter Ryan's weight and height into the corresponding Weight and Height fields as follows:

Click in the field below the label "Weight" and type **150**.

Click (or tab to) the next field below the label "Height" and type **69**.

### Step 19

As you have done in previous exercises, locate the Physical Exam section and click the **N** check box next to **head injury**. The finding will turn blue.

### Step 20

Locate the Assessment section.

Locate and click the **Y** check box next to **vasoconstrictor withdrawal from caffeine**. The finding will turn red.

### Step 21

Locate the Therapy section and click the **Y** check box next to the clinical concept **regular exercise.**

Locate and click on the clinical concept **avoid caffeinated beverages**. The finding will turn red.

Locate and click the Actions button on the toolbar, and then click Details in the drop-down menu, which will open the Details entry pop-up window.

Click in the Note field and type **stop taking pep pills**.

Confirm you have typed the note correctly, and then click the OK button to close the pop-up and add the information to the finding. The finding on your screen should now read "avoid caffeinated beverages stop taking pep pills."

### Step 22

Locate the Counseling and Education section and click on the clinical concept **abstinence from alcohol**. The finding will turn red.

Locate and click the Actions button on the toolbar, and then click Details in the drop-down menu, which will open the Details entry pop-up window.

Locate and click the down-arrow in the Prefix field. A drop-down list will appear. Locate **continue** in the list and click on it. The prefix field should now read "continue."

Confirm you have the prefix field set correctly, and then click the OK button to close the pop-up and add the information to the finding. The finding on your screen should now read "continue abstinence from alcohol."

### Step 23

Locate and click on the clinical concept **abstinence from recreational drugs**. The finding will turn red.

Locate and click the Actions button on the toolbar, and then click Details in the drop-down menu, which will open the Details entry pop-up window.

Locate and click the down-arrow in the Prefix field. A drop-down list will appear. Locate **continue** in the list and click on it. The prefix field should now read "continue."

Confirm you have the prefix field set correctly, and then click the OK button to close the pop-up and add the information to the finding. The finding on your screen should now read "continue abstinence from recreational drugs."

Locate the clinical concept **maintain a healthy diet** and click the **Y** check box next to it. The finding will turn red.

### Step 24

Locate and click the blue Quippe icon button on the toolbar. Select the option Create PDF on the drop-down menu. A PDF of your encounter note will open in a new window.

Note, Figure 3-44 shows everything on one page. Your PDF may create two pages. Compare the findings you entered, not the number of pages. If everything is correct, proceed to step 25. If there are any differences other than paging, review the preceding steps and correct your errors.

**Figure 3-44** PDF of the completed encounter note for Ryan Poole.

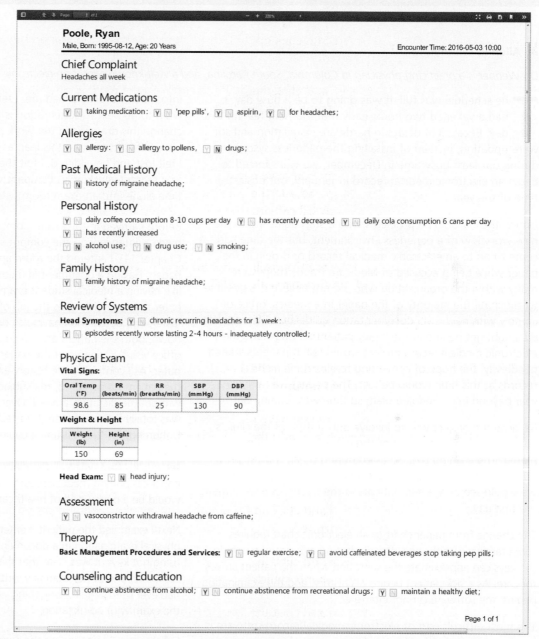

If wish to print a copy of your completed encounter notes for yourself or because your instructor requires you to turn them in, print or download the PDF at this time.

**Step 25**

The final step in every exercise is to submit your completed work for a grade.

Locate and click the blue Quippe icon button on the toolbar to display the drop-down menu, and then select the menu option Submit for Grade. This will complete Exercise 3F.

# Real-Life Story

## Paperless in Less Than a Day

**By Allen R. Wenner, M.D.[1]**

*Dr. Wenner is a practicing physician in Columbia, South Carolina, and a well-known expert on electronic health records.*

The schedule was full. It was going to be a busy day. I had awakened two hours early that morning fearing this day. Because of delays in hardware installation and software updating, instead of installing the paperless system during our least busy time in December, we were forced to begin an electronic medical record in January, our busiest time of the year.

I knew there would be problems with a staff adjusting to the new workflow of a paperless environment, but the time had come to go to an electronic medical record or drown in the paper while being accused of Medicare fraud. There were many within the organization who did not believe it is possible to eliminate the majority of the paper in a medical office or comply with new CMS documentation guidelines. I feared that we might get behind in the heavy patient schedule and the electronic medical record project would fail. If patients waited needlessly, the hope of converting to electronic medical records at this time would be lost. The project was already a year beyond my scheduled plan, so time was running out.

Because the project was to involve only a third of the clinic's patients, only brief training of three employees was completed. The training had occurred during breaks on the previous day and was not well structured. It was anticipated that we would see only a few patients in the paperless environment the first day.

The change from paper chart to an electronic chart requires some familiarity with the software, but no amount of touching the keys can approximate the sensation when the patient arrives for care. As a sick patient begins his history, and the examination begins, the software cannot interfere.

The most difficult part of electronic medical record software is the new capability of software. Having multiple windows open in electronic chart is like seeing several things at once. This is a stark contrast to the familiar one or two sheets that can be viewed in the paper record. Arranging the multiple windows in a way that is most appropriate for one's use in a real clinical examination requires time to think about and experience. On the first day of my actual use, the lack of familiarity with this new capability caused a decrease in my productivity as the information overwhelmed me. I felt lost at times not knowing what to do next. Disorientation is to be expected with any change this dramatic in the work process. All physicians will have difficulty making this leap as just I did that first morning. I felt lost and bewildered. I felt the same uncertainty I first felt as a second-year medical student when I walked for the first time alone into an exam room with a live patient.

Before I arrived in the exam room, each patient completed a medical interview on the computer (described further in Chapter 11). I entered the room and the clinical examination began. Having a documented medical history on each patient is like having a medical student examine the patient before you enter the room. It makes the job of gathering the data easier, faster, and better than having to do it entirely yourself. As I sat down, both the patient and I recognized a new format of the office visit—a triangle of the patient, the doctor, and the computer. As I confirmed the history and briefly edited the data that the patient had entered, the subjective note was completed without me dictating a word. Over half of my documentation was totally finished before I started the physical examination. Unhurried, for the first time I could ask my patients open-ended questions about how their illness was affecting their life. I could see quickly that when all the pieces of the computer-based paperless patient medical record functioned together, this would be a new world of healthcare delivery.

Next I examined the patient. I entered the objective data for the physical examination in a documentation-by-exception fashion using hot keys. It was clear that this system was far faster, more complete, and better than any written or dictated method that I had ever used. Again, everything was complete by the end of the exam with no dictation.

Subsequently, I noticed on the computer screen the appointment schedule online in real time. I had never seen it before. I never knew how many patients were actually waiting to see me, what time they had arrived, and why they were coming. It was immediately apparent that having the schedule of patients and their presenting complaints was helpful to the workflow. As patients arrived, I had the ability to order tests and procedures in advance of seeing them. This hastened workflow and saved the patient

---

[1] Allen R. Wenner MD, Primetime Medical, Inc.

waiting time. Throat cultures were taken of all patients presenting with sore throats. I could look at the names and complaints of familiar patients and order studies from another exam room. This increased my efficiency.

The other remarkable part of the first morning was a consistency in the presentation of data. The nursing staff checked the vital signs and medications in a uniform fashion. Heretofore, because of any changes in staff necessitated by a large organization, sometimes information was omitted or documented differently in the paper format by various staff members. The computerized format made everything the same. Because the medications were located in a consistent place on the screen, medication review was easier. This increased productivity slightly.

Laboratory, therapeutic, and radiological ordering were next in the workflow. Software streamlined this process and productivity was again enhanced. Electronic prescription writing was faster than any paper equivalent. Coding was frustrating. Coding is a process that is normally performed by the front office staff. Provider coding will enhance coding accuracy. Provider coding is a necessity to avoid rejected insurance claims and to prevent accusations of fraud under Medicare law. Diagnosis coding was difficult because ICD codes weren't created with the practicing physicians in mind as its user. Procedural coding seemed easier, yet still more trouble than writing a five-digit number or circling a super bill entry. I slowed down coding. My neck began to hurt as I realized that I had the keyboard at the wrong height and the mouse was on the wrong side.

I felt lost at many times during the first day, even if only for a moment. Despite my computer skills, I could not remember where I was within the office visit. It was a horrible feeling of not only trying to determine what was wrong with the patient, but also trying to document it appropriately without a scrap of paper. Although the first day was only to be for practice, I had to have the documentation for the legal medical record and I was no longer dictating.

In an electronic system, disposition, instructions, patient education, and referral are all different. The process is markedly different yet more complete. A learning curve is required.

We were late going to lunch as we tried to get the last patients through the system. The first morning we had had a 10% loss of efficiency, but I had expected much worse. At lunch the staff discussed what was happening to other employees. Soon they began to check in our afternoon patients because we missed most of our lunch. Throughout the afternoon minor delays occurred as the originally trained staff members began to show other employees how the system worked. The technical support staff graciously taught other staff how to use the system in brief lessons. Twice the anticipated number used the system by the first afternoon. Less hectic patient flow in the afternoon allowed for more comfort with the software.

Adequate on-site technical support prevented any hardware failures until the last hour, when a computer failure prevented data entry. Aside from that computer hiccup, the day went surprisingly well. Nobody was abandoned in the waiting room unseen for hours. No patient was left in an exam room asleep. No patient departed without a prescription. Indeed, most were given a patient education handout. Patients were favorably impressed that they could see their medical record appearing before their eyes.

The day had gone much better than I had anticipated. My neck hurt as I arrived home. I self-diagnosed a job-related injury from twisting toward the screen on my ill-positioned stool. I denied that my neck pain was tension from the stress of taking a medical office paperless in less than a day. I knew how the Wright brothers felt a hundred years ago. I went to bed early, contemplating the day, knowing we would never go back again. We had left the world of the paper medical record forever.

The advantage of the system is clear. The paperwork is finished at the time the patient leaves the exam room. Patient education is possible. The software assures full documentation of the visit as it is happening. But the most amazing part of it all was that I spent 100% of my day sitting next to my patients. I never left them once!

## Chapter Three Summary

In this chapter you have learned about the Student Edition software: the toolbar buttons and their respective drop-down menus, the workspace (entry and concise views), and the encounter navigation bar located below the workspace. You have also learned how to generate a PDF of the encounter note for printing or download.

As you continue through the course, you can refer to the exercises in this chapter when you need to remember how to perform a particular task.

| Task | Exercise / Step | Page # |
|---|---|---|
| Selecting a patient | 3A | 74 |
| Setting an encounter date | 3A | 74 |
| Record findings using Yes No check boxes | 3A | 78 |
| Create PDF for printing or download | 3A step 15 | 79 |
| Restarting an exercise using New Encounter option | 3B step 2 | 83 |
| Navigating Medcin clinical concepts hierarchy | 3B | 84 |
| Expand and collapse hierarchical tree structure | 3B | 85 |
| Add clinical concepts to workspace | 3B | 85 |
| Removing clinical concept or finding from encounter note | 3B step 24 | 89 |
| Switching workspace between Entry and Concise views | 3C step 10 | 94 |
| Adding details to findings | | |
|     Adding a value and setting unit | 3D step 4 | 98 |
|     Adding free text | 3D step 5 | 98 |
|     Adding onset and episode | 3D step 6 | 99 |
|     Adding Status and Duration | 3D step 7 | 99 |
|     Adding a modifier | 3D step 11 | 100 |
|     Adding a prefix | 3F step 21 | 110 |
| Recording the Chief complaint | 3E | 102 |
| Recording Vital Signs, weight and height | 3E | 103 |

EHR software allows clinicians to document the patient exam by selecting clinical concepts for symptoms, history, physical examination, tests, diagnoses, and therapy.

The Quippe Student Edition software has been specially created for this course. Therefore it will be different in some aspects from EHR systems you will encounter when working in a medical office. Nonetheless, the concepts, skills, and familiarity with EHR systems that you will acquire by practicing with the Student Edition will transfer directly into the workplace.

To more easily understand the Student Edition software, we divided the screen into four sections and discussed each of them.

1. **The Toolbar** located at the top of the application.

   The Toolbar consists of a row of buttons, each containing a small picture called an *icon* and, except for the first button, a brief label. The purpose of the Toolbar is to allow quick access to menus and commonly used functions. Clicking a button on the Toolbar invokes a drop-down menu or activates a function. The toolbar also contains a textbox used for search.

   The toolbar buttons are as follows:

   ◆ Quippe icon button – invokes the application menu containing options: New Encounter, Open Encounter, Quit Encounter, Create PDF, and Submit for Grade.

   ◆ Search is a textbox with a button used to search for concepts in the Medcin nomenclature that match terms typed into the box. Search will be covered in a subsequent chapter.

- **Browse button** – invokes a drop-down list of Concepts (used to add clinical concepts into the workspace), and Sample Custom Content (used to select Forms and Lists), covered in subsequent chapters.

- **Prompt button** – invokes an Intelligent Prompt function to add clinical concepts related to a diagnosis to the workspace.

- **View button** – invokes a menu of options to vary what is displayed in the workspace. Entry view displays both entered and unentered findings. Concise view displays only entered findings. Outline view displays expandable headings for sections that have recorded findings.

- **Tools button** – contains an option to invoke the E&M code calculator.

- **Actions button** – invokes a drop-down menu with options of open a pop-up window to add Details to a finding, Duplicate a finding, Prompt, based on a finding, or Delete a finding. The Actions button is enabled only when a clinical concept, finding, or text macro is selected. The Actions menu can be invoked by a right-click mouse button.

2. **The Workspace** is the large pane in the center of the left side of the application.

   The workspace is the area where clinical documentation takes place. This portion of the screen typically contains section headings under which are listed clinical concepts relevant to the heading; for example, past medical history items under the heading Past History.

   Clinical concepts (unrecorded findings) may already be in the workspace when the exercise template is loaded, or may be added into the workspace from the list of Medcin concepts invoked by the Browse button on the toolbar.

3. **The Navigation bar** is the narrow strip located below the workspace containing links to section headings in the workspace. Clicking on a link in the navigation bar scrolls the workspace pane and selects the section belonging to that heading.

4. **The Content pane** is located along the right side of the application window. The content pane displays information about the patient, sources, and orders.

   **The Encounter Note.** The first step in creating the encounter note is to select the patient from an alphabetical list in the New Encounter window. This window also allows you to set the date and time of the encounter. Certain exercises require you to set a specified date so that historical patient data will be accurately displayed. In exercises that do not require a date you may use the current date if you choose; however, the patient's age displayed in your content pane may not match the figures or case studies in the book.

   **Findings.** Findings are medical data relevant to the patient visit recorded in the encounter note. Findings are broadly categorized as being subjective, objective, assessment, or plan. Subjective findings are symptoms and history reported by the patient. Objective findings are physical measurements and observations made by the clinician. For example, patient complains of a fever is a subjective finding reported by the patient. Oral temperature of 102°F as measured by the medical assistant is an objective finding. After reviewing subjective symptoms and history, and performing objective physical examination, the clinician makes an assessment and a plan of treatment. Assessment findings are diagnoses, syndromes, or conditions. Plan findings include orders for tests, therapy, medication, counseling, and education.

   Findings are recorded in the EHR by clicking on clinical concepts, which then turn red or blue, or by clicking on a check box adjacent to the finding. Clinical concepts that are gray are unentered and, although displayed in the workspace, will not appear in the completed encounter note unless they are recorded as a finding.

The state of a finding can be changed by clicking the opposite check box from the one currently selected. A finding can be changed back to an unentered clinical concept by clicking on the check box currently checked, which will uncheck it. Findings without check boxes have three states, unentered, positive, negative, and will cycle through the three states by successive clicks.

**The Medcin Nomenclature.** In this chapter you learned to navigate the Medcin nomenclature to locate and add clinical concepts to the encounter note workspace. The nomenclature is accessed by clicking the Browse button on the toolbar and clicking the Concepts book icon. This opens a drop-down list, which you can pin open by clicking the small red stickpin icon in the upper right corner of the list.

Medcin clinical concepts are organized in a hierarchy of six domains, each identified with a colored block letter and the domain name: S (symptoms), H (history), P (physical examination), T (tests), D (diagnosis, syndromes, and conditions), and R (therapy or plan).

The clinical concepts are displayed in a hierarchical *tree* structure where buttons with small plus symbols indicate more detailed clinical concepts are available. Clicking the small plus symbol next to a clinical concept expands the list further, like branches on a tree. When the tree is expanded, the button changes from a small plus symbol to a small minus sign. If the button with the small minus sign is clicked, the expanded list collapses to its previous level.

Clinical concepts are added to the encounter note in the workspace by locating and clicking on a desired clinical concept in the tree structure. Clicking on the concept name highlights it. Clicking the Add to Note button at the top of the concept list adds the highlighted item to the workspace. You can close the list by clicking the Browse button again, or by clicking anywhere in the application outside the drop-down list.

In the Student Edition, *highlight* means that a colored rectangle appears around a clinical concept, finding, or section of the workspace.

**Details.** When the clinician clicks a clinical concept, it becomes a finding and part of the encounter note. The clinician may then add details to the finding to provide additional data or even alter the meaning of the finding. Details may be added to a finding at any time by selecting the finding (which highlights it), clicking the toolbar Actions button, and selecting the Details option in the drop-down menu, which opens a pop-up window. Details that may be added or set in this window are Prefix, Modifier, Status, Value, Unit (of measure), Note (free text), Onset, Duration, and Episodes. Details recorded with a finding modify the narrative text of the note. For example, headache becomes headache inadequately controlled when the status field is set accordingly.

Both unentered clinical concepts and recorded findings can be removed from the encounter note workspace by using the delete option found on the Actions drop-down menu.

**Text fields.** The ideal EHR contains very little free text, as codified findings are preferable. However, free text is used to record the Chief Complaint, to explain or enhance some detail of a finding, and, in text macros, to add blocks of text that may be required to narrate a procedure or document informed consent. Text macros will be introduced in Chapter 4.

**Completing Exercises.** The final step in every Quippe exercise is to check your work by using the concise view option and/or creating a PDF. Once you have verified that everything is correct, you submit your work for a grade using the Submit for Grade option on the application menu.

If you wish to print or download a copy of the PDF, it is important to do so before clicking the Submit for Grade button, as that will end the exercise.

It is important to remember while working on an exercise not to close or refresh your web browser before clicking Submit for Grade, as you will lose all work you have done on the exercise. However, if you need to restart an exercise or quit without completing it, use one of two options on the Quippe icon application menu. The New Encounter option will restart the exercise without exiting Quippe. The Quit Encounter option will quit the exercise and return you to MyHealthProfessionsLab. Understand that by using either the New Encounter or the Quit Encounter option, you will lose whatever work you have done on the exercise.

## Testing Your Knowledge of Chapter 3

### Step 1

Log in to MyHealthProfessionsLab following the directions printed inside the cover of this textbook.

Locate and click on Chapter 3 Test.

### Step 2

Answer the test questions. When you have finished, click the Submit Test button.

## Testing Your Skill Exercise 3G: Another Cause of Headache

Now that you have performed all the exercises in Chapter 3 this exercise will help you and your instructor evaluate your acquired skills. Use the information in the case study and the features of the software you already know to document the patient's encounter.

### Case Study

Carla Lopez is a 27-year-old female whose chief complaint is monthly headaches. She tells the clinician she gets chronic recurring headaches just before her period. She adds that this makes her highly irritable and she can't concentrate. She takes medications for pain, but denies her headache episodes are recently worse or that she gets depressed.

Carla has no allergies, and no history of migraines, or family history of migraines. She drinks 1–2 cups of coffee in the morning and has a cup of tea in the evening. Her alcohol use is moderate. She does not smoke or use recreational drugs.

Here are Carla's vital signs:

| | |
|---|---|
| Temperature: | 98.6 |
| Pulse: | 65 |
| Respiration: | 20 |
| SBP: | 118 |
| DBP: | 76 |
| Weight: | 130 |
| Height: | 64 |

The clinician performs a head exam and finds no evidence of injury. The clinician's diagnosis is premenstrual headache syndrome, and recommends she continue analgesics, maintain a healthy diet, and get regular exercise.

### Step 1

Start a supported web browser program and follow the steps listed inside the cover of this textbook to log in to the MyHealthProfessionsLab for this course.

Locate and click on the link **Exercise 3G**. This will open the Quippe software window with the New Encounter window displayed in the center.

### Step 2

Locate and click on the patient name, and then click the OK button. In this exercise, you do not need to set the date or time of the encounter.

Read the case study *carefully*.

### Step 3

Use the case study information above to record vital signs and other findings, adding Value, Units, Prefix, or Modifier details where appropriate.

*Hint*: You will have to Browse and add to the note concepts for taking medication and to add the diagnosis. The diagnosis is in the "benign" tree. Before Browsing for the diagnosis click any white space in the encounter pane that does not highlight a finding or section heading.

Once you have documented all the information provided in the case study, proceed to step 4.

### Step 4

If wish to print a copy of your completed encounter notes for yourself or because your instructor requires you to turn them in, use the Create PDF option, and then print or download the PDF at this time.

Submit your completed work for a grade using the Submit for Grade option on the application menu. This will complete Exercise 3G.

# Chapter Four

# Increased Familiarity with EHR Software

**4**

## Learning Outcomes

*After completing this chapter, you should be able to:*

◆ Document a patient visit with increased proficiency

◆ Set and clear the Prefix field for a finding

◆ Learn eight methods EHR systems use to record findings

◆ Use a text macro

## Applying Your Knowledge

In this chapter, you will practice documenting patient visits using the Student Edition software. One of the goals in this chapter is to increase your familiarity with the software and thereby increase your speed of data entry. Another is to learn how similar EHR systems document encounter notes so you can more easily transition skills acquired in this course into a work environment.

In Chapter 3, you learned the basic layout of the screen and the concepts of creating an encounter note, adding findings, editing findings, and adding details to findings. Detailed instructions for scrolling and navigating the lists, which were provided in the previous chapter, should no longer be necessary. From this point forward, simplified instructions will guide you in areas where you are already familiar with the program.

Exercises in this book are intended to provide conceptual learning experiences with the software. The encounter notes you will produce will be similar to documents you would create in a medical office. However, they are not intended to represent full and complete medical exams. The exercises, although medically accurate, have been purposely shortened to ensure you can complete the exercise in a class period.

## Documenting a Brief Patient Visit

The next exercise will allow you to evaluate your knowledge of the software by using only the features you have learned in Chapter 3. If you have any difficulty with this exercise, you should review the exercises in Chapter 3 before continuing with this chapter.

### Guided Exercise 4A: Documenting a Visit for Common Cold

Using what you have learned so far, document Mr. Baker's brief exam.

**Case Study**

Patient Harold Baker feels like he has caught some sort of bug. Like many patients who have a cold, he wants to see his doctor, and so the medical office has scheduled a brief 10-minute office visit for him.

**Step 1**

Start a supported web browser program and follow the steps listed inside the cover of this textbook to log in to the MyHealthProfessionsLab for this course.

Locate and click on the link **Exercise 4A**. This will open the Quippe software window with the New Encounter window displayed in the center.

**Step 2**

Patients are listed in alphabetical order by last name. Locate and click on the patient named **Baker, Harold**. In this exercise, you do not need to set the date and time of the encounter. Once you have selected the patient as shown in Figure 4-1, click the OK button.

**Step 3**

Click in the blank space under the heading Chief Complaint as you have in previous exercises, and type **Patient reported cold or flu** as shown in Figure 4-2.

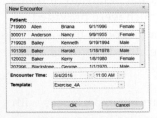

**Figure 4-1** Select Harold Baker from the New Encounter window.

**Figure 4-2** Chief complaint: Patient reported cold or flu.

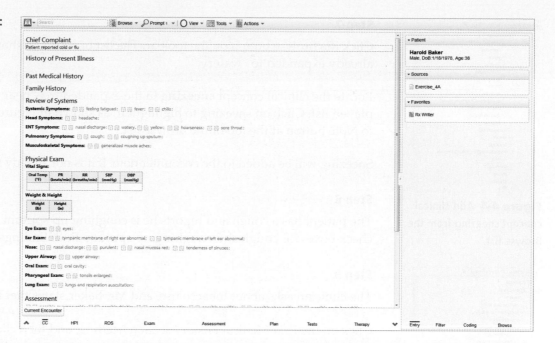

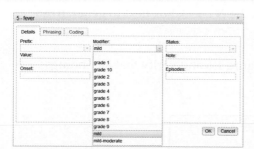

**Figure 4-3** Select "mild" from the Modifier drop-down list.

## Tip for Right-click Mouse Button

A computer mouse typically has at least two buttons—the "left-click" and "right-click" buttons. In normal usage you click with the left mouse button. In Quippe you can *right-click* on a finding to invoke the Actions drop-down menu, the same as if you had clicked the Actions button on the toolbar. This is a better method of invoking the Actions menu because clicking a second time on a finding that is already set can change its state.

If you are using a touchscreen or stylus that does not have a right-click function, continue to use the Actions button on the toolbar as you have been; just make sure the finding is in the correct state after closing the Detail pop-up window.

### Step 4

The patient states he has a mild fever.

Locate and click the **Y** check box for fever. The finding will turn red.

*Right-click* on the finding (or click the Actions button on the toolbar), and select Details from the Actions drop-down menu.

### Step 5

In the Details pop-up window, locate and click the Modifier field. Locate and click on **mild** in the drop-down list as shown in Figure 4-3.

Click OK to close the Detail window. The description should now read "mild fever."

### Step 6

The patient reports a headache, runny nose, and sneezing.

Locate and click the **Y** check boxes for **headache**, **nasal discharge**, and **watery**. All three findings should turn red.

Sneezing is not in the workspace; you will have to add it.

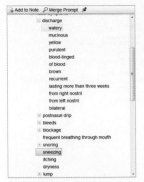

**Figure 4-4** Add clinical concept sneezing from the Browse list.

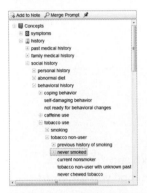

**Figure 4-5** Add the clinical concept never smoked from the expanded behavioral history tree.

**Figure 4-6** Portion of the workspace showing Chief Complaint, History, and Review of System findings.

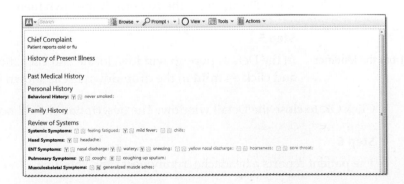

### Step 7

Click the Browse button on the toolbar. The list of concepts should open with the tree already expanded to "watery."

Locate the clinical concept **sneezing** in the expanded tree, near the bottom of the displayed list. Click on sneezing to highlight it, as shown in Figure 4-4, and click the Add to Note button at the top of the browse list.

Sneezing will be added to the encounter note. If it is not already red, click the **Y** check box.

### Step 8

The patient has a cough and reports he is coughing up sputum. Locate and click the **Y** check boxes for **cough** and **coughing up sputum**. Both findings should turn red.

### Step 9

The clinician asks about tobacco use, and Mr. Baker states that he has never smoked.

Click on the Past Medical History section heading, and then click the Browse button on the toolbar.

Click the small plus symbols next to the Concepts book icon and the History domain.

Locate and click the small plus symbols next to social history, behavioral history, tobacco use, and tobacco non-user, as shown in Figure 4-5.

Locate the clinical concept **never smoked** in the expanded tree, and click on it to highlight it. Click the Add to Note button at the top of the browse list.

Locate and click the **Y** check box to record the finding never smoked.

### Step 10

Mr. Baker has not been experiencing any muscle aches. Return to the Review of Symptoms section of the note to locate and click the **N** check box next to **generalized muscle aches.** The finding should turn blue.

Compare the upper portion of your screen to Figure 4-6 and verify that all findings recorded in steps 3–10 are correct.

### Step 11

Chapter 3 described four functional areas of the Quippe screen: the toolbar, the workspace, the content pane, and the navigation bar (defined previously in Figure 3-3). By using the navigation bar to quickly reposition the Physical Examination section to the top of screen you will be able to easily locate and enter findings for the rest of the encounter note.

Locate the navigation bar at the bottom of your screen and click on the **Exam** link (it has a blue line above it in Figure 4-7). This will automatically scroll your window and position Physical Examination at the top of the workspace pane.

**Figure 4-7** Exam link on the Navigation bar.

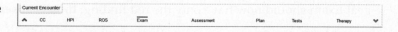

### Step 12

Before the clinician begins the physical examination, the medical assistant or nurse takes the patient's vital signs and records them. Enter Mr. Baker's vital signs in the corresponding fields as follows:

| | |
|---|---|
| Temperature: | **99.7** |
| Pulse: | **65** |
| Respiration: | **25** |
| SBP: | **120** |
| DBP: | **80** |

When you have entered all of the vital signs, enter weight and height. Mr. Baker weighs **175** pounds and is 6 feet tall (entered as **72** inches).

### Step 13

The clinician examines the patient's eyes and ears, which are normal.

Locate and click the **N** check boxes for the findings **eyes**, **tympanic membrane of right ear**, and **tympanic membrane of left ear**. All three findings should turn blue.

### Step 14

The clinician observes that the nasal membranes are inflamed, and discharge is present, but not purulent. Mr. Baker's sinuses were tender to palpation. Record the findings as follows:

✓  **Y** nasal discharge

✓  **N** purulent

✓  **Y** nasal mucosa red

✓  **Y** tenderness of sinuses

### Step 15

The clinician examines the upper airway and oral cavity, which are normal. Mr. Baker's tonsils were removed as a child.

Locate and click the **N** check boxes for **upper airway**, **oral cavity**, and **tonsils enlarged**. All three findings should turn blue.

### Step 16

Click the Browse button on the toolbar. The concepts list should open on enlarged (under tonsils). Scroll the list upward until you can see tonsils at the top of the list (as

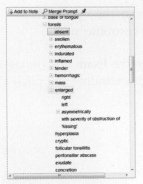

**Figure 4-8** Adding "absent" from the expanded tree of the concept tonsils.

shown in Figure 4-8). Locate and click on the clinical concept "absent" to highlight it, and then click the Add to Note button.

Tonsils absent will be blue. Click the **Y** check box to change it to red.

Click on tonsils enlarged again, and then click the Actions button on the toolbar and select Delete from the Actions drop-down menu. The finding will be deleted. Pharyngeal Exam should now have only the red finding: **tonsils absent**.

### Step 17

The clinician listens to Harold's lungs and records that they sound normal.

Locate and click the **N** check box for **lungs and respiration auscultation**. The finding turns blue.

### Step 18

The clinician's diagnosis is that Harold Barker had a common cold.

Proceed to the Assessment section, where you will notice many possible diagnoses of upper respiratory conditions. Locate and click the **Y** check box for **possible common cold**. The finding will turn red.

Since the clinician is certain of the diagnosis, remove the prefix "possible" by *right-clicking* on the finding (or click the Actions button on the toolbar) and select Details from the Actions drop-down menu.

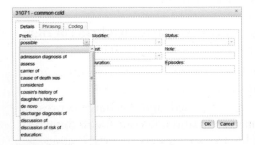

**Figure 4-9** Details pop-up window with Prefix list.

### Step 19

Locate and click the down-arrow next to the Prefix field in the Details pop-up window. A list of prefixes will be displayed. Prefixes, like modifier and status, change the meaning and description of a finding. Notice that the first row in the drop-down list is a blank. The blank (when present) is used to clear a previously set entry.

Locate and click on the blank row in the drop-down list of prefixes, as shown in Figure 4-9, and then click on the OK button. The pop-up window should close and the diagnosis should now read "common cold."

### Step 20

The doctor recommends that Harold drink plenty of fluids and get bed rest.

Locate and click on the **Y** check boxes for **fluid**s and **bed rest** in the Therapy section. Both findings will turn red.

### Step 21

Locate and click the View button on the toolbar, and then select Concise from the drop-down menu.

Compare your screen to Figure 4-10. If everything is correct, proceed to step 22. If there are any differences, click the View button on the toolbar, select the Entry option on the drop-down menu, and then correct your work according to the preceding steps.

**Figure 4-10** Concise view of Harold Baker's completed encounter note.

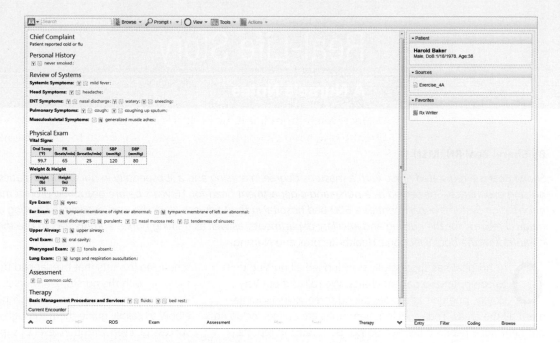

## Step 22

If you wish to print a copy of your completed encounter notes for yourself or because your instructor requires you to turn them in, locate and click the blue Quippe icon button on the toolbar. Select the option Create PDF on the drop-down menu and then download or print the resulting PDF. Do this before clicking Submit for Grade in Step 23.

## Step 23

The final step in every exercise is to submit your completed work for a grade.

Locate and click the blue Quippe icon button on the toolbar, and then select the Submit for Grade option from the drop-down menu. This will complete Exercise 4A.

Having successfully completed this exercise, you should be comfortable with the general process of locating findings and expanding the tree to view additional findings. Future exercises in this book will instruct you to expand the tree by listing multiple findings for which you will click the small plus signs.

# Visually Different EHR Styles

The Quippe Student Edition software has been specially modified for this course. Therefore, it may differ in some aspects from EHR systems you will encounter when working in a medical facility, but the concepts, skills, and familiarity with EHR systems you will acquire by practicing with the Student Edition will transfer directly into the workplace.

Many EHR software packages are based on the Medcin nomenclature. Each vendor has created a unique visual style, and although there is a common nomenclature, the EHR may look quite different.

One difference is the look of the buttons. Instead of the Y and N buttons you have used thus far, many systems use round or square buttons that do not contain letters. But

# Real-Life Story

**By Sharyl Beal RN, MSN**

*Sharyl Beal is a registered nurse with a master's degree in nursing and a subspecialty in nursing informatics. Sharyl has over 40 years nursing experience. She served as a nurse and a department head for 16 years before becoming project manager for the Clinical Information Systems department at a 500-bed hospital in the Midwest. Here she was involved in creating and implementing electronic medical records for the nursing and ancillary departments, as well as training nurses and doctors to use the clinical systems. She is co-author of the book* Electronic Health Records and Nursing.

Our hospital has successfully transitioned all nursing units to computerized patient charts. We rolled it out very slowly, one unit at a time, taking three years to implement all the areas. Today, all inpatient units are online, including our behavioral health units. We do not print nursing reports—everyone works online. These are some of my experiences and observations from this project.

We did med/surg first because it is the broadest definition and fits the majority of patients. When that model was in operation, we went to the next unit and asked, "With this as a model, what do we need to do to make it work for you?" We did a fair amount of redesign as we added units, but sometimes they were minor changes like adding descriptors that had not been necessary for another unit.

The first thing we did for all departments was to spend considerable time flowcharting all their processes; how they get their patients, how they communicate about their patients, with whom, what it looks like. We created a "life in the day of" scenario for every skill level in the unit; then we designed their charting based on their patient population.

The last unit to go online was Behavioral Health. Behavioral Health was challenging because this department's charts contain more abstract observations describing mental reactions, emotional reactions, and so on. But the most problematic unit was the Obstetrics (OB) Department.

OB charting is not difficult, but it is very meticulous. Our OB Department had a lot of rules and regulations about what had to be charted and how it was to be worded. The hospital legal department had to review all of our designs before the nurses could begin using them; they then reviewed samples of what was actually being documented once the department went online. We had to do some redesign to let the nurses better describe things, but we finally got it to everyone's satisfaction.

That was our design process; implementation was another matter. Our methodology of bringing one unit online at a time allowed us to provide plenty of support when the unit went online. I think that was key. Clinical Informatics personnel were

scheduled in shifts that overlapped the nursing shifts. We were in the unit, with the nurses, 24 hours a day for the first two weeks. Whenever new users were struggling, someone was right at their elbow to calmly guide them through, to make sure they were successful. Even with that level of support, there were some concerns that remained constant through the last unit of the rollout.

Nurses are very accustomed to being in control, confident in their expertise and their skills; when their department becomes computerized, all of a sudden everything they know has to be translated through the limitations of a computer. The most common reaction when we rolled out charting into a new unit was that the nurses were extremely apprehensive their first day of charting. The universal complaint was that they could not sleep the night before.

My experience was that at the end of the first day they were still not feeling good about it, but when they came back the second day they had figured out how to get through it and they had very few questions. By the third day, they were usually doing very well. They still did not feel confident about finding the information, but they knew they could do it.

The nurses' biggest fear was that they would spend all their time taking care of the computer instead of their patients. They verbalized that idea for months afterwards, but that really is not reality. Research has repeatedly shown that nurses spend 50 to 70% of their time documenting. In short, nurses already spend an enormous amount of their work life documenting, but it takes them a long time to feel like they are spending less time on the computer than on their patients.

The real issue was that they felt like they were cut off from the information; they could not just flip open a chart and see what they were looking for. They had to remember how to find it and that was time out of their day. I have had them cry; I have had them yell, venting their frustration. But the good part was that they were all in the same boat together, so their peers readily understood what they were going through because they were all going through it together.

The nurses who had the easiest time transitioning were nurses who were accustomed to taking the time to write everything down as they went through their workday. The majority of nurses do not do that. Most nurses have notes stuffed in their pockets and tons of information in their head. They tend to store it up and write it all down when they come back from lunch or at the end of their shift. When they try to follow that same model with a computer, but they are not yet comfortable with the computer; it is twice as hard because they have a lot to remember and they have to figure out what to do with it. Nurses who normally charted as their day progressed did not have to remember as much so they seem to learn faster.

In nursing school students have to chart as it happens—instructors insist on it. This meant that nurses who just came out of nursing school had an advantage because they came to the job with good habits. Additionally, most of the new nurses grew up with computers and were more familiar with them.

We found that the ancillary departments—respiratory therapy, physical therapy, dietary, and so on—were also easy to implement. Their documentation is much more concrete, limited in its focus, so it was much easier to adapt from paper to computer. They were almost self-sufficient from the very beginning.

The doctors, however, were another story. You have to spend time up front making sure the doctors can get the information, and most doctors cannot give up enough time in their day to learn a computer. The nurses trained for 8 hours for the computer but the doctors only for about 15 minutes. We balanced this by trying to be attentive to any doctor who came on the floor. We would often say, "Let me help you find the information. The nurses are now charting on the computer. As of today you are not going to find that information on a piece of paper." We don't print anything. The doctors have adapted to the readily available information so well that on the rare occasion when we have downtime, it is usually the physicians who are the most upset.

One thing I think is important is for the nursing leadership to dedicate time to learning the system so its members are fully on board with why the switch to computers is happening and what the benefits are. Then when their staff is apprehensive or when the physicians are frustrated because the nurses have not charted, there is reinforcement from the management that computerized charting is an expectation.

This point was illustrated in two of the units we rolled out. In one unit, the leadership was very computer savvy and expected the staff to do well. Leadership members held reinforcing in-service programs every 10 days and they would have us talk about specific areas where they thought their staff was weak in charting. Because the nurse manager was so proactive, that whole area adapted very easily and as a result the physicians adapted very easily.

In another unit where the nurse manager was not very computer savvy, the manager's apprehension reinforced that of the staff. For that reason, our team found it necessary to support them. Although this unit has been online for long time, there is still a core group of nurses who just do not understand it, because their leaders do not require them to do it.

One final benefit of an involved leadership is that it results in better charting. When we did the first units, the implementation team spent a lot of time reading the documentation for quality, seeing if the nurses forgot to chart something, and so on. However, as the rollout continued throughout the hospital, the implementation team could not really spend a lot of time reviewing. You really need the people who know the patient population of the unit, the leaders, the managers, or supervisors to be spending some time each day randomly selecting charts created by their nurses, reading them, and helping their nurses understand if they are not doing it thoroughly enough. This not only improves the quality of the charts but also helps the staff get better at it quickly.

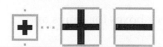

**Figure 4-11** Alternative style of buttons used to record findings in another EHR system.

when clicked to record a finding, the buttons turn red or blue, just as the findings have done in the preceding exercises. An example was shown in Figure 3-5. One EHR goes further and uses a large plus symbol and a large minus sign similar to those shown in Figure 4-11 to record findings as normal or abnormal. It is also possible to record findings by putting a check mark in a box.

As you learned in previous exercises, most Quippe findings can be selected by clicking on the words of the clinical concept, allowing template designers to dispense with buttons altogether.

Although various EHR vendors present different user interfaces, the functionality of quickly documenting a patient encounter by clicking on clinical concepts instead of typing extensive amounts of free text is common to most of them. By becoming familiar with the Student Edition software, you should have no trouble transitioning to any Medcin-based EHR in your job.

# Guided Exercise 4B: Recording Findings Using Alternate Methods

While it is unlikely any EHR system would use all the methods of recording findings presented in this exercise, the exercise will allow you to experience eight of the most common approaches EHR systems use to record findings.

### Case Study

Franklin Jones is a 77-year-old male who is experiencing some arthritic pain and swelling in his left knee. He is also having mild seasonal allergy symptoms. He is a long-term smoker and moderate drinker. His adult daughter has accompanied him to the doctor's office and provides patient information to the medical assistant.

### Step 1

Start a supported web browser program and follow the steps listed inside the cover of this textbook to log in to the MyHealthProfessionsLab for this course.

Locate and click on the link **Exercise 4B**. This will open the Quippe software window with the New Encounter window displayed in the center.

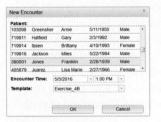

**Figure 4-12** Selecting Franklin Jones from the patient list in the New Encounter window.

### Step 2

Patients are listed in alphabetical order by last name. Locate the scroll bar on the right edge of the patient list and scroll the list until you locate the patient named **Jones, Franklin**. Click on his name. In this exercise, you do not need to set the date and time of the encounter. Once you have selected the patient as shown in Figure 4-12, click the OK button.

### Step 3

Click in the blank space under the heading Chief Complaint, as you have in previous exercises, and type **knee pain**.

### Step 4

Locate Allergies under the heading Past Medical History. These findings use the Yes/No style of check boxes with which you are familiar. Click the **Y** check boxes for **allergy** and **allergy to pollens**. Both findings will turn red.

Mr. Jones is not allergic to drugs or anesthetics. Click the **N** check boxes for **drugs** and **reaction to anesthetics**. Both findings will turn blue.

### Step 5

Proceed to the next group, Reported Medical History, which documents serious medical conditions patients may have currently or had previously. This section uses a check list style to select findings.

Locate and click the box next to the clinical concept **essential hypertension**. A check mark will appear and the finding will turn red.

Click the box again and the finding returns to an unentered state. In previous exercises findings had three states: unentered (gray), yes (red), and no (blue). In a check list style, there are only two states: yes or unentered. Putting a check in a box indicates the patient reported having had the condition. Conditions that the patient never had are simply left unchecked.

Mr. Jones has essential hypertension. Check the box again and confirm the finding is red.

**Step 6**

Proceed to the next group, Family History, which documents serious medical conditions that closely related family members may have had. These are conditions that tend to run in families and therefore may be predictors of the patient's health. They are usually documented in tandem with the patient's medical history.

Applying what you learned in step 5, put check marks beside the findings **family history of heart disease** and **family history of cancer**. Both findings will turn red.

Compare your screen to Figure 4-13. The findings selected in steps 2–6 should match the figure.

**Figure 4-13** Partially completed encounter showing Chief complaint, Past History, and Family History findings.

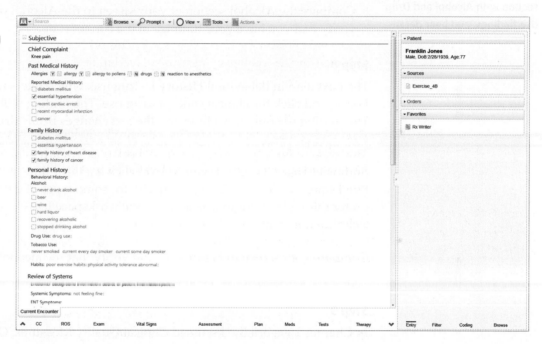

**Step 7**

Locate Behavioral History, which documents a patient's lifestyle choices such as the use of alcohol, recreational drugs, and tobacco, as well as diet and exercise habits. Mr. Jones says he drinks about a six-pack of beer a week.

In documenting his alcohol use you will discover unique characteristics of this section.

First, click on the clinical concept **never used alcohol** (obviously incorrect for this patient). You will notice that the box has an X instead of a check mark. Click the box again and the finding returns to the unentered state (gray) similar to the check list style in steps 5–6, except it uses an X.

Since Mr. Jones drinks beer, locate and click on the box next to **beer**. The box now has an X and the finding turns red, but something else has happened: An entry field for the number of bottles of beer per week appeared. Type **6** in the field.

Notice that bottles per week has a small down-arrow to the right of it. This indicates that a drop-down list is available. Click on it to see the choices available, but make sure you select **bottles per week** and not bottles per day.

These are, in fact, the same Details fields (Value and Unit) as in the Details pop-up window. This method, however, accepts the data when the finding is selected, saving the clinician the extra steps of clicking the toolbar Actions button, opening the pop-up, and closing it after recording the details.

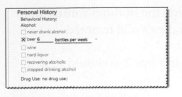

**Figure 4-14** Personal History section with Alcohol and Drug Use findings, and beer details.

In addition to value and units, another feature is available with this style of finding. Locate and click the box next to **stopped drinking alcohol as of**. This time the detail field accepts a date. Locate and click the down-arrow to the right of the date field and a pop-up calendar will appear. Of course, this information is incorrect; Mr. Jones has not stopped drinking. Click on the box with the X again so the clinical concept will return to an unentered state.

Compare the Alcohol section of your screen to the Alcohol portion of Figure 4-14 to verify that you have your findings in the correct state.

### Step 8

The next item in Behavioral History is drug use, which refers to recreational drugs. Locate and click the clinical concept **drug use**. The finding will turn red. Click it again. The finding not only turns blue, but the text changes from "drug use" to "no drug use."

This style of finding does not require check boxes of any type. Simply clicking on the finding changes its state. If you were to click it a third time, it would return to its unentered state. While check boxes are useful for some types of data entry, many physicians prefer this style of finding, as it makes the workspace less cluttered and reads more like a clinical note without all the check boxes.

Compare your screen to Figure 4-14 and verify that the alcohol and drug use findings are set correctly.

### Step 9

In Chapter 1 we briefly discussed Clinical Quality Measures. One of those measures is to ask patients about their tobacco use and to assist patients in quitting. Mr. Jones states he been smoking a pack a day for the last 50 years.

Locate Tobacco Use, and click on the clinical concept **current every day smoker**. A new row of clinical concepts appears to allow you to document the form of tobacco he is smoking.

Even though the findings do not have X boxes, the method of entry for the Tobacco use section is similar to alcohol use in that there are only two states, red (yes) or gray (unentered). If you were to click current every day smoker again, the finding would turn gray, but unlike drug use, this style of finding does not have a blue (no) state.

Make sure current every day smoker is red, and then locate and click on the clinical concept **cigarettes**. Similar in behavior to the finding for beer, a value field will appear to allow you to enter pack-years. Unlike the beer finding, there is not a drop-down menu to change the unit.

The length of time and quantity of cigarettes smoked is reported in a standard unit called *pack-years*. A pack-year is calculated as 20 cigarettes a day for 1 year. If a patient

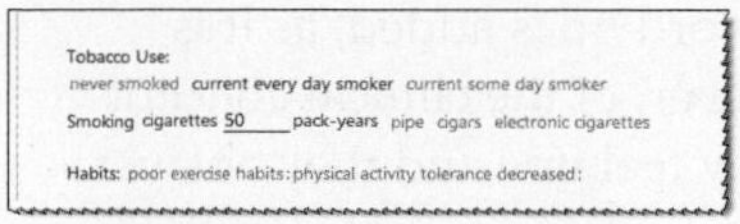

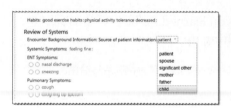

**Figure 4-15** Personal History, Tobacco Use section with findings and details.

smoked two packs a day for 15 years, the calculated result would be 30 pack-years. If a patient smoked half a pack a day for 10 years, the calculated result would be 5 pack-years.

Mr. Jones reports smoking a pack a day for 50 years. Type **50** into the field.

Compare the Tobacco Use portion of your screen to Figure 4-15.

### Step 10

Next, document Mr. Jones' exercise habits. These clinical concepts behave similar to the drug use finding, in that they have three states and do not use check boxes. Mr. Jones reports that he has **good exercise habits** but his **physical activity tolerance has decreased** due to painful arthritis in his knee.

Apply what you learned in step 8; locate the two clinical concepts adjacent to the label "Habits," and click on them until their descriptions match the bold text in the previous paragraph.

### Step 11

In most cases the patient tells the clinician their history, family history, social history, and symptoms, but sometimes that information is provided by someone accompanying the patient. For example, in a pediatric practice the information is almost always provided by a parent or other caregiver, as the patients are too young to give reliable information. Elderly patients like Mr. Jones are sometimes accompanied by their spouse or adult child. Therefore, many clinics record who provided the information documented in the encounter.

Previous exercises in this chapter used drop-down lists to select prefixes, modifiers, and units. This step demonstrates a method of recording a finding by selecting it from a drop-down list.

**Figure 4-16** Selecting child as source of information from the drop-down list; figure also shows correct findings for the Habits section.

Proceed to the Review of Systems section and locate the label "Source of patient information." Notice the blue finding "patient." Locate and click the down-arrow to the right of it. The drop-down list shown in Figure 4-16 will appear. Select **child** from the drop-down list.

Note: Figure 4-16 will also help you verify that you set the patient exercise habits correctly in step 10.

### Step 12

Begin this step by using the navigation bar to quickly position Review of Systems at the top of the workspace.

Locate the navigation bar at the bottom of your screen and click on the **ROS** link (it has a blue line above it in the figure). This will automatically scroll your workspace and position Review of Systems at the top as shown in Figure 4-17. The content of your workspace will not fully match this figure until you have recorded additional findings in subsequent steps, but you can compare the first item in the figure to verify that you have set the finding correctly in step 11.

### Step 13

The next finding, adjacent to the label "Systemic Symptoms," is something of an anomaly. For most clinical concepts, the negative state represents the normal condition.

For example, when the finding headache turns blue, the word no is added, as it is normal *not* to have a headache. The opposite is true, however, of the clinical concept **feeling fine**. If the medical assistant asks the patient if they feel fine and they answer yes, then that is normal. But thus far, the positive state of a finding represented the abnormal condition. So, for this finding (and a few others like it) the software adds no or not to the red state instead of the blue state.

This is a three-state finding that will change color each time you click it. Click on **feeling fine** to see the descriptions change, but leave it set to **not feeling fine** when you are through.

### Step 14

Locate the ENT Symptoms group of clinical concepts. ENT stands for Ears, Nose, and Throat.

Notice that the concepts in this group are preceded by two round buttons. The left button is used to set the finding positive or abnormal. The right button is used to set the finding negative or normal.

Locate **nasal discharge** and click the right button. Both the finding and the button will turn blue. Now, click the left button. Both the finding and the button will turn red.

Locate **sneezing** and click the left button. Both the finding and the button will turn red.

### Step 15

Proceed to the Pulmonary Symptoms group of clinical concepts.

Mr. Jones has a nonproductive cough. Apply what you learned in the previous step to set the finding **cough** positive and the finding **coughing up sputum** negative.

Compare your findings in the ENT and Pulmonary groups to the corresponding portions of Figure 4-17.

**Figure 4-17** Review of Systems at the top; shows recorded findings for Systemic, ENT, Pulmonary, and Musculoskeletal symptoms.

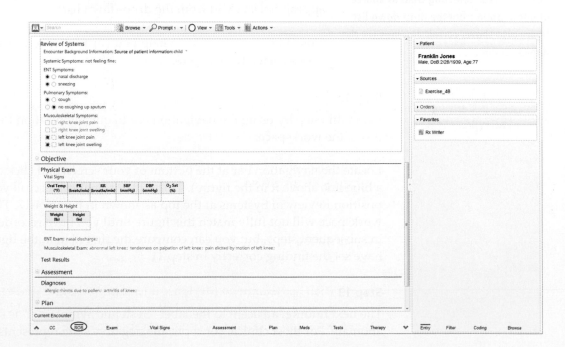

## Step 16

Proceed to the Musculoskeletal Symptoms group of clinical concepts. Notice that the concepts in this group are preceded by two squares. These squares are not check boxes, though; they are buttons to select findings and behave similar to the round buttons in the previous two steps. The left button is used to set the finding positive or abnormal. The right button is used to set the finding negative or normal.

In this style it is not necessary to click buttons for every finding, only the findings that we want to record. In this case, Mr. Jones reports pain and swelling in his left knee. Therefore, skip the clinical concepts that concern the right knee.

Locate and click the left buttons for each of the left knee findings:

- left knee joint pain
- left knee joint swelling

Both the findings and their buttons will turn red. The right knee findings should be left in the gray, unentered state.

Compare your screen to Figure 4-17. All findings recorded in steps 11–16 should match the figure.

## Step 17

Proceed to the Physical Exam section and enter Mr. Jones's vital signs as listed below. Notice that one new measurement, **O$_2$ Sat**, has been added to the vital signs. This stands for Oxygen Saturation. In medicine, this is the percentage of hemoglobin filled with oxygen molecules relative to the total hemoglobin in the body. Typically, in a medical office, this is measured by placing a small device called a pulse oximeter on the patient's finger, as shown in Figure 4-18.

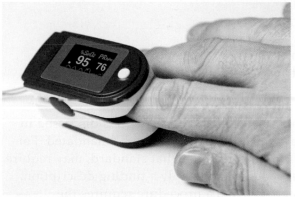

Courtesy Juan R. Velasco/Shutterstock

**Figure 4-18** Pulse oximeter measuring patient's oxygen saturation and pulse.

Enter Mr. Jones's vital signs into the corresponding fields. They are as follows:

| | |
|---|---|
| Temperature: | 97.6 |
| Pulse: | 76 |
| Respiration: | 20 |
| SBP (systolic) | 125 |
| DBP (diastolic) | 85 |
| O$_2$ Sat: | 95 |

Mr. Jones weighs **147** pounds and is 5′ 7″ (**67** inches) tall. Enter his weight and height in the corresponding fields.

## Step 18

The remaining findings in the Physical Exam section have three states: neutral (gray), abnormal (red), and negative or normal (blue.)

The clinician has examined Mr. Jones and observed **nasal discharge, abnormal left knee, tenderness on palpation of left knee**, and **pain elicited by motion of the left knee**. Locate and click each of these concepts until the finding turns red.

## Step 19

Proceed to the Assessment section and enter the clinician's diagnoses by clicking on **allergic rhinitis due to pollen**, and **arthritis of knee**. Both findings should turn red.

Compare your screen to Figure 4-19. All findings recorded in steps 11–19 should match Figure 4-19.

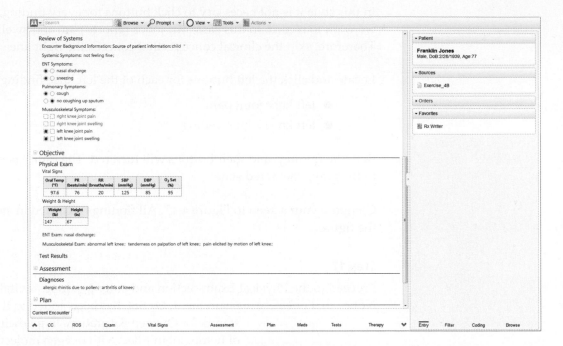

**Figure 4-19** Recorded findings for Review of Systems, Objective, and Assessment sections.

## Step 20

Locate the navigation bar at the bottom of your screen and click on the Therapy link. This will scroll your screen so that you can see the Plan section more clearly.

Although codified medical records are the ideal for all the reasons discussed in Chapter 2, sometimes more than a few words of free text may be mandated. For example, surgical notes for a procedure, though somewhat standard, may require a more detailed description of the procedure than simply a finding description. Another example, as shown in this step, is when a procedure requires the patient's consent and the clinic requires specific language in the encounter note. Rather than retype the entire consent statement in as free text every time it is needed, a text macro can be created to paste a block of text into the note. If there are clinical findings that need to be part of the text, the macro can include fields for selecting them.

The doctor is going to give Mr. Jones an injection in his left knee to relieve his pain and reduce the swelling. At the beginning of the encounter note, the medical assistant confirmed that Mr. Jones is not allergic to anesthetics; however, the office requires the clinician to document the patient's informed consent to the procedure.

Locate **Authorization given for joint injection** and click the **Y** check box. A block of text will be inserted into the encounter note, as shown in Figure 4-20. Notice that four places in the text are highlighted: select, joint, 22 (gauge needle), and 4 (mL). These are fields in which you can select Medcin findings and enter details.

**Figure 4-20** Therapy section with Authorization checked and macro text displayed.

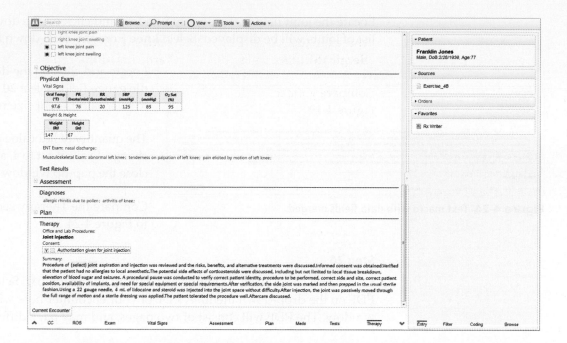

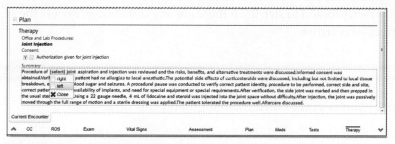

**Figure 4-21** Click highlighted "select" field to set laterality "left" from the drop-down list.

**Figure 4-22** Actions menu option Data Field Entry used for text macros.

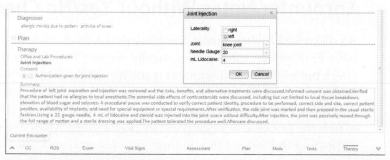

**Figure 4-23** Pop-up window for text macro data field entry; select knee joint and 20 gauge needle.

### Step 21

Locate and click on the word **(select)** at the beginning of the paragraph. A drop-down list will display as shown in (Figure 4-21), allowing you to record laterality (right or left). Select **left,** as the injection was to Mr. Jones' left knee.

### Step 22

When using text macros, the toolbar Actions button has a different drop-down menu. Locate and click the Actions button on the toolbar. The drop-down menu shown in Figure 4-22 will be displayed. Click on the Data Field Entry option. The pop-up window shown in Figure 4-23 will be displayed.

### Step 23

The pop-up window allows you to set all the findings used in the text macro at once, saving the effort of clicking and setting each of the highlighted fields individually.

The laterality has already been set to the left in step 21. The needle size and quantity injected have the default values highlighted in the text, but these can be changed in the Data Field Entry pop-up.

Locate the joint field in the pop-up window and click on the down-arrow next to it. A list of joints will be displayed. Select **knee** from the drop-down list.

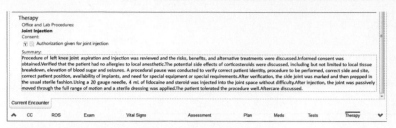

**Figure 4-24** Text macro with data fields merged.

Locate and click on the down-arrow for the needle gauge field. Select **20** from the drop-down list to select a different size needle.

The quantity of lidocaine administered did not change. Leave it set to 4, and click the OK button to close the pop-up window and record the findings.

Compare the Therapy section of your workspace to Figure 4-24.

### Step 24

Locate and click the blue Quippe icon button on the toolbar. Select the option Create PDF on the drop-down menu. A PDF of your encounter note will open in a new window. The PDF will consist of two pages, and may page differently from the figure.

Compare your PDF to Figure 4-25a and Figure 4-25b. You will need to scroll the PDF to see all of it. If everything is correct, proceed to step 25. If there are any differences, review the preceding steps and correct your errors.

### Step 25

If you wish to print a copy of your completed encounter notes for yourself or because your instructor requires you to turn them in, then print or download the PDF at this time.

The final step in every exercise is to submit your completed work for a grade.

Locate and click the blue Quippe icon button on the toolbar to display the drop-down menu, and then select the Submit for Grade menu option. This will complete Exercise 4B.

## Encounter Notes Without Yes/No Check Boxes

As discussed earlier, many clinicians prefer to document without check boxes or have EHR systems that automatically remove them from the final note. Without check boxes the final document reads more like a doctor's clinical note. The following exercise uses a template that omits check boxes except in the Alcohol section. As you record findings, they will change color and the narrative text will change to match the positive or negative state. Remember, Medcin concepts have three colors indicating the state of the finding: gray (neutral and unentered), red (positive or abnormal), and blue (negative or normal).

## Additional Exercises

The following exercises provide additional opportunities for you to practice using features of the software with which you have become familiar. Exercises in Chapter 3 and this chapter covered each feature used in these exercises. If you have difficulty at any step during these exercises, refer to the corresponding exercise for that feature in Chapter 3 or the preceding two exercises in this chapter. Remember that findings set

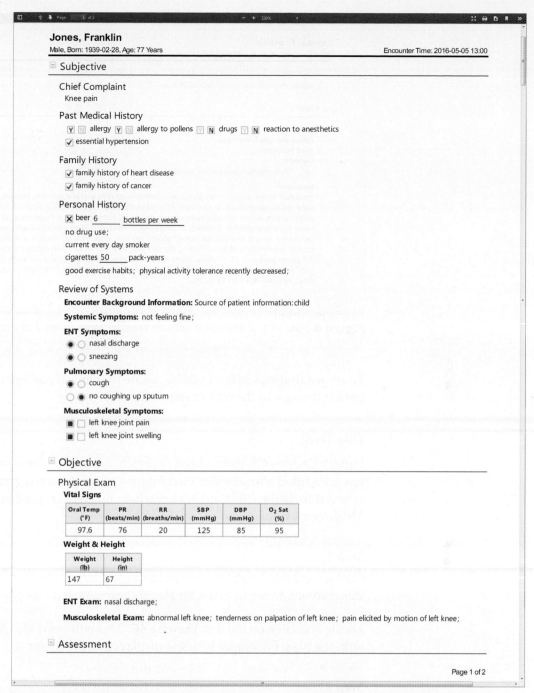

**Figure 4-25a** PDF of encounter note for Franklin Jones (page 1 of 2. See overleaf for page 2).

to negative/normal change their descriptions when recorded. To assist you in matching the desired state of recorded findings, red and blue bullets are provided in the exercise steps. However, because the text of findings changes as their state changes, findings in the exercise steps are given with their *unentered* descriptions so that you can locate them in the encounter pane.

## Critical Thinking Exercise 4C: A Patient with Sinusitis

This exercise will help you evaluate how well you can apply the previous exercises to create an encounter note. The exercise provides step-by-step instructions, but does not provide screen figures for reference.

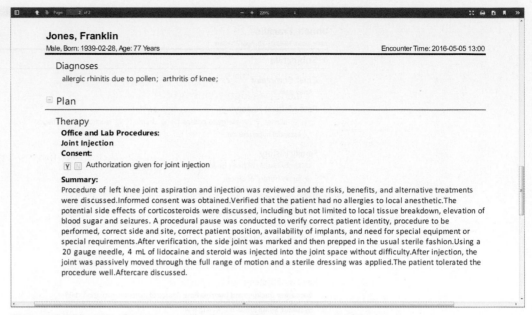

**Jones, Franklin**
Male, Born: 1939-02-28, Age: 77 Years                                   Encounter Time: 2016-05-05 13:00

Diagnoses
  allergic rhinitis due to pollen;  arthritis of knee;

⊟ Plan

Therapy
  **Office and Lab Procedures:**
  **Joint Injection**
  **Consent:**
    ☐Y ☐N Authorization given for joint injection

  **Summary:**
  Procedure of left knee joint aspiration and injection was reviewed and the risks, benefits, and alternative treatments were discussed.Informed consent was obtained.Verified that the patient had no allergies to local anesthetic.The potential side effects of corticosteroids were discussed, including but not limited to local tissue breakdown, elevation of blood sugar and seizures. A procedural pause was conducted to verify correct patient identity, procedure to be performed, correct side and site, correct patient position, availability of implants, and need for special equipment or special requirements.After verification, the side joint was marked and then prepped in the usual sterile fashion.Using a 20 gauge needle, 4 mL of lidocaine and steroid was injected into the joint space without difficulty.After injection, the joint was passively moved through the full range of motion and a sterile dressing was applied.The patient tolerated the procedure well.Aftercare discussed.

**Figure 4-25b** PDF of encounter note for Franklin Jones (page 2 of 2 pages).

To record findings in this exercise, locate the clinical concept and click on it repeatedly until it changes to the correct state and color.

**Case Study**

Patient Charles Green has been experiencing stuffy sinus pain. The medical office has scheduled a brief office visit for him to see the nurse practitioner (hereafter referred to as the clinician). Using what you have learned so far, document Mr. Green's brief exam.

**Step 1**

Start a supported web browser program and follow the steps listed inside the cover of this textbook to log in to the MyHealthProfessionsLab for this course.

Locate and click on the link **Exercise 4C**. This will open the Quippe software window with the New Encounter window displayed in the center.

**Step 2**

Locate the scroll bar on the right edge of the patient list and scroll the list until you locate the patient named **Green, Charles**. Click on his name, and then click the OK button. In this exercise, you do not need to set the date and time of the encounter.

**Step 3**

Click in the blank space under the Chief Complaint heading as you have in previous exercises, and type **Stuffy sinus**.

**Step 4**

The patient reports sinus pain, stuffy nose (nasal passage blockage), and nasal discharge.

Locate the Review of Systems section and record the following findings by clicking on their descriptions until they turn red.

- sinus pain
- nasal discharge
- nasal passage blockage

## Step 5

The patient says he has not had a fever. Locate and click the clinical concept fever until it turns blue.

- fever

The description will change to no fever.

## Step 6

The patient reports he has been taking over-the-counter cold medication.

Locate the Past Medical History section and click on the clinical concept for reported medication history:

- taking OTC cold medication

OTC is an acronym for over-the-counter.

## Step 7

The clinician asks the patient about his behavioral habits.

Mr. Green admits smoking a pack of cigarettes a day for about 12 years. The clinician counsels the patient to stop smoking. Record these findings in the Personal history section:

- current every day smoker

Additional clinical concepts will appear. Click on the following additional findings:

- cigarettes
- Patient education on smoking cessation

A value field will appear for cigarettes: ____ pack-years. Type **12** in the field.

## Step 8

Mr. Green says he drinks a couple of bottles of beer a week and does not use recreational drugs.

Locate and click the check box next to **beer**. A value field will appear. Type the number **2**, and then click the down-arrow next to bottles per day and select **bottles per week** from the drop-down list.

Locate and click the clinical concept **drug use** until it turns blue.

- drug use

**Step 9**

Proceed to the Physical Exam section and enter Mr. Green's vital signs in the corresponding fields as follows:

| | |
|---|---|
| Temperature: | **96.7** |
| Pulse: | **67** |
| Respiration: | **27** |
| SBP: | **120** |
| DBP | **88** |
| O$_2$ Sat: | **92** |

Enter his weight and height. Charles Green weighs **177** pounds and is **68** inches tall.

**Step 10**

The clinician examines the patient's head, eyes, and ears, all of which are normal. Click on each of the following findings until they turn blue:

- head injury
- eyes
- tympanic membrane of right ear
- tympanic membrane of left ear

**Step 11**

Examining the patient's nose, the clinician observes nasal discharge and tenderness of sinuses. Locate and click the following findings:

- nasal discharge
- tenderness of sinus

**Step 12**

The clinician examines the inside of his mouth, listens to his lungs, and finds that everything is normal. Locate and click on each of the following findings until they turn blue:

- upper airway
- oral cavity
- pharyngeal exam
- lungs and respiration auscultation
- chest percussion abnormal

The descriptions will change.

**Step 13**

The clinician concludes that the patient has acute sinusitis that is already improving.

Locate and click on Assessment in the navigation bar below the work space.

Notice that the possible diagnoses in the Assessment section do not include acute sinusitis.

Locate and click the Browse button on the toolbar, and click the plus symbol next to Concepts to open the list of Medcin concepts.

Locate the plus symbol for the domain heading Diagnoses, syndromes and conditions.

Locate and click on the small plus symbol next to "ENT disorder."

Locate and click on the small plus symbol next to "nose."

Locate and click on the small plus symbol next to "sinusitis."

Locate and click on the word "acute" to highlight it, and then click on the Add to Note button at the top of the list.

Locate and click on acute sinusitis until it is red.

- acute sinusitis

*Right-click* on the finding (or click the Actions button on the toolbar) and select Details from the Actions drop-down menu.

Locate and click the down-arrow next to the **status** field in the Details pop-up window, and select **improving** from the drop-down list. Click on the OK button to close the pop-up window.

The diagnosis will change to read "acute sinusitis – improving."

## Step 14

The nurse practitioner advises Mr. Green to continue taking over-the-counter antihistamines, rest, drink plenty of fluids, and to abstain from smoking.

Locate and click on the following findings in the Therapy section:

- fluids
- bed rest
- antihistamines/decongestants

*Right-click* on the antihistamines/decongestants toolbar and select Details from the Actions drop-down menu.

In the Details pop-up window, locate the **Prefix** field and notice that it says "ordered." Click the down-arrow next to it, then locate and click the prefix **continue** in the drop-down list.

Click in the Details Note field and type **OTC**.

Click on the OK button to close the pop-up window.

The description should now read "continue antihistamines/decongestants OTC."

## Step 15

Locate and click on the following finding in the Counseling and Education section:

- abstinence from smoking

## Step 16

Locate and click the View button on the toolbar, and then select Concise from the drop-down menu.

Compare your screen to Figure 4-26. (You may have to scroll your screen to see the entire encounter note.)

**Figure 4-26** Concise view of Charles Green's completed encounter note.

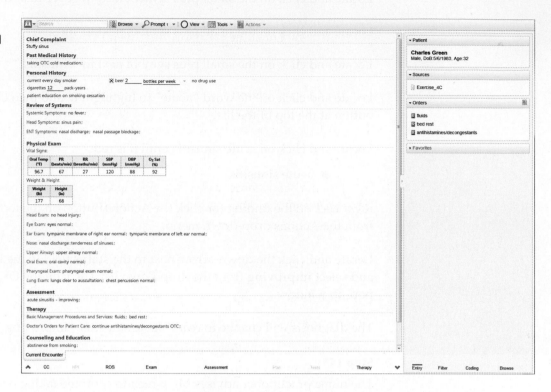

If everything is correct proceed to step 17. If there are any differences, click the View button on the toolbar, select the Entry option on the drop-down menu, and then correct your work according to the preceding steps.

## Step 17

If you wish to print a copy of your completed encounter notes for yourself or because your instructor requires you to turn them in, print or download the PDF at this time.

The final step in every exercise is to submit your completed work for a grade.

Locate and click the blue Quippe icon button on the toolbar to display the drop-down menu, and then select the Submit for Grade menu option. This will complete Exercise 4C.

## Critical Thinking Exercise 4D: Patient with Urinary Problem

In this exercise, you use the skills you have acquired to document this exam. The template for this exercise is more specific to female patients, and typical of one that might be used at an OB/GYN office.

### Case Study

Carrie Cook is a 35-year-old mother of a 6-year-old. She recently has been having difficulty urinating; feeling that she needs to go frequently, but not much comes out; and the urine is cloudy. She is on birth control and is not pregnant. Carrie has decided to see her gynecologist about this instead of her family doctor.

### Step 1

Start a supported web browser program and follow the steps listed inside the cover of this textbook to log in to the MyHealthProfessionsLab for this course.

Locate and click on the link **Exercise 4D**. This will open the Quippe software window with the New Encounter window displayed in the center.

### Step 2

Locate the scroll bar on the right edge of the patient list and scroll the list until you locate the patient named **Cook, Carrie**. Click on her name, and then click the OK button. In this exercise, you do not need to set the date and time of the encounter.

### Step 3

Click in the blank space under the heading Chief Complaint as you have in previous exercises, and type **Difficult, painful urination.**

### Step 4

Begin the visit by recording Carrie's vital signs and medical history.

Enter Carrie's vital signs in the corresponding fields as follows:

| | |
|---|---|
| Temperature: | **101** |
| Pulse Rate: | **70** |
| Respiration Rate: | **20** |
| SBP: | **120** |
| DBP: | **80** |
| Weight: | **125** |
| Height: | **65** |

When you have finished, check your work. If it is correct, proceed to step 5.

### Step 5

Scroll to the top of the encounter and record the patient's allergy information. Carrie has no allergies.

Locate and click on the following findings until they turn blue and the descriptions change.

- allergy
- allergy drugs

### Step 6

Gynecologist offices typically document past pregnancies. Carrie has one child. Locate **pregnancy** in the last line of the Past Medical History, Diagnoses group and click on it until it turns red:

- pregnancy

*Right-click* on the finding and select Details from the Actions drop-down menu. In the pop-up window, click in the Onset field, type **2010**, and then click the OK button. Verify that your finding is red and reads "pregnancy 2010."

**Step 7**

Proceed to Current Medications and document Carrie's birth control.

- birth control using oral contraceptives

**Step 8**

Proceed to Personal History and click the following findings until they turn blue and their descriptions change.

- tobacco use
- drug use
- poor exercise habits
- not in a monogamous relationship

**Step 9**

Carrie is sexually active and drinks an occasional glass of wine. Locate and click on the following findings until they turn red:

- sexually active
- alcohol use

Various forms of alcohol use will be displayed. Click wine.

- wine

Type **1** in the **glasses per week** field.

**Step 10**

Proceed to Review of Systems. Locate and click on the following symptoms until they turn red. (All findings except the first one are located in GU Symptoms.)

- fever
- urine is cloudy
- increased urinary frequency
- frequent small amounts of urine
- urinary urgency
- incomplete emptying of bladder
- pain during urination

**Step 11**

Proceed to the Physical Exam section. Locate the Gastrointestinal Exam and Genitourinary Exam sections. Locate and click on the following findings until they turn red.

- abdominal tenderness
- urinary bladder
- tender
- urethra
- tenderness

**Step 12**

A urinalysis was performed, and the results have been merged into the encounter note. The doctor reviews the results. Locate and click on **performed urinalysis** in the Test Results section to highlight it. Click the Action button on the toolbar and select Details from the drop-down menu. In the Details pop-up window, change the prefix from performed to **reviewed**, and then click the OK button. The finding description should change to "reviewed urinalysis." Verify that the finding is still red.

**Step 13**

Proceed to the Diagnoses section, and locate and click on the finding **urinary tract infection** until it turns red.

- urinary tract infection

**Step 14**

Proceed to the Plan section, and locate and click on the finding **antibacterials** until it turns red.

- antibacterials

**Step 15**

Locate the Navigation bar at the bottom of your screen and click on the label Therapy to highlight that section.

Click the Browse button on the toolbar and the plus symbol next to Concepts and then click on the small plus symbol next to the domain heading Therapy.

Locate and click on the small plus symbol next to **basic management procedures and services.**

Scroll the drop-down list downward to locate the clinical concept **education and instructions**. (It is located almost at the end of the indented section of basic management procedures and services.) Click the small plus symbol next to the clinical concept **education and instructions** and then expand the concept **instructions for patient** (located immediately below "education and instructions").

Scroll the expanded tree downward until you locate **abstinence from alcohol.** (The concept is located quite far down the expanded tree of "instructions for patient.") Refer to Figure 3-26 in Chapter 3 if you need assistance locating it.

Once you locate it, click on the words "abstinence from alcohol" to highlight the concept and then click the Add to Note button.

**Step 16**

Locate and click on the following Counseling and Education and Therapy findings until they turn red.

- abstinence from alcohol
- fluids
- cranberry juice

**Step 17**

Locate and click the View button on the toolbar, and then select Concise from the drop-down menu.

Compare your screen to Figure 4-27. (You may have to scroll your screen to see the entire encounter note.)

**Figure 4-27** Concise view of Carrie Cook's completed encounter note.

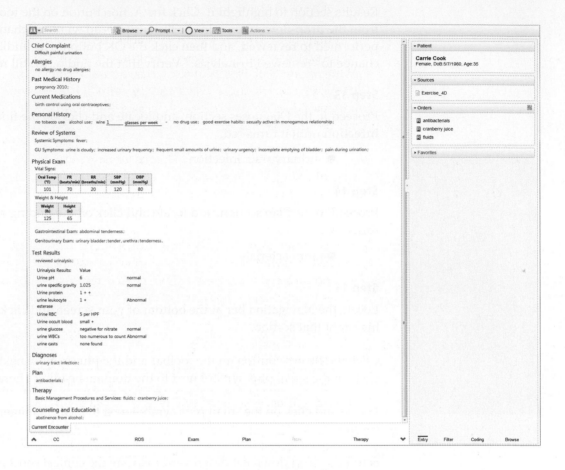

If everything is correct, proceed to step 18. If there are any differences, click the View button on the toolbar, select the Entry option on the drop-down menu, and then correct your work according to the preceding steps.

**Step 18**

If wish to print a copy of your completed encounter notes for yourself or because your instructor requires you to turn them in, print or download the PDF at this time.

The final step in every exercise is to submit your completed work for a grade.

Locate and click the blue Quippe icon button on the toolbar to display the drop-down menu, and then select the Submit for Grade menu option. This will complete Exercise 4D.

## Chapter Four Summary

In this chapter you have performed exercises intended to increase your familiarity with the Student Edition software and thereby increase your speed of data entry. You have also learned how to record findings without check boxes, delete and modify prefixes, and use text macros.

Text macros not only add text to the note, but can contain drop-down fields for merging findings into the block of text. Findings are selected in text macros by clicking on highlighted portions of the text or by clicking the toolbar Actions button and selecting the Data Field Entry option.

The Actions button on the toolbar is enabled only when a heading, finding or text macro is selected, and in the case of text macros the menu option Details is replaced with the option Data Field Entry. If your mouse or computing device has a right-click function, you can right-click on a finding to invoke the Actions drop-down menu. If your device does not have right-click, continue to use the Actions button on the toolbar where the instructions say "right-click."

In these and many subsequent exercises you are permitted to use the current date instead of setting it to a specific date. Remember that when you do that, the date of the encounter and the patient's age will differ from the samples given in the book. However, all of the other items in your printout or file should match the figure in the book.

As you continue through the course, you can refer to the Exercises in the table below if you need to remember how to use a particular feature you learned in this chapter. You should not proceed with the remainder of the text until you feel you can perform the exercises in this chapter with ease.

| Task | Guided Exercise(s) | Page # |
|------|--------------------|--------|
| Clearing the Prefix field | 4A step 19 | 124 |
| Modifying the Prefix | 4C step 14 | 141 |
| Recording findings without checkboxes | 4B step 8 | 130 |
| Recording findings from a drop-down list | 4B step 11 | 131 |
| Using the Navigation bar | 4B step 13 | 131–32 |
| Adding findings in a text macro | 4B step 21 | 135 |

## Testing Your Knowledge of Chapter 4

### Step 1

Log in to MyHealthProfessionsLab following the directions printed inside the cover of this textbook.

Locate and click on Chapter 4 Test.

### Step 2

Answer the test questions. When you have finished, click the Submit Test button to close the window.

## Testing Your Skill Exercise 4E: An Asthma Patient Who Sleeps with a Dog

Now that you have performed all the exercises in Chapter 4 this exercise will help you and your instructor evaluate your acquired skills. Use the information in the case study and the features of the software you already know to document the patient's encounter.

**Case Study**

John Lewis is a 33-year-old established patient who comes to the office with a chief complaint of wheezing and short of breath.

John has allergies and is allergic to pollens and dust. His past medical history includes asthma and hay fever, which have been treated with corticosteroids in the past. John says asthma runs in his family.

John does not smoke or use drugs, but works around dust and with people who smoke cigarettes. He has a dog that he keeps in the house. He usually drinks 3 beers with the guys from work on Friday nights.

The clinician asks the patient about his symptoms. John says he hasn't had fever, chills, or sinus pain, but has been sneezing. He complains of wheezing and awakening at night short of breath.

John's vital signs are as follows:

| | |
|---|---|
| Temperature: | 98.8 |
| Pulse Rate: | 68 |
| Respiration Rate: | 22 |
| SBP: | 120 |
| DBP: | 80 |
| $O_2$ Sat | 94 |
| Weight: | 175 |
| Height: | 71 |

The clinician listens to John's lungs and hears wheezing, but respiratory movements are normal and no rhonchi or rales are heard. The clinician's assessment is that John has mild intermittent asthma.

The clinician's Therapy orders include environmental control measures, and avoid exposure to allergens. The clinician suggests that John avoid pollen by keeping the air conditioning running in recirculating mode, and tells him to avoid letting his dog sleep with him.

**Step 1**

Start a supported web browser program and follow the steps listed inside the cover of this textbook to log in to the MyHealthProfessionsLab for this course.

Locate and click on the link **Exercise 4E**. This will open the Quippe software window with the New Encounter window displayed in the center.

**Step 2**

Locate and click on the patient name, and then click the OK button. In this exercise, you do not need to set the date or time of the encounter.

**Step 3**

Use the case study information just presented to record vital signs and other findings. Read the case study *carefully* and document only the findings mentioned. Although the template contains many concepts that do not apply to John's case, it does not contain every finding you will need. Here are some hints to help you add them.

*Hint*: Browse Concepts and add dust to the note as soon as you record John's allergy to pollen.

*Hint*: While documenting Review of Systems, Browse ENT symptoms to locate and add sneezing to the note.

*Hint*: After recording the Assessment of asthma, Browse the list of concepts, and expand asthma, and mild, to locate intermittent and add it to the note.

Once you have documented all the information provided in the case study, proceed to step 4.

### Step 4

If you wish to print a copy of your completed encounter notes for yourself or because your instructor requires you to turn them in, use the Create PDF option, and then print or download the PDF at this time.

Submit your completed work for a grade using the Submit for Grade option on the application menu. This will complete Exercise 4E.

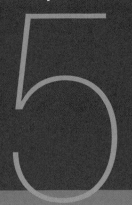

# Data Entry at the Point of Care

## Learning Outcomes

*After completing this chapter, you should be able to:*

◆ Use Lists to speed up data entry

◆ Describe Review of Systems

◆ Be able to quickly record pertinent negatives using Otherwise Normal

◆ Understand and use Forms

◆ Use Lists and Forms together

## Why Speed of Entry Is Important in the EHR

A survey of nurses conducted by Jackson Healthcare[1] found that nurses in a hospital setting spent 25 percent of their time on indirect patient care activities. The report stated that the majority of that time was spent on documentation. In Chapter 2, EHR expert Dr. Allen Wenner estimated that in a medical office "up to 67% of the nurse or clinician's time with the patient is spent entering the patient's symptoms into the visit documentation."

There is no question that symptoms, history, orders, observations, assessments, and all other aspects of patient care must be documented. The accuracy of documentation and efficiency of workflow can be improved by documenting at the time of the encounter, not after the clinician has left the patient. Previous chapters have referred to this as point-of-care or real-time data entry—that is, to document the visit completely during the face-to-face encounter, before the patient ever leaves the office.

Speed of entry is important because the less time it takes to record the provider's notes, the more time a provider has available for patient care. Real-time data entry is important because the chart is always up-to-date. Accuracy is improved because nothing is

---

[1]Jackson Healthcare, "Hospital Nurses Study 2010 Summary of Findings," Jackson Healthcare, LLC, Alpharetta, GA, 2010.

forgotten. Documenting at the point of care allows the nurse to ask the patient to elaborate or clarify any point of concern. Best of all, when the provider leaves the patient's room, the notes are done. No longer will the doctor or nurse spend the final hours of every day finishing up paperwork. Most importantly, health information about the patient is available for other caregivers instead of in the provider's memory or dictation system.

To document in real time, a provider must be able to quickly navigate and enter findings. To help the clinician accomplish this, an EHR needs to present the finding the provider needs when it is needed. In this chapter we are going to look at several approaches EHR vendors use to help the healthcare professional accomplish that.

## Templates, Lists, and Forms Speed Data Entry

Exercises in the previous chapters documented relatively simple encounters with findings that were fairly easy to locate. However, completely documenting a full encounter could take quite a bit of time, especially when clinical concepts have to be added to the workspace. Additionally, patients often have multiple problems, with more complex history and symptoms. For example, it is not unusual for an obese patient to have both diabetes and hypertension.

Is there a faster way to document findings than Browsing the Concept list, expanding the trees, and adding clinical concepts to the note? Yes!

EHR vendors work constantly with EHR users to devise means to locate and present clinical concepts when they are most likely needed. Tobacco Use, for example, presents additional concepts for the clinician to document when a patient is identified as a smoker.

There are three methods that are used extensively in EHR systems to expedite point-of-care data entry. Templates, Lists, and Forms are different approaches to solve the problem of displaying clinical concepts that a provider uses most frequently for cases typical to that clinician's specialty.

## Shortcuts That Speed Documentation of Typical Cases

Both inpatient and outpatient facilities see a lot of patients with similar conditions. There are several reasons for this:

◆ The top 10 diseases cause the highest proportion of patients to be hospitalized.

◆ Geographic location may cause a facility to see more cases of a particular nature than similar facilities in another region.

◆ Seasonal increases of certain illnesses such as influenza and other upper respiratory infections may occur.

◆ The specialty of the clinic or hospital may focus on a single type of disease or patient. For example, an oncology center sees only cancer patients, or a children's hospital focuses on children's diseases.

◆ In outpatient clinics the specialty of the physicians often means patients are seeing them for similar reasons. For example, pulmonary specialists see primarily respiratory cases, nephrologists see patients with kidney problems, and a pediatric clinic sees children.

◆ When nurses document admissions and create care plans for patients with similar ailments they tend to need similar sets of findings based the patients' conditions.

Facilities have discovered that for similar cases, clinicians tend to perform the same type of exam, look for the same findings, order the same tests, and prescribe from a short list of treatments recommended for the condition. Therefore, it is logical to create shorter, quicker methods of entering the data. This is frequently based on the admitting diagnosis or type of ailment.

## The Concept of Templates

Templates determine how headings and clinical concepts are organized in the workspace, and ultimately in the clinician's note. They also determine the visual presentation of concepts in the workspace, such as using a table for entering vital signs instead of using Detail entry. Templates are utilized by EHR vendors to customize the EHR to meet the documentation needs of different medical specialties. Templates allow clinicians to document as suits their workflow.

Each of the exercises in this textbook uses a template specially created for that exercise. The flexibility of templates allows the exercises to look and behave differently, so students become familiar with a broad range of documentation styles and methods. While a medical practice might have several templates that could be used for different clinicians or specialties within the practice, only one template is used per encounter note. Unlike lists and forms, which we will discuss later, templates cannot be merged into an encounter note.

As you have seen in previous exercises, templates are not limited to section headings and tables, but can also contain the clinical concepts most likely to be needed, saving the clinician from having to browse for them and add them to the note. However, if a template were to contain every possible clinical concept a clinician might need across a diverse range of patients, the workspace would become cluttered and difficult to navigate.

## The Concept of Lists

You may not have heard the term *Lists* used in the context of an EHR, but the concept should be very familiar to you because you have been scrolling and navigating the list of concepts since Chapter 3. Now, imagine that you are a pediatrician who treats many children with earaches (otitis media) and that each time the patient's chief complaint is an earache, the system could magically present the findings that you typically used to document the visit. That is the idea behind lists. Of course, lists do not magically appear. They are created by clinicians or their staff for the many types of exams and conditions seen at their practice. However, the time spent making each list is saved again and again when subsequent patients are seen for the same or similar reasons.

The advantage of using these short lists is that they save repeatedly browsing the full Medcin concept tree. A list adds a desired subset of the nomenclature to the workspace with one click. The list can (and usually does) contain concepts in every domain. This means that time savings are realized all the way through the exam. If certain therapies or certain drugs are used for a particular condition, then when the clinician clicks the mouse on the Therapy section, those items are already present. When using a list, if there is a finding that is needed, but is not on the list, the provider can still browse the full hierarchy of Medcin concepts and add it. If the clinician finds the list is missing a concept that is frequently needed, the list can be easily modified.

Although lists are sometimes limited to one particular condition such as otitis media, this is not a rule; it is a convenience factor because shorter lists mean less clutter in the workspace. Lists are flexible and can contain as many findings as necessary to document a typical visit. For example, an adult upper respiratory infection (URI) could be the result of rhinitis, sinusitis, or bronchitis, but diagnosing any of these diseases involves documenting similar body system symptoms and physical examination findings. Therefore, rather than create a list for each diagnosis, one comprehensive list containing the clinical concepts common to various types of upper respiratory infections will have what the clinician needs the majority of the time.

Conversely, when diagnoses are not related to the same body systems, it is better to create separate lists, even if patients frequently have both conditions. Unlike templates, multiple lists *can* be used in a single encounter. So, while many patients have both hypertension and diabetes, some patients have only one condition or the other. Therefore, rather than create a combined diabetes-hypertension list, the clinician can simply add both the diabetes list and the hypertension list to the workspace for patients who have both conditions.

Over time, a practice creates lists for any medical condition that it sees regularly. If clinicians differ in how they would document a particular exam, they can create a copy of the list in their personal folder and tailor it to their style of medicine.

> **NOTE**
>
> ## Alternate Instructions for Right-click function
>
> Exercises in this and subsequent chapters will direct you to invoke the Actions drop-down menu for a finding by right-clicking on the finding. If you are using a touchscreen or stylus that does not have a right-click function, you may click the Actions button on the toolbar as an alternative method. If you do, be certain the finding is still in the correct state after you have completed the action step.

## Guided Exercise 5A: Using an Adult URI List

This exercise uses the template for a hypothetical Family Practice clinic. Family practice physicians see a broad range of patients, so the template includes clinical concepts the clinician uses frequently for most patients; but the template does not contain all the concepts a doctor would need for every condition. When additional concepts are needed to document particular conditions, a list is a good way to quickly add the relevant clinical concepts.

A good example of a multiple diagnosis type of list is the one used in the following exercise for adult URI (an acronym for upper respiratory infection). During the cold and flu season, medical clinics and primary care physicians often see many patients with URI.

In the course of the exercise you will learn to use the List feature to quickly add concepts necessary to document a patient presenting with an URI. You will see how a list speeds up the documentation process considerably.

## Case Study

Kerry Baker comes to the office complaining of sinus pain, stuffiness, and a runny nose. She says she has caught her husband's bug. The medical practice has created a List of Medcin concepts to use for this type of visit and have named it Adult URI.

### Step 1

Start a supported web browser program and follow the steps listed inside the cover of this textbook to log in to the MyHealthProfessionsLab for this course.

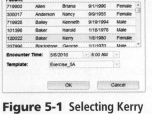

Locate and click on the link **Exercise 5A**. This will open the Quippe software window with the New Encounter window displayed in the center.

**Figure 5-1** Selecting Kerry Baker from the New Encounter window patient list.

### Step 2

Locate and click on the patient named **Baker, Kerry**. In this exercise, you do not need to set the date and time of the encounter. Once you have selected the patient as shown in Figure 5-1, click the OK button.

### Step 3

Click in the blank space under the heading Chief Complaint, as you have in previous exercises, and type **Patient reported cold or flu** as shown in Figure 5-2.

**Figure 5-2** Chief complaint for "patient reported cold or flu" in the family practice template.

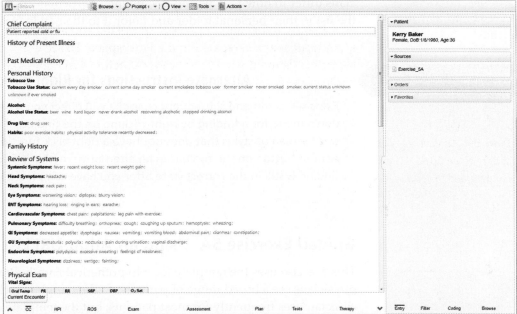

### Step 4

Scroll the workspace and study the template. Notice there are concepts for each body system in Review of Systems and Physical Exam sections. The Assessment section contains diagnoses for many of the conditions a family practice clinic treats.

The patient states she has sinus pain.

Locate the "Head Symptoms" heading in the Review of Systems section. This is where the clinical concept for the symptom sinus pain would normally be found. Since it is not there, you will have to add it to the workspace.

If a finding has focus (is still highlighted), clicking the Browse button opens the concept list within the domain of the currently highlighted finding. This is useful when adding multiple findings of the same type. If, instead, you want the Browse button to start with just the Concepts and Sample Custom Content book icons, click on any whitespace in the encounter pane that does not cause a concept or heading to have focus, *before* you click the Browse button. If you forget and the Browse list opens in concepts, scroll to the top of the list and click the small minus sign next to Concepts to collapse the concept list.

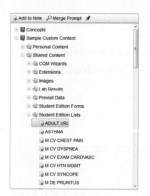

**Figure 5-3** Select Adult URI from Student Edition Lists (invoked by the Browse button).

Click any white space in the encounter pane that does not highlight a heading or clinical concept. Now, click the Browse button on the toolbar as you have in previous exercises, but this time when the drop-down menu is displayed, click the plus symbol next to the Sample Custom Content book icon. When the tree is expanded, locate and click on the plus symbol next to Shared Content and Student Edition Lists. The drop-down list displays the various Lists available to providers in the practice.

Locate and click on the List named Adult URI to highlight it (as shown in Figure 5-3) and then click on the Add to Note button.

### Step 5

The clinical concepts in the Adult URI list are merged with the family practice concepts already present in the workspace. However, there is no duplication. For example, fever was already in the family practice template, and although it is also in the Adult URI list, a duplicate was not created in the workspace. To see which findings have been added, locate the Content pane (identified as section 4 in Figure 3-3). Locate and click on the name of the list, Adult URI in the Content pane (circled in red in Figure 5-4). Concepts that are part of the Adult URI list will become highlighted.

**Figure 5-4** Clinical concepts added from the Adult URI list are highlighted in yellow.

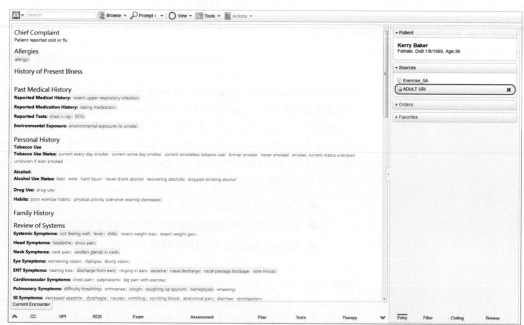

This step is informational only and not a necessary one in using a list. Click again on Adult URI in the Content pane to turn the highlights off.

### Step 6

Locate the label "Head Symptoms" in the Review of Systems section, where you will now see the clinical concept **sinus pain** has been added. Click on the finding until it turns red.

- sinus pain

The patient reports she has had a mild fever. Locate Systemic Symptoms and click on the finding until it turns red.

- fever

*Right-click* on fever and select Details from the Actions drop-down menu.

In the Details pop-up window, locate and click the Modifier field, and then select **mild** from the drop-down list (as shown previously in Figure 4-3). Click OK to close the Details window. The description should now read "mild fever."

### Step 7

Kerry complains her nose feels stuffed up even though she is experiencing nasal discharge.

Locate ENT Symptoms, and click on the following symptom findings, which will turn red:

- nasal discharge
- nasal passage blockage

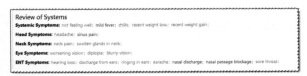

Compare the Review of Systems portion of your screen to Figure 5-5.

**Figure 5-5** Review of the Systems portion of the encounter with Kerry's symptoms in red.

### Step 8

Return to the top of the encounter note to enter the patient's history. Kerry denies having allergies and is not currently taking medications, but has had a recent URI.

You will recall from previous exercises, the history domain had many levels of the tree, which had to be expanded. In this case, because you are using a list, those items related to Adult URI are already displayed. This makes documenting history relevant to URI quicker. Locate and click on the following History findings until they turn the color indicated by the bullets. Remember, the descriptions below are the ones you see before you click the concept.

- (blue) Allergies
- (red) recent upper respiratory infection
- (blue) taking medications

### Step 9

Proceed to the Personal History and record Kerry's behavioral habits. Kerry has never smoked, drinks a glass of wine once a week, and exercises regularly. Locate and click on the following findings until they turn red:

- Never smoked
- Wine

Type **1** in the Glasses per week field.

Locate and click on the following concepts until they turn blue. Their descriptions will change.

- drug use
- poor exercise habits

Compare the Allergy and History sections of your screen to Figure 5-6.

**Figure 5-6** Chief Complaint, Allergies, and History sections of Kerry's encounter note.

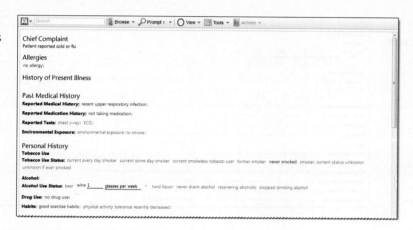

### Step 10

Proceed to the Physical Exam section of the encounter note and enter Kerry's vital signs in the corresponding fields as follows:

| | |
|---|---|
| Temperature: | 99 |
| Pulse: | 78 |
| Respiration: | 16 |
| SBP: | 120 |
| DBP: | 80 |
| $O_2$ Sat: | 95 |

When you have entered all the vital signs, enter her weight and height. Ms. Baker weighs **100** pounds and is 5 feet tall (entered as **60** inches).

### Step 11

The clinician examines Kerry's ears, nose, and throat, and checks her lymph nodes.

Locate Ear Exam and click on the following concept until it turns blue. The description will change from abnormal to normal.

- tympanic membranes abnormal

Locate the label Nose, and click on the following findings until they turn red:

- nasal discharge
- purulent
- tenderness of sinuses

Proceed to the next two items in the physical exam and record the following findings as normal:

- pharyngeal exam
- enlarged lymph nodes

Both findings should turn blue, and their descriptions will change.

Compare the Physical Exam section of your screen to Figure 5-7.

**Figure 5-7** Findings recorded in the Physical Exam portion of the workspace.

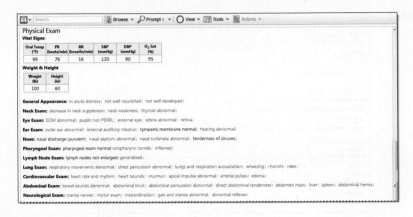

## Step 12

The clinician has determined that the patient has acute sinusitis. Proceed to the Assessment section.

Locate and click on acute sinusitis until it turns red.

- acute sinusitis

## Step 13

The clinician recommends that Kerry drink plenty of fluids and use a cool mist vaporizer at night. Proceed to the Therapy section.

Locate and click on the following concepts. Both findings will turn red.

- cool mist vaporizer
- fluids

## Step 14

Locate and click the View button on the toolbar, and then select Concise from the drop-down menu.

Compare your screen to Figure 5-8. If everything is correct, proceed to step 15. If there are any differences, click the View button on the toolbar, select the Entry option on the drop-down menu, and then correct your work according to the preceding steps.

## Step 15

If you wish to print a copy of your completed encounter notes for yourself or because your instructor requires you to turn them in, use the Create PDF option, and then print or download the PDF at this time.

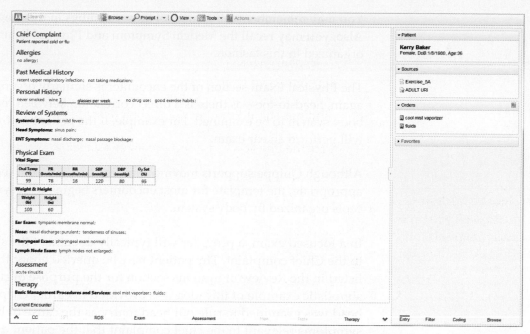

**Figure 5-8** Concise view of correctly completed encounter for Kerry Baker.

The final step in every exercise is to submit your completed work for a grade.

Locate and click the blue Quippe icon button on the toolbar, and then select the Submit for Grade option from the drop-down menu. This will complete Exercise 5A.

# Review of Systems and Pertinent Negatives

**Review of Systems (ROS)** is a way of organizing reported symptoms by the body systems, starting from the head to the toes, and is often called head-to-toe. You may be familiar with the body systems from anatomy and physiology or other medical classes. The body systems in a standard ROS are:

◆ Constitutional symptoms

◆ HEENT (head, eyes, ears, nose, mouth, throat)

◆ Cardiovascular

◆ Respiratory (Pulmonary)

◆ Gastrointestinal

◆ Genitourinary

◆ Musculoskeletal

◆ Integumentary (skin and/or breast)

◆ Neurological

◆ Psychiatric

◆ Endocrine

◆ Hematologic/lymphatic

◆ Allergic/immunologic

You may remember seeing some of these headings in the previous exercise templates. Also, you may recall the Medcin Symptom and Physical Examination domains are organized in this fashion.

The Physical Exam section of the encounter is similarly organized by body system— again, head-to-toe—as there is a direct correlation between reported symptoms and the body system to be examined. For example, if the patient reports earache, the clinician will perform an ear exam.

Although Quippe supports moving a finding to a different section of the note when appropriate, the template for most encounters begins with symptoms and exam concepts organized by body system.

In a focused exam, a provider will typically document the symptoms directly related to the Chief complaint. The patient may be queried about the remaining symptoms listed in the Review of Systems section for the purpose of ruling out other causes. A simplistic example of this idea was provided in earlier chapters where the patient's head was examined to rule out head injury as the cause of headaches. Documenting symptoms relevant to the chief complaint that the patient does *not* present is sometimes equally important in determining the diagnosis. These findings are called **pertinent negatives**.

The same idea applies in the Physical Exam, where by documenting body systems that were examined and found normal, the clinician narrows the range of probable diagnoses. To expedite documentation, clinicians often record the abnormal findings first and the remaining clinical concepts as "Otherwise Normal."

Think of a time when you visited a doctor or clinic for something minor, like a cold. The clinician looked in your ears and the back of your throat, felt the glands in your neck, and listened to your chest with a stethoscope. The clinician did not pause at each step of the exam and document the finding, but instead completed the exam, and then documented everything in the physical exam section at once.

Because this is the way clinicians typically review symptoms and document examination findings, it is useful to have an EHR feature to perform this function. In Quippe, the function is called *Otherwise Normal*. In other EHR systems it may be called *Auto-negative, Auto-normal,* or *Within Normal Limits (WNL)*. The purpose of this function is to set all unentered clinical concepts in a selected group to normal with a simple click of the Otherwise Normal option. It does not alter or affect findings in the group, which are already set to either a positive or a negative state.

As you can imagine, this feature can greatly speed up documentation, but it works best when used with a list or form so the unentered clinical concepts in the selected section are limited to those that are typically used for conditions related to the chief complaint. If a clinician were to use the Otherwise Normal feature on a template such as the full family practice template used in Exercise 5A, the findings would indicate that the clinician had examined every body system. This might be true for an annual physical, but the family practice template would likely record too many findings for a patient with sinusitis.

The otherwise normal feature is helpful to quickly document pertinent negatives of symptoms and body systems that the clinician actually reviewed and examined. It should never be used to document findings that the clinician did not perform.

# Guided Exercise 5B: Using Lists and Otherwise Normal

In this exercise you will apply what you have learned about lists in the previous exercise and learn to use the Otherwise Normal feature. Instead of beginning with the family practice template, which contained clinical concepts for all types of patients the clinic sees, this exercise uses a template that contains only major section headings and the behavioral history items that the practice asks every patient. When the list is added to the note, the concepts in the list will automatically group under the relevant headings.

### Case Study

In Chapter 4, you documented a visit for an adult URI for Kerry's husband Harold. On the following Monday he returns to the clinic, as his condition has not improved. You are going to document a visit very similar to his previous visit, but this time using a list and the Otherwise Normal feature.

### Step 1

Start a supported web browser program and follow the steps listed inside the cover of this textbook to log in to the MyHealthProfessionsLab for this course.

Locate and click on the link **Exercise 5B**. This will open the Quippe software window with the New Encounter window displayed in the center.

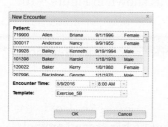

**Figure 5-9** Selecting Harold Baker from the New Encounter window patient list.

### Step 2

Locate and click on the patient named **Baker, Harold**. In this exercise, you do not need to set the date and time of the encounter. Once you have selected the patient as shown in Figure 5-9, click the OK button.

### Step 3

Click in the blank space under the Chief Complaint heading as you have in previous exercises, and type **Return visit for a cold**.

### Step 4

The medical assistant begins the encounter by taking Harold's vital signs.

Locate the Physical Exam section and enter the measurements listed below in the corresponding fields of the Vital Signs table.

| | |
|---|---|
| Temperature: | **99.9** |
| Pulse: | **75** |
| Respiration: | **25** |
| SBP: | **130** |
| DBP: | **90** |
| $O_2$ Sat: | **95** |

When you have entered all the vital signs, enter his weight and height. Mr. Baker weighs **175** pounds and is 6 feet tall (entered as **72** inches).

### Step 5

Notice that except for Personal History, other sections do not have clinical concepts. When the Adult URI list is added, only concepts pertinent to respiratory infections will be in the workspace.

Click any whitespace in the encounter pane that does not highlight a heading or finding, and then click on the Browse button in the Toolbar. Click the plus symbol next to the Sample Custom Content book icon. When the tree is expanded, locate and click on the plus symbol next to Shared Content and Student Edition Lists.

Locate and click on the list named Adult URI to highlight it (as shown previously in Figure 5-3) and then click on the Add to Note button.

Clinical concepts from the list will populate the workspace.

### Step 6

Harold states he was seen at the clinic last week for the same ailment, which has not improved.

Begin with the patient's Past Medical History.

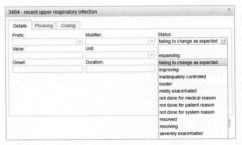

**Figure 5-10** Selecting Status "failing to change as expected."

Locate and click on recent **upper respiratory infection**, which will turn red. *Right-click* on the finding and select Details from the Actions drop-down menu.

In the Details pop-up window, click in the Status field and select "failing to change as expected" from the drop-down list, as shown in Figure 5-10. Click the OK button to close the Details window.

The finding description should read: "Recent upper respiratory infection–failing to change as expected."

### Step 7

Harold states he is not on any prescription medications and that he has never smoked.

Locate and click **taking medications** until the finding turns blue. The description will change as well.

Locate **never smoked** in the Tobacco use section and click on it. The finding will turn red.

Compare the Chief Complaint and History sections of your screen to Figure 5-11.

**Figure 5-11** Portion of encounter note showing chief complaint and history findings recorded for Harold Baker.

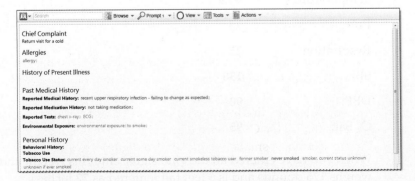

### Step 8

The clinician asks Harold about his symptoms, and Harold says he is not feeling well, has a mild fever, headache, sinus pain, nasal discharge, and stuffiness, and is coughing up phlegm.

Locate and click on the following findings, which will turn red:

- not feeling well
- fever
- headache
- sinus pain
- nasal discharge
- nasal passage blockage
- coughing up sputum

Compare your recorded findings to those shown in Figure 5-12.

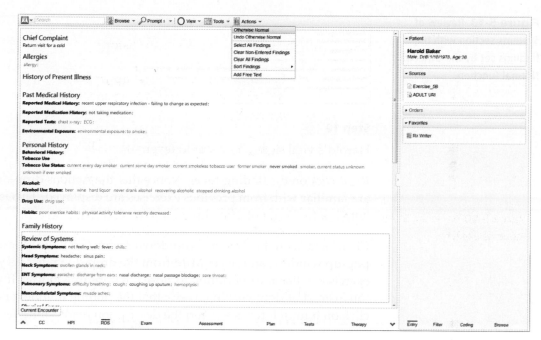

**Figure 5-12** Actions button drop-down menu when Review of Systems section is selected; also shows ROS abnormal findings (in red).

### Step 9

The clinician asks if he has had chills, swollen glands, earaches, sore throat, difficulty breathing, or achy muscles. Harold says he has had none of those. Record these normal findings by using the Otherwise Normal feature.

Begin by locating and clicking on the Review of Systems heading label. This will outline the entire Review of Systems section as shown outlined (in yellow) in Figure 5-12.

As noted earlier, findings already recorded or those outside this selected group will not be affected by the Otherwise Normal function. Also, the group does not have to be an entire section. A smaller group such as pulmonary Symptoms could be selected instead. The only criteria are that some level of heading is selected to define the intended group of clinical concepts to be recorded as normal.

Locate and click the Actions button on the toolbar, and the drop-down menu shown at the top of Figure 5-12 will be displayed. Note that the menu options for the Actions button change according to the type of item that has focus. When a finding is selected, the Details option is presented; when a text macro is selected, the Data Field Entry option is available; but when a heading or subheading is selected, the options pertain to setting or unsetting all findings within the selected group. These include:

◆ Otherwise Normal

◆ Undo Otherwise Normal

◆ Select All Findings

◆ Clear Non-entered Findings

◆ Clear All Findings

Click in the drop-down menu and select the option **Otherwise Normal**. Compare the Review of Systems section of your screen to Figure 5-13.

**Figure 5-13** Review of Systems section with blue findings set by the Otherwise Normal function.

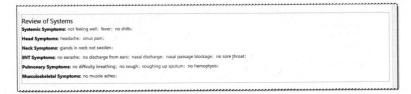

### Step 10

Harold's vital signs show a mild fever.

*Right-click* on the finding **fever.** Notice that the Actions drop-down menu options you are familiar with from previous exercises are displayed. This is because the selected item is a finding, not a heading.

Click Details on the Actions drop-down menu. Click the Modifier field in the Details pop-up window, and select **Mild** from the drop-down list, as you have in previous exercises. Click the OK button to close the pop-up window. If you used the Actions button instead of right-clicking, verify that the finding mild fever is still red. If it is not, click on it until it turns red and the description reads "mild fever."

### Step 11

Proceed to the physical exam.

Locate and click on the following Physical Exam findings until they turn red.

● nasal discharge
● purulent
● tenderness of sinuses
● chest percussion abnormal
● lungs and respiration auscultation

Compare the Physical Exam section of your screen to Figure 5-14 and verify that your physical exam findings are set correctly.

**Figure 5-14** Red findings recorded in the Physical Exam portion of the note.

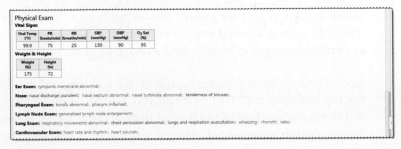

## Step 12

Now locate and click on the Physical Exam heading. Verify that the section is outlined in a box similar to the one in Figure 5-15. Next, click the Actions button on the Toolbar, and select Otherwise Normal from the drop-down menu.

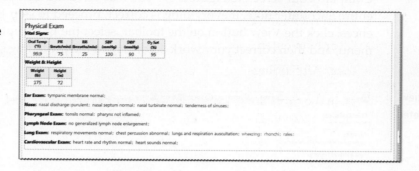

**Figure 5-15** Physical Exam portion of the encounter note after invoking the Otherwise Normal function.

Compare the Physical Exam section of your screen to Figure 5-15 and confirm your normal (blue) findings match the figure.

## Step 13

The clinician has determined that Harold has a common cold.

Proceed to the Assessment section, and then locate and click on the following finding:

- common cold

## Step 14

Since Harold is not improving, the clinician decides to order amoxicillin, but notices the allergy information is not recorded in the encounter note. Harold says he's not allergic to antibiotics, but the fact must be documented in the medical record.

Scroll to the top of the workspace, locate the clinical concept **allergy**, and click it until it turns blue and the description changes to "no allergy."

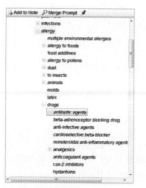

**Figure 5-16** Clinical concept tree for Allergy with antibiotic agents highlighted.

Locate and click the Browse button on the toolbar. The expanded tree of concepts should automatically display the allergy section of the history domain, as shown in Figure 5-16.

Locate and click on the small plus symbol next to "Drugs," and then in the expand tree click on "antibiotic agents" to highlight the concept. Locate and click the Add to Note button at the top of the Concept list.

The finding **no allergy to antibiotic agents** should be recorded in the allergy section. If it is not blue, click on it until it turns blue.

## Step 15

Locate the Navigation bar at the bottom of the workspace pane and click on the link "Plan." Your screen will scroll to the plan section.

Locate **amoxicillin** and click it until it turns red.

Proceed to the Therapy section, and there, locate and click on the following findings:

- cool mist vaporizer
- fluids

**Step 16**

Locate and click the View button on the toolbar, and then select Concise from the drop-down menu.

Compare your screen to Figure 5-17. You may have to scroll your screen to see the entire encounter note. If everything is correct, proceed to step 17. If there are any differences, click the View button on the toolbar, select the Entry option on the drop-down menu, and then correct your work according to the preceding steps.

**Figure 5-17** Concise view of Harold Baker's completed encounter note.

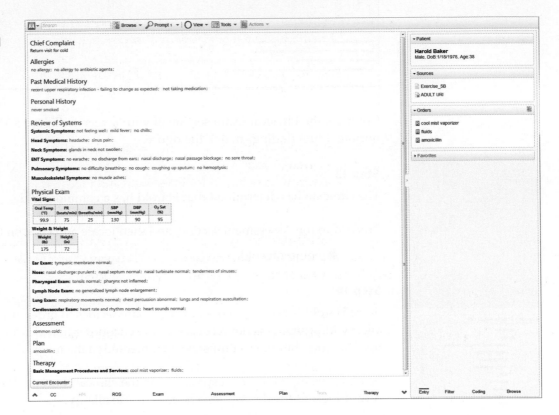

**Step 17**

If wish to print a copy of your completed encounter notes for yourself or because your instructor requires you to turn them in, use the Create PDF option, and then print or download the PDF at this time.

The final step in every exercise is to submit your completed work for a grade.

Locate and click the blue Quippe icon button on the toolbar, and then select the Submit for Grade option from the drop-down menu. This will complete Exercise 5B.

In this exercise, you have practiced using lists and learned to use the Otherwise Normal feature to quickly complete Review of Systems and Physical Exam sections.

## Critical Thinking Exercise 5C: Using Syncope List for a TIA Case

Now that you have learned that the Lists and Otherwise Normal features can help you enter EHR data more quickly, prove it to yourself with this exercise. In this exercise you will apply what you have learned, by using a different list for a different type of condition.

## Case Study

Victoria Mayhew is an 82-year-old female admitted for syncope (fainting) and what was probably a TIA or Transient Ischemic Attack. The patient experienced a sudden loss of consciousness for less than 5 minutes, as reported by her daughter who accompanied her to the hospital. For approximately 20 minutes following this episode, she experienced mild confusion and difficulty talking, and now doesn't recall the incident at all. There don't seem to be any residual effects except mild confusion as to the situation.

### Step 1

Start a supported web browser program and follow the steps listed inside the cover of this textbook to log in to the MyHealthProfessionsLab for this course.

Locate and click on the link **Exercise 5C**. This will open the Quippe software window with the New Encounter window displayed in the center.

### Step 2

Patients are listed in alphabetical order by last name. Locate and click on the patient named **Mayhew, Victoria**. Once you have selected the patient, click the OK button. In this exercise, you do not need to set the date and time of the encounter.

### Step 3

Click in the blank space under the heading Chief Complaint as you have in previous exercises, and type **Patient fainted without warning while sitting in a chair, followed by 20 minutes of confusion with difficulty talking**.

### Step 4

Begin the encounter by recording Victoria's vital signs.

Enter Victoria's vital signs and weight and height in the corresponding fields as follows:

| | |
|---|---|
| Oral Temperature: | **98.2** |
| Pulse rate: | **72** |
| Respiration: | **18** |
| SBP: | **140** |
| DBP: | **96** |
| $O_2$ Sat | **95** |
| Weight: | **99** |
| Height: | **60** |

### Step 5

Victoria is accompanied by her daughter, who is providing the information about the incident. Proceed to the Review of Systems section and locate the label "Source of patient information." Locate the down-arrow at the end of the line. A drop-down list will appear. Select **child** from the drop-down list.

### Step 6

Because her daughter reported that Victoria fainted, we will use a List created for documenting this type of incident (syncope).

Click on any whitespace in the workspace that does not cause a concept or heading to have focus. Locate and click on the Browse button in the Toolbar at the top of your screen, and then click the plus symbol next to the Sample Custom Content book icon. When the tree is expanded, locate and click on the plus symbols next to "Shared Content" and "Student Edition Lists."

Scroll downward to the end of the lists to locate and click on the name **M CV Syncope** to highlight it, and then click on the Add to Note button.

Clinical concepts from the list will populate the workspace.

### Step 7

Locate and click on the following symptoms until they turn red:

- fainting
- speech disturbance

*Right-click* speech disturbance and select Details from the Actions drop-down menu.

In the Details pop-up window, locate and click on the Status field, and then select **improving** from the drop-down list. Click on the OK button to close the pop-up window.

The description should change to "Speech disturbance – improving."

### Step 8

Locate and click on the Review of Systems section heading. The entire section should become outlined.

Locate and click the Actions button on the toolbar and select Otherwise Normal from the drop-down menu.

### Step 9

Scroll to the top of the workspace and document the patient's past medical history.

Locate and click on the following history finding until it turns red:

- cardiac problems

*Right-click* on the finding and select Details from the Actions drop-down menu.

In the Details pop-up window, locate and click in the Onset field, and then type **5 years**. Click on the OK button to close the pop-up window.

The finding should be red and its description should read "cardiac problems 5 years ago."

Locate and click on the Past Medical History section heading. The entire section should become outlined.

Locate and click the Actions button on the toolbar and select Otherwise Normal from the drop-down menu.

The remaining history items will be recorded as normal except for murmur, which will remain unentered. This is because murmur could be part of her cardiac problems, so it is not automatically set normal.

**Step 10**

Proceed to Personal History, which has one finding. Click on it until it turns red.

- a history of coronary artery disease

**Step 11**

Victoria's daughter says her mother has never smoked, and stopped drinking alcohol 20 years ago. Proceed to Behavioral History and click each of the following findings until they turn red.

- never smoked
- stopped drinking alcohol

Victoria's daughter doesn't know the precise date, so just type **1986** in the date field. The field will display January 1, 1986 (as 1/1/86).

**Step 12**

Victoria does not use recreational drugs, and her activity has not recently decreased.

Locate and click on the following findings until they turn blue:

- drug use
- physical activity tolerance recently decreased

The descriptions will change.

**Step 13**

Proceed to the Physical Exam section.

Locate **Neurological Exam** and click on the finding until it turns blue.

Locate and click the Browse button on the toolbar. The Concepts list should automatically open to neurological exam. Click on the red stickpin to hold the list open.

Click the small plus symbols next to the following concepts to expand the tree: "level of consciousness decreased," "cognitive functions diminished," "orientation," and "disoriented." By expanding the tree first it will be easier to add multiple findings to the note.

Beginning beneath "level of consciousness decreased," work your way down the expanded tree. Locate each of the following findings, click on it, and click the Add to Note button. Add the following neurological findings:

- drowsy
- confusion
- to time, place, and person
- to date
- to situation

Click the Browse button on the toolbar to close the list.

Because the finding "neurological exam" was blue when we added the neurological concepts, the additional findings were also recorded as normal (blue) as well.

### Step 14

However, all is not normal; the patient is confused as to where she is and states she doesn't remember the incident ever happening. Modify three findings.

Click on the finding "neurological exam normal" until it turns red and reads: **neurological exam**

Click on the finding "oriented to situation" until it turns red and reads **disoriented to situation**.

*Right-click* disoriented to situation and select Details from the Actions drop-down menu. Click in the Note field in the Details pop-up window and type **patient doesn't recall incident**.

Click the OK button to close the pop-up window. The description should now read "disoriented to situation patient doesn't recall incident."

Click on the finding "no confusion" until it turns red and reads **confusion**, then *right-click* and select Details from the Actions drop-down menu. In the Details pop-up window locate and click in the Modifier field, and select **mild** from the drop-down list of modifiers.

Click the OK button to close the pop-up window. The description should now read "mild confusion."

### Step 15

Locate and click on the Physical Exam section heading. The entire section should become outlined.

Locate and click the Actions button on the toolbar and select Otherwise Normal from the drop-down menu.

All physical exam findings not previously recorded will be set as normal except three: tachycardia, heart sounds, and murmur, which should remain unentered.

### Step 16

Proceed to the Assessment section.

Locate and click on the finding **transient ischemic attack** until it turns red.

### Step 17

The doctor has told the nurse he is going to admit Ms. Mayhew for overnight observation and orders a CT scan of her head.

Proceed to the Tests section, and locate and click on the finding **CT scan of head** until it turns red.

Proceed to the Therapy section, and locate and click on the finding **hospitalization** until it turns red.

### Step 18

Locate and click View button on the toolbar, and then select Concise from the drop-down menu.

Compare your screen to Figure 5-18. (Note: the screen in the figure is elongated; you will need to scroll your screen to compare all of it.) If everything is correct, proceed to step 19. If there are any differences, click the View button on the toolbar, select the Entry option on the drop-down menu, and then correct your work according to the preceding steps.

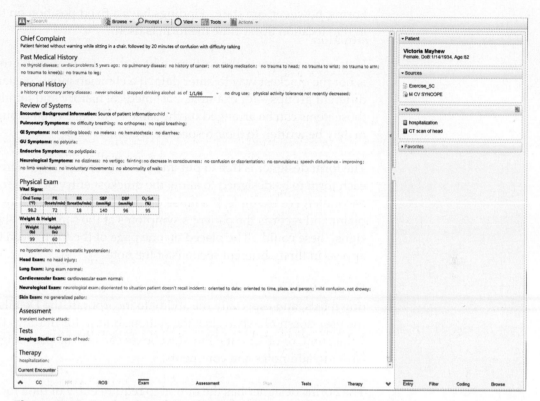

**Figure 5-18** Concise view of completed encounter note for Victoria Mayhew.

### Step 19

If wish to print a copy of your completed encounter notes for yourself or because your instructor requires you to turn them in, use the Create PDF option, and then print or download the PDF at this time.

The final step in every exercise is to submit your completed work for a grade.

Locate and click the blue Quippe icon button on the toolbar, and then select the Submit for Grade option from the drop-down menu. This will complete Exercise 5C.

## The Concept of Forms

In this chapter, you experienced the value of using predesigned lists for specific types of exams such as Adult URI and Syncope. Another feature that can speed up data entry is called a **Form**.

Forms are pop-up windows that display a desired group of clinical concepts in a consistent position every time. Forms enable quick entry of positive and negative findings, as well as finding Details such as value or onset date.

## Comparison of Lists and Forms

The value of lists is that they are dynamic and expand as necessary. A side effect of this is that sometimes findings do not appear in the same place in the workspace. This is because the addition of findings from the list has pushed them further down the screen, so the user must scroll the workspace to find them.

Forms, however, are static. Findings have a fixed position on the form and will remain in that location every time the form is used.

Lists add concepts to the sections where they are normally grouped. But sometimes this is not the quickest way to enter data. If a clinician must constantly move between two different groups—for example, past medical history and family medical history—then those items can be arranged on the same form page even though the findings will ultimately be written to their respective sections.

The form designer is free to put any clinical concept anywhere on the form. This allows each form to be designed to allow the quickest entry of data for a particular type of encounter. For example, if a nurse or medical assistant routinely enters the Chief complaint and records the patient's symptoms at the same time she or he takes the vital signs, these could all be placed on one page of the form, even though the findings will appear in three different sections of the note.

Forms offer many additional features to the designer. These include check boxes, drop-down lists, and especially the ability to incorporate the Details fields in the design, so the user doesn't have to click the Actions button for findings that consistently require value, unit, or other data. Free-text boxes can also be pre-assigned in a form, making it easier to add notes and comments.

The Forms designer has the option to require entry of data for certain findings before the form can be closed, as well as to decide on which pages the Otherwise Normal feature may be used.

# Initial Intake Form for an Adult

The intake form used in the following exercise provides an example of the different designs and features that are possible with forms. These include the unique ability to record two types of history at once, the Otherwise Normal feature, and other features you will explore during the exercise.

Figure 5-19 is an example of a form that might be found in a medical facility that uses paper medical records. You have probably seen a similar form at your own doctor's office. As you complete the following exercise, notice the similarities to the design of the EHR form. Electronic forms are one of the easiest ways to use an EHR.

### Guided Exercise 5D: Using Forms

In this exercise, you will use an EHR form to record symptoms, history, and a physical exam. The EHR form, in this case, has been abridged to shorten the time it takes a student to complete the exercise; a full version of the form like the one used in a medical office would have much more detail. A short intake form might be used by a nurse or medical assistant for prescreening.

## Memorial Hospital
## Anytown, USA

Date: _____

Patient Name: _____
Date of Birth: _____
❑ Male    ❑ Female

Race: _____

What is the reason you are here today?

_____

Please check any of the following conditions which you have had

**General**
❑ Serious Infections
  (e.g. pneumonia)
❑ Diabetes Mellitus
❑ Rheumatic fever
❑ HIV Infection
❑ Cancer

**Cardiovascular**
❑ High Blood Pressure
❑ Congestive Heart failure
❑ Heart Murmur
❑ Heart Valve Disease
❑ Angina
❑ Heart Attack
❑ High Cholesterol
❑ Abnormal Heart Rhythm
❑ Blood Clot in Veins
❑ Blocked Arteries in Neck
❑ Blocked Arteries in Legs

**HEENT**
❑ Glaucoma
❑ Allergies "hay fever"
❑ Frequent Ear Infections
❑ Frequent Sinus Infections

**Respiratory**
❑ Asthma
❑ Emphysema
❑ Blood Colt in Lungs
❑ Sleep Apnea

**Musculoskeletal /
Extremities**
❑ Osteoporosis
❑ Rheumatoid Arthritis
❑ Degenerative Joint Disease
❑ Fibrmyalgia
❑ Neck Pain (herniated disk)
❑ Back Pain (herniated disc)

**GI/GU**
❑ Stomach Ulcers
❑ Ulcerative Colitis
❑ Crohns Disease
❑ Bleeding from Intestines
❑ Diverticulitis
❑ Colon Polyps
❑ Irritable Bowel Disease
❑ Hepatitis
❑ Cirrhosis of the liver
❑ Liver Failure
❑ Pancreatitis
❑ Gallstones
❑ Kidney Stones
❑ Kidney Failure
❑ Prostate Disease
❑ Endometriosis
❑ Sex Transmitted Infection

**Lymphatic / Hematologic**
❑ Thyroid Goiter
❑ Over Active Thyroid
❑ Under Active Thyroid
❑ Transfusions
❑ Anemia

**Skin / Breast**
❑ Acne
❑ Eczema
❑ Psoriasis
❑ Fibrocystic Breast Disease

**Neurological / Psychiatric**
❑ Chronic Vertigo (Meniere's)
❑ Peripheral Nerve Disease
❑ Migraine Headaches
❑ Stroke
❑ Multiple Sclerosis
❑ Depression
❑ Anxiety

Please check any of the following major illnesses in your family members:

❑ Tuberculosis
❑ Emphysema
❑ Heart Disease
❑ High Blood Pressure
❑ Osteoporosis

❑ Diabetes Mellitus
❑ Thyroid Disease
❑ Anemia
❑ Hemophilia
❑ Other _____

❑ Kidney Disease
❑ Epilepsy
❑ Neurological Disorder
❑ Liver Disease
❑ Other _____

❑ Breast Cancer
❑ Ovarian Cancer
❑ Colon Cancer
❑ Prostate Cancer
❑ Other _____

If you have had surgery please indicate the year:

| Year | Surgery | Year | Surgery | Year | Surgery | Year | Surgery |
|------|---------|------|---------|------|---------|------|---------|
| ____ | Angioplasty | ____ | Colonoscopy | ____ | Neurosurgery | ____ | Tubal ligation |
| ____ | Appendectomy | ____ | Coronary Bypass | ____ | Sinus Surgery | ____ | C-Section |
| ____ | Back or Neck Surgery | ____ | Ear Surgery | ____ | Stomach Surgery | ____ | Hysterectomy |
| ____ | Bladder Surgery | ____ | Gallbladder | ____ | Thyroid Surgery | ____ | Ovary Removed |
| ____ | Carotid Artery Surgery | ____ | Hip Surgery | ____ | Tonsillectomy | ____ | Breast Surgery |
| ____ | Carpal Tunnel Surgery | ____ | Inguinal Hernia | ____ | Trauma Related Surgery | ____ | Thyroid Surgery |
| ____ | Chest/lung Surgery | ____ | Knee Surgery | ____ | Vascular Surgery | ____ | Other |

Please indicate when you had the following preventative services:

| Date | Immunizations | Date | Tests | Date | Tests / Exams | Date | Tests / Exams |
|------|---------------|------|-------|------|---------------|------|---------------|
| ____ | Flu Vaccine | ____ | Chest X-ray | ____ | Colon Cancer Stool Test | ____ | Breast Exam |
| ____ | Hepatitis Vaccine | ____ | EKG | ____ | Flexible Sigmoidoscopy, | ____ | Mammogram |
| ____ | Pneumonia Vaccine | ____ | Echocardiogram | ____ | Rectal Exam | ____ | Pap Smear |
| ____ | Tetanus Booster | ____ | Stress Test | ____ | Barium Enema | ____ | Bone Density Test |
| ____ | Other | ____ | Cardiac Angiogram | ____ | Prostate Cancer Blood Test | ____ | Date of last Physical Exam |

### Personal Habits

**Tobacco**
❑ Never
❑ Previous user
❑ Current user
# packs per day _____

**Alcohol**
❑ Never
❑ Previous user
❑ Current user
# drinks per day _____

**Caffeine**
❑ Never
❑ Previous user
❑ Current user
# cups per day _____

**Illicit Drugs**
❑ Never
❑ Previous user
❑ Current user

**Figure 5-19** Sample of a paper intake form to be completed by the patient.

**Case Study**

Terry Chun is a 32-year-old female complaining of an excruciating headache lasting more than one week. She is being admitted for status migrainosus.

**Step 1**

Start a supported web browser program and follow the steps listed inside the cover of this textbook to log in to the MyHealthProfessionsLab for this course.

Locate and click on the link **Exercise 5D**. This will open the Quippe software window with the New Encounter window displayed in the center.

**Step 2**

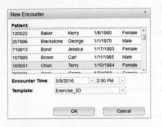

**Figure 5-20** Selecting Terry Chun from the Patient Selection window.

In the New Encounter window patient list, locate and click on **Chun, Terry** as shown in Figure 5-20, and then click the OK button. In this exercise, you do not need to set the date and time of the encounter.

**Step 3**

Click in the blank space under the Chief Complaint heading as you have in previous exercises, and type **Severe headaches**

You can compare your Chief Complaint to the upper left portion of Figure 5-21.

**Figure 5-21** Chief complaint "Severe headaches"; also showing the drop-down menu for selecting the Short Intake form.

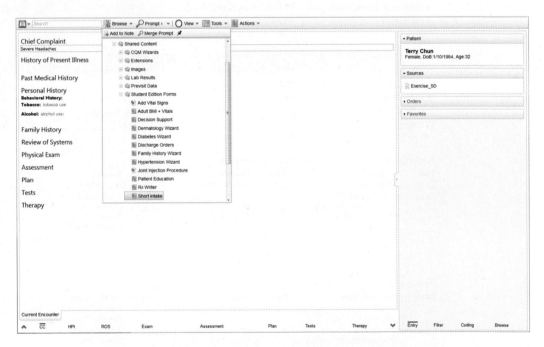

**Step 4**

Click anywhere in the workspace pane that does not highlight a finding or a heading, and then click the Browse button on the Toolbar at the top of the screen.

Locate and click the plus symbol next to the Sample Custom Content icon on the drop-down menu. When the tree is expanded, locate and click on the plus symbols next to "Shared Content" and "Student Edition Forms." The drop-down menu displays the various forms available to providers in the practice.

Locate and click on the form named Short Intake to highlight it (as shown in Figure 5-21) and then click on the Add to Note button.

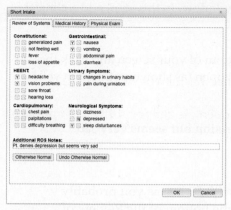

**Figure 5-22** Short Intake form, Review of Systems tab (before invoking Otherwise Normal).

The Short Intake form will be displayed. It will resemble Figure 5-22 except that none of your findings will have Y or N checked yet and Additional ROS notes will be blank.

### Step 5

Take a few minutes to study the form on your screen.

Note that at the top of the form there are tabs labeled Review of Systems, Medical History, and Physical Exam. This form has three pages on which you may enter data. In subsequent steps, you will use each of these pages to record findings from this form.

At the bottom of the form are OK and Cancel buttons. When you are finished using the form, clicking the OK button records the form data into the encounter note. Some forms require you to complete certain components or pages before the OK button is enabled. This form does not; the OK button can be clicked on any page.

Remember, even though the form looks different than the encounter note, you really are adding and removing findings on the note when you work with the form.

### Step 6

The Review of Systems tab uses Y/N checkboxes, which you are familiar with from earlier exercises.

The patient reports that she has severe headaches, causing vision problems, nausea, vomiting, and trouble sleeping.

Begin in the HEENT section of the form. Remember, HEENT stands for head, eyes, ears, nose, and throat. Locate and click in the **Y** check boxes for the following findings:

✓ **Y** headache

✓ **Y** vision problems

### Step 7

Locate the Gastrointestinal section of the form, and click in the **Y** check boxes for the following findings:

✓ **Y** nausea

✓ **Y** vomiting

Proceed to the Neurological Symptoms section of the form, and click the indicated check boxes for the following findings:

✓ **N** depressed

✓ **Y** sleep disturbances

Confirm that the Y/N check boxes on your screen match those in Figure 5-22.

## Step 8

Forms also allow entry of free-text notes right on the form. This saves the clinician the time it takes to add notes using the Details popup window. In this step, add a clinical impression to the ROS findings.

Locate the Additional ROS Notes section at the bottom of your screen and click the blank space just below it. A free-text entry box will open (as shown outlined in yellow in Figure 5-22).

In the box type the following text: **Pt. denies depression but seems very sad**.

## Step 9

The Otherwise Normal feature can also be used with forms, as you probably inferred from the presence of the two buttons at the bottom of the Review of Systems page.

First, observe and remember which findings have check boxes set to Y or N. Then, click the Otherwise Normal button. Notice that all findings on the page that were not previously set have been set to normal.

Click the Undo Otherwise Normal button. The findings should return to the state they were in Figure 5-22).

Locate the Neurological symptom "depressed" and notice the N check box is still set. Because the N box was set by the clinician, neither the Otherwise Normal nor the undo button altered the state of the finding.

Click the Otherwise Normal button once more to again set unentered findings to normal.

The Otherwise Normal functions are different between lists and forms. When a list is used, Otherwise Normal becomes available when any section or group is selected (by clicking its heading). In forms, the Otherwise Normal function applies to the entire tab page. Sections or group titles cannot be clicked individually in a form to limit the function. Also, the decision whether the Otherwise Normal and Undo buttons are available on a given tab is made by the form designer. This is because, as you will see in the next step, a form can mix findings from many different sections and groups on a single tab page.

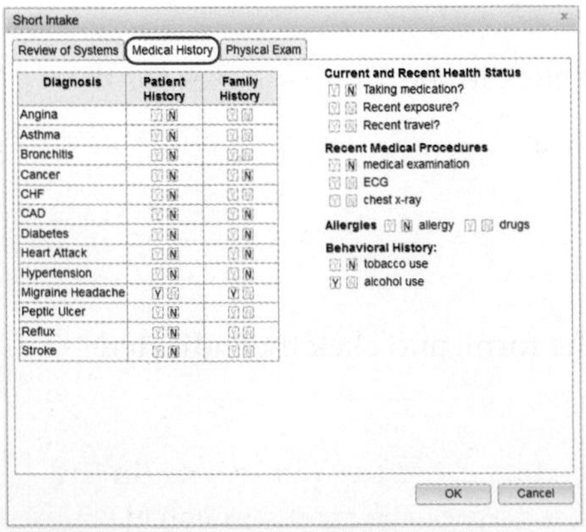

## Step 10

Locate the Medical History tab (circled in red in Figure 5-23) at the top of the form, and click on it.

This page illustrates another advantage of forms. Normally, when you do an intake history on a patient, you go through many items twice: "Have you ever had a heart attack? Has anyone in your family ever had a heart attack?" On this page, the form has been designed to save the clinician time, by making it easy to record answers to either personal, family history, or both types of history questions in adjacent columns. Compare the information on this tab of the EHR form with the paper form in Figure 5-19.

**Figure 5-23** Short Intake form, Medical History tab (correctly completed).

**Step 11**

Sometimes patients do not know the medical history of other family members; therefore, you will only record findings the patient is sure about. As the medical assistant asks Ms. Chun the history questions, the patient will know the answer to only some of them.

Enter the Patient History and Family History only for the following items:

| Diagnosis | Patient History | Family History |
|---|---|---|
| Angina | ✓ N | |
| Asthma | ✓ N | |
| Bronchitis | ✓ N | |
| Cancer | ✓ N | ✓ N |
| CHF (congestive heart failure) | ✓ N | |
| CAD (coronary artery disease) | ✓ N | ✓ N |
| Diabetes | ✓ N | ✓ N |
| Heart Attack | ✓ N | ✓ N |
| Hypertension | ✓ N | ✓ N |
| Migraine headache | ✓ Y | ✓ Y |
| Peptic Ulcer | ✓ N | |
| Reflux | ✓ N | |
| Stroke | ✓ N | |

**Step 12**

Terry tells the nurse that she is not currently taking medication and has not had a recent medical examination. She does not have allergies and does not smoke, but does drink a couple of glasses of wine a week.

Complete the rest of her medical history in the right side of the form page by locating and clicking on the Y and N check boxes as shown in the following table:

| | |
|---|---|
| Taking Medication | ✓ N |
| Medical Examination | ✓ N |
| Allergy | ✓ N |
| Tobacco use | ✓ N |
| Alcohol use | ✓ Y |

Carefully compare your screen to Figure 5-23 before proceeding. Verify that you have checked only the boxes indicated.

**Step 13**

Locate the Physical Exam tab (circled in red in Figure 5-24) at the top of the form, and click on it.

The first thing you will notice about this page is that it includes the Vital Signs (in the upper left corner of the page). Recording vital signs as part of the intake physical saves time. This page illustrates how forms can combine many different elements to make data entry more convenient.

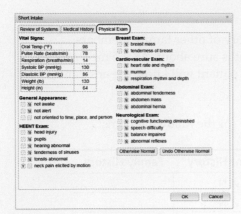

**Figure 5-24** Short Intake form, Physical Exam tab (correctly completed).

Enter the following vital signs for Terry Chun:

| | |
|---|---|
| Oral Temperature: | 98 |
| Pulse Rate: | 78 |
| Respiration: | 14 |
| Systolic BP: | 130 |
| Diastolic BP: | 86 |
| Weight: | 133 |
| Height: | 64 |

### Step 14

During the physical, the nurse observes the patient has neck pain elicited by motion. Locate the finding **Neck pain on motion** and click the check box for **Y**.

Everything else appears normal. Locate the Otherwise Normal button at the bottom of the second column, and click on it.

All Physical Exam findings with check boxes should have Y or N checked *except* **not oriented to time, place, and person**, which should have neither Y nor N checked. As you will recall from the previous exercise, this clinical concept is within the tree of cognitive functioning; since this finding was left unentered, the parent concept was not abnormal.

Compare your screen to Figure 5-24. If everything is correct, locate and click the OK button on the bottom of the form.

When the form closes, the encounter note now contains findings that were entered on the form. Notice that the findings do not have check boxes. One advantage of forms is that check boxes used for data entry can be omitted from the encounter note. As discussed earlier, many clinicians believe encounter notes without boxes look more professional when printed or sent to a colleague.

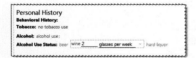

**Figure 5-25** Behavioral History portion of Terry Chun's encounter note.

### Step 15

Locate the Personal history section and notice that answering the question about alcohol use in the form invoked the additional alcohol questions required to document the patient's alcohol consumption.

Locate and click on **wine**, and then type **2** in the value field for glasses per week, as shown in Figure 5-25.

### Step 16

Compare your screen to Figure 5-26. Notice the Past Medical History and Family History sections. Although the clinical concepts in the form were in adjacent columns, the findings in the encounter note are automatically positioned in their assigned sections.

Similarly, other items recorded on the form Medical History page are now located in the Allergies, Reported Medical History, Reported Medication History, and Behavioral History groups.

### Step 17

Even though check boxes are only used in the form, the state of the recorded findings in the encounter note can be changed by clicking on the finding description (as you have done in previous exercises).

**Figure 5-26** Allergies, Histories, and ROS findings entered in encounter via Short Intake form.

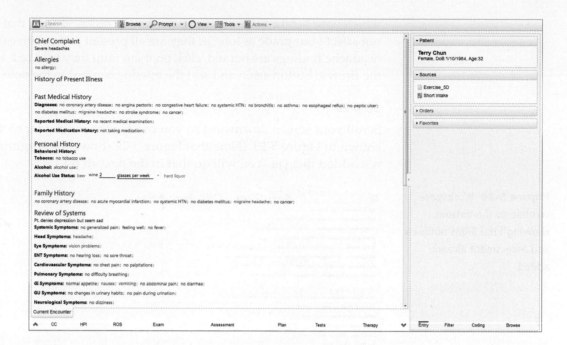

Locate Head Symptoms in the Review of Systems section, and click on **headache**. The finding will change to blue and its description to "no headache." Click it again, and it will turn gray (unentered). Click it one more time, and it turns red.

### Step 18

The patient says her headaches are excruciating, the worst she has ever had. They have been unremitting for over a week and are keeping her from sleeping.

With the (red) finding "headache" highlighted, click the Browse button on the toolbar. The list of concepts should automatically open to headache symptoms.

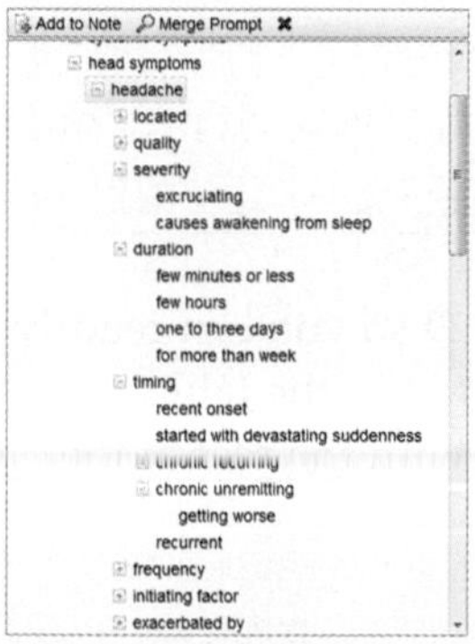

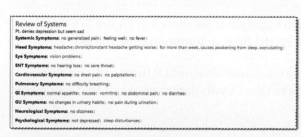

**Figure 5-27** Expand the trees for severity, duration, timing, and chronic unremitting, showing concepts to add to note.

Locate and click the red stickpin in the upper right corner of the list to hold the list open.

Expand the tree for "Headache" by clicking on the small plus symbols next to "Severity," "Duration," "Timing," and "Chronic/Unremitting." The expanded tree should look like Figure 5-27.

Locate and click on **excruciating** to highlight it and then click the Add to Note button.

Locate and click on **causing awakening from sleep** to highlight it and then click the Add to Note button.

Locate and click on **for more than a week** to highlight it and then click the Add to Note button.

Locate and click on **getting worse** to highlight it and then click the Add to Note button.

Click on the Browse button to close the list of concepts.

### Step 19

Because headache was already red, the four new findings will probably be added in the red state. Compare your group of Head Symptoms to those in Figure 5-28. Note that the sequence in

**Figure 5-28** Review of Systems portion of encounter with additional headache symptoms.

which your headache findings appear may be different from that in the figure. This will not affect your grade as long as they are all present and positive (red). If any of the headache findings are not red, click on them until they turn red. If any are missing, click the Browse button again and add the missing concept to the note.

**Step 20**

Scroll your screen downward so you can see the remainder of the encounter note as shown in Figure 5-29. (Note that Figure 5-29 shows the admitting diagnosis. We have not added this yet. You will do that in the next step.)

**Figure 5-29** Workspace scrolled to the bottom, showing Vital Signs outlined and assessment already added.

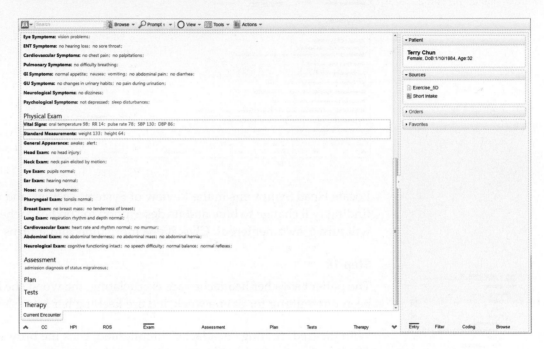

Vital Signs and Standard Measurements are outlined in Figure 5-29 so you can readily locate them. Notice that vital signs, weight, and height are not listed in the table format of previous exercises, but in a narrative format consistent with the rest of the encounter note.

**Step 21**

Ms. Chun is being admitted for overnight observation.

Locate and click the Assessment heading, and then click the Browse button on the toolbar. Click on the plus symbols next to Concepts and the domain Diagnoses, Syndromes and Conditions.

Scroll the list to locate "Neurologic Disorders." Click the small plus symbols to expand the tree for neurologic disorders, headache syndromes, and migraine.

Locate and click on **status migrainosus** to highlight it (as shown in Figure 5-30, and then click the Add to Note button. Click on the Browse button to close the list.

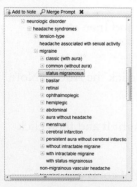

**Figure 5-30** Expanded tree of neurologic disorder, headache syndromes, and migraine with status migrainosus highlighted.

Locate and click status migrainosus in the encounter note until it turns red, and then click the Actions button on the toolbar. Select the Details option on the drop-down menu.

**Step 22**

Locate and click in the Prefix field in the Details pop-up window. Select "Admission diagnosis of" from the drop-down list of prefixes, as shown in Figure 5-31. Click the OK

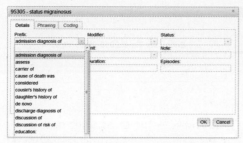

**Figure 5-31** Detail pop-up window with Prefix "admission diagnosis of" selected.

button to close the pop-up window. The description should change to "Admission diagnosis of migraine headache."

Compare your Assessment section to the one at the bottom of Figure 5-29.

### Step 23

Locate and click the blue Quippe icon button on the toolbar. Select the option Create PDF on the drop-down menu. A PDF of your encounter note will open in a new window.

The PDF will consist of two pages. You may need to scroll the PDF to see all of it. Compare your PDF to Figure 5-32a and Figure 5-32b. If everything

**Figure 5-32a** PDF of encounter note for Terry Chun (Page 1 of 2). See overleaf for page 2.

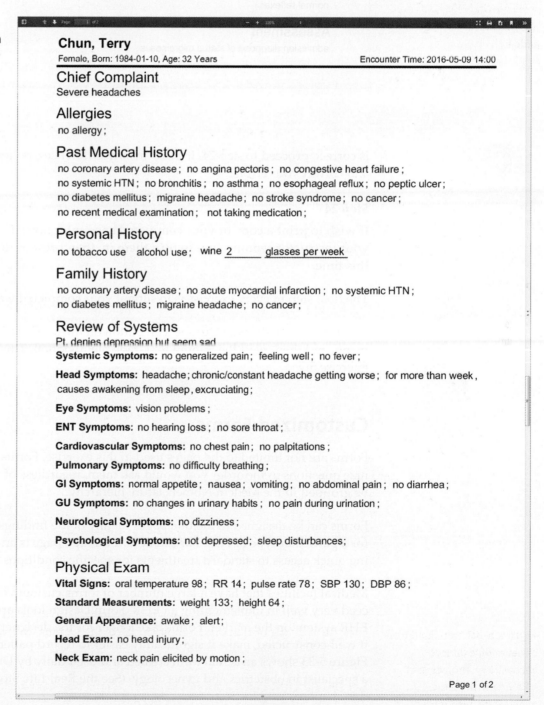

**Chun, Terry**
Female, Born: 1984-01-10, Age: 32 Years          Encounter Time: 2016-05-09 14:00

### Chief Complaint
Severe headaches

### Allergies
no allergy ;

### Past Medical History
no coronary artery disease ;  no angina pectoris ;  no congestive heart failure ;
no systemic HTN ;  no bronchitis ;  no asthma ;  no esophageal reflux ;  no peptic ulcer ;
no diabetes mellitus ;  migraine headache ;  no stroke syndrome ;  no cancer ;
no recent medical examination ;   not taking medication ;

### Personal History
no tobacco use    alcohol use ;    wine 2_____ glasses per week

### Family History
no coronary artery disease ;  no acute myocardial infarction ;  no systemic HTN ;
no diabetes mellitus ;  migraine headache ;  no cancer ;

### Review of Systems
Pt. denies depression but seem sad

**Systemic Symptoms:** no generalized pain ;  feeling well ;  no fever ;

**Head Symptoms:** headache ; chronic/constant headache getting worse ;  for more than week ,
causes awakening from sleep , excruciating ;

**Eye Symptoms:** vision problems ;

**ENT Symptoms:** no hearing loss ;  no sore throat ;

**Cardiovascular Symptoms:** no chest pain ;  no palpitations ;

**Pulmonary Symptoms:** no difficulty breathing ;

**GI Symptoms:** normal appetite ;  nausea ;  vomiting ;  no abdominal pain ;  no diarrhea ;

**GU Symptoms:** no changes in urinary habits ;  no pain during urination ;

**Neurological Symptoms:** no dizziness ;

**Psychological Symptoms:** not depressed ;  sleep disturbances ;

### Physical Exam
**Vital Signs:** oral temperature 98 ;  RR 14 ;  pulse rate 78 ;  SBP 130 ;  DBP 86 ;

**Standard Measurements:** weight 133 ;  height 64 ;

**General Appearance:** awake ;  alert ;

**Head Exam:** no head injury ;

**Neck Exam:** neck pain elicited by motion ;

Page 1 of 2

**Figure 5-32b** PDF of encounter note for Terry Chun (Page 2 of 2).

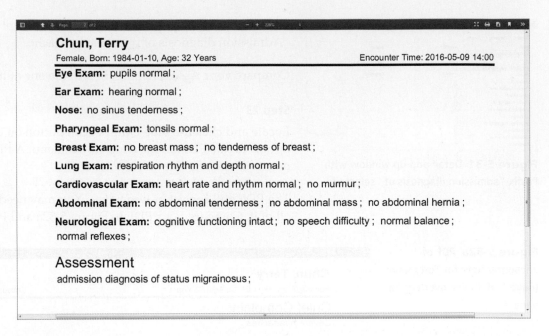

**Chun, Terry**
Female, Born: 1984-01-10, Age: 32 Years                    Encounter Time: 2016-05-09 14:00

**Eye Exam:** pupils normal ;

**Ear Exam:** hearing normal ;

**Nose:** no sinus tenderness ;

**Pharyngeal Exam:** tonsils normal ;

**Breast Exam:** no breast mass ;  no tenderness of breast ;

**Lung Exam:** respiration rhythm and depth normal ;

**Cardiovascular Exam:** heart rate and rhythm normal ;  no murmur ;

**Abdominal Exam:** no abdominal tenderness ;  no abdominal mass ;  no abdominal hernia ;

**Neurological Exam:** cognitive functioning intact ;  no speech difficulty ;  normal balance ;
normal reflexes ;

## Assessment
admission diagnosis of status migrainosus ;

is correct, proceed to step 24. If there are any differences, review the preceding steps, and correct your errors.

**Step 24**

If wish to print a copy of your completed encounter notes for yourself or because your instructor requires you to turn them in, then print or download the PDF at this time.

The final step in every exercise is to submit your completed work for a grade.

Locate and click the blue Quippe icon button on the toolbar to display the drop-down menu, and then select the Submit for Grade menu option. This will complete Exercise 5D.

## Customized Forms

Forms are not limited to the pages used in this exercise. Forms also allow you to organize questions in the order you would ask them, regardless of where the findings may be grouped in the Medcin Nomenclature hierarchy.

Forms can be designed to include pages for any of the findings expected to be needed for a particular type of visit. For example, a therapy page is an excellent means of having quick access to standard treatments for specific conditions.

Medical facilities that have a large number of forms customized for their providers succeed very well in implementing an EHR. Form Design tools are a part of almost every EHR system on the market. Forms take longer for the designer to create than Lists, but, if well-constructed, make it significantly easier to record patient exams as they happen. Figure 5-33 shows an actual form created and used daily by Dr. Michael Lukowski, MD, a specialist in obstetrics and gynecology. (See the Real-Life Story by Dr. Lukowski in this chapter.)

**By Michael Lukowski, MD**

*Michael Lukowski is a specialist in obstetrics and gynecology. He has been practicing more than 25 years. He uses an EHR in his practice, enters his own data, and has designed his own EHR forms.*

I started using forms right away. When the trainer told me about forms, I thought, "This is the way to go." It slows you down if you have to search a lot. Forms gave me a discrete window into the database so that I could pick out things that I use day in and day out.

I try to put much of my exam in as data points (findings) rather than just free text. I use free text only as a comment to a finding. To me the whole idea of this is to have retrievable information that I can analyze over time. So I always try to use the (nomenclature) database as my main way to construct a note and then add free text to that if I have to. I find that I use less and less free text because I can pick out findings that say pretty much what I need to say.

## Workflow

Using forms, I do what I have always done. My nurse puts in the vital signs; we do some simple lab tests like a hematocrit. The patient is sitting in the exam room when I go in. I sit down and talk with her. As we are talking, I am filling in her history using a tablet computer, just like I used to do with a paper chart. When I am done with that part of the exam, I call my nurse in and do the physical exam.

When the physical exam is finished, I leave and come back to my office. While the patient gets dressed, I finish filling out the rest of the encounter. The patient comes to my office once she is dressed and we talk a little bit more; I finalize her note and write any prescription. If the patient has a pharmacy that receives electronic prescriptions, I transmit them directly to the pharmacy. If the pharmacy does not, I print it on paper and the staff brings it to me to sign.

## Forms

I use four forms: Gyn, Post-partum, Pre-op, and then one that contains all the procedures I do, which is still a work in progress, but it covers a lot.

I have a number of tabs within each form. For instance, the Gyn form starts with the intake page. My assistant fills in the menstrual history, pap smear, mammograms, methods of birth control, and so on.

I move through the rest of the tabs, except at the right side of the form; I use three different tabs for assessment so that I

can have all the diagnoses I normally use available without searching.

Figure 5-33 shows one of the forms I use every day. The Tabs are: Intake info, VS and Off Labs, Pain Hx, V & V, GI and UTI Sx, Meno & PMS, Fertility Eval, BC Counseling, Soc Hx, Med Hx, and three tabs for assessment.

The tabs are not necessarily in the order I use them but, rather, the order I made the form in—but I know where everything is. If I do want to browse, I have a search box right at the top of my form. I can type in a term I want and hit my search button.

This system—I'm in love with it. It takes either the same time or less time than it used to on paper and I get a note that is 10 times better.

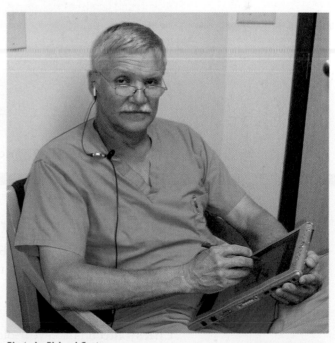

**Photo by Richard Gartee**

**Dr. Lukowski enters data in the exam room on a Tablet using an EHR form he designed.**

*(continued)*

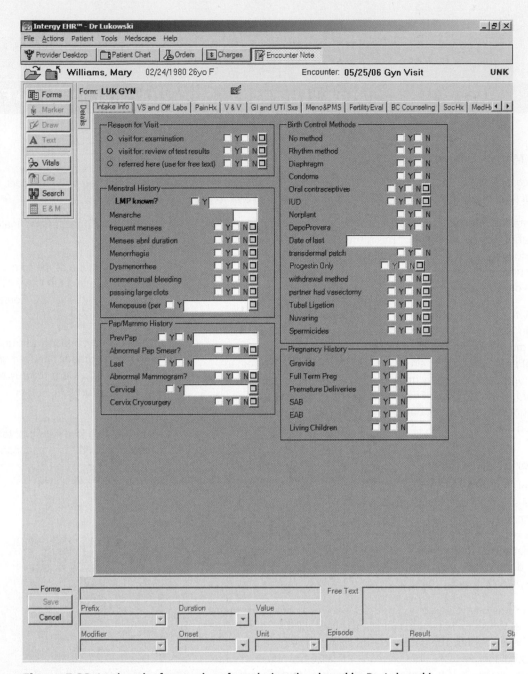

**Figure 5-33** Intake tab of gynecology form designed and used by Dr. Lukowski.

## Critical Thinking Exercise 5E: Using a Form and a List

In this exercise you will use both the form and the list from the previous exercises. Applying what you have learned so far, document Mr. Green's hospital admission.

### Case Study

Charles Green is a 33-year-old male with a complaint of a new-onset frequent cough that is progressively worse, especially at night. His chest hurts when he coughs, and he sometimes vomits because of the coughing. The patient was previously seen at his doctor's office and diagnosed with acute sinusitis. His condition has deteriorated. He is being admitted to the hospital for pneumonia.

**Step 1**

Start a supported web browser program and follow the steps listed inside the cover of this textbook to log in to the MyHealthProfessionsLab for this course.

Locate and click on the link **Exercise 5E**. This will open the Quippe software window with the New Encounter window displayed in the center.

**Step 2**

In the New Encounter window patient list, locate and click on **Green, Charles**.

Locate the date field and type **05/10/2016** or use the drop-down calendar to set the date to **May 10, 2016**. You do not need to set the time of the encounter.

Click the OK button.

**Step 3**

Click in the blank space under the Chief Complaint heading as you have in previous exercises, and type **Recurrent cough and dyspnea.**

**Step 4**

Click anywhere in the workspace pane that is not a finding or a heading, and then click the Browse button on the Toolbar at the top of the screen.

Locate and click the plus symbol next to the Sample Custom Content icon on the drop-down menu. When the tree is expanded, locate and click on the plus symbols next to Shared Content and Student Edition Forms. The drop-down menu displays the various forms available to providers in the practice.

Locate and click on the form named Short Intake to highlight it (as shown previously in Figure 5-21) and then click on the Add to Note button.

The Short Intake form will be displayed.

**Step 5**

The patient reports that he is feeling poorly, and has a fever, headaches, difficulty breathing, and trouble sleeping, but no chest pain.

On the Review of Systems tab locate and click in the check box next to the letter shown in bold typeface for the following findings:

✓ **Y** not feeling well

✓ **Y** fever

✓ **Y** headache

✓ **N** chest pain

✓ **N** palpitations

✓ **Y** difficulty breathing

✓ **Y** vomiting

✓ **Y** sleep disturbance

*Do not* click the Otherwise Normal button.

### Step 6

Locate and click the Medical History tab at the top of the form.

Enter the Patient History and Family History only for the following items:

| Diagnosis | Patient History | Family History |
|---|---|---|
| Bronchitis | ✓ Y | |
| Cancer | ✓ N | ✓ N |
| CHF (congestive heart failure) | ✓ N | ✓ N |
| CAD (coronary artery disease) | ✓ N | ✓ N |
| Diabetes | ✓ N | ✓ N |
| Heart Attack | ✓ N | ✓ N |
| Hypertension | ✓ N | |
| Migraine headache | ✓ N | |
| Peptic Ulcer | ✓ N | |
| Reflux | ✓ N | |
| Stroke | ✓ N | |

### Step 7

Locate **Taking Medication** and click the **Y** check box.

Locate **medical examination** and click the **Y** check box. A date field will open next to the finding. Type **05/06/2016** or use the drop-down calendar to set the date to May 6, 2016.

Locate **chest x-ray** and click the **N** check box.

Locate **allergy** and click the **N** check box.

Locate **tobacco use** and click the **Y** check box.

Locate **alcohol use** and click the **Y** check box.

### Step 8

Locate and click on the Physical Exam tab at the top of the form.

Enter Mr. Green's vital signs in the corresponding fields as follows:

| | |
|---|---|
| Oral Temperature: | **101** |
| Pulse Rate: | **88** |
| Respiration: | **26** |
| Systolic BP: | **130** |
| Diastolic BP: | **86** |
| Weight: | **174** |
| Height: | **68** |

**Step 9**

On the Physical Exam tab, locate and click in the check box containing the letter **Y** for the following findings:

✓ **Y** tenderness of sinuses

✓ **Y** neck pain on motion

✓ **Y** respiration rhythm and depth

Everything else is normal. Click on the Otherwise Normal button. Every item on the Physical Exam tab should now have data *except* "not oriented to time, place, and person."

Locate and click on the OK button at the bottom of the form to return to the encounter note.

**Step 10**

Locate Reported Medication History and click on the finding taking medication until it turns red.

Locate and click the Browse button on the toolbar. The list of concepts should open to medications in the history domain.

Scroll the list of Medcin concepts downward to locate "over-the-counter medications," and then click the plus symbol next to it to expand the tree. Locate and click on **for colds** to highlight it, and then click the Add to Note button. If the Concepts list does not close automatically, click on the Browse button to close it.

Verify that both findings—taking medication and taking OTC cold medication—are red.

**Step 11**

Proceed to Behavioral History and record Mr. Green's tobacco and alcohol use. You may recall from his previous visit, Mr. Green has been smoking a pack of cigarettes a day for twelve years and drinks two beers a week.

Locate and click on **current every day smoker**.

Additional clinical concepts will appear. Click on **cigarettes** and type: **12** in the pack-years field.

Locate Alcohol Use Status and click on **beer**. Type the number **2** in field for **bottles per week**.

**Step 12**

Click anywhere in the workspace pane that is not a finding or a heading, and then click the Browse button on the Toolbar at the top of the screen.

Locate and click the plus symbol next to the Sample Custom Content icon. When the tree is expanded, locate and click on the plus symbols next to Shared Content, and then on the plus symbol next to Student Edition Lists. Locate and click on the list named **Adult URI** to highlight it (refer to Figure 5-3) and then click on the Add to Note button.

**Step 13**

Begin in the Past Medical History section. Locate the clinical concept **recent upper respiratory infection** and click until it turns red.

**Step 14**

Proceed to the Review of Systems section. Locate and click on the following symptom findings until they turn red:

- sinus pain
- cough
- coughing up sputum

**Step 15**

Locate and click the Browse button on the toolbar. The concept list should open to "coughing up sputum." Locate "cough" just above it, and click on the small plus sign next to cough to expand the tree. Click the red stickpin icon to hold the list open.

Locate and click the concept **worse at night** to highlight it, and then click the Add to Note button.

Locate and click the concept **causing awakening from sleep** to highlight it, and then click the Add to Note button.

Click the Browse button to close the list. Two new findings, "cough causing awakening from sleep" and "cough worse at night," should be red. If not, click them until they turn red.

**Step 16**

Locate and click on the Review of Systems heading. The entire section should become outlined.

Locate and click on the Actions button on the toolbar, and then select Otherwise Normal from the drop-down menu.

**Step 17**

Proceed to the Physical Exam section and locate Lung Exam.

Locate and click on the following Lung Exam findings until they turn red:

- respiratory movements abnormal
- chest percussion abnormal
- wheezing
- ronchi

Locate and click on the Physical Exam heading. The entire section should become outlined.

Locate and click on the Actions button on the toolbar, and then select Otherwise Normal from the drop-down menu.

**Step 18**

Proceed to the Assessment section. Locate and click on the diagnosis **pneumonia** until it turns red.

*Right-click* on pneumonia and then select Details from the Actions drop-down menu.

Locate and click in the Prefix field in the Details pop-up window. Select "Admission diagnosis of" from the drop-down list of prefixes, as shown previously in Figure 5-31. Click the OK button to close the pop-up window.

The description should change to "Admission diagnosis of pneumonia."

### Step 19

The doctor orders a chest x-ray.

Proceed to the Tests section. Locate and click on **CXR with PA and lateral views** until it turns red.

### Step 20

Locate and click the blue Quippe icon button on the toolbar. Select the option Create PDF on the drop-down menu. A PDF of your encounter note will open in a new window.

The PDF will consist of two pages. You may need to scroll the PDF to see all of it. Compare your PDF to Figure 5-34a and Figure 5-34b. If everything is correct, proceed to step 21. If there are any differences, review the preceding steps and correct your errors.

**Figure 5-34a** PDF of encounter note for Charles Green's hospital intake (page 1 of 2). See overleaf for page 2.

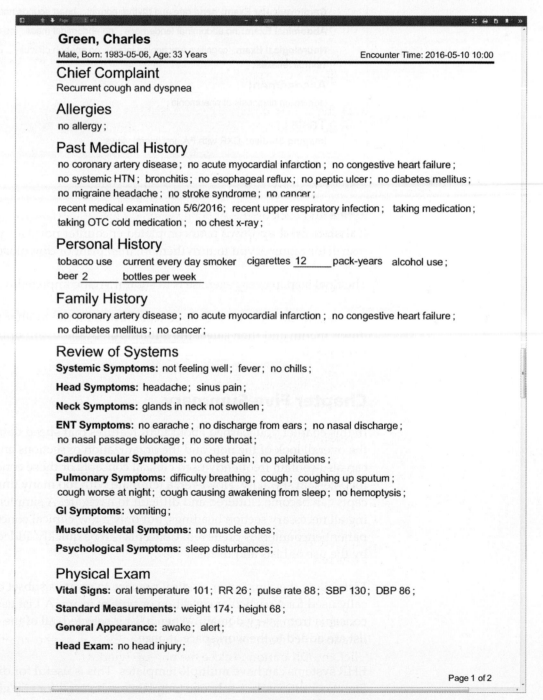

Green, Charles
Male, Born: 1983-05-06, Age: 33 Years                    Encounter Time: 2016-05-10 10:00

**Chief Complaint**
Recurrent cough and dyspnea

**Allergies**
no allergy;

**Past Medical History**
no coronary artery disease; no acute myocardial infarction; no congestive heart failure; no systemic HTN; bronchitis; no esophageal reflux; no peptic ulcer; no diabetes mellitus; no migraine headache; no stroke syndrome; no cancer; recent medical examination 5/6/2016; recent upper respiratory infection; taking medication; taking OTC cold medication; no chest x-ray;

**Personal History**
tobacco use    current every day smoker    cigarettes 12 ____ pack-years    alcohol use; beer 2 ____ bottles per week

**Family History**
no coronary artery disease; no acute myocardial infarction; no congestive heart failure; no diabetes mellitus; no cancer;

**Review of Systems**
**Systemic Symptoms:** not feeling well; fever; no chills;
**Head Symptoms:** headache; sinus pain;
**Neck Symptoms:** glands in neck not swollen;
**ENT Symptoms:** no earache; no discharge from ears; no nasal discharge; no nasal passage blockage; no sore throat;
**Cardiovascular Symptoms:** no chest pain; no palpitations;
**Pulmonary Symptoms:** difficulty breathing; cough; coughing up sputum; cough worse at night; cough causing awakening from sleep; no hemoptysis;
**GI Symptoms:** vomiting;
**Musculoskeletal Symptoms:** no muscle aches;
**Psychological Symptoms:** sleep disturbances;

**Physical Exam**
**Vital Signs:** oral temperature 101; RR 26; pulse rate 88; SBP 130; DBP 86;
**Standard Measurements:** weight 174; height 68;
**General Appearance:** awake; alert;
**Head Exam:** no head injury;

Page 1 of 2

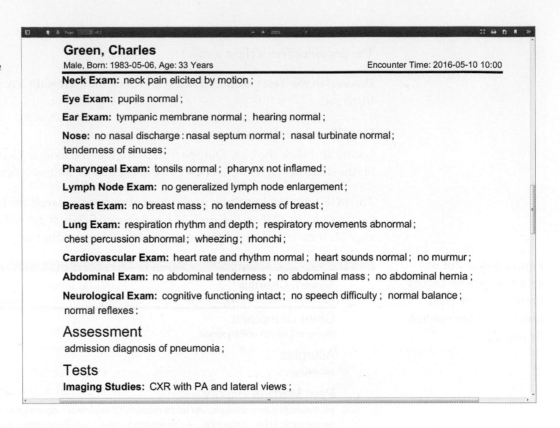

**Green, Charles**

Male, Born: 1983-05-06, Age: 33 Years        Encounter Time: 2016-05-10 10:00

**Neck Exam:** neck pain elicited by motion ;

**Eye Exam:** pupils normal ;

**Ear Exam:** tympanic membrane normal ;  hearing normal ;

**Nose:** no nasal discharge : nasal septum normal ;  nasal turbinate normal; tenderness of sinuses ;

**Pharyngeal Exam:** tonsils normal ;  pharynx not inflamed ;

**Lymph Node Exam:** no generalized lymph node enlargement ;

**Breast Exam:** no breast mass ;  no tenderness of breast ;

**Lung Exam:** respiration rhythm and depth ;  respiratory movements abnormal ; chest percussion abnormal ;  wheezing ;  rhonchi ;

**Cardiovascular Exam:** heart rate and rhythm normal ;  heart sounds normal ;  no murmur ;

**Abdominal Exam:** no abdominal tenderness ;  no abdominal mass ;  no abdominal hernia ;

**Neurological Exam:** cognitive functioning intact ;  no speech difficulty ;  normal balance ; normal reflexes ;

## Assessment
admission diagnosis of pneumonia ;

## Tests
**Imaging Studies:** CXR with PA and lateral views ;

## Step 21

If wish to print a copy of your completed encounter notes for yourself or because your instructor requires you to turn them in, then print or download the PDF at this time.

The final step in every exercise is to submit your completed work for a grade.

Locate and click the blue Quippe icon button on the toolbar to display the drop-down menu, and then select the Submit for Grade menu option. This will complete Exercise 5E.

## Chapter Five Summary

In this chapter you learned about EHR features that speed data entry. Templates define the overall look of the note and the organization of sections and headings. Templates can also contain frequently used clinical concepts or those concepts likely to be needed for a certain specialty. However, a template with too many unnecessary clinical concepts can become cluttered and difficult to navigate. A simpler template design containing all necessary section headings, but only a few clinical concepts required for most patient encounters is preferred. Concepts can be quickly added and findings recorded by the use of Lists and forms.

**Lists** allow the clinician or medical practice to create a subset of the nomenclature typically used for a particular condition or type of exam. A List usually contains clinical concepts from every domain. When a list is selected, all of the clinical concepts in the list are added to the workspace at once.

EHR systems can have multiple templates. This is useful for different providers or different conditions, but only one template can be used for any given encounter. Unlike templates, multiple lists (and forms) *can* be used in the same encounter. This is useful if a patient has multiple conditions.

Because using lists lessens the need to Browse for clinical concepts, lists are a sure way to speed up data entry of routine exams and increase adoption of the EHR by clinicians in the practice. Over time, medical practices should build up a library of Lists covering the medical conditions that are frequently seen at their practice.

A List is accessed by clicking the Browse button on the Toolbar, expanding the folders Sample Custom Content, Shared Content, and Student Edition Lists. Once the list is located, click it to highlight it and then click the Add to Note button at the top of the drop-down menu.

**Forms** display a desired group of findings in a presentation that allows for quick entry of not only positive and negative findings but of any Details fields such as value or dates. The form can also set prefixes as well. Forms provide some features that lists cannot; for example:

1. Forms are static; findings have a fixed position on Forms and will consistently remain in that position every time the form is opened.

2. Clinical concepts belonging to different sections of the encounter can be arranged on the same page of the form in any manner that will enable the quickest data entry.

3. Forms may include any Details fields, and a free-text box, eliminating the need for the pop-up window to record additional data.

4. Forms can use check boxes and drop-down lists for ease of data entry, yet omit them in the encounter note for a more readable presentation.

5. Forms can control which findings are required and which are optional; every question on a Form does not have to be answered for every visit.

6. Lists add all clinical concepts in the list to the workspace. Forms add only recorded findings to the workspace, skipping form items that were not entered.

A form is accessed by clicking the Browse button on the Toolbar, expanding the folders Sample Custom Content, Shared Content, and Student Edition Forms. Once the form is located, click it to highlight it and then click the Add to Note button. A pop-up window containing the form will be invoked. Clicking OK in the form window will record the findings in the note.

**Otherwise Normal** is another function that speeds up data entry. After recording abnormal findings, a clinician can quickly document normal findings by selecting a section or group heading and clicking Otherwise Normal on the Actions button drop-down menu. All unentered findings in the selected section or group are set to normal (except findings already set by the user and concepts whose parent finding is abnormal).

Otherwise Normal works best with lists, because the concepts added by lists to various sections are likely to be relevant to the current condition and therefore pertinent negatives.

Otherwise Normal may or may not be available on a form, as that decision is under the control of the form designer. If it is available, a button will present on the form page. On a multipage form, Otherwise Normal only sets findings on the current tab (page).

After completing this chapter, you should be comfortable with the general process of locating concepts and expanding the tree to view additional concepts, adding concepts using Lists, locating and using Forms, and using the Otherwise Normal feature.

| Task | Exercise | Page # |
|------|----------|--------|
| Locate the folder of lists and add a list to an encounter note | 5A | 155 |
| Locate and use Otherwise Normal | 5B | 163–164 |
| Locate the folder of forms and use a form to record findings | 5D | 174–175 |
| Use Otherwise Normal on a form | 5D | 176 |

## Testing Your Knowledge of Chapter 5

### Step 1

Log in to MyHealthProfessionsLab following the directions printed inside the cover of this textbook.

Locate and click on Chapter 5 Test.

### Step 2

Answer the test questions. When you have finished, click the Submit Test button to close the window.

## Testing Your Skill Exercise 5F: A Patient with Dyspnea

Now that you have performed all the exercises in Chapter 5 this exercise will help you and your instructor evaluate your skill at documenting a patient encounter. Use the features of the software you have practiced thus far in the course.

### Case Study

Howard Cook is an established patient who presents with dyspnea, a medical term for shortness of breath.

Howard's chief complaint is difficulty breathing. He is allergic to pollens and has a past medical history of asthma, but has not had a recent URI. He has had a recent chest x-ray that was normal. He does not smoke any more, but he formerly smoked a pack of cigarettes a day for four years.

He says he hasn't had a fever, and denies having any cardiovascular symptoms. Mr. Cook is having difficulty breathing, and is wheezing, but states that his difficulty breathing is not accompanied by chest pains. He reports awakening in the night short of breath.

When the clinician examines Howard's lungs she hears wheezing and observes Howard using accessory muscles during expiration. The findings of the cardiovascular exam are "otherwise normal." The clinician's assessment is asthma, but the concept is missing from the assessment section, and you will have to add it.

The clinician orders Howard a bronchodilator to ease his breathing and relieve the wheezing.

Howard's vital signs are as follows:

| | |
|---|---|
| Oral Temperature: | **98.6** |
| Pulse Rate: | **88** |
| Respiration: | **30** |
| Systolic BP: | **130** |
| Diastolic BP: | **90** |
| Weight: | **175** |
| Height: | **69** |

### Step 1

Start a supported web browser program and follow the steps listed inside the cover of this textbook to log in to the MyHealthProfessionsLab for this course.

Locate and click on the link **Exercise 5F**. This will open the Quippe software window with the New Encounter window displayed in the center.

### Step 2

Locate and click on the patient name, and then click the OK button. In this exercise, you do not need to set the date or time of the encounter.

### Step 3

Read the case study *carefully* and create an encounter note from the information provided in the case study.

*Hint*: Locate a list with the name of his presenting problem and add it to the note before you start.

*Hint*: Use the Add Vital Signs form to enter Howard's vital signs and standard measurements.

*Hint:* The diagnosis, asthma, is a respiratory disorder, in pulmonary obstructive disorders.

Once you have documented all the information provided in the case study, proceed to step 4.

### Step 4

If wish to print a copy of your completed encounter notes for yourself or because your instructor requires you to turn them in, use the Create PDF option, and then print or download the PDF at this time.

Submit your completed work for a grade using the Submit for Grade option on the application menu. This will complete Exercise 5F.

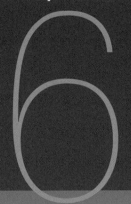

# Chapter Six

# Understanding
# Electronic Orders

## Learning Outcomes

*After completing this chapter, you should be able to:*

◆ Discuss the importance of electronic orders and results

◆ Search for a clinical concept

◆ Move a finding to a different encounter section

◆ Understand and use the Prompt feature

◆ Name the nine laboratory sciences and three areas of pathology

◆ Record orders for tests

◆ Explain the workflow of electronic orders and results

◆ Describe the workflow of radiology orders and reports

◆ Use a diagnosis to find protocols

◆ Order tests to confirm or rule out a diagnosis

◆ Use a CPOE to write a prescription

◆ Discuss Closed Loop Safe Medication Administration

◆ Name the five rights of medication administration

◆ Order medications using a quick-pick list

## The Importance of Electronic Orders and Results

As you learned in Chapter 1, computerized provider order entry, or CPOE, is viewed by IOM, Leapfrog, and others as one of the key features of an EHR that can improve quality of care, patient safety, and clinician efficiency.

According to the IOM report[1] CPOE systems can improve workflow processes by:

◆ Preventing lost orders

◆ Eliminating ambiguities caused by illegible handwriting

◆ Reducing the medication errors of dose and frequency, drug–allergy, and drug–drug interactions

◆ Monitoring for duplicate orders

◆ Reducing the time to fill orders

◆ Automatically generating related orders

◆ Improving clinician productivity

Computerized results improve workflow processes because:

◆ They can be accessed more easily than paper reports by the clinician at the time and place they are needed.

◆ They reduce lag time, allowing for quicker recognition and treatment of medical problems.

◆ Automated display of previous test results makes it possible to reduce redundant and additional testing.

◆ They allow for better interpretation and for easier detection of abnormalities, thereby ensuring appropriate follow-up.

◆ Access to electronic consults and patient consents can establish critical linkages and improve care coordination among multiple providers, as well as between provider and patient.

All types of treatments and care events are the result of provider orders. Examples include labs, x-rays, other diagnostic tests, medications, oxygen, diet, therapy, and even home medical devices such as a walker or wheelchair. As the IOM report suggests, when care is ordered electronically, the care is expedited and the workflow process is improved to the benefit of the patient.

CPOE is used by many types of healthcare providers. Some examples include licensed nurse practitioners, physician assistants, registered nurses, and other types of doctors such as osteopaths, dentists, and chiropractors.

## Recording Orders in the Student Edition

In this chapter, we will discuss several types of orders, the effect of an EHR on the process, and the workflow. In subsequent exercises you will have the opportunity to record orders and view test results. Although you may not be a provider who writes orders, there are a number of reasons we include orders in this course:

1. Orders are an essential component of any patient chart and a key objective for the IOM, Leapfrog, the HITECH Act, and the CMS "meaningful use" criteria.

2. Charts that include electronic orders and results offer the student a more realistic view of the complete EHR workflow.

---

[1] R. S. Dick and E. B. Steen, *The Computer-based Patient Record: An Essential Technology for Health Care* (Washington, DC: Institute of Medicine, National Academy Press, 1991, revised 1997, 2000).

3. Nurses, medical assistants, clinical coordinators, unit clerks, and other allied health professionals often enter verbal orders into an EHR on behalf of the ordering clinician.

4. Nurses or other allied health professionals may enter their own patient orders directly in the EHR within their particular scope of practice. This is a necessary step when creating the nursing plan of care.

5. Nurse practitioners and physician assistants in nearly all states are licensed to write prescriptions and thus will use an electronic prescription writer. Nurse practitioners order laboratory, radiology, and other diagnostic tests with the same authority as their physician counterparts.

6. In some critical care units a nurse will act as a scribe for the *code* team, documenting the emergency care as it is being delivered, including the ordering of stat tests and meds (as described in the Real-Life story in this chapter).

7. Physicians in some medical offices utilize scribes to enter EHR documentation (including orders) on their behalf.

You will learn to record orders for lab tests in the EHR, and later exercises will simulate the process of ordering and tracking lab results on a computer. However, the Student Edition software does not contain a working electronic lab order system. You cannot use the Student Edition software to write or send actual orders to a lab, as this ability would be inappropriate in a student edition.

Similarly, exercises later in the chapter include a simulation of writing prescriptions electronically. Again, the Student Edition software does not contain a real electronic prescription system. You cannot use it to write or send actual prescriptions to a pharmacy; this also would be inappropriate in a student edition.

## Learning to Use the Search and Prompt Features

As you learned in Chapter 2, medical nomenclatures such as SNOMED-CT and Medcin have hundreds of thousands of clinical concepts. The challenges with large clinical vocabularies include:

◆ How can you locate a concept among hundreds of thousands?

◆ Does the nomenclature use the same term for the concept as you do?

◆ Which domain do you start in?

◆ Where are other related clinical concepts?

The Search feature provides a quick way to locate a desired clinical concept in the nomenclature. Search produces a list of the findings almost instantly. Medcin addresses semantic differences in medical terms in several ways:

1. Search performs automatic word completion, so if you search for knee but the concept is "knees," search will still find it.

2. Search will begin when you pause typing, but pressing the Enter key will cause it to search without waiting.

3. Medcin includes an extensive list of synonyms that are used in an alternate word search. For example, if you search for knee injury, the search results will also

include knee burns, knee trauma, and fractured patella, as these are all forms of knee injury.

4. Search identifies clinical concepts in all six domains so that when you search for a word or phrase the results list displays in all domains.

## How Search Works

Search is not designed to find every instance that contains the words being searched because the search results will often have too many findings. Instead, Search finds and displays the highest level match but you can click the plus symbol to expand the tree below it.

For example, in Chapter 3 you did an exercise with Headache during which you expanded the tree to show many types of headache. If you searched for Headache, the search results would display the finding "Headache" with a small plus symbol next to it. If you wanted to peruse the various types of headaches, you would click on the plus symbol to expand the next level of the tree. If, however, you were searching for "migraine headache," the search results would show migraine headache, without needing to expand the tree.

## Guided Exercise 6A: Using Search and Prompt, and Ordering Tests

When patients are referred for diagnosis or follow-up care, a battery of diagnostic tests may be ordered to be done before the patient's scheduled appointment so the results can be available when the clinician sees the patient. This is especially true of tests that require more time to result or require the capabilities of an outside lab or radiology center.

Having the results ready when the clinician sees the patient allows the results to be considered during the exam, used to determine or confirm the assessment, and used to educate and counsel the patient.

In this exercise, you will learn to use the Search and Prompt features as well as how to move a clinical concept or finding from one section to another. The exercise will not produce a very thorough exam note, but it will give you experience using the features.

### Case Study

The patient, Gary Yamamoto, has been referred to the cardiology clinic with suspected angina. The patient did not seem in any immediate danger when he was seen by his family physician at the time of the referral and has been given an appointment at the clinic later this week. In the meantime, we are going to enter orders for some tests to be done prior to a scheduled appointment so the results will be available when he arrives for his clinic visit.

### Step 1

Start a supported web browser program and follow the steps listed inside the cover of this textbook to log in to the MyHealthProfessionsLab for this course.

Locate and click on the link **Exercise 6A**. This will open the Quippe software window with the New Encounter window displayed in the center.

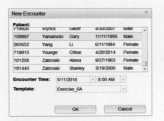

**Figure 6-1** Selecting Gary Yamamoto from the New Encounter window.

### Step 2

Patients are listed in alphabetical order by last name. Scroll to the end of the list to locate and click on the patient named **Yamamoto, Gary**. In this exercise, you do not need to set the date and time of the encounter. Once you have selected the patient as shown in Figure 6-1, click the OK button.

### Step 3

Click in the blank space under the heading Chief Complaint as you have in previous exercises, and type **Pt. referred with suspected angina** as shown in the upper left corner of Figure 6-2.

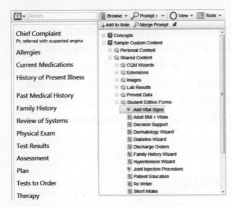

**Figure 6-2** Selecting Add Vital Signs form; figure also shows chief complaint.

### Step 4

Typically at this step a medical assistant or nurse enters the vital signs. This template doesn't contain the predefined vital signs table, but it can be added to the encounter.

Click anywhere in the workspace pane that does not highlight a finding or a heading, and then click the Browse button on the Toolbar at the top of the screen.

Locate and click the plus symbol next to the Sample Custom Content book icon on the drop-down menu. When the tree is expanded, locate and click on the plus symbols next to Shared Content and Student Edition Forms. The drop-down menu displays the various forms available to providers in the practice.

Locate and click on the form named **Add Vital Signs** to highlight it (as shown in Figure 6-2) and then click on the Add to Note button.

The data entry table for vital signs will be added to the encounter as shown in Figure 6-3 except it will not yet contain the vitals data (added in the next step).

**Figure 6-3** Vital Signs entered for Gary Yamamoto.

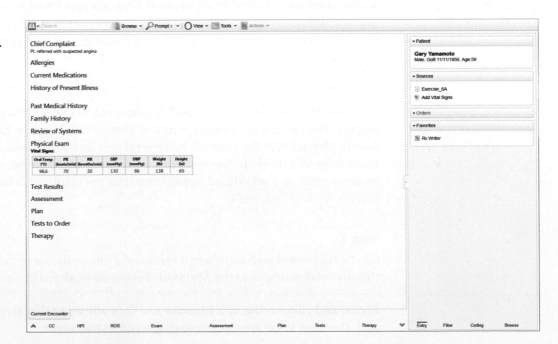

### Step 5

Enter Gary Yamamoto's vital signs in the corresponding fields as follows:

| | |
|---|---|
| Temperature: | **98.6** |
| Pulse: | **70** |
| Respiration: | **20** |
| SBP: | **130** |
| DBP: | **86** |
| Weight: | **138** |
| Height: | **65** |

Compare your screen to Figure 6-3.

### Step 6

A medical technician performs an electrocardiogram (ECG) on Mr. Yamamoto and saves the results for the doctor. The nurse records in the chart that the ECG has been performed. Rather than browse the entire Medcin nomenclature to locate the test, you can quickly locate and add the desired clinical concept using the Search function.

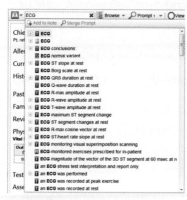

**Figure 6-4** Search results for ECG. Select Test ECG and click the Add to Note button.

Locate and click in the Search box on the Toolbar near the top of the screen. Type **ECG** and then press the Enter key on your keyboard. A list of clinical concepts containing the search term will be displayed as shown in Figure 6-4. Notice that each concept is preceded by a block letter showing the Medcin domain in which it is located. As discussed earlier in this section, the Search result displays results in any domain that has a concept that matches the search string. For example, the second item in Figure 6-4 is ECG History as indicated by the block letter "H", and near the bottom of the list is an item for ordering ECG monitored exercise in the R (therapy) domain.

The one we want is ECG in the Test domain. Locate and click the ECG that is the item at the top of Figure 6-4. This will highlight the clinical concept as shown in the figure. With the clinical concept highlighted, locate and click the Add to Note button at the top of the search list.

This will add the ECG to the section Tests to Order.

The problem here is that the concept has been added to the default section for ordered tests; however, the technician has already performed the ECG.

## Moving Concepts and Findings to a Different Section

### Step 7

You are probably familiar with the concept of dragging and dropping files and folders in your operating system or other software. Similarly, Quippe allows you to drag a clinical concept or finding from one section of the encounter note to another.

Position your mouse pointer over ECG. Click and hold your left mouse button as you drag the finding ECG upward to the Test Results section. The dotted arrow in Figure 6-5 shows the direction you should move the finding. A green arrow will temporarily appear over the finding as you move it. When the green arrow and finding are on the Test Results section heading, release the left mouse button.

**Figure 6-5** Drag ECG upward from Tests to Order, and drop on the Test Results section.

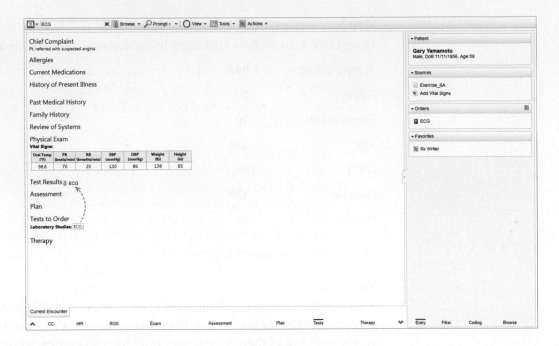

Ordered ECG should now be in the Test Results section. If it is not, or if it dropped into the Physical Exam or Assessment section, repeat the drag and drop using more care or precision.

### Step 8

Once ECG has been moved to the Test Results section, change the prefix from ordered to performed.

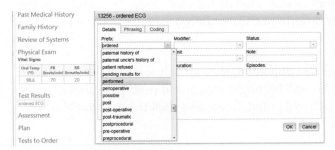

**Figure 6-6** Select "performed" from the prefix drop-down list in the ECG Details pop-up window.

With ECG still selected, *right-click* on ECG, and then select Details from the Actions drop-down menu. The Details pop-up window will be displayed.

Click on the down-arrow next to the Prefix field and scroll the list of prefixes to locate and select the prefix **performed** as shown in Figure 6-6.

Click the OK button to close the pop-up window. The finding should read "performed ECG." If it is not red, click on it until it changes to red.

## Merge Prompt—Intelligent Prompting

### Step 9

At this point Mr. Yamamoto's encounter note consists of vital signs, the chief complaint, and the performed ECG test. What history and symptoms should the nurse or medical assistant inquire about? Lists and forms provide guidance in this area, but it would be impractical for clinics to create a list or form for every possible ailment.

Chapter 2 described the millions of index relationships between concepts in the Medcin knowledge base. Using this relational data, the Prompt feature can locate and present related clinical concepts across all six domains, much like a list would, except the concepts added to the encounter by the Merge Prompt function are determined based on a key finding such as a diagnosis or condition.

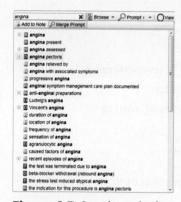

**Figure 6-7** Search results for angina. Select angina pectoris. Click the Merge Prompt button.

In this case, we see from the chief complaint that the patient is referred for suspected angina.

Click your mouse on the X in the Search box on the toolbar, or delete ECG with the backspace key. Type the medical term **angina** and then press the Enter key on your keyboard. The list of concepts shown in Figure 6-7 should appear. If it does not, verify that you have spelled angina correctly.

You will notice this time that search returned results for angina in many different domains. In the drop-down list, locate **angina pectoris** (preceded by the block letter D indicating the diagnoses domain). Click on angina pectoris to highlight it, and then click the Merge Prompt button at the top of the search list.

Compare your screen to Figure 6-8, ignoring for the moment the circled items. Scroll the encounter pane downward to observe that unentered clinical concepts have been added to every section. The full name of the feature is "Prompt with current finding." This feature adds concepts to the encounter pane similar to the way a list would, except the added concepts are all clinically related to the finding currently highlighted. The added concepts all have some bearing on determining or documenting a patient who may have angina pectoris. Toward the bottom of the encounter pane are listed numerous tests that the clinician might order to determine the nature of the patient's heart problem. Also notice in the Assessment section, there are additional diagnoses that the clinician might wish to consider, as these conditions can present some of the same symptoms as angina.

**Figure 6-8** Clinical concepts added to the encounter pane by Merge Prompt. Circled findings are to be recorded in step 10.

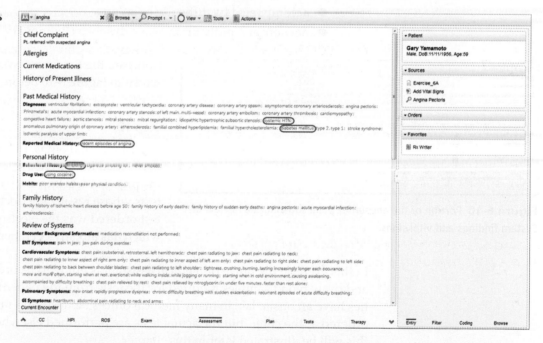

Turn your attention to the content pane on the right where the two sources that have added content to the encounter note are identified: Add Vital Signs and the Angina Pectoris prompt (preceded by a magnifying glass icon). Earlier you may have noticed ECG in the content pane orders; that disappeared when you changed ordered ECG to performed ECG.

**Step 10**

The patient does not smoke, and denies any history of angina, high blood pressure, or diabetes. Scroll the encounter pane to the top and record the patient's history findings. Since the Past Medical History section contains a lot of clinical concepts, the ones you will record in this step have been circled in Figure 6-8 to help you locate them.

Locate and click on the following history items until they turn blue. The descriptions will change after you click them.

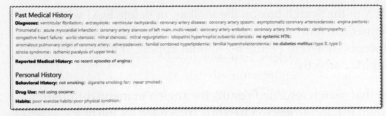

**Figure 6-9** Portion of the encounter pane showing history findings.

- systemic HTN (hypertension)
- diabetes mellitus
- recent episodes of angina
- smoking
- using cocaine

Compare the history portion of your screen to Figure 6-9.

### Step 11

The patient complains that he has pain in his jaw during exercise. Proceed to the Review of Systems section, and locate and click on the following finding until it turns red.

- jaw pain during exercise

The nurse or medical assistant asks Mr. Yamamoto if he has chest pain or difficulty breathing (dyspnea). The patient says no. Locate Cardiovascular Symptoms and click on the following findings until they turn blue. The descriptions will change.

- chest pain
- accompanied by difficulty breathing
- new onset rapidly progressive dyspnea (Pulmonary Symptom section)

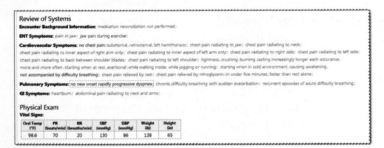

**Figure 6-10** Portion of the encounter pane showing the Review of System findings and vital signs.

Compare the Review of Systems portion of your screen to Figure 6-10 before proceeding.

### Step 12

Except for Vital Signs, the physical exam is not performed in this encounter because the purpose of the pre-visit workup is to order and perform some tests whose results the doctor will analyze. The first test ordered was the electrocardiogram (ECG), which has already been performed.

In this exercise the nurse or medical assistant is going to record orders for three lab tests and draw blood samples required for the tests from the patient. Although some facilities have an onsite lab, in many medical offices lab tests and radiology procedures are ordered at the clinic, but the actual tests are performed elsewhere. The workflow for this will be illustrated later in this chapter.

Proceed to the Tests to Order section, and click on the following blood tests:

- comprehensive metabolic panel
- lipid panel
- total serum creatine kinase level
- cardiac troponin T

Locate and click on the following imaging study:

- P-A and lateral

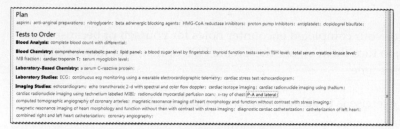

```
Plan
aspirin; anti-anginal preparations; nitroglycerin; beta adrenergic blocking agents; HMG-CoA reductase inhibitors; proton pump inhibitors; antiplatelet; clopidogrel bisulfate;

Tests to Order
Blood Analysis: complete blood count with differential;

Blood Chemistry: comprehensive metabolic panel; lipid panel; a blood sugar level by fingerstick; thyroid function tests;serum TSH level; total serum creatine kinase level;
MB fraction; cardiac troponin T; serum myoglobin level;

Laboratory-Based Chemistry: a serum C-reactive protein;

Laboratory Studies: ECG; continuous ecg monitoring using a wearable electrocardiographic telemetry; cardiac stress test;echocardiogram;

Imaging Studies: echocardiogram; echo transthoracic 2-d with spectral and color flow doppler; cardiac isotope imaging; cardiac radionuclide imaging using thallium;
cardiac radionuclide imaging using technetium labelled MIBI; radionuclide myocardial perfusion scan; x-ray of chest; P-A and lateral ;
computed tomographic angiography of coronary arteries; magnetic resonance imaging of heart morphology and function without contrast with stress imaging;
magnetic resonance imaging of heart morphology and function without then with contrast with stress imaging; diagnostic cardiac catheterization; catheterization of left heart;
combined right and left heart catheterization; coronary angiography;
```

**Figure 6-11** Plan portion of the encounter pane showing ordered tests in the Test to Order section.

Compare your Test to Order section with Figure 6-11.

### Step 13

The laboratory requires a diagnosis code for orders; however, the actual diagnosis will not be determined until the clinician completes the note. The way most offices work around this requirement is to add a prefix such as "possible," "suspected," or "rule-out" to the diagnosis. In this case, because we have a referral, we can use the prefix "referral diagnosis."

Locate **angina pectoris** in the Assessment section and click on it until it turns red.

*Right-click* angina pectoris, and then select Details from the Actions drop-down menu. The Details pop-up window will be displayed.

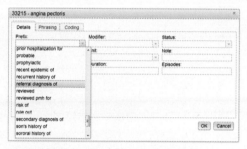

**Figure 6-12** Select the prefix "referral diagnosis of" in the angina pectoris Details pop-up window.

Click on the down-arrow next to the Prefix field and scroll the list of pre-fixes to locate and select the prefix "referral diagnosis of" as shown in Figure 6-12.

Click the OK button to close the pop-up window. The finding should read "referral diagnosis of angina pectoris."

### Step 14

This completes Mr. Yamamoto's pre-visit orders. Locate and click the View button on the toolbar, and then select Concise from the drop-down menu.

Compare your screen to Figure 6-13. If everything is correct, proceed to step 15. If there are any differences, click the View button on the toolbar, select the Entry option on the drop-down menu, and then correct your work according to the preceding steps.

**Figure 6-13** Concise view of the completed encounter note with angina orders for Gary Yamamoto.

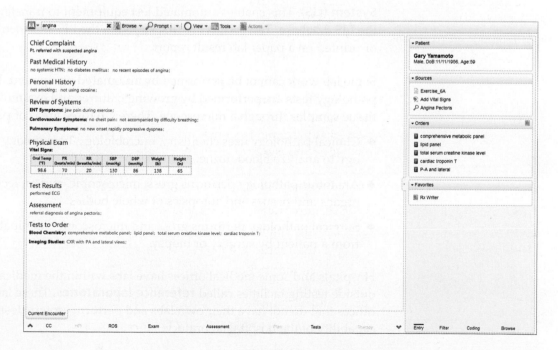

**Step 15**

If wish to print a copy of your completed encounter notes for yourself or because your instructor requires you to turn them in, use the Create PDF option, and then print or download the PDF at this time.

The final step in every exercise is to submit your completed work for a grade.

Locate and click the blue Quippe icon button on the toolbar, and then select the Submit for Grade option from the drop-down menu. This will complete Exercise 6A.

## Lab Orders and Reports

Laboratory and other diagnostic tests are ordered to determine the health status of the patient, and to confirm, or to rule out, a suspected diagnosis. The order is assigned a unique ID called a requisition or accession number.

Laboratory services consist of nine sciences:

◆ Hematology

◆ Chemistry

◆ Immunology

◆ Blood bank (donor and transfusion)

◆ Pathology

◆ Surgical pathology

◆ Cytology

◆ Microbiology

◆ Flow cytometry

Many laboratory tests use automated instruments to analyze blood and other samples. These instruments typically have an electronic interface to the Laboratory Information System (LIS). This enables automated test equipment to transfer test results directly to the LIS database. Test results are first stored in the LIS and then transferred to the EHR or printed on a paper lab result report.

Some lab work cannot be performed by automated equipment. For example, some pathology tests are performed by growing cultures and examining them, or examining tissue samples through a microscope. There are three areas of pathology:

◆ Clinical pathology uses chemistry, microbiology, hematology, and molecular pathology to analyze blood, urine, and other body fluids.

◆ Anatomic pathology performs gross, microscopic, and molecular examination of organs and tissues and autopsies of whole bodies.

◆ Surgical pathology performs gross and microscopic examination of tissue removed from a patient by surgery or biopsy.

Hospitals and some medical offices have labs within the medical facility. There are also outside testing facilities called reference laboratories. These labs process tests for offices that do not have their own labs and perform esoteric tests that are beyond the capability of the hospital laboratory.

There are also medical tests that do not have to be performed in a laboratory. Certain tests may be performed by handheld instruments at the patient's bedside or even the patient's home. This is called **point-of-care testing**. One example of such an instrument is a *glucose monitor*. The glucose monitor measures the amount of a type of sugar in a patient's blood. The results of this test can be electronically transferred from the glucose monitor device to the EHR. In a hospital, the data is usually transferred via the LIS.

The fluid or tissue to be examined is called the **specimen**. The specimen may be collected from the patient at the medical facility and then transported to the laboratory, or the patient may be sent to the laboratory to have his or her blood drawn there.

Here are various ways in which a sample for a blood test might be obtained:

◆ A nurse in the emergency department may draw blood from a patient, but a different person may carry the sample to the hospital laboratory.

◆ A laboratory at an inpatient hospital may send a phlebotomist to the patient's room to draw the blood required for ordered tests.

◆ A surgery patient may be directed to the hospital laboratory during preadmission, where a phlebotomist or laboratory technician may draw the sample before the patient is admitted.

◆ A physician's office may have a small laboratory where certain tests can be performed in the office.

◆ A physician's office may draw the blood but send the specimen to an outside reference lab. In this case a courier will collect the specimens from the medical office and transport them to the lab.

◆ A physician's office may give a written lab requisition to the patient and send them to the outside reference lab. When the patient arrives at the lab, a phlebotomist employed by the lab company will draw the blood.

Whether blood is drawn at a medical office, laboratory, or in a hospital at the patient's bedside, a phlebotomist or nurse will collect a specified amount of blood from the patient in one or more vials.

A provider usually only collects the specimen when it is part of the exam or procedure—for example, taking a swab for a throat culture, or removing a mole that is to be sent to pathology.

If a test requires a urine sample or stool specimen, this might be obtained from the patient at the medical facility or might be brought by an outpatient to his or her appointment.

Certain tests may not be covered by the patient's insurance and the patient must sign an acknowledgment that he or she has been advised that the test will not be paid by insurance. This is called an *Advance Beneficiary Notice*, or *ABN*. An example of the ABN form required by CMS is shown in Figure 2-23.

If the clinician's diagnosis or plan of treatment is dependent on the outcome of the test, then timeliness is important. In such a case, the patient cannot be treated until the provider receives and reviews the results. Similarly, tissue samples need to be examined for certain surgical pathologies and the results made available to the surgeon during the surgery. Although many of the steps are the same, electronic lab orders enable the provider to begin treatment sooner because the provider is aware of the results sooner.

The results of tests that are performed by automated equipment are communicated to the LIS, which assigns codes and records values for each component of the test. The lab system computer then compiles the results into a report that includes the information from the original requisition, test codes, codes for each component of the test, as well as standard reference ranges for each component associated with the actual value measured with the component. Additional notes, such as whether the value is considered outside the reference range (high or low) and whether the results were verified by repeat testing, also are merged into the report data.

When the report is complete, it is reviewed by the pathologist before being sent to the ordering clinician. The ordering clinician will review the results of the test and take appropriate action.

From the beginning of the order to completion of the review by the clinician, the status of the order is important. If too much time elapses between when the patient needs the test and a treatment is given based on that test's results, the patient's condition could deteriorate.

To determine how much time has elapsed, the medical office must know which patients have tests pending results and when they were ordered. The office is then in a position to follow up on the test by calling the lab or the patient.

Orders are tracked in an EHR from the moment they are entered in the system. If a patient fails to show up for a test, the lab can inform the medical office because the lab received the requisition electronically and is expecting the patient.

In the EHR system, all orders have a status. Lab orders that have been sent but have no results are referred to as *pending*. A report of pending orders is always available.

Labs may sometimes send preliminary results to give the clinician an early indication of the test and then send final results once the test has been repeated for verification. For example, a bacterial culture's preliminary results may appear after 24 hours, but the culture may be monitored for 72 hours before the final results.

EHR systems may connect to the lab system frequently as new orders are written or at predefined intervals throughout the day. Whenever a connection is established between the two systems, all available results for all of the clinic's patients are downloaded to the EHR. When lab results are received, most systems merge the data instantly into the patient's chart. Software matches each result to the original requisition order.

The status will then be preliminary, final, or corrected, as designated by the lab.

With an electronic order system, the patient's results are usually available the same day or the next morning. The clinician is notified as soon as results are ready. The clinician may order follow-up tests, a follow-up visit, send a task to have the patient called, add comments or annotations to the test, and compare the results to previous similar test results. The EHR system also keeps track of which results have not yet been reviewed by the clinician.

An important tool clinicians use to care for their patients is trending, which is comparing the change of certain test components or vital signs over a period of time.

In a paper chart, the trend is observed by paging through past tests, locating the desired component on each report, and making a mental comparison. However, when the lab results are stored as data in the EHR, the computer can instantly find all instances of any component the clinician wishes to consider. Additionally, with computerized data, graphs and charts can be easily created for any finding that has numerical results. Figure 2-19 and Figure 2-20 showed two examples of trending lab results.

Paper lab results are generally scanned into the EHR. As discussed in Chapter 2, this does not facilitate trending. The benefit of electronic lab results is that the codified data is merged into the EHR. Without an electronic laboratory interface, the provider and the patient both miss the advantages that codified lab data provides.

Electronic lab orders and results benefit both the patient and the practice. Waiting for the results of an important test is stressful to patients. Electronic laboratory interfaces help expedite the process, ensuring the provider knows about the results as soon as they are ready at the lab. Whether the patient is subsequently contacted by the phone or has access to lab results via the web, the waiting time (and accompanying anxiety) is reduced.

## Workflow of Electronic Lab Orders and Results

EHR systems allow the clinician to order a test while the clinician is creating the encounter note. The order is automatically documented as part of the encounter note (in the Plan section) as you did in Guided Exercise 6A. Ordering tests from the EHR typically will invoke a window in which you create the electronic lab order and send it to the lab. An actual lab interface is not present in the Quippe Student Edition, as order transmission capability would be inappropriate in a classroom setting. The workflow below will serve to illustrate the omitted functionality.

Figure 6-14 illustrates the workflow of electronic lab orders and results. In this scenario the clinician wants additional information about the patient's health that can be obtained by analyzing the patient's blood. The provider orders a blood test. Implied within the order is a request for a nurse, phlebotomist, or other medical personnel to draw a sample of the patient's blood. Follow the workflow figure as you read the following:

**①** The workflow begins when the provider orders a lab test. Using an EHR at the point of care, the provider can create the order from within the EHR.

The electronic order system compares the test codes on the order to coverage rules for the patient's insurance and automatically alerts the user if a signed ABN is required.

CPOE systems also display a list of recent and pending orders for the patient. This serves two purposes. First, it prevents unintentional duplicate orders, as the clinician is aware if another provider has already ordered the same or similar test. Second, the clinician is made aware of regular preventative or health maintenance tests for which the patient is due.

**②** In CPOE systems the provider does not complete the actual requisition form. The lab order initiates a task for a nurse, medical assistant, or phlebotomist to act on. The task involves at least two actions: completing the requisition and obtaining a specimen.

A nurse, phlebotomist, or other staff person will complete the electronic requisition in a computer. The patient's demographic and insurance information is populated automatically, eliminating mistakes caused by retyping.

Uniquely numbered labels are automatically printed as part of the electronic requisition process.

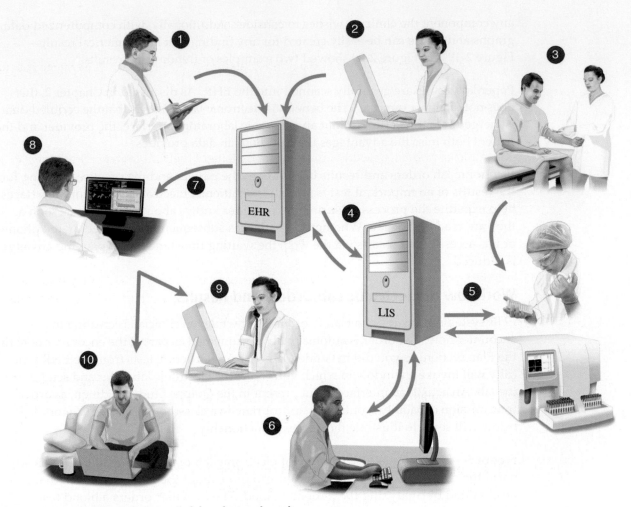

**Figure 6-14** Workflow of electronic lab orders and results.

**3** The specimen of the patient's blood is drawn. The labels are attached to the specimen vial or container.

**4** The requisition is transmitted electronically to the lab system computer and contains the information required to process the test. Electronic orders are transmitted to the lab either in real time as each requisition is completed or in batches throughout the day.

Specimens obtained at the medical office for tests performed at an outside lab are picked up by a courier and transported to the lab one or more times a day.

If the patient is sent to an outside lab for the blood to be drawn, the requisition is already waiting in the lab system when the patient arrives because it was sent electronically.

**5** The lab performs the requested tests and communicates the results through the Laboratory Information System (LIS).

**6** As soon as any results are ready at the lab, they are reviewed by the pathologist and made available to the medical facility's EHR.

**7** The results are returned electronically and merged into the patient's EHR.

The EHR will alert the clinician that the results are ready.

**8** The clinician will review the results on screen. Access to other components of the EHR allows easy comparison of current results with previous tests and allows the clinician to determine trends. The clinician can then order the treatments and follow-up tests, send messages to the staff or the patient, and do it all from their EHR.

**9** In an outpatient setting, a nurse or other staff member receives an electronic task to call the patient.

**10** Alternatively, some facilities allow the patient to view the test results online via a secure web site.

Electronic lab orders are assigned a status the moment they are created. This means it is easy for a clinician to see that a test has already been ordered by another provider. It also means that the order is not buried in some paper chart, but electronically tracked so the clinic is alert to missing or overdue results.

## Guided Exercise 6B: Ordering an X-Ray

In this exercise, you will apply what you have learned in the previous exercise, using the Search and Merge Prompt features, and dragging and dropping findings from one section to another. You will also learn about the Merge Prompt feature.

### Case Study

Patient Manuel Lopez has injured his knee and is examined by a nurse practitioner, who will order an x-ray. Using what you have learned in previous exercises, document his visit and the nurse practitioner's orders.

### Step 1

Start a supported web browser program and follow the steps listed inside the cover of this textbook to log in to the MyHealthProfessionsLab for this course.

Locate and click on the link **Exercise 6B**. This will open the Quippe software window with the New Encounter window displayed in the center.

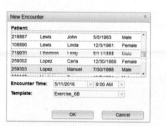

**Figure 6-15** New encounter window with Manuel Lopez selected.

### Step 2

Scroll the list of patients to locate and click on the patient named **Lopez, Manuel**. In this exercise, you do not need to set the date and time of the encounter. Once you have selected the patient as shown in Figure 6-15, click the OK button.

### Step 3

Click in the blank space under the heading Chief Complaint, and type **Sprained his left knee**.

### Step 4

Add Vital Signs to the template. Click any white space in the encounter pane that does not highlight a finding or a heading, and then click the Browse button on the Toolbar at the top of the screen.

Locate and click the plus symbol next to the Sample Custom Content icon on the drop-down menu. When the tree is expanded, locate and click on the plus symbols next to Shared Content and Student Edition Forms. The drop-down menu displays the list of forms shown previously in Figure 6-2.

Locate and click on the form named **Add Vital Signs** to highlight it and then click on the Add to Note button.

The data entry table for vital signs will be added to the encounter pane.

**Step 5**

Enter the patient's vital signs as listed below.

| | |
|---|---|
| Temperature: | **98.8** |
| Pulse: | **75** |
| Respiration: | **25** |
| SBP: | **120** |
| DBP: | **88** |
| Weight: | **164** |
| Height: | **68** |

Compare your screen with Figure 6-16.

**Figure 6-16** Upper portion of encounter showing Chief Complaint and Vital Signs.

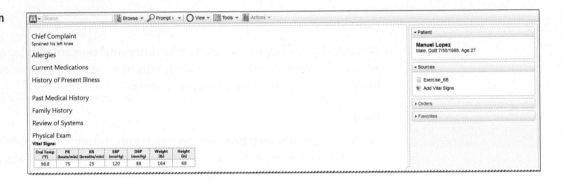

**Step 6**

Click anywhere in the workspace pane that does not highlight a finding or a heading, and then click your mouse in the Search box on the toolbar at the top of the screen.

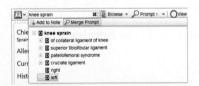

**Figure 6-17** Search results for knee sprain. Expand the tree. Select "left." Click the Merge Prompt button.

Type **knee sprain** and press the Enter key on your keyboard. Note: Search will sometimes start automatically after you stop typing, but pressing the Enter key ensures that search does not wait to start when you have a slow Internet connection.

The search function will return a drop-down list with the diagnosis knee sprain. Click the plus symbol next to it to expand the tree as shown in Figure 6-17.

In the expanded tree for knee sprain locate and click on **left** to highlight it and then click the Merge Prompt button at the top of the list.

Clinical concepts related to knee sprain will be added to your encounter pane.

**Step 7**

Locate Sources in the content pane on the right and notice that there is now an instance of "knee sprain left." Click on the magnifying glass icon and concepts in the encounter pane that were added by the merge prompt become highlighted.

In Figure 6-18 they are highlighted yellow. The color may be different on your screen.

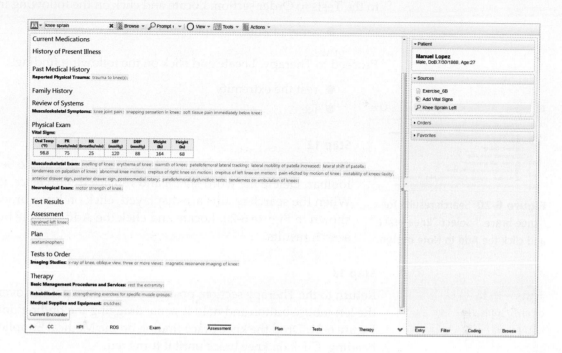

**Figure 6-18** Clinical concepts added to the encounter pane by Merge Prompt are highlighted yellow in the figure.

Click on the magnifying glass again to turn off the highlights.

### Step 8

Since the patient's chief reason for the visit is a knee injury, you will want to move it from Past Medical History to History of Present Illness.

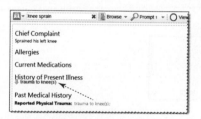

**Figure 6-19** Drag "trauma to knee(s)" upward from Past Medical History, and drop on the History of Present Illness section.

Position your mouse pointer over **trauma to knee(s)** in the Past Medical History section. Click the left mouse button and hold it down as you drag the clinical concept upward as shown in Figure 6-19. When it is positioned over the section label History of Present Illness, release the mouse button and drop the concept into the new section. Click on **trauma to knee(s)** until it turns red.

### Step 9

Proceed to Review of Systems. Locate and click on the following symptoms until they turn red:

- knee joint pain
- soft tissue pain immediately below the knee

### Step 10

Proceed to the Physical Exam, Musculoskeletal Exam group. Locate and click on the following findings until they turn red:

- swelling of knee
- tenderness on palpitation of knee
- pain elicited by motion of knee

Proceed to the Assessment section and click on the following diagnosis until it turns red:

- sprained left knee

**Step 11**

To be certain there is no further damage, the nurse practitioner orders an x-ray. Proceed to the Tests to Order section. Locate and click on the following imaging study:

● x-ray of knee, oblique view, three or more views

Proceed to Therapy. Locate and click on the following findings:

● rest the extremity
● ice

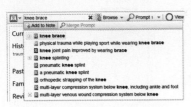

**Figure 6-20** Search results for "knee brace." Select "knee brace" and click the Add to Note button.

**Step 12**

The nurse practitioner orders a knee brace. Click in the Search box on the toolbar. Delete the word *sprain* and replace it with *brace*. (Search for knee brace.) When the search results are displayed, click on **knee brace** to highlight it, as shown in Figure 6-20. Locate and click the Add to Note button at the top of the search results.

**Step 13**

Return to the Therapy section, position your mouse pointer over knee brace, and click the left mouse button and hold it while dragging the finding downward as shown in Figure 6-21. Drop the knee brace finding on the Medical Supplies and Equipment heading. Click on knee brace until it turns red.

● knee brace

**Figure 6-21** Drag "knee brace" downward, and drop into the Medical Supplies and Equipment group.

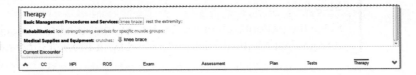

**Step 14**

A merge prompt instance listed in the content pane can also be used to remove unentered clinical concepts that were added by the merge prompt. Locate and click on the instance of "knee sprain left" in the content pane; an X appears at the right end of the label, as shown circled in Figure 6-22. Click on the X at the end of the instance of knee sprain, and unentered concepts added by the knee sprain merge prompt will be removed.

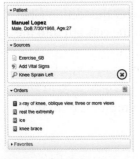

**Figure 6-22** Source instance of Knee Sprain Left; click X (circled in red) to remove unentered concepts.

**Step 15**

Compare your screen to Figure 6-23. If everything is correct, proceed to step 16. If there are any differences, correct your work according to the preceding steps.

**Step 16**

If you wish to print a copy of your completed encounter notes for yourself or because your instructor requires you to turn them in, use the Create PDF option, and then print or download the PDF at this time.

The final step in every exercise is to submit your completed work for a grade.

Locate and click the blue Quippe icon button on the toolbar, and then select the Submit for Grade option from the drop-down menu. This will complete Exercise 6B.

**Figure 6-23** Correctly completed encounter note for Manuel Lopez.

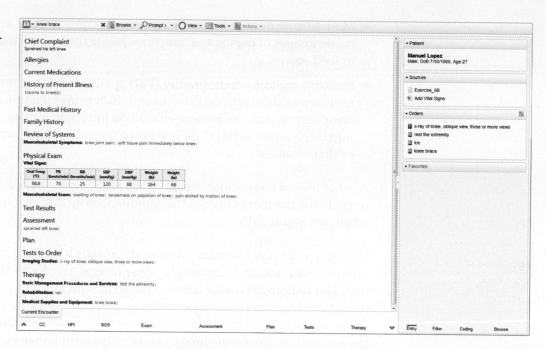

# Radiology Orders and Reports

When diagnostic information is needed, the provider may order an x-ray or other radiology study. Most acute care hospitals have radiology departments. Radiology departments typically have a **radiology information system (RIS)**, a **picture archiving and communication system (PACS)** for storing diagnostic images, and a dictation/transcription or voice recognition system for reports. Medical offices may perform some imaging studies such as ultrasound, or even have x-ray equipment on site, but patients requiring CAT scans and MRI are usually referred by a medical office to an outside imaging facility or a hospital radiology department.

CPOE systems in hospitals may send electronic orders directly to the radiology department RIS system. Radiology orders may also be transmitted electronically from a provider in a medical office to the radiology department or an outpatient imaging facility. Whatever the origin of the order, virtually all radiology orders are entered into the RIS to track the order for the remainder of the process.

Many of the diagnostic imaging devices used in the radiology department are capable of receiving order and patient data electronically from the RIS system. Patient data is then incorporated in the image data. Once the image is captured, it will transfer electronically into the PACS.

Traditional x-rays used to be taken on photographic film. To be stored in a PAC system, the film then had to be digitized using a scanner. Today, x-ray systems can record the image on a special plate that captures the image digitally, eliminating the steps of developing the film and then scanning it. In addition to x-rays, other types of diagnostic images studied by radiologists include:

◆ **Computerized axial tomography (CAT)** systems use x-rays to see into the patient's body and capture thousands of digital images. Using computer software, the system then constructs a view of cross sections of the body from the digital images. In some facilities this is also referred to as *CT* or *computed tomography*.

◆ **Magnetic resonance imaging (MRI)** uses magnetic fields and pulses of energy to create images of organs and structures inside the body that cannot be seen by x-ray or CAT scan.

◆ **Positron emission tomography (PET)** combines CT and nuclear scanning using a radioactive substance called a *tracer*, which is injected into a patient's vein. A computer records the tracer as it collects in certain organs, then converts the data into three-dimensional (3-D) images of the organs. PET can be used to detect or evaluate cancer.

A set of related images interpreted by the radiologist is called a *study*; a *hanging protocol* refers to the number of images that simultaneously display on the radiologist's monitor (shown in Figure 2-15).

Once the x-ray, CAT scan, or other study images have been captured, a radiologist interprets the results. Increasingly, these images are stored and read in a digital format. The radiologist uses a computer system with much higher resolution than standard computer screens to view the images. Special software not only displays the image but also allows the radiologist to manipulate it, zooming in and out, changing the contrast, reversing the image colors, and offering many other capabilities that help the radiologist.

Radiology reports are rarely available as codified EHR data, except for radiological observations related to the size and stage of tumors; those are codified.

When the report is complete and reviewed by the radiologist, it is sent to the ordering provider. Radiology reports almost always originate in an electronic text format at the radiologist's office. The ordering clinician may receive radiology results as a text file, fax, or paper report (which can be scanned as a document image). Any of these forms of the report may then be imported into the EHR.

If the ordering clinician and radiologist are within the same organization or hospital, the ordering provider may have direct access to the images studied by the radiologist and located on the hospital's PAC server (described in Chapter 2). If the radiology order came from an outside medical practice, copies of the radiology images may accompany the report sent to the ordering provider.

Electronic transmission of images uses a national standard called *DICOM*, which stands for Digital Imaging and Communications in Medicine. Electronic orders, results, and other data may be communicated between the hospitals and other systems using the HL-7 standard. Both DICOM and HL7 were discussed in Chapter 2.

## Workflow of Radiology Orders

EHR systems allow the clinician to order imaging studies while the clinician is creating the encounter note. The order is automatically documented as part of the encounter note (in the Plan section) as you did in Guided Exercises 6A and 6B. Ordering imaging studies from the EHR typically will invoke a window in which you create the electronic order and send it to the radiology facility. In Student Edition software the transmission screen is omitted.

Figure 6-24 illustrates the workflow of electronic radiology orders and results. In this scenario the clinician wants additional information about the patient's lungs that can be

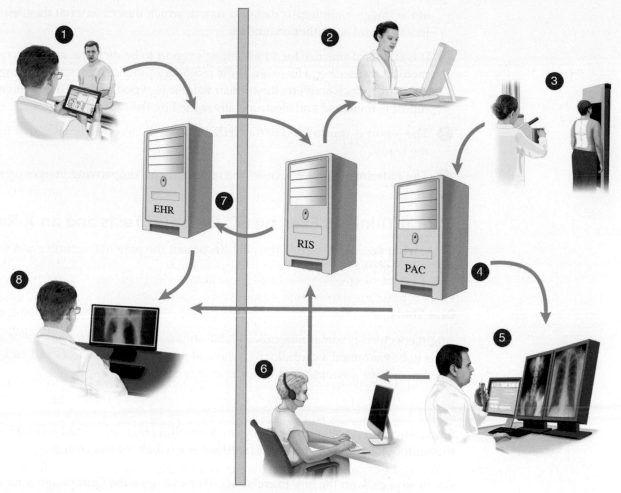

**Figure 6-24** Workflow of electronic radiology orders and image studies results.

obtained by an x-ray. The provider orders a "chest P-A and lateral," which consists of three x-rays of the chest: posterior, anterior, and lateral views. Follow the workflow figure as you read the following:

**1** The workflow begins when the provider orders an imaging study. Using an EHR at the point of care, the provider can create the order from within the EHR.

The EHR transmits the order to the Radiology Information System or RIS.

**2** The patient goes to the radiology department or outpatient radiology facility, where a radiology technician retrieves the order.

**3** The x-ray, CAT scan, or other type of radiology image is digitally captured, stored in the PAC system, and linked to the order in the RIS system. The images are queued for the radiologist to read.

**4** The radiologist opens the RIS record for the study, and the associated images are retrieved from the PAC and displayed on a high-definition monitor in the radiologist's preferred order (hanging protocol).

**5** Because radiologists use computer controls to manipulate and control the image, their observations are seldom keyed by them into an EHR program. While looking at the image, radiologists dictate a report, which describes what they see, its size, location, and any other comments.

**6** It is standard practice for a radiologist's report to be dictated, and then typed by a medical transcriber. However, some radiology practices use speech recognition software, which converts the human voice into typed reports. In either case, the report is reviewed and electronically signed by the radiologist.

**7** The report is transmitted to the EHR, which will alert the clinician that the results are ready.

**8** The ordering provider reviews the report and accompanying images on screen.

## Critical Thinking Exercise 6C: Ordering Tests and an X-Ray

Using what you have learned thus far, document the patient encounter and the clinician's orders.

### Case Study

Angina pectoris is sometimes called stable angina. Paul Mitsuhiro has stable angina. He is to be examined a cardiologist, who will need preliminary tests and an x-ray. Document Paul's symptoms, history, and orders.

### Step 1

Start a supported web browser program and follow the steps listed inside the cover of this textbook to log in to the MyHealthProfessionsLab for this course.

Locate and click on the link **Exercise 6C**. This will open the Quippe software window with the New Encounter window displayed in the center.

### Step 2

Patients are listed in alphabetical order by last name. Scroll the list to locate and click on the patient named **Mitsuhiro, Paul**. In this exercise, you do not need to set the date and time of the encounter. Once you have selected the patient, click the OK button.

### Step 3

Click in the blank space under the heading Chief Complaint as you have in previous exercises, and type **Pt. with stable angina**.

### Step 4

Click anywhere in the workspace pane that does not highlight a finding or a heading, and then click the Browse button on the Toolbar at the top of the screen.

Locate and click the plus symbol next to the Sample Custom Content icon on the drop-down menu. When the tree is expanded, locate and click on the plus symbols next to Shared Content and Student Edition Forms. The drop-down menu displays the various forms available to providers in the practice.

Locate and click on the form named **Add Vital Signs** to highlight it, and then click on the Add to Note button. Refer to Figure 6-2 for assistance in locating the form.

The data entry table for vital signs will be added to the encounter pane.

**Step 5**

Enter Paul Mitsuhiro's vital signs in the corresponding fields as follows:

| | |
|---|---|
| Temperature: | **98.6** |
| Pulse: | **78** |
| Respiration: | **28** |
| SBP: | **110** |
| DBP: | **68** |
| Weight: | **168** |
| Height: | **68** |

**Step 6**

A medical technician performs an electrocardiogram (ECG) on Mr. Mitsuhiro and saves the results for the doctor.

Locate and click in the Search box on the Toolbar near the top of the screen. Type **ECG** and then press the Enter key on your keyboard. A list of clinical concepts containing the search term ECG will be displayed.

Locate and click the ECG that is in the Test domain. This will highlight the clinical concept. Refer to Figure 6-4 for assistance in locating the test. With the clinical concept highlighted, locate and click the Add to Note button at the top of the search list.

This will add the ECG to the Tests to Order section.

**Step 7**

Position your mouse pointer over ECG in the Tests to Order section. Click and hold your left mouse as you drag the finding ECG upward to the Test Results section. When the finding is on the Test Results section heading, release the left mouse button to drop it there.

The ordered ECG should now be in the Test Results section. If it is not, or if it dropped into the Physical Exam or Assessment section, repeat the drag and drop using more care or precision.

**Step 8**

Once the ECG has been moved to the Test Results section, change the prefix from ordered to performed.

*Right-click* ECG and then select Details from the Actions drop-down menu. The Details pop-up window will be displayed.

Click on the down-arrow next to the Prefix field, scroll the list of prefixes to locate and select the prefix **performed**, and then click the OK button to close the pop-up window.

The finding should read "performed ECG." If it is not red, click on it until it changes to red.

### Step 9

As stated in the case study, stable angina is another term for angina pectoris.

Click your mouse in the Search box on the toolbar, and delete ECG with the backspace key. Type the medical term **stable angina** and then press the Enter key on your keyboard. The diagnosis stable angina should appear in the drop-down list of concepts. If it does not, verify you have spelled the search term correctly.

Click on stable angina to highlight it, and then click the Merge Prompt button at the top of the search list.

Clinical concepts associated with stable angina should populate the encounter pane, and the content pane should list two sources below the exercise: Add Vital Signs and Stable Angina.

### Step 10

The patient has a history of angina, including recent episodes, but does not have high blood pressure, diabetes, or other heart conditions.

Locate **angina pectoris** in the Past Medical History section, Diagnoses group, and click it until it turns red.

Proceed to the Reported Medical History group, and position your mouse pointer over **recent episodes of angina**. Click and hold your left mouse as you drag it upward and drop the concept on the History of Present Illness section. Click on the finding until it turns red.

### Step 11

The patient has smoked a pack of cigarettes per day for 20 years.

Proceed to the Personal History section, and locate and click the following finding so it turns red:

- cigarette smoking for

*Right-click* on the finding and select Details from Actions the drop-down menu.

Click in the Value field and type **20**. Click on the down-arrow in the Unit field and select **pack-years** from the drop-down list. Click the OK button to close the pop-up window.

The finding description should read "cigarette smoking for 20 pack-years."

### Step 12

The patient complains that he has pain in his jaw during exercise and when cold. He has a prescription for nitroglycerin tablets, which he takes whenever his pain is not relieved by a few minutes rest.

Proceed to the Review of Systems section, and locate and click on the following findings until they turn red.

- jaw pain during exercise
- chest pain radiating to back between shoulder blades
- while jogging or running

- starting when in a cold environment
- chest pain relieved by rest
- chest pain relieved by nitroglycerin

### Step 13

The laboratory requires a diagnosis code for orders. Proceed to the Assessment section and click on the finding until it turns red:

- stable angina

### Step 14

Proceed to the Tests Ordered section. Locate and click on the following blood tests:

- complete blood count with differential

Locate and click on the following imaging study:

- P-A and lateral

### Step 15

This completes Mr. Mitsuhiro's orders. Locate and click the View button on the toolbar, and then select Concise from the drop-down menu.

Compare your screen to Figure 6-25. If everything is correct, proceed to step 16. If there are any differences, click the View button on the toolbar, select the Entry option on the drop-down menu, and then correct your work according to the preceding steps.

**Figure 6-25** Concise view of the completed encounter note for Paul Mitsuhiro.

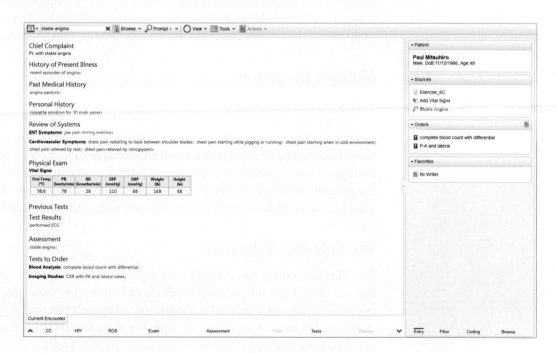

### Step 16

If you wish to print a copy of your completed encounter notes for yourself or because your instructor requires you to turn them in, use the Create PDF option, and then print or download the PDF at this time.

The final step in every exercise is to submit your completed work for a grade.

Locate and click the blue Quippe icon button on the toolbar, and then select the Submit for Grade option from the drop-down menu. This will complete Exercise 6C.

## Protocols Based on Diagnosis

Disease-based protocols can help the clinician write the orders and document the exam more quickly. Instead of searching through a list of a thousand prescription drugs, the clinician can access a short list of drugs that are regularly prescribed for a particular type of infection. These lists can be created for individual prescribing clinicians, for the practice as a whole, or by some recognized authority such as a medical association.

Similarly, the clinician can create a specific group of orders used to test for certain conditions. When a diagnosis is suspected, the list can be quickly located and the clinician can order tests, consults, or imaging studies all at once.

### Primary and Secondary Diagnoses

The concept of the primary diagnosis is also important. The **primary diagnosis** is the reason why the patient came to the office or hospital. Other conditions that are addressed during the visit are listed as **secondary diagnoses** (also called **comorbidity**). In a hospital, secondary diagnoses are classified as POA, present on admission, or HAC, hospital acquired condition.

Any conditions that exist concurrently with the primary diagnosis should be reviewed, examined, or treated and documented in the exam note. Often this is facilitated by a problem list, which is a summary of ongoing or previous conditions. The problem list helps the clinician keep track of the patient's needs beyond the scope of the chief complaint for today's visit. You will see an example of a problem list in Chapter 7.

### Multiple Diagnoses

Multiple diagnoses occur mainly in patients with ongoing or chronic conditions requiring regular visits. It is correct and appropriate to continue to use diagnosis codes from past visits for as long as the patient continues to have the illness or condition and that condition is clearly documented in the record. For example, a patient with diabetes mellitus—poorly controlled might be seen regularly. With this disease, on some visits the patient will likely have other problems as well. Therefore, the diagnosis "Diabetes Mellitus" should be included in every visit note and on insurance claims for those visits.

### The Rule-Out Diagnosis

The diagnosis for a patient may take more than one visit to be determined or confirmed, but the outpatient billing guidelines do not allow for "possible," "probable," "suspected," "rule-out," or similar diagnoses. Although the prefix "possible" may be appropriate and necessary in the exam note, the insurance claim for an outpatient visit should not be coded with a diagnosis for the suspected disease.

This creates a dilemma when ordering diagnostic tests from outside facilities. Reference laboratories cannot bill for tests unless there is a diagnosis. Only the clinician ordering the test is allowed to assign the diagnosis; the reference lab cannot. Therefore, labs require an order for a test to include a diagnosis code, even though the purpose of the test is only to determine if the patient in fact has the disease. Guided Exercise 6D provides an example of a rule-out diagnosis.

# Using Symptoms and History to Prompt for Findings

It is not unusual during the course of an office visit for a patient to bring up additional problems or to provide a piece of information to the clinician that suddenly brings focus on another area of the patient's health.

In this exercise you will learn to use prompt to add multiple lists of concepts and to create different sets of orders based on symptoms and history findings.

## Guided Exercise 6D: Patient With Multiple Diagnoses

### Case Study

Alena Zabroski is a 53-year-old female who complains of jaw pain. She has been to her dentist, who has found nothing wrong. The clinician initially suspects angina based on her family history and orders tests to confirm or rule out the diagnosis.

### Step 1

Start a supported web browser program and follow the steps listed inside the cover of this textbook to log in to the MyHealthProfessionsLab for this course.

Locate and click on the link **Exercise 6D**. This will open the Quippe software window with the New Encounter window displayed in the center.

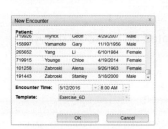

**Figure 6-26** New Encounter window with Alena Zabroski selected.

### Step 2

Scroll to the bottom of the list of patients to locate and click on the patient named **Zabroski, Alena**. In this exercise, you do not need to set the date and time of the encounter. Once you have selected the patient as shown in Figure 6-26, click the OK button.

### Step 3

Click in the blank space under the heading Chief Complaint as you have in previous exercises, and type **Patient reports jaw pain**.

### Step 4

In this exercise, the medical assistant will begin the visit by taking Alena's vital signs.

Enter Alena's vital signs in the corresponding fields of the encounter as follows:

| | |
|---|---|
| Temperature: | **98.1** |
| Pulse: | **70** |
| Respiration: | **21** |
| SBP: | **114** |
| DBP: | **70** |
| O$_2$ Sat: | **95** |
| Weight: | **150** |
| Height: | **70** |

Compare your screen to Figure 6-27 to verify you have entered the Chief Complaint and Vital Signs correctly.

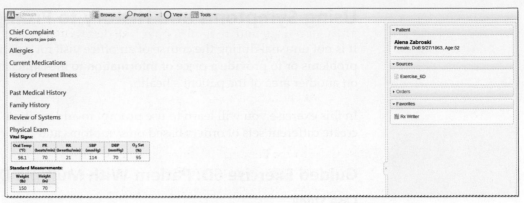

**Figure 6-27** Chief complaint and Vital Signs measurements for Alena Zabroski.

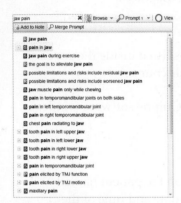

**Figure 6-28** Search results for jaw pain. Select the symptom "pain in jaw" and click the Add to Note button.

## Step 5

As you learned in the previous exercises, prompt provides a convenient way to load a group of relevant clinical concepts for which there is not a list.

Since the patient reports jaw pain, click in the Search box located on the toolbar, type **jaw pain**, and press Enter.

A list of search results similar to Figure 6-28 will be displayed.

Jaw pain is a symptom, so locate and click on the concept **pain in jaw**, which is preceded by a block letter S (for symptom). With pain in jaw highlighted, as shown in Figure 6-28, click the Add to Note button.

Locate the ENT Symptoms group, and click on the finding until it turns red.

- pain in jaw

Locate and click the Prompt button on the toolbar. Intelligent Prompt will be listed in the sources section of the content pane, and the encounter pane will be filled with a substantial quantity of clinical concepts. This is because jaw pain could be a symptom of many different conditions, as you will see if you scroll down to the Assessment section. Note if clicking the Prompt button alone does not immediately generate the list of clinical concepts, click the down-arrow on the Prompt button and select 1: Small from the drop-down menu.

## Step 6

The patient denies ever having had a cardiac arrest, high blood pressure, or diabetes. She hasn't sustained any injury to her head or jaw that could be causing her pain.

Scroll back up to the Past Medical History section and begin documenting Alena's history in the Past Medical History diagnoses group. Locate and click the following findings until they turn blue. The descriptions will change.

- cardiac arrest
- angina pectoris
- systemic HTN
- diabetes mellitus

Proceed to the Reported Physical Trauma and Other groups. Locate and click the following findings until they turn blue. The descriptions will change.

- trauma to head
- to jaw
- animal bite

**Step 7**

Proceed to the Personal History section. The patient has recently been undergoing emotional stress. She does not smoke, use cocaine, or birth control pills. She does not exercise and is in poor physical condition.

Locate and click on the following finding until it turns red.

- recent emotional stress

Locate and click the following findings until they turn blue. The descriptions will change.

- smoking
- using cocaine
- birth control using oral contraceptives

Locate the Habits group and click on the following findings until they turn red.

- poor exercise habits
- poor physical condition

The patient reports there is a history of angina in her family. Locate the following finding in the Family History section, and click on it until it turns red.

- angina pectoris

Compare your screen to Figure 6-29. If there are any differences, review the preceding steps and correct your errors. You may have to scroll your screen to see all the sections.

**Figure 6-29** History sections of the encounter pane with the findings correctly set.

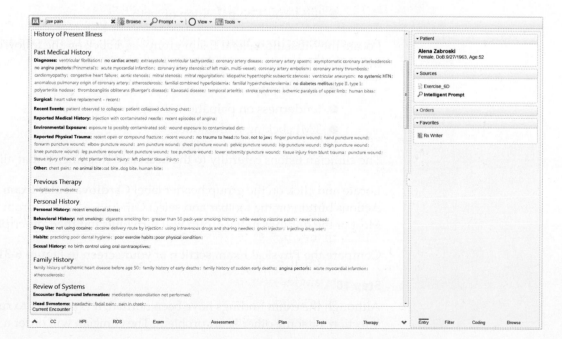

## Step 8

Proceed to the Review of Systems section, and locate and click on the following findings until they turn blue. The descriptions will change.

- headache
- Neck pain

Locate the ENT Symptoms group, and click on the following finding until it turns red.

- jaw pain during exercise

Locate the Cardiovascular Symptoms group, and click on the following findings until they turn red.

- while walking up steps and hills
- accompanied by difficulty breathing

Compare the Review of Systems portion of your screen to Figure 6-30.

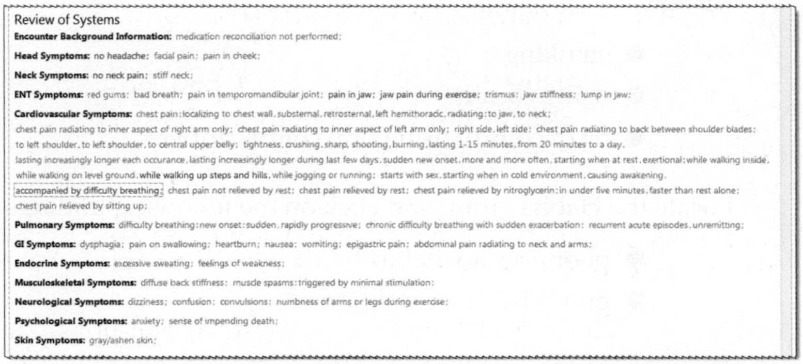

**Figure 6-30** Portion of the encounter pane showing the Review of System findings correctly set.

Review of Systems

**Encounter Background Information:** medication reconciliation not performed;

**Head Symptoms:** no headache; facial pain: pain in cheek;

**Neck Symptoms:** no neck pain; stiff neck;

**ENT Symptoms:** red gums; bad breath; pain in temporomandibular joint; pain in jaw; jaw pain during exercise; trismus: jaw stiffness; lump in jaw;

**Cardiovascular Symptoms:** chest pain: localizing to chest wall, substernal, retrosternal, left hemithoracic, radiating: to jaw, to neck;
chest pain radiating to inner aspect of right arm only; chest pain radiating to inner aspect of left arm only; right side, left side; chest pain radiating to back between shoulder blades;
to left shoulder, to left shoulder, to central upper belly; tightness, crushing, sharp, shooting, burning, lasting 1-15 minutes, from 20 minutes to a day,
lasting increasingly longer each occurance, lasting increasingly longer during last few days, sudden new onset, more and more often, starting when at rest, exertional, while walking inside,
while walking on level ground, while walking up steps and hills, while jogging or running; starts with sex, starting when in cold environment, causing awakening,
accompanied by difficulty breathing; chest pain not relieved by rest; chest pain relieved by rest; chest pain relieved by nitroglycerin; in under five minutes, faster than rest alone;
chest pain relieved by sitting up;

**Pulmonary Symptoms:** difficulty breathing: new onset: sudden, rapidly progressive; chronic difficulty breathing with sudden exacerbation; recurrent acute episodes, unremitting;

**GI Symptoms:** dysphagia; pain on swallowing; heartburn; nausea; vomiting; epigastric pain; abdominal pain radiating to neck and arms;

**Endocrine Symptoms:** excessive sweating; feelings of weakness;

**Musculoskeletal Symptoms:** diffuse back stiffness; muscle spasms: triggered by minimal stimulation;

**Neurological Symptoms:** dizziness; confusion; convulsions; numbness of arms or legs during exercise;

**Psychological Symptoms:** anxiety; sense of impending death;

**Skin Symptoms:** gray/ashen skin;

## Step 9

The clinician performs the physical exam looking for possible causes of jaw pain, but all four of the findings are normal.

Scroll your screen so you can see the Physical Exam section. Locate the ENT Exam group, and click on the following finding until it turns blue. The description will change.

- tenderness on palpation of teeth

Locate the Musculoskeletal Exam group, and click on the following findings until they turn blue. The descriptions will change.

- head injury
- tenderness on palpation of angle of jaw
- TMJ clicking with motion

The clinician listens carefully to the heart and documents that all findings are normal.

Locate and click on the group header label **Cardiovascular Exam** to highlight it. Click the Actions button on the toolbar and select Otherwise Normal from the drop-down menu. Most of the findings in the group will turn blue and their descriptions will change.

Compare the Physical Exam section of your screen to Figure 6-31.

## Step 10

Although the exam findings have been normal, it is prudent to rule out angina, an infection, or some other heart problem. The clinician will order a lab test and chest x-ray.

**Figure 6-31** Portion of the encounter pane showing the correctly set findings in the Physical Exam section.

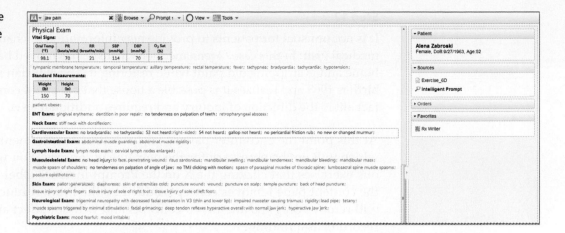

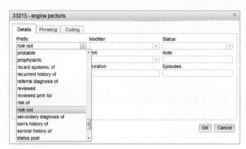

**Figure 6-32** Select "rule out" from the prefix drop-down list in the angina pectoris Details pop-up window.

An ECG will be performed in the office, and the patient will be given a continuous ECG monitor device to wear for 24 hours, similar to the Holter monitor shown in Figure 1-17.

In the Assessment section, locate and click on **angina pectoris** until it turns red. *Right-click* the finding and then select Details from the Actions drop-down menu. The Details pop-up window will be displayed.

Click on the down-arrow next to the Prefix field and scroll the list of prefixes to locate and select the prefix **rule out** as shown in Figure 6-32.

Click the OK button to close the pop-up window. The finding should read "rule out angina pectoris." Verify that the diagnosis is red.

### Step 11

Proceed to the Tests to Order section. Locate and click on the following tests to order them:

- a serum C-reactive protein
- ECG
- continuous ECG monitoring using a wearable electrocardiograph telemetry
- P A and lateral

Verify that all the findings in the Assessment and Tests to Order sections of your screen match those in Figure 6-33.

**Figure 6-33** Assessment and Tests to Order sections of the encounter pane with the findings correctly set.

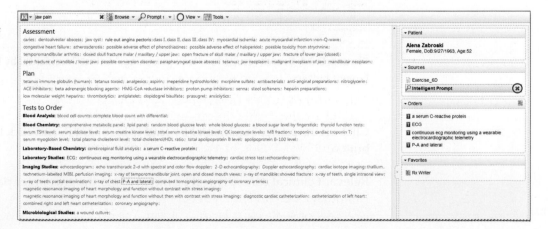

## Step 12

It is not unusual for patients to provide new information or change topics during their medical visit. In this case, Alena mentions that she has moved back to her childhood home and is stripping old paint while restoring it. The clinician notes that her date of birth is 1963 and realizes it is possible a house that old could contain lead paint. This fact alters the direction of inquiry and requires additional tests.

At this point the encounter pane is fairly cluttered with unentered clinical concepts, which will not be necessary for the new line of inquiry. You will recall from previous exercises that clicking the X on the Prompt instance label in the source section of the content pane removes concepts added by the Prompt function. However, this will remove only the unentered concepts and will not affect any concept already recorded as a finding.

Locate and click on the label Intelligent Prompt under Sources in the Content pane to highlight it. Locate and click the X on the right end of the label (circled in Figure 6-33). Only unentered concepts will be removed.

## Step 13

Click in the Search box located on the toolbar, type **lead poisoning**, and press Enter. When the search results are displayed, locate and click the plus symbol next to "poisoning by lead" as shown in Figure 6-34.

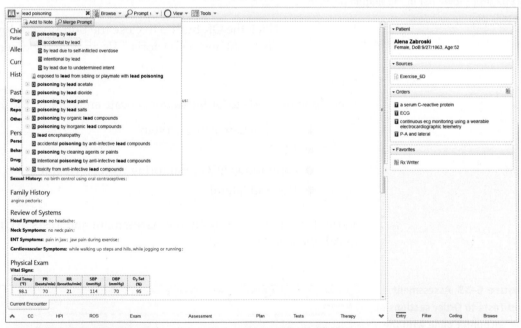

**Figure 6-34** Search results for "lead poisoning." Select "accidental by lead" and click the Merge Prompt button.

Click on the concept **accidental by lead** to highlight it, and click the Merge Prompt button.

Relevant clinical concepts will be merged into the encounter pane.

## Step 14

The clinician is going to first record this new piece of information in the Past Medical History, Environmental Exposure group. Locate and click on the following finding until it turns red.

- exposure to lead

In Personal History, locate and click on the following finding until it turns red.

- house has peeling lead based paint

## Step 15

Proceed to the Review of Systems section. Locate and click on the following findings until they turn blue. Their descriptions will change.

- nausea
- vomiting
- confusion
- disorientation
- generalized convulsions

Compare the Past Medical History, Personal History, and Review of Systems sections of your screen to Figure 6-35 to verify that you have recorded the findings in steps 14 and 15 correctly.

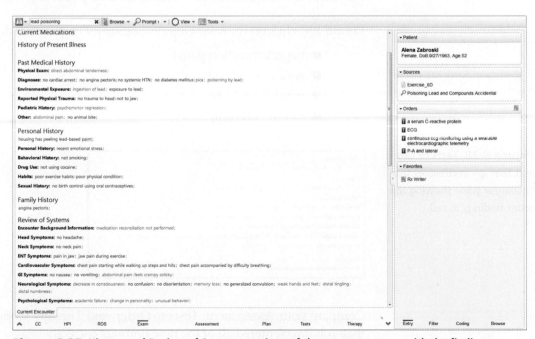

**Figure 6-35** History and Review of Systems sections of the encounter pane with the findings correctly set.

## Step 16

Scroll your screen until the Physical Exam section is at the top of the encounter pane.

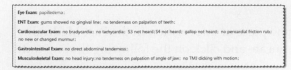

Figure 6-36 Physical Exam section of the encounter pane showing the findings correctly set.

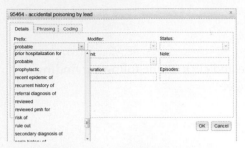

Figure 6-37 Select "probable" from the prefix drop-down list in the Details window for accidental poisoning by lead.

Locate and click on the following findings until they turn blue. The descriptions will change.

- Gums showed Gingival Line
- Direct abdominal tenderness

Figure 6-36 shows a portion of the Physical Exam section. Compare your screen to it and verify that you have added all of the above findings correctly.

### Step 17

Proceed to the Assessment section. Locate and click on the following finding until it turns red.

- accidental poisoning by lead paint

*Right-click* on the finding and then select Details from the Actions drop-down menu. In the pop-up window, click in the Prefix field and select **Probable** from the drop-down list as shown in Figure 6-37.

Click the OK button to close the pop-up window. The diagnosis should now read "Probable accidental poisoning by lead paint."

### Step 18

The clinician orders several lab tests and is also concerned about others who might be in the home and will need to be screened for lead poisoning as well.

Locate and click on the following findings until they turn red.

- hepatic function panel
- serum lead level
- urine lead, 24 hr
- family screening

Figure 6-38 Tests to Order and Therapy sections of the encounter pane showing the order findings in red.

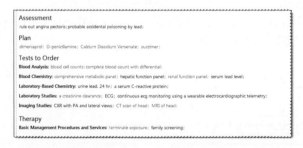

Compare your Assessment, Tests to Order, and Therapy sections to Figure 6-38 to verify that you have entered all of the new findings correctly.

### Step 19

This completes Ms. Zabroski's encounter note. Locate and click the View button on the toolbar, and then select Concise from the drop-down menu.

Compare your screen to Figure 6-39. The textbook figure has been elongated to show the entire encounter. You will likely need to scroll your screen to compare your entire encounter.

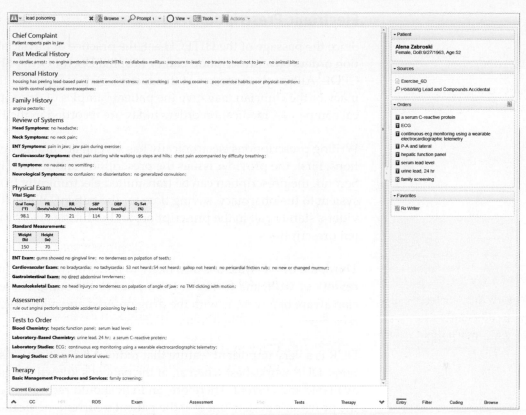

**Figure 6-39** Completed encounter note for Alena Zabroski in concise view.

If everything is correct, proceed to step 20. If there are any differences, click the View button on the toolbar, select the Entry option on the drop-down menu, and then correct your work according to the preceding steps.

### Step 20

If wish to print a copy of your completed encounter notes for yourself or because your instructor requires you to turn them in, use the Create PDF option, and then print or download the PDF at this time.

The final step in every exercise is to submit your completed work for a grade.

Locate and click the blue Quippe icon button on the toolbar, and then select the Submit for Grade option from the drop-down menu. This will complete Exercise 6D.

## Medication Orders

The most common type of order is for medication. Ever since the IOM report revealed that high numbers of deaths have occurred because of preventable medical errors, hospitals have increased their focus on patient safety. Hospitals' efforts have included CPOE, computerizing the pharmacy, and using positive identification systems to correctly match the medication with the patient, thus ensuring the right patient receives the right medication. In ambulatory settings, electronic prescription writers are incorporated into EHR software and include drug utilization review and formulary checking functions (described in Chapter 2 and below).

## Electronic Prescriptions

Since the passage of the HITECH act, the practice of physicians hand-writing medication orders on a prescription pad or hospital Doctor Order Sheet has been replaced with CPOE. Although a member of the doctor's staff may phone the prescription to the pharmacy or the clinician may give the patient samples of drugs provided by pharmaceutical companies, medication orders today are recorded in the EHR.

Writing prescriptions electronically has several advantages over the old paper prescriptions. First, the provider issues the prescription and records it in the chart in one step. Second, the prescription can be transmitted electronically from the provider's computer system to the pharmacy, saving time for the patient, eliminating the need for the provider's staff to call in the prescription, and reducing errors caused by illegible handwritten prescriptions.

Third, the CPOE system is also likely to perform two other functions: **drug utilization review or DUR**, and **formulary compliance checking**. These functions make the clinician aware of any issue with the drug ordered and allow the prescription to be corrected prior to sending it to the pharmacy.

DUR is a very important feature that reduces the patient's risk of adverse drug reactions. DUR works best when all of the patient's known drugs and allergy information is available and current. Therefore, an EHR should record not only prescriptions issued by the provider's system but also the patient's current medications even if prescribed elsewhere. These are usually reported by the patient during the intake interview or during the exam. The current medications list should be updated each visit before the provider issues any prescriptions. Figure 2-21 in Chapter 2 shows a DUR screen in a commercial electronic prescription system.

Formulary compliance was discussed earlier in Chapter 2 as an example of decision support. Formularies are lists of drugs that will be covered by the patient's insurance plan. Prescribing drugs that are not on the formulary means the patient will have to pay the entire cost. If the drug is too expensive, the patient may choose not to fill the prescription and thus not receive the therapeutic benefit of the drug. Figure 2-22 in Chapter 2 shows a formulary compliance screen in a commercial electronic prescription system.

When the patient goes to the pharmacy to have the prescription filled, the pharmacist will retrieve the order in the pharmacy computer system. As an additional safety measure the pharmacy system will perform DUR again, as the pharmacy may have records of prescriptions from other providers about which the patient failed to inform the doctor.

Formulary compliance is again checked by the pharmacy. Formulary lists are usually per insurance plan, and because there are so many different plans, the physician's system may not have had access to all of them. The pharmacy system checks the formulary by electronically communicating with an intermediary company called a **pharmacy benefit manager**. This provides information used by the pharmacy to determine the copay amount for the prescription.

The patient's insurance may require that a generic or less costly drug be substituted for a brand-name drug on the prescription. Unless the provider has indicated **DAW or "Dispense As Written"** on the prescription, it is very likely that the pharmacist will substitute a medically equivalent drug for the one prescribed by the provider. Most prescriptions allow substitution of a less costly generic drug when available. Prescriptions marked DAW may require approval from the insurance company's pharmacy benefit manager and medical justification from the ordering provider on why a brand name drug must be used.

If the pharmacy formulary checking, the DUR check, or a DAW order indicates a problem with filling a prescription, the pharmacist must contact the prescribing provider to change the order. Often the call from the pharmacist comes when the provider is with another patient, so a message is left and the call is returned at a later time. This creates a delay for the patient and pharmacist and consumes extra time for the provider, who has to return the phone calls.

The CPOE component of an EHR can provide additional benefits to both the clinician and the patient. Because each medication is automatically recorded in the medications list as the prescription is created, a current and recent medications list is available to the clinician when writing the prescription. This reduces prescribing errors.

EHR systems also shorten the time it takes to write a prescription by maintaining a list of prescriptions the clinician writes frequently. This speeds up the writing of prescriptions for common ailments seen at the practice. Physicians of patients with chronic diseases frequently write renewals for existing prescriptions; with EHR systems, physicians perform this task with a few clicks of the mouse. Additional time is saved because all FDA-approved drugs are listed in the prescription writer, eliminating the need to use a drug reference book to find less frequently prescribed drugs. An example of an EHR prescription writer will be used in Exercise 6E.

## Closing the Loop on Safe Medication Administration

Hospital EHR systems help protect patients by closing the loop on medication administration. This safety initiative starts with an electronic medication prescription from CPOE to the pharmacy computer system, where the order is checked and approved by the pharmacist for dispensing to the nurse. The nurse can then use an electronically documented process to ensure the five patient rights of medication administration safety. Before administering the medication, a handheld scanner device is used to read a barcode on the patient's armband to ensure the medication is being given to the right patient. Next, the nurse scans the barcodes on each medication or intravenous solution and the computer program checks the electronic order and warns the nurse of any discrepancies. If the medication dose, route, and time match the order for the patient, the nurse can then administer the medication to the patient. In some electronic systems a repeat scan of the patient's armband or a scan of the nurse's identification badge completes the documentation, confirming that the medication has been administered.

### Medication Administration—The Five Rights

1. Right patient
2. Right time and frequency
3. Right medication
4. Right dose
5. Right route of administration

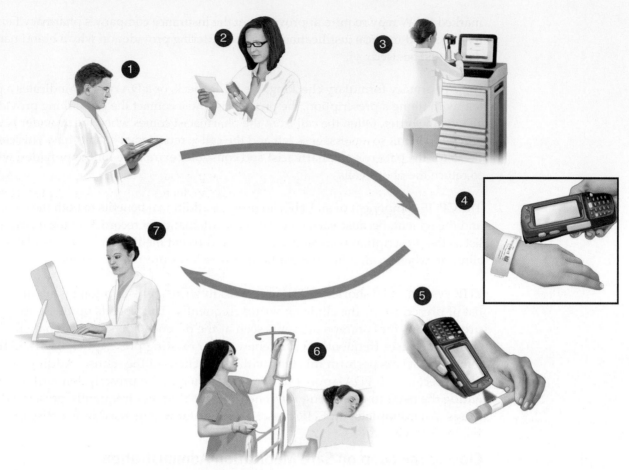

**Figure 6-40** Medication safety—the closed loop process.

Follow the numbers in Figure 6-40 as you read the following:

**1** Clinician writes the prescription using CPOE.

**2** Prescription is checked and approved by the pharmacist.

**3** Nurse receives the order electronically and removes the vial from the medication-dispensing system.

**4** A handheld scanner device is used to read a barcode on the patient's armband to ensure the medication is being given to the right patient.

**5** Nurse scans the barcodes on each medication or intravenous solution and the computer program checks the electronic order and warns the nurse of any discrepancies.

**6** Nurse administers the medication to the patient.

**7** Nurse documents the patient's chart. (In some hospital systems a repeat scan of the patient's armband or a scan of the nurse's identification badge completes the chart documentation, without manual entry.)

## Guided Exercise 6E: Writing Prescriptions in an EHR

In this exercise you will learn to use the Student Edition prescription writer to enter orders a nurse has received by phone from the doctor. It is necessary for the nurse to enter the prescription, because the patient needs to start taking the antibiotic immediately and this doctor does not have remote access to her EHR to write the prescription herself.

## Case Study

You will recall from the previous chapter that Kerry Baker was recently seen for an upper respiratory infection. It has been 10 days since her last visit and her condition has not improved. She would like a prescription for an antibiotic, but the physician has already left for the day. The nurse contacts the physician, who verbally orders amoxicillin. The nurse will write the prescription and the doctor will cosign the order later, usually within 24 hours.

### Step 1

Start a supported web browser program and follow the steps listed inside the cover of this textbook to log in to the MyHealthProfessionsLab for this course.

Locate and click on the link **Exercise 6E**. This will open the Quippe software window with the New Encounter window displayed in the center.

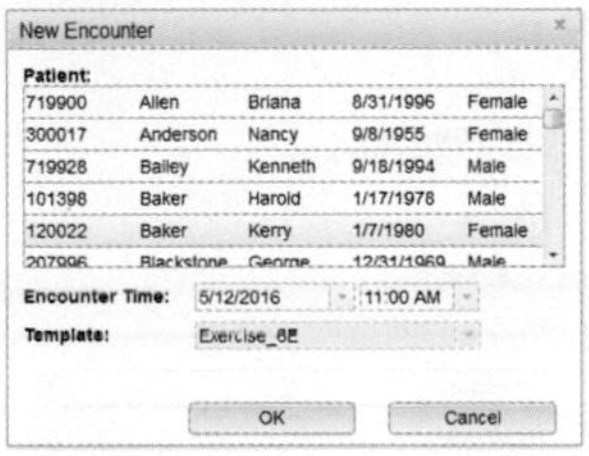

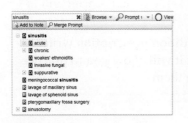

**Figure 6-41** Select patient Kerry Baker in the New Encounter window.

### Step 2

Locate and click on the patient named **Baker, Kerry.** In this exercise, you do not need to set the date and time of the encounter. Once you have selected the patient as shown in Figure 6-41, click the OK button.

### Step 3

Click in the blank space under the heading Chief Complaint as you have in previous exercises, and type **Medication request from patient**.

Note: the correctly entered Chief Complaint can be seen in Figure 6-44.

### Step 4

The patient reports that her acute sinusitis has not improved and requests an antibiotic. The nurse contacts her physician, who is out of the office without access to the EHR. The doctor and nurse review Ms. Baker's previous encounter, and the doctor gives the nurse a verbal order for the medication. First, document the reason.

Locate and click in the Search box on the Toolbar near the top of the screen. Type **sinusitis** and then press the Enter key on your keyboard. A list of clinical concepts containing the search term sinusitis will be displayed.

Locate the diagnosis sinusitis that is preceded with the block letter D and click the small plus symbol to expand it.

Locate and click **acute** to highlight the clinical concept as shown in Figure 6-42. With the clinical concept highlighted, locate and click the Add to Note button at the top of the search list.

**Figure 6-42** Search results for sinusitis. Expand the diagnosis "sinusitis." Select "acute" and click the Add to Note button.

### Step 5

Proceed to the Assessment section and click on the finding until it turns red.

- acute sinusitis

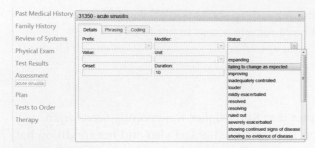

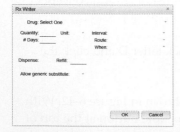

**Figure 6-43** Select "failing to change as expected" from the Status drop-down list in the Details window for acute sinusitis.

*Right-click* on the finding and then select Details from the Actions drop-down menu. In the pop-up window, click in the Duration field and type **10**.

Next, click in the Status field and select **failing to change as expected** from the drop-down list as shown in Figure 6-43.

Click the OK button to close the pop-up window. The diagnosis should now read "acute sinusitis for 10 days – failing to change as expected," as shown in Figure 6-44.

**Step 6**

You will now enter the medication order using the prescription writer.

In the content pane, locate the label Favorites and if Rx Writer is not showing click on it to display the list of favorites as shown circled in red in Figure 6-44.

**Figure 6-44** Encounter pane showing the correct Chief Complaint and Assessment.

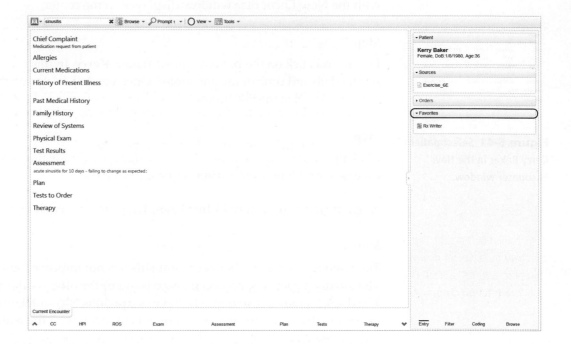

Locate and *double-click* **Rx Writer** to invoke the Student Edition prescription writer shown in Figure 6-45. This is not a full CPOE system, but it will allow you to practice entering medication orders without actually transmitting them.

**Step 7**

A simple prescription writer window will be invoked, as shown in Figure 6-45.

Although clinicians usually have personal order sets that allow them to quickly pick from a list of frequently prescribed drugs, you do not have access to this doctor's list. Therefore you will use a drop-down list to locate the ordered drug.

**Figure 6-45** Rx Writer screen.

Locate the Drug field, click on the "Select one" label, and the drop-down list shown in Figure 6-46 will be displayed.

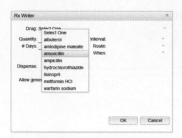

**Figure 6-46** Select Drug "amoxicillin" from the drop-down list.

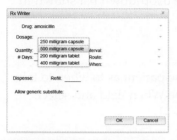

**Figure 6-47** Select Dosage "500 milligram capsule" from the drop-down list.

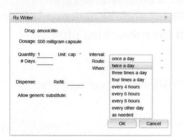

**Figure 6-48** Type 1 in the Quantity field, select cap for Unit, and select "twice a day" from the Interval drop-down list.

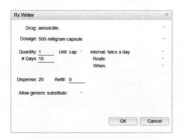

**Figure 6-49** Type 10 in the Days field. Dispense amount is automatically calculated. Refills are zero.

Click on **amoxicillin**.

After you click on amoxicillin, the Dosage field becomes available. Dosage includes the strength of the drug and the form such as capsule or tablet.

### Step 8

Locate and click your mouse on the Dosage field, and from the drop-down list, select **500 milligram capsule**, which is highlighted in Figure 6-47.

### Step 9

Next we will complete the "Sig"[2] information that the pharmacist will include on the label. It consists of the quantity of capsules to take each time, the number of times per day, the number of days to take the drug, the total quantity the pharmacist is to dispense, the number of refills allowed, and any special instructions to the patient about when to take the medication such as "before meals" or "at bedtime." The clinician also indicates if a generic is allowed to be substituted. Drop-down lists of available Sig choices make writing the prescription very fast. This feature is found in virtually all commercial EHR prescription systems.

Locate and click in the Quantity field and type **1**. The doctor wants the patient to take one capsule at a time.

Click Unit field and select the form **cap** for capsule from the drop-down list. If the order is a liquid or injectable, for example cough syrup, the clinician would set unit to teaspoon, tablespoon, or milliliter. Proceed to the next field.

The Interval field indicates how often the patient is to take the medication. Locate and click on the Interval field, and the drop-down list shown in Figure 6-48 will be displayed.

Select **twice a day** from the drop-down list.

### Step 10

Locate and click in the Days field and type **10**. The doctor wants the patient to take one capsule twice a day for ten days as shown in Figure 6-49.

Once the Days field is entered, the number of capsules to dispense is automatically calculated by multiplying quantity times interval (twice means 2) times days ($1 \times 2 \times 10 = 20$). However, the provider can change the dispense amount. This is necessary because for certain orders the clinician must specify the amount to dispense. For example, the interval for a headache medication used occasionally would be "as needed" (PRN). In that case, the provider would enter the number of pills to be dispensed.

### Step 11

The number of times the prescription may be refilled is entered in the Refill field. For this prescription the doctor does not want it refilled unless the patient comes in for a follow-up visit.

---

[2]Sig, from the Latin *signa*, are instructions for labeling a prescription.

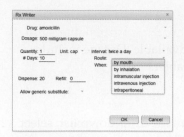

**Figure 6-50** Route: select "by mouth" from the drop-down list.

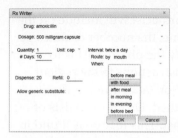

**Figure 6-51** Select "with food" from the drop-down list in the When field.

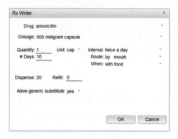

**Figure 6-52** Set Allow generic substitute to "yes." The figure shows the correctly completed prescription.

**Figure 6-53** Encounter pane showing the amoxicillin prescription in the Plan section.

Locate and click in the Refill field. Type **0**; there are no refills.

Compare your screen to Figure 6-49.

### Step 12

The next two fields are Route and When.

Route, like Unit, is usually determined by the form of the dosage selected. A capsule, tablet, or liquid is taken by mouth, but drugs that are injected may be administered by intramuscular, intravenous, or intraperitoneal route. Since the form of amoxicillin being prescribed is a capsule, the route is "by mouth." Click the down-arrow for Route and select **by mouth** from the drop-down list shown in Figure 6-50.

### Step 13

The When field is used to provide further instruction to the patient as to when to take the medication. Locate and click on the down-arrow for the When field and select "with food" from the drop-down list as shown in Figure 6-51.

### Step 14

Locate and click the down-arrow next to "Allow generic substitute" and select **yes**. This indicates the pharmacist is allowed to substitute a generic drug for a name brand if available. Yes is the correct setting for most prescriptions. If no is selected, the prescription is marked DAW, meaning "Dispense As Written," and the patient's insurance company may require medical justification from the prescribing physician or may require the patient to pay for the drug.

Compare your prescription to Figure 6-52. If there are any differences, correct your error. When everything is correct, click on the OK button.

The prescription information will be written into your patient encounter note as shown in Figure 6-53.

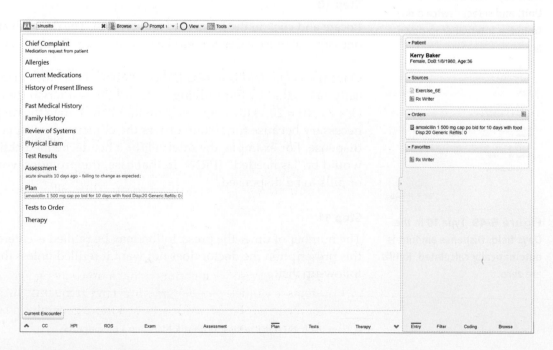

| | |
|---|---|
| qd | every day |
| q1d | once a day |
| bid | twice a day |
| tid | three times a day |
| q8h | every 8 hours |
| qid | four times a day |
| q6h | every 6 hours |
| q4h | every 4 hours |
| qod | every other day |
| prn | as needed |
| mg | milligram |
| ml | milliliter |
| cc | cubic centimeter |
| po | by mouth |
| IM | intramuscular |
| IV | intravenous |

Standard acronyms are routinely used in prescriptions. Locate the amoxicillin prescription in the encounter pane and decode the sig information using the abbreviations listed in *Sig Shorthand*.

### Step 15

The nurse now documents the doctor's instructions.

Locate and click in the Search box on the Toolbar, type **verbal orders**, and press the Enter key on your keyboard.

Locate and click on "Verbal orders to change plan of care were received from" to highlight it as shown in Figure 6-54, and then click the Add to Note button.

Locate the finding in the Therapy section of the encounter, and click on it until it turns red.

● Verbal orders to change plan of care were received from

### Step 16

*Right-click* on the finding and then select Details from the Actions drop-down menu. In the pop-up window, click in the Note field and type **Dr. Thomas** as shown in Figure 6-55.

Click the OK button to close the pop-up window. The finding should now read "Verbal orders to change plan of care were received from: Dr. Thomas."

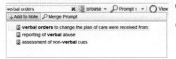

**Figure 6-54** Search results for verbal orders.

### Step 17

Compare your screen to Figure 6-56. Notice that the Content pane on the right lists two orders.

If everything on your screen matches Figure 6-56, proceed to step 18. If there are any differences, review the preceding steps and correct your work.

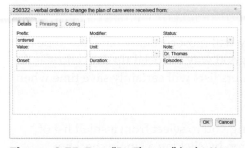

**Figure 6-55** Type "Dr. Thomas" in the Note field of the verbal order finding Details window.

### Step 18

If you wish to print a copy of your completed encounter notes for yourself or because your instructor requires you to turn them in, use the Create PDF option, and then print or download the PDF at this time.

The final step in every exercise is to submit your completed work for a grade.

Locate and click the blue Quippe icon button on the toolbar, and then select the Submit for Grade option from the drop-down menu. This will complete Exercise 6E.

## Quick Access to Frequent Orders

In the previous exercise we mentioned that a time-saving feature that is typical in all CPOE systems is a quick-pick list of a clinician's frequently used orders. These may take the form of diagnosis-based order sets, or a more generalized list of the prescriptions the clinician writes most frequently.

**Figure 6-56** Completed encounter note for Kerry Baker's prescription request.

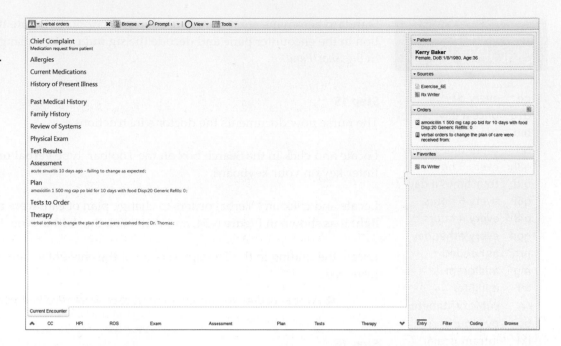

With thousands of tests that could be ordered and thousands of drugs to choose from, a clinician does not have the time to go through a search of medications or tests to write a prescription or order a lab. Many clinicians find that they order a fairly narrow range of tests (appropriate to their specialty and patient population) and write prescriptions for only a small group of medications.

It makes sense for clinicians to keep a list of the items they most frequently use from which they can select when writing the order. Commercial EHR systems handle this in different ways; some automatically create the list by memorizing what the clinician has been ordering, whereas other systems allow the clinicians to build their own lists. Most EHR systems offer a combination of both.

The EHR system you will use in a medical facility will most certainly have this type of feature. Making use of the feature is definitely a good way to speed up data entry at the point of care. Creating or customizing Rx and orders lists will certainly save time when the clinician is with the patient.

The next exercise emulates this feature by allowing you to select from a small list of medications and write the complete sig information by clicking a single checkbox.

## Guided Exercise 6F: Ordering Medications Using Discharge Orders

In this exercise you will record discharge orders using a quick-pick list to enter multiple medication orders that are part of a standard discharge protocol for patients with congestive heart failure (CHF).

### Case Study

Nancy Anderson is a 60-year-old female who was admitted to the hospital for congestive heart failure. She is to be discharged today, and the doctor's orders for her discharge medications and follow-up instructions are similar for most patients who

# Real-Life Story

## When Orders and Results Are Critical

**by Marney Thompson RN**

*Marney Thompson is a registered nurse working in the critical care unit of a large hospital.*

When I was in nursing school I did a 16-week rotation in a critical care setting and I loved it. Since then I have always worked in medical intensive care, or critical care units. I like the challenges of that type of nursing where you have an intensive patient with multiple needs and you are managing all the complications that come along with the acute phase—so you can get that patient to the next phase, which is recovery. I feel a strong sense of purpose being part of the team who responds when there is a patient who is coding.

I have been fortunate that all the hospitals I have worked in used electronic records. The patient's vital signs, CVP (cerebral vascular pressure) monitoring, heart rate, oxygenation, blood pressure—all transfer directly into our charts electronically. Our hospital EHR also has CPOE, so all lab and medication orders are electronic. The lab results are also electronic, which means the intensivist and I can both be looking at a patient's most recent results at the same time, even though the doctor might be in a different part of the hospital.

In addition, our hospital pharmacy is computerized, which means that when a situation is critical I can order meds on behalf of the doctor; the pharmacist can then review them and communicate with the Pyxis Medstation in the nursing unit to dispense them. Here is a situation that happened recently.

This patient was on BIPAP (bilevel positive airway pressure) and his respirations were *agonal looking*. He was not responsive—had not been responsive since coming to the unit—but he started to look like he was going downhill. I contacted the doctor (our intensivist), who ordered some stat lab tests: a BMP (basic metabolic panel), a CBC (complete blood count), and a magnesium level—pretty standard stuff for any patient who is crashing. We drew the specimens and sent them to the lab stat. The BMP takes about 45 minutes to be processed. In the meantime, I noticed that his QRS intervals started to widen. I suspected that it was related to possible electrolyte imbalances because his urine output had significantly decreased despite fluid boluses. I got an EKG, which confirmed it. I, another nurse, and an RT (respiratory therapist) were in the room trying to get an ABG (arterial blood gas) from the femoral artery, when suddenly none of us could feel a pulse. Basically, he was in PEA (pulseless electrical activity). Of course at that point we called the code.

The code team arrived. We had started CPR (cardio-pulmonary resuscitation) and shortly after starting CPR we got a pulse back. We still had to intubate the patient because of his respiratory status. While the CRNA (Certified Registered Nurse Anesthesiologist)

was intubating, I was able to bring up his lab results so we could get a bigger picture. At that time his potassium was extremely high. The doctor was at the bedside assessing the patient, assisting with intubation and calling out orders. I was at the computer looking at the labs and entering orders.

The doctor said, "Let's go ahead and push an amp of D-50 (dextrose) and ten units of insulin. Then we'll push an amp of calcium chloride after that. His bi-carb is low—push 2 amps of bi-carb and put an order in for another ABG right away."

The doctor was ordering this in rapid succession, while I entered the orders and transmitted them to the pharmacist, who cleared them very quickly; my co-worker went to pull the meds from the Pyxis machine. Literally in a matter of minutes, people were handing the drugs through the door, scanning and administering them. It was over and done, just that quick.

Our hospital policy supports the closed loop medication administration safety initiative, which you will read about elsewhere in this chapter. Let me describe how that works. When the doctor was giving me verbal orders, I was entering them in the CPOE. The medication orders were automatically sent to the pharmacy. The pharmacist interacted with that order on the pharmacy system, validated that the orders were safe and ready to dispense, and sent an order to the dispensing system. When the nurse went to the drawer to pull it out of the machine, the order was in there and allowed her to get it. Then she gave it to the nurse in the room, who scanned the patient's armband, scanned the medication, and then administered it. The system also documented it. So there is no transcription error, no misinterpretation of the orders errors—it is all electronically one order moving through the systems. I love it. I feel like I am getting double-checked five times. The pharmacist is also getting double-checked because when the order goes to the Pyxis machine it also comes up on my order list screen, highlighted in yellow for the nurse to confirm this is in fact the correct order for the correct patient. I know instantly what the pharmacist is dispensing. If there is any miscommunication, the nurse will have the ability to catch any error from the pharmacy.

When the crisis is over and the doctor has time to get into his own CPOE system, there is a button there labeled "cosign." He can click the cosign button and it will show him all the verbal orders that he has given—that someone else has entered for him. He can select them and cosign them at that time. Also, each doctor has a work folder in the EHR, so if he does not cosign them at that time they will show up in his work folder as items he needs to attend to. Most of the intensivists on our unit cosign their orders before the end of their shift.

Even when we are not in a code situation, there are times throughout the night when nurses are entering orders. For example, last night I had a patient come in who was already on a dopamine drip at 20 micrograms. The patient was tachycardic; blood pressure was 70 and 80 systolic. The doctor was at the bedside speaking with the surgeon when the anesthesiologist came to intubate. I said to the doctor, "Can I have Levophed?" and entered the order. I got the Levophed hanging, but the patient's pressure was still dumping. Because the physicians were evaluating the patient for septic versus cardiogenic shock, I asked, "How about some dobutamine?" The doctor told me to go ahead with the order.

Even with all three of those hanging, the patient still was not improving, and the anesthesiologist was requesting a better BP before sedation for intubation. I asked, "What else do we want to hang to get some blood pressure—can I have some vasopressin?" The doctors preferred to have me enter the orders in the computer while they continued to confer about the patient. By me entering the orders at the bedside, pharmacy was able to get the drugs to me more quickly as well.

I enjoy working in the CCU. You are responsible for almost every aspect of your patient's care. You have to be an advocate for your patient, someone who can handle herself in stressful situations, and think quickly in crisis.

have been admitted for CHF. Following a discharge protocol ensures all items in the hospital guidelines are considered and makes writing medication orders quick work.

### Step 1

Start a supported web browser program and follow the steps listed inside the cover of this textbook to log in to the MyHealthProfessionsLab for this course.

Locate and click on the link **Exercise 6F**. This will open the Quippe software window with the New Encounter window displayed in the center.

### Step 2

Locate the patient named **Anderson, Nancy** in the patient list and click on her name.

### Step 3

In this exercise, you will need to set the date and time of the encounter. There are two ways of doing this. You can click in the date field and type over the date using the format MM/DD/YYYY. The alternative method is to select the date from a pop-up calendar, which is invoked by clicking on the small down-arrow next to the date field.

Locate the date field, and use either method to set the date to **May 12, 2016.**

### Step 4

In this step you set a specific time of the encounter. There are two methods for doing this. You can click the down-arrow in the time field to invoke a drop-down list of times at fifteen-minute intervals, and then scroll the list to locate and click on the designated time to select it. Alternatively, time can also be set by typing directly into the time field using the HH:MM format and including either AM or PM.

Locate the time field, and use either method to set the time to **4:00 PM.**

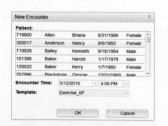

**Figure 6-57** Select patient Nancy Anderson, set the date to 5/12/2016, and set the time to 4:00 PM in the New Encounter window.

### Step 5

Compare your screen to Figure 6-57. Verify that Nancy Anderson is the selected patient, the date field displays 5/12/16, and the time field displays 4:00 PM, and then locate and click the OK button.

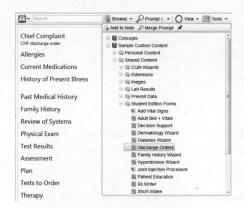

**Figure 6-58** Select Discharge Orders from Student Edition Forms in the drop-down list.

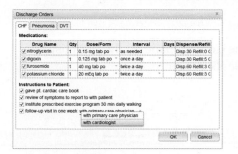

**Figure 6-59** Select "with cardiologist" in the otherwise completed CHF Discharge Orders screen.

When the encounter template is displayed in the workspace, locate and click in the blank space located just below the Chief Complaint heading and type the following text: **CHF discharge order.**

Note: the correctly entered Chief Complaint is visible in the upper left corner of Figure 6-58.

### Step 6

Click anywhere in the workspace pane that does not highlight a finding or a heading, and then click the Browse button on the Toolbar at the top of the screen.

Locate and click the plus symbol next to the Sample Custom Content icon on the drop-down menu. When the tree is expanded, locate and click on the plus symbols next to Shared Content and Student Edition Forms. The drop-down menu displays the various forms available to providers in the practice.

Locate and click on the form named **Discharge Orders** to highlight it (as shown in Figure 6-58) and then click on the Add to Note button.

A pop-up window containing discharge orders will be displayed. It will resemble Figure 6-59 except none of your findings will be checked yet.

### Step 7

The hospital has standard discharge protocols for various conditions. These conditions are listed in tabs across the top of the pop-up window. Since Ms. Anderson was hospitalized for congestive heart failure, use the CHF tab, which is already displayed.

Medications routinely ordered for CHF patients are listed with the prescription information already filled out. Detail entry fields and drop-down lists allow the prescriptions to be adjusted to the needs of the patient before writing the order, but they are preset to the dosage, quantity, and interval typically used. Simply clicking the checkbox next to an order will write the prescription.

Locate and click the checkboxes next to the following medications:

✓ nitroglycerin 1 0.15 mg tab po as needed Disp.30 Refill:0

✓ digoxin 1 0.125 mg tab po once a day Disp.30 Refill:5

✓ furosemide 1 40 mg tab po twice a day Disp.60 Refill:3

✓ potassium chloride 1 20 mEq tab po twice a day Disp.60 Refill:3

### Step 8

Proceed to the Instructions to Patient section.

The doctor gives the patient a booklet on cardiac care prepared by the hospital and reviews with the patient symptoms that should be reported immediately if they occur. Locate and click the two items to document them.

✓ gave pt. cardiac care book

✓ review of symptoms to report with patient

### Step 9

The doctor advises the patient to follow a prescribed exercise program of walking thirty minutes a day. Locate and click the checkbox next to the exercise order.

✓ institute prescribed exercise program 30 min daily walking

### Step 10

The doctor also wants the patient to follow up with a cardiologist in one week. The follow-up finding defaults to "with primary care physician," but a drop-down list permits the instruction to be easily modified.

Locate and click the checkbox next to **follow-up visit in one week** and then click the down-arrow next to "with primary care physician." Select "with cardiologist" from the drop-down list as shown in Figure 6-59.

If everything on your screen is checked as in Figure 6-59, click the OK button to close the Discharge Orders window and write the orders to the encounter note.

### Step 11

Compare your screen to Figure 6-60. Notice that the Content pane on the right lists the orders as though you had written each one with the Rx Writer.

**Figure 6-60** Completed encounter with Nancy Anderson's discharge orders.

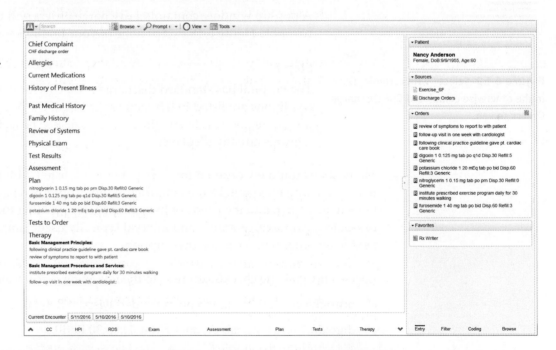

If everything on your screen matches Figure 6-60, proceed to step 12. If there are any differences, review the preceding steps and correct your work.

### Step 12

If you wish to print a copy of your completed encounter notes for yourself or because your instructor requires you to turn them in, use the Create PDF option, and then print or download the PDF at this time.

The final step in every exercise is to submit your completed work for a grade.

Locate and click the blue Quippe icon button on the toolbar, and then select the Submit for Grade option from the drop-down menu. This will complete Exercise 6F.

# Chapter Six Summary

This chapter introduced two new functions on the Quippe Toolbar: the Search and Prompt features. You also learned to use the Rx Writer and a quicker way of recording orders using the Discharge Order form, which demonstrates a type of quick-pick list.

**Search** provides a quick way to locate a desired finding in the nomenclature. Medcin addresses semantic differences in medical terms in three ways:

1.  Search performs automatic word completion, so if you search for knee but the concept is "knees," search will still find it.

2.  Search will begin when you pause typing, but pressing the Enter key will cause search to start immediately.

3.  Medcin includes an extensive list of synonyms that are used in an alternate word search. For example, if you search for knee injury, the search results will also include knee burns, knee trauma, and fractured patella, as these are all forms of knee injury.

Search identifies clinical concepts in all six domains so that, when you search for a word or phrase, the results list displays for all domains.

Search is not designed to find every instance that contains the words being searched because the search results will often have too many findings. Instead, Search finds and displays the highest level match, but you can click the plus symbol to expand the tree below it.

**Prompt** is short for "prompt with current finding." Prompt generates a list of concepts that are clinically related to the finding currently highlighted.

The **Rx Writer** can be used to add a prescription for a medication order. Nurses and other medical personnel frequently enter orders based on a physician's verbal order. The Student Edition Rx Writer cannot transmit or issue legal prescriptions; its purpose is to allow you to practice entering medication orders in an encounter.

A quick-pick list or form is a popular method of quickly writing medication orders for frequently ordered prescriptions, as all of the fields are preset, although they can be changed before saving the order.

Multiple diagnoses can be assigned to a single encounter. This occurs mainly because patients with ongoing or chronic conditions require regular visits. It is correct and appropriate to continue to use diagnosis from past visits for as long as the patient continues to have that illness or condition.

As you continue through the course, you can refer to the Guided Exercises in this chapter when you need to remember how to perform a particular task.

| Task | Exercise | Page # |
| --- | --- | --- |
| Search for a finding in the nomenclature | 6A | 199 |
| Merge Prompt (add concepts related to highlighted finding) | 6A | 201 |
| Drag and drop findings to a different section | 6B | 211 |
| Order tests based on diagnosis | 6D | 225 |
| Use the prescription writer | 6E | 234–237 |
| Use a quick-pick list to write prescriptions and discharge orders | 6F | 241–242 |

## Testing Your Knowledge of Chapter 6

### Step 1

Log in to MyHealthProfessionsLab following the directions printed inside the cover of this textbook.

Locate and click on Chapter 6 Test.

### Step 2

Answer the test questions. When you have finished, click the Submit Test button to close the window.

## Testing Your Skill Exercise 6G: Discharging a Patient with Deep Vein Thrombosis

Now that you have performed all the exercises in Chapter 6 this exercise will help you and your instructor evaluate your acquired skills. Use the information in the case study and the features of the software you already know to document the hospital discharge instructions.

### Case Study

Irene Smith is an 81-year-old female who was hospitalized for right leg pain that started after a recent visit to her daughters, which included a prolonged cross-country airline flight. The diagnosis was deep venous thrombosis, and the chief complaint is DVT. Now Ms. Smith is ready to be discharged.

She has been on the anticoagulant heparin during her hospital stay, but that is to be discontinued. Instead she is being given a prescription for Warfarin sodium, 1 milligram tablet. At home she is to take 1 tab twice a day for 30 days, 3 refills, generic.

When she was admitted she had erythema with swelling and edema of the right calf, conditions that the clinician observes are no longer present, and there is no tenderness on palpation. Ms. Smith's vital signs are normal as well. The test results of an ultrasound are normal, but since she has been on a blood thinner, the clinician orders an INR blood test.

The clinician follows the hospital protocol and uses the Discharge Orders for DVT/VTE, clicking all the items on the checklist.

Having already written her prescription with Rx Writer, the clinician is aware that patients on warfarin must have a blood test performed regularly and orders a prothrombin time test in two weeks and also tells her to see her primary care physician in the same time frame.

The clinician prescribes exercise and provides patient education as part of her discharge plan.

### Step 1

Start a supported web browser program and follow the steps listed inside the cover of this textbook to log in to the MyHealthProfessionsLab for this course.

Locate and click on the link **Exercise 6G**. This will open the Quippe software window with the New Encounter window displayed in the center.

**Step 2**

Locate and click on the patient name, and then click the OK button. In this exercise, you do not need to set the date or time of the encounter.

**Step 3**

Read the case study *carefully*. Use the case study information above to record relevant findings, but not every concept in the template applies to her situation.

*Hint*: Use the forms mentioned in the case study to complete the encounter.

Once you have documented all the information provided in the case study, proceed to step 4.

**Step 4**

If wish to print a copy of your completed encounter notes for yourself or because your instructor requires you to turn them in, use the Create PDF option, and then print or download the PDF at this time.

Submit your completed work for a grade. This will complete Exercise 6G.

# Comprehensive Evaluation of Chapters 1–6

This comprehensive evaluation will enable you and your instructor to determine your understanding of the material covered so far. Complete both the online test and the two exercises provided below. Depending on the time provided, it may be necessary to do this in two separate sessions. Your instructor will advise you. Do not begin the Part III exercise if there will not be enough class time to complete it.

## Part I–Testing Your Knowledge of Chapters 1–6

### Step 1

Log in to MyHealthProfessionsLab following the directions printed inside the cover of this textbook.

Locate and click on Comprehensive Evaluation Test 1.

### Step 2

Answer the test questions. When you have finished, click the Submit Test button.

## Part II–Guided Exercise CE1: Document Image Retrieval

Use the document image simulation program to retrieve scanned documents and locate the answers to five questions from information contained in them.

### Case Study

Raj Patel is an 80-year-old male who arrives in the emergency department accompanied by his daughter. His daughter informs the triage nurse that Mr. Patel was previously an inpatient at this hospital.

Using what you have learned in Chapter 2, find the information the triage nurse needs about Mr. Patel's previous stay.

### Step 1

You will need paper and a pen or pencil for this exercise.

Start a supported web browser program and follow the steps listed inside the cover of this textbook to log in to the MyHealthProfessionsLab for this course.

### Step 2

Locate and click on the link Comprehensive Evaluation Exercise 1.

The Document/Image System program you previously used in Guided Exercise 2A will be displayed.

**Step 3**

Locate and click "Select" in the Menu bar at the top of the screen, and then click "Patient" in the drop-down list.

Locate and click on the patient name **Raj Patel** in the patient selection window.

**Step 4**

The catalog list of Mr. Patel's documents will display.

Locate and click on the catalog entry for his Admission Face Sheet.

Locate and write down the following information:

1. What was the date of admission?
2. What was the date of discharge?
3. What was the admitting diagnosis?
4. What was the name of the attending physician?

**Step 5**

Locate and click on the catalog entry for his Discharge report.

Locate and write down the following information:

5. To where was the patient discharged?

**Step 6**

Locate and click the Exit button in the Document Image program toolbar.

A page asking you a series of questions about Mr. Patel's previous admission will be displayed.

Answer the questions using the information you have written on your paper. When you have finished, click the Submit Quiz button.

**Save the paper on which you wrote Mr. Patel's information, as you will need it for the next exercise.**

## Part III–Critical Thinking Exercise CE2: ER Visit for Shortness of Breath

The following exercise will use features of the software with which you have become familiar. Complete each step in sequential order using the instructions and other information provided.

Do not begin this exercise unless there is enough class time to complete it.

### Case Study

Raj Patel is an 80-year-old male who presents with shortness of breath and possible severe asthma. He reports awakening in the night short of breath. Mr. Patel does not smoke, but he is exposed to secondhand smoke and has pets in the house.

### Step 1

Start a supported web browser program and follow the steps listed inside the cover of this textbook to log in to the MyHealthProfessionsLab for this course.

### Step 2

Locate and click on the link Comprehensive Evaluation Exercise 2.

In the New Encounter window, locate and click on **Patel, Raj**.

Set the date to **05/13/2016** and time to **5:00 AM**.

Verify that the date and time are set correctly, and then click the OK button.

### Step 3

Locate and click in the blank space below the label Chief Complaint, and type **Pt. reports awakening short of breath.**

### Step 4

Begin by recording Mr. Patel's vital signs in the corresponding fields as follows:

| | |
|---|---|
| Temperature: | **98.8** |
| Pulse Rate: | **80** |
| Respiration Rate: | **28** |
| SBP: | **145** |
| DBP: | **90** |
| $O_2$ Sat: | **95** |
| Weight: | **139** |
| Height: | **66** |

When you have finished, check your work. If it is correct, proceed to step 5.

### Step 5

Locate and click in the Search box on the toolbar. Type **awakening short of breath** and press the Enter key.

Click on "awakening at night short of breath" in the search results list, and then click on the Add to Note button.

### Step 6

Document the reported symptom.

Locate the finding in the Review of Systems, Pulmonary symptoms group, and click on the finding until it turns red.

- awakening at night short of breath

Locate and click the down-arrow on the Prompt button on the toolbar and select 1:Small from the drop-down menu. The encounter pane will fill with related concepts.

### Step 7

The first thing the ER will do is rule out a heart attack. Mr. Patel denies any chest pain or heart palpitations.

Locate Cardiovascular symptoms and click the following findings until they turn blue. The descriptions will change.

- chest pain
- palpitations

### Step 8

Tests are ordered and performed to rule out a heart attack.

Proceed to the Tests to Order tests section. Locate and click each of the following tests. Once you have clicked a test, use the toolbar Action button, Details option to change its prefix from ordered to **performed**. After clicking OK to close the Details window, drag the test upward and drop it in the Test Results section. Repeat this procedure until all four tests are in Test Results.

Blood Chemistry tests:

- CK isoenzyme levels
- cardiac tropin I
- cardiac tropin T

Laboratory Studies:

- ECG

### Step 9

Locate and click on the group heading Cardiovascular Exam in the Physical Exam section. Click the Actions button on the toolbar and select "Otherwise Normal" from the drop-down list.

### Step 10

Scroll to the top of the encounter, locate the Past Medical History section and click on the following findings until they turn blue. The descriptions will change.

- coronary artery disease
- angina pectoris
- acute myocardial infarction
- cardiomyopathy

### Step 11

Locate the Assessment section and click on the following findings until they turn blue. The descriptions will change.

- possible atrial fibrillation
- cardiomyopathy

With cardiomyopathy still selected, click the Actions button, select Details from the drop-down menu, and set the Prefix field to "possible."

**Step 12**

Now that the ER doctor has decided that Mr. Patel has not had a heart attack, eliminate the unentered findings cluttering the screen by locating and clicking on the prompt instance in the Content pane Sources section: "Intelligent Prompt." When it is highlighted, locate and click the X at the right end of the instance.

**Step 13**

Take the patient's medical history by using the Short Intake form. Click the Browse button on the toolbar and expand the appropriate drop-down lists to locate the Short Intake form in Student Edition Forms, and then click the Add to Note button.

When the Short Intake form is displayed, locate and click on the Medical History tab.

Enter the Dx History and Family History by clicking on the Y (yes) check box or the N (no) check box for the findings that are checked in the following table. Some findings are already entered. *Do not change those.*

| Diagnosis | Dx Hist | Family Hist |
|---|---|---|
| Angina | ✓ N | ✓ N |
| Asthma | ✓ Y | ✓ Y |
| Bronchitis | ✓ Y | ✓ N |
| Cancer | ✓ N | ✓ N |
| Congestive Heart Failure | ✓ N | ✓ N |
| Coronary Artery Disease | ✓ N | ✓ N |
| Diabetes | ✓ N | ✓ N |
| Heart Attack | ✓ N | ✓ N |
| Hypertension | ✓ N | ✓ N |
| Migraine Headache | | |
| Peptic Ulcer | | |
| Reflux | | |
| Stroke | ✓ N | ✓ N |

Complete the rest of his medical history on the right side of the form by locating and clicking on the check boxes as follows:

| | |
|---|---|
| Taking Medication | ✓ N |
| Recent Exposure (Contagious Disease) | ✓ N |
| Recent Travel | ✓ N |
| Recent Medical Examination | ✓ Y |
| Recent ECG | ✓ Y |
| Recent Chest X-Ray | ✓ N |
| Allergies | ✓ Y |
| Allergy to Drugs | ✓ N |
| Tobacco | ✓ N |
| Alcohol | ✓ N |

When you clicked the Y checkbox for ECG, a date field became available. Click in the date field next to ECG and type **5/13/2016**.

When you have finished, check your work. If it is correct, click on the OK button to close the pop-up window.

### Step 14

The nurse inquires about Mr. Patel's allergies and is informed he is allergic to pollen.

Locate the Allergy section and click on the following finding until it turns red.

- allergy to pollens

### Step 15

The triage nurse explores the possibility his difficulty is related to his asthma.

Click on any white space in the encounter pane that is not a section label or finding, and then click the Browse button on the toolbar. Expand the appropriate drop-down lists to locate the Asthma list in Student Edition Lists, and then click the Add to Note button.

### Step 16

Locate the Review of Symptoms section and click on the following finding until it turns red.

- medication reconciliation not performed

### Step 17

Click the Browse button on the toolbar. The drop-down list should open to concepts related to the currently selected finding. If it does not, expand the Concept list, Symptoms domain, Encounter background information.

Locate the concept "Source of patient information" and, if necessary, click the plus symbol to expand it, then expand the tree for family member. Locate and click on "child" to highlight it, and then click the Add to Note button. Verify that "child" is red.

### Step 18

Locate and click on the following symptom findings until they turn red:

- difficulty breathing
- recurrent acute episodes
- wheezing

Locate and click on the heading Review of Systems. Click the Action button on the toolbar and select "Otherwise Normal."

### Step 19

Scroll upward to the Past History section to add additional history. Note that many history findings were already set via the Short Intake form.

Locate and click on the following history findings until they turn blue:

- previous hospitalization for pulmonary problem
- previous emergency room visit for pulmonary problem

Locate and click on the following history findings until they turn red:

- secondhand tobacco smoke in the home
- exposure to dust
- contact with pets or other animals

## Step 20

A coworker brings the nurse the information from his scanned medical records (the information that you retrieved in the previous exercise).

Locate and click the X in Search box on the toolbar to clear the field. Type **Surgical History** and press the Enter Key.

Locate "Surgical / Procedural History" in the search results and click the small plus symbol to expand the tree. Click on **prior surgery** to highlight it, and then click the button "Add to Note."

Locate the finding that has been added to the Reported Prior Surgical / Procedural History group and click on it until it turns red. Click the Action button on the toolbar and select Details from the drop-down menu.

In the Details pop-up window locate and click in the Onset field. Type the date of admission you wrote down in the previous exercise. Use the MM/DD/YYYY format.

Locate and click in the Duration field. Count the number of days from the date of admission to the date of discharge. Count the admission date, but not the discharge date. Type your answer followed by the word **days** in the Duration field.

Locate the note field and click in it. Type **Spinal surgery and post op**.

When you are satisfied everything is correctly entered, click the OK button.

## Step 21

The ER doctor returns, listens to the patient's lungs, and examines his nasal passages.

Proceed to the Physical Exam section. Locate "Nose" and click the finding **intranasal polyp** until it turns red, and then click the Actions button on the toolbar and select Details from the drop-down menu.

In the Details window, locate and click in the Value field. Type the numeric value **0.2** (two tenths).

Locate and click the down-arrow in the Unit field, and select **cm** from the drop-down list.

Click OK and verify that the finding description reads "intranasal polyp 0.2 cm."

## Step 22

Locate the Lung Exam group and click on the following findings until they turn red:

- accessory muscles used during expiration
- wheezing
- expiratory
- prolonged expiratory time

Locate the Physical Exam heading, click the Action button on the toolbar, and select "Otherwise Normal" on the drop-down menu.

**Step 23**

Locate asthma in the Assessment section and click on it until it turns red.

- asthma

**Step 24**

Proceed to the Plan section and order the following tests:

- complete blood count with differential
- peak flow
- CXR with PA lateral view

**Step 25**

Click on Favorites, and then *double-click* on Rx Writer. The prescription writer window will be invoked.

Click on the Drug field and select **Albuterol** from the drop-down list.

Click on the Dosage field and select **90 microgram puffs** from the drop-down list.

Click in the Quantity field and type **2**.

Click on the Interval field and select **four times a day** from the drop-down list.

Click in the Days field and type **prn**.

Click on the Route field and select **by inhalation** from the drop-down list.

Locate and click in the Dispense field. Type **1**.

Click in the Refill field and type **3**.

Click the down-arrow next to "Generic substitute allowed" and select **yes** from the drop-down list.

When the prescription is correct, locate and click on the OK button.

**Step 26**

A reference figure is not provided for the Comprehensive Exercise. It is recommended you use the Create PDF option to print or download a PDF at this time.

Compare your PDF to the previous steps and verify that you have entered all the required data.

If everything is correct, proceed to step 27. If there are any differences, correct your work according to the preceding steps.

**Step 27**

The final step in every exercise is to submit your completed work for a grade.

Locate and click the blue Quippe icon button on the toolbar, and then select the Submit for Grade option from the drop-down menu. This will complete Comprehensive Evaluation Exercise CE2.

# Problem Lists, Lab Results, and Body Mass Index

## Learning Outcomes

*After completing this chapter, you should be able to:*

◆ Understand and use Problem Lists

◆ Create problem sections in a problem-oriented chart

◆ Copy and cite information from previous visits in a new encounter

◆ Retrieve pending test results

◆ Review lab test results

◆ Calculate Body Mass Index

### Important Information About the Exercises in This Chapter

The exercises thus far have permitted you to skip setting the encounter date and time. In the next few chapters, you will work with patients' complete medical history using information from several previous encounters. In certain exercises it will be necessary to match the encounter date and time exactly as instructed in the exercise in order to maintain the correct chronology of the patient's data. If you need to review how to set the date and time when creating a new encounter, see Chapter 3, Guided Exercise 3A.

## Longitudinal Patient Records to Manage Patients' Health

One of the differences between inpatient and outpatient charts identified in Chapter 1 is the time span covered in the patient chart. Inpatient charts typically concern a particular inpatient stay or episode of care. In a medical office the electronic health record is a longitudinal record encompassing numerous encounters over an extended period of time. This is also true for hospital-operated specialty clinics focusing on problematic diagnoses—for example, diabetes, asthma, or hypertension. These clinics maintain longitudinal records as well.

Providers in a specialty clinic or primary care practice come to know their regular patients, helping to monitor and hopefully improve the patient's health. To do so, the clinician must review the records from the patient's past encounters and recheck previous problems on every visit.

Providers also must keep track of what medications the patient is currently taking and if any dosages have changed, which tests have results, and any other orders that have been issued. A clinician will always check the medications list before writing a new prescription, as well as to renew any that were about to expire.

Before the EHR, current medications and current problems were copied by hand to a list in the front of the paper chart or the clinician simply remembered them while skimming the chart, keeping a mental list as he or she read the chart.

In a codified electronic chart, the software itself can dynamically locate the necessary information and organize it for quick review. Additionally, the clinician can note the items reviewed, make updates to the problems, and then record them in the current encounter. The clinician does not have to search for findings in the system because the findings are already identified in the previous encounter notes.

The exercises in this chapter will allow you to experience some of the benefits of the longitudinal record. Although commercial EHR vendors use national standard nomenclatures such as Medcin, they differentiate their software with unique visual styles. Software you will use in a clinic or medical office will have features to aid the clinician in managing patients' health similar in concept to those in the Student Edition, but the presentation of the information is likely to have a different appearance.

## Understanding Problem Lists

A Problem List provides an up-to-date list of the diagnoses and conditions that affect an individual patient's care. Clinicians of all levels are trained to work with Problem Lists and depend on the information contained in them when providing care. Furthermore, maintaining a Problem List is a requirement for accreditation by organizations such as the Joint Commission (JCAHO) and one of the Meaningful Use criteria discussed in Chapter 1.

Problem Lists are used to track both acute and chronic conditions related to the care of the patient. Most clinical information recorded in the chart will be related to one or more problems. Clinic staff should be able to easily see the active problems for a patient and view the history of problems.

The relationship between diagnoses and problems is very close, often synonymous. If you have taken a medical billing course you may think this is similar to the billing concept of primary and secondary diagnosis; however, it is not. Although diagnoses are required for billing, the concept of primary and secondary does not apply in a Problem List. While chronic diseases that are poorly controlled or malignancies take precedence in clinical decision making over mild conditions that are not life threatening, the idea of a Problem List is to make sure everyone who touches the patient knows what conditions are present.

In many EHR systems, a problem is added to the Problem List either manually or automatically from the assessment in the encounter note. Most clinicians prefer to add the problems manually so that diagnoses for "possible" and "rule-out" conditions do not appear on the Problem List until the diagnosis is confirmed. Manually adding a problem to the Problem List is especially useful when the condition is being treated by a specialist at another office (and thus there is not an assessment in the primary clinician's note), but the clinician wants to remain aware of the condition. It is also possible to manually add findings to the Problem List that would normally be in the Past Medical History section of the encounter.

Problems usually have an onset date, indicate Chronic or Acute, and show whether or not the problem is active. Problems are usually removed from the list manually once the patient is "cured" or the problem is "resolved." Some problems have a natural period of time in which they normally resolve themselves. These problems are called **acute self-limiting**, and some EHR systems offer the option of setting the status of acute self-limiting problems to inactive after a designated period of time.

The status of the problem is updated at each visit, and if resolved, may be set as inactive or deleted. The following are typical of the types of status assigned to active problems:

◆ Resolved

◆ Resolving

◆ Improving

◆ Well controlled

◆ Unchanged

◆ Inadequately controlled

◆ Mildly exacerbated

◆ Failing to change as expected

◆ Expanding

◆ Worsening

◆ Severely exacerbated

Problem Lists are also used by health maintenance and preventative screening software within the EHR to inform the provider and patient of measures that should be taken for persons with conditions on the problem list. Health maintenance software also generates recommendations for preventative screening tests based on the age and sex of the patient, called *wellness conditions*. Wellness conditions are intended to keep healthy patients healthy. Both disease conditions and wellness conditions have measures that are typically performed for patients with that health condition. An example of a health maintenance preventive screening program was shown in Chapter 2, Figure 2-24.

The following examples show preventive care recommendations for two disease conditions and two wellness conditions:

◆ an annual EKG for a person with a history of congestive heart failure

◆ a quarterly blood sugar test for a patient with diabetes

◆ a mammogram for a healthy woman over 35

◆ immunizations for a healthy infant

## The Problem-oriented Chart

Lawrence Weed, MD, father of the **problem-oriented chart**, devised a note structure corresponding to the problem list for documenting patients with multiple problems. His concept of a "problem-oriented" view is to organize entries in a patient record by problem. Rather than lump all diagnoses under assessment, all orders under plan, and all tests under tests, the problem-oriented chart links test orders, therapy, and prescriptions to the respective problem. This problem-oriented view allows the clinician to quickly see not only the patient's problems, but also what has been done for them. The next exercise will illustrate a problem-oriented chart.

## Guided Exercise 7A: Working With a Problem-oriented Chart

In this exercise you are going to start a new encounter, and if you set the date correctly the system will automatically retrieve and display tabs for previous encounters at the bottom of the encounter note pane. Clinical concepts in the current encounter note that have corresponding findings in previous notes will be underlined by the software to identify them for follow-up by the clinician.

### Case Study

Juan Garcia, an outpatient who has been treated previously, is returning for a follow-up visit.

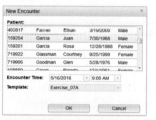

**Figure 7-1** Selecting Juan Garcia and setting the date to May 16, 2016 9:00 AM in the New Encounter window.

### Step 1

Start a supported web browser program and follow the steps listed inside the cover of this textbook to log in to the MyHealthProfessionsLab for this course.

Locate and click on the link Exercise 7A.

### Step 2

In the New Encounter window, locate and click on **Garcia, Juan**.

Set the date to **05/16/2016** and time to **9:00 AM** as shown in Figure 7-1.

Verify that the date and time are set correctly, and then click the OK button.

### Step 3

Located at the bottom of the workspace pane are four tabs as shown in Figure 7-2. The first tab is Current Encounter, and the next three are labeled with dates. These tabs contain encounter notes from previous visits.

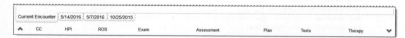

**Figure 7-2** Tabs located below the encounter pane show previous encounter dates.

### Step 4

Locate and click on the tab displaying the date **5/7/2016** at the bottom of the pane. The encounter note from Mr. Garcia's May 7, 2016 visit will be displayed as shown in Figure 7-3.

Reading the encounter note we see that Juan Garcia came to the clinic on May 7, 2016, with a fever, sinus pain, stuffiness, purulent nasal discharge, and sinus tenderness. Scroll the pane downward to read the rest of the encounter. We see that the clinician

**ALERT**

If your screen does not display the date tabs shown in Figure 7-2 you did not set the correct date. Locate and click the Quippe menu button on the toolbar, select New Encounter from the drop-down menu, and then repeat step 2. If you need help, review Chapter 3, Guided Exercise 3A.

**Figure 7-3** Encounter note for May 7, 2016.

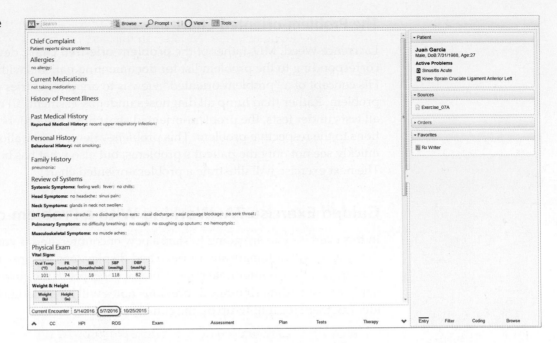

diagnosed the patient with acute sinusitis, ordered a sinus culture for bacteria, and prescribed an antibiotic.

**Step 5**

Locate and click on the tab containing the date **5/14/2016** at the bottom of the pane to display the encounter note from that visit.

While recovering from sinusitis, Mr. Garcia twisted his knee, resulting in a sprain. Review the encounter note from May 14, 2016, noting that antibiotics ordered in the May 7 encounter are documented in Current Medications, and recent upper respiratory infection is documented in Past Medical History.

Scroll the encounter pane downward to see the rest of the note. Compare your screen to Figure 7-4.

**Figure 7-4** Problem-oriented note for May 14, 2016 encounter.

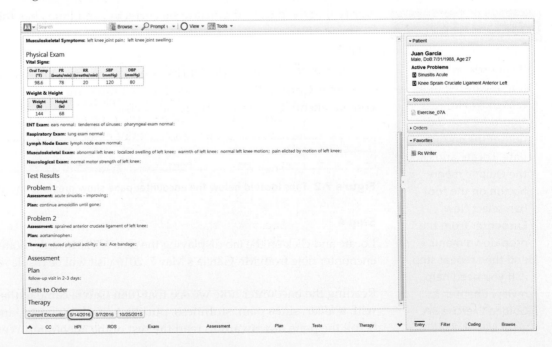

On May 14, 2016, Mr. Garcia had two active problems: acute sinusitis and sprained anterior cruciate ligament of left knee. In this encounter we see an example of the problem-oriented chart discussed earlier in this chapter. Notice that, instead of a single assessment section, there are sections labeled "Problem 1" and "Problem 2." In each section the diagnosis, plan, and therapy are listed. Had there been test orders, they would also be grouped with the diagnosis for which they were ordered.

Juan was seen on a Saturday and was instructed to come back to the office Monday for a follow-up.

### Step 6

Now that you have reviewed the two previous notes, locate and click on the Current Encounter tab at the bottom of the workspace.

Locate and click in the blank space below the label Chief Complaint, and type **Knee injury follow-up**.

Compare your screen to the portion of the screen shown in Figure 7-5. Note that the word "allergy" is underlined. This feature of Quippe informs the clinician that the concept was documented for this patient in one or more previous encounters.

**Figure 7-5** Portion of current encounter showing the Chief Complaint with the Active Problems list on the right.

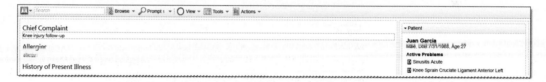

Click on either the 5/7/2016 or the 5/14/2016 tab at the bottom of the pane and determine how the allergy finding was set on previous encounters. Click the Current Encounter tab and click on **allergy** until it is set the same as it was in the previous encounters.

### Step 7

There are easier ways to record information from previous encounter notes into the current encounter. While you cannot edit or add any findings in the previous encounter records, you can copy them into the current encounter, where they can then be modified or updated.

Locate and click on the tab labeled 5/7/2016.

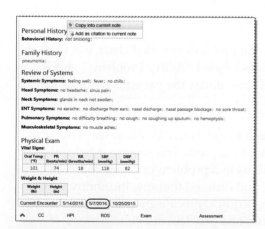

**Figure 7-6** Copying "not smoking" from the 5/7/2016 encounter into the current note.

Locate and click on the Behavioral History finding **not smoking**. A dropdown menu will appear over the finding similar to Figure 7-6. Click on the option Copy into current note.

The other option, Add as a citation to current note, will be explained later.

### Step 8

Locate and click on the Current Encounter tab. Locate the Personal History section and notice that "not smoking" has been copied into the current encounter.

Using what you have learned in previous chapters, move the finding into the Tobacco use group. Click on **not smoking** and hold the left mouse button down while you drag upward and drop it on the label

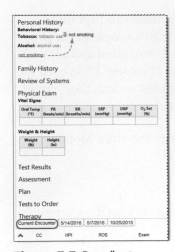

**Figure 7-7** Drag "not smoking" upward and drop onto Tobacco use.

"Tobacco," as illustrated by the arrow Figure 7-7. Make certain you do not accidently change the state of the finding while dragging and dropping it.

**Step 9**

The Copy into current note feature is not limited to single findings, but whole groups or sections of findings can be copied in this manner.

Locate and click on the 5/14/2016 tab.

Scroll the workspace pane to the bottom to locate and click on the Problem 1 heading. The entire section will be outlined and the drop-down menu will appear over the heading as shown in Figure 7-8. Click on the Copy into current note option.

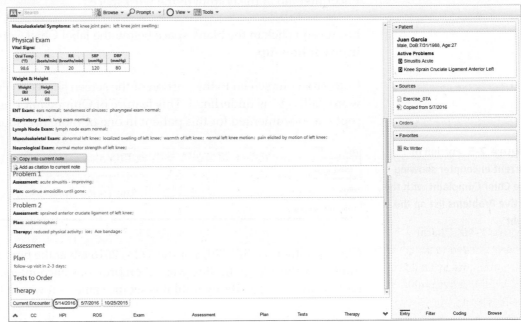

**Figure 7-8** Copy the Problem 1 section into the current note (from the 5/14/2016 encounter).

Now locate and click on the Problem 2 heading, and then select the Copy into current note option when the drop-down menu appears.

Locate and click on the Current Encounter tab and compare your screen to Figure 7-9. Verify that problem sections with their previous findings have been added.

**Step 10**

The problem sections in the note are examples of a problem-oriented chart, but they are not the problem list. The problem list in Quippe is labeled "Active Problems" and is located in the upper-right corner of the content pane under the patient's name as shown in Figure 7-9.

In Quippe a clinician can prompt on any problem in the Active Problem list, similar to the merge prompt feature you learned in previous chapters. This feature is helpful during follow-up visits. Since the problem sections in a problem-oriented chart are comprised only of Assessment, Plan, ordered tests, and ordered therapy, the ability to prompt on active problems allows the clinician to quickly locate and document history, symptoms, and exam findings, while focusing on one problem at a time.

Locate the list of **Active Problems** and *double-click* on **Sinusitis Acute**.

**Figure 7-9** Current encounter note after copying two problem sections from 5/14/2016.

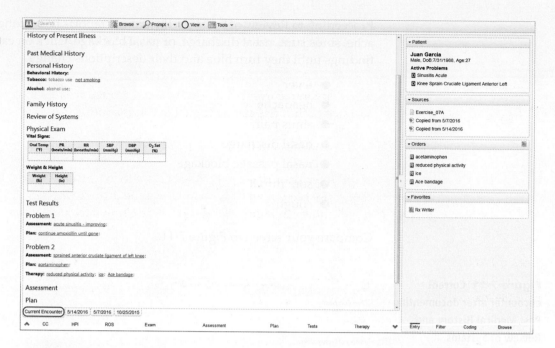

## Step 11

Compare your screen to Figure 7-10. Clinical concepts related to acute sinusitis have populated the encounter pane. Also notice Sources in the Content pane displays a merge prompt instance of Sinusitis Acute (with magnifying glass icon).

**Figure 7-10** Clinical concepts added to the current encounter note by double-clicking the active problem Sinusitis Acute.

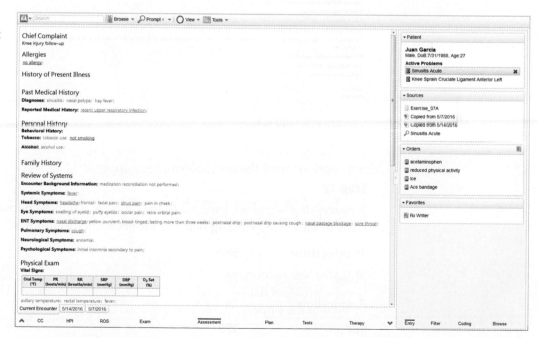

In this case the clinician did not want to copy the old findings forward, but rather to reexamine the patient. Underlined concepts identify findings documented in previous visits, which the clinician will certainly want to recheck. Begin in Past Medical History. It is evident from the problem list that the patient was diagnosed with sinusitis and has had a recent upper respiratory infection. Locate and click both findings until they turn red.

- sinusitis
- upper respiratory infection

Proceeding to Review of Systems, the patient reports he no longer has a fever, headache, sinus pain, nasal discharge, or nasal blockage. Click on each of the underlined findings until they turn blue and their descriptions change.

- fever
- headache
- sinus pain
- nasal discharge
- nasal passage blockage
- sore throat
- cough

Compare your screen to Figure 7-11.

**Figure 7-11** Current encounter after documenting Past Medical History and Review of Systems.

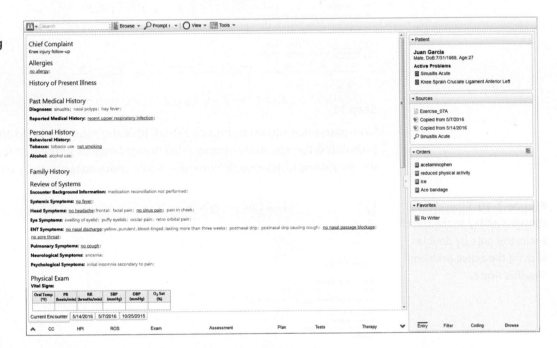

### Step 12

If everything is correct, proceed to the Physical Exam section and record Juan's vital signs in the corresponding fields of the encounter as follows:

| | |
|---|---|
| Temperature: | 98.6 |
| Pulse: | 78 |
| Respiration: | 20 |
| SBP: | 120 |
| DBP: | 80 |
| O₂ Sat: | 99 |
| Weight: | 144 |
| Height: | 68 |

The clinician reexamines all of the previous physical exam findings and determines that the patient's sinusitis has been resolved. As you did in the previous step, locate and click each of the underlined physical exam findings until they turn blue and their descriptions change.

- nasal discharge
- purulent
- nasal turbulent swollen
- tenderness of sinuses

### Step 13

Proceed to the Problem 1 section and click on acute sinusitis – improving until it turns blue.

*Right-click* on the finding and select Details from the Actions drop-down menu.

In the Details pop-up window, click in the Status field, and select Resolved from the drop-down list. Click the OK button. The description should now read "no acute sinusitis – resolved."

### Step 14

The patient confirms he has taken all of the prescribed amoxicillin.

Locate **amoxicillin** in Problem 1, *right-click* on it to invoke the Actions drop-down menu, and then select Delete. The finding will be deleted. Compare the Physical Exam and Problem 1 sections of your screen to Figure 7-12. If everything is correct, proceed to the next step.

**Figure 7-12** Current encounter note showing Vital Signs, Physical Exam, and Problem 1 resolved.

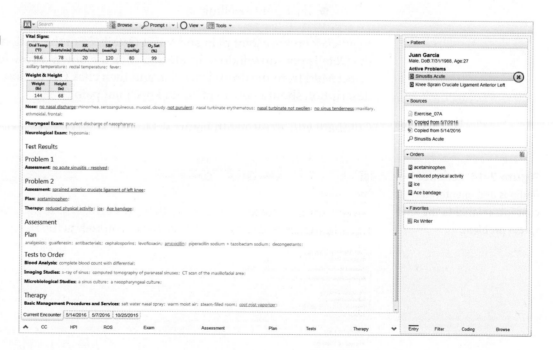

### Step 15

Since Mr. Garcia's sinusitis problem has been resolved, remove it from the problem list.

Locate **Sinusitis Acute** in the Active Problems listed under the patient's name. Locate and click the X at the right end of the item (circled in red in Figure 7-12). Sinusitis Acute will be deleted from the problem list, but this will not affect the diagnosis in the encounter pane.

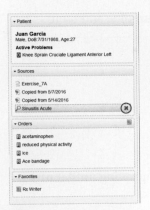

**Figure 7-13** Sources section of the content pane; click X (circled in red) to delete unentered concepts.

### Step 16

Next, clean up unentered concepts. Locate the Sources section in the content pane and click on the prompt instance labeled "Sinusitis Acute." Locate and click the X at the right end of the item (circled in red in Figure 7-13). Unused concepts related to sinusitis will be removed from the encounter pane.

### Step 17

Using what you have learned in the previous steps, document the findings for the second problem. Locate Active Problems in the content pane and *double-click* on **Knee Sprain Cruciate Ligament Anterior Left** in the problem list. Clinical concepts related to Mr. Garcia's knee sprain will populate the workspace pane.

Notice that there is now only one date tab at the bottom of the pane. This is because there was only one previous encounter for the knee injury. Since we have already copied the problem into the current note in step 9 it is not necessary to click on it.

### Step 18

Scroll the pane upward to Past Medical History to begin documenting history and Review of Systems symptoms related to the current problem. Mr. Garcia suffered a trauma to his knee. He is still experiencing some mild joint pain and swelling.

Locate and click on the following findings until they turn red.

- trauma to knee
- knee joint pain
- knee joint swelling

*Right-click* on knee joint pain and select Details from the Actions drop-down menu. In the Details pop-up window, locate and click the down-arrow for the Modifier field. Select Mild from the drop-down list, and then click OK to close the window. The description should now read "mild knee joint pain."

Compare your screen with Figure 7-14.

**Figure 7-14** Recorded findings and unentered concepts related to the knee sprain problem.

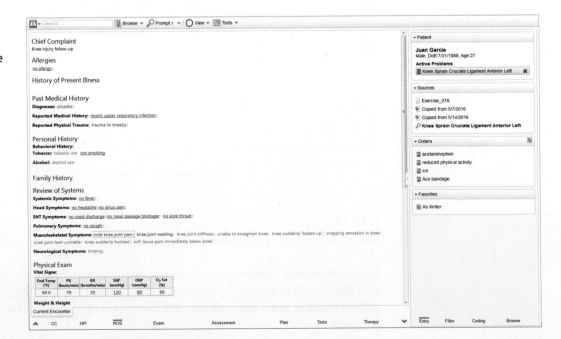

### Step 19

Proceed to the Musculoskeletal Exam in the Physical Exam section. Locate and click the following findings until they turn red.

- swelling of knee
- tenderness on palpation of knee

The clinician believes the condition is improving. Proceed to the Problem 2 section, *right-click* on the assessment **sprained anterior cruciate ligament of left knee** to invoke the Actions drop-down menu, and select Details.

In the Details pop-up window, click in the Status field and select **improving** from the drop-down list, and then click OK to close the window. Make certain the finding is still red after you are finished.

### Step 20

Click the View button on the toolbar and select Concise from the drop-down menu. Compare your screen to Figure 7-15. If everything on your screen matches the figure, proceed to step 21. If there are any differences, review the preceding steps and correct your work.

**Figure 7-15** Concise view of correctly completed encounter for Juan Garcia.

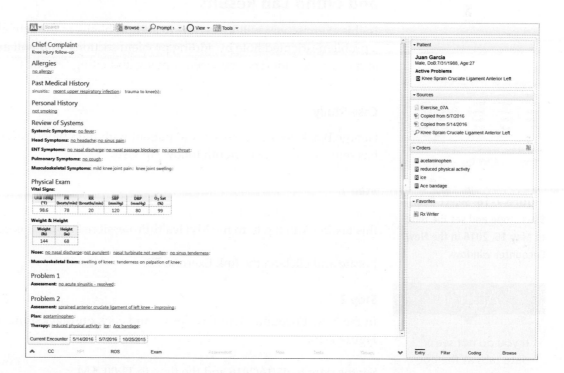

### Step 21

If you wish to print a copy of your completed encounter notes for yourself or because your instructor requires you to turn them in, use the Create PDF option, and then print or download the PDF at this time.

The final step in every exercise is to submit your completed work for a grade.

Locate and click the blue Quippe icon button on the toolbar, and then select the Submit for Grade option from the drop-down menu. This will complete Exercise 7A.

## Citing Previous Encounter Data

Presenting the information in a problem-oriented view and copying findings from previous encounters enables the clinician to quickly document the reexamination of each area examined during the previous visits. However, copying findings makes them part of the current exam. There are times when the clinician wishes to include for review previous findings without merging the findings in the current visit note. For example, a clinician might want to compare a current lab report with an older lab report.

Quippe offers two options for documenting previous findings in the current encounter. Copying merges the selected data into the current note as findings. Citation places the selected data at the bottom of the current encounter in a report format that is visible, but not as part of the actual findings in the note.

The difference can be important. For example, a clinician might want to include a review of a previously resolved problem section, without causing the problem to be documented as a current problem, which it is not. The next exercise will illustrate how previous data is cited into a current encounter.

## Guided Exercise 7B: Adding Problems, Retrieving and Citing Lab Results

In this exercise you will learn how to add problems to the active problem list, and create a problem-oriented note by adding problem sections. You will also retrieve lab results and learn the difference between copying and citing findings.

### Case Study

George Blackstone is a 46-year-old patient with high blood pressure and diabetes. He has returned for a two-month follow-up visit.

### Step 1

Start a supported web browser program and follow the steps listed inside the cover of this textbook to log in to the MyHealthProfessionsLab for this course.

Locate and click on the link Exercise 7B.

### Step 2

In the New Encounter window, locate and click on **Blackstone, George** as shown in Figure 7-16.

Set the date to **05/16/2016** and the time to **11:00 AM**.

Verify that the date and time are set correctly, and then click the OK button.

### Step 3

Locate and click in the blank space below the label Chief Complaint, and type **Two month follow-up**.

Click on any white area of the encounter pane that does not cause a heading or finding to have focus. The three date tabs should reappear at the bottom of the encounter pane. If you do not see them, click another white area of the encounter pane.

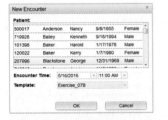

**Figure 7-16** Select George Blackstone and set the date to May 16, 2016 in the New Encounter window.

ALERT

If you do not see date tabs at the bottom of the encounter pane, you have not set the date correctly. Click the Quippe Icon button on the toolbar and select New Encounter from the drop-down menu, and then repeat step 2.

## Step 4

Locate the tab containing the date **3/15/2016** at the bottom of the encounter pane and click on it. A note from Mr. Blackstone's March 15, 2016 visit will be displayed.

Locate and click on the Current Medications heading so that it is highlighted and the copy menu is displayed as shown in Figure 7-17.

**Figure 7-17** Copy Current Medications from 3/15/2016 into the current note.

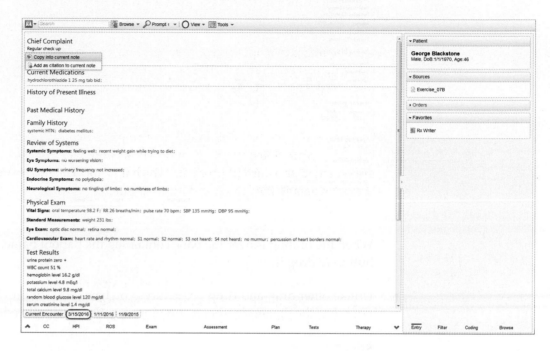

Click on the option Copy into Current Note.

## Step 5

Scroll the pane downward if necessary to locate and click on the Assessment heading so that it is highlighted and the copy menu is displayed as shown in Figure 7-18.

**Figure 7-18** Copy the Assessment section from 3/15/2016 into the current note.

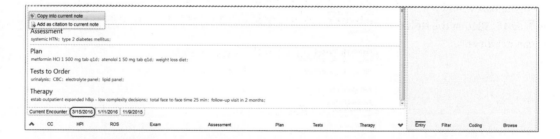

Click on the option Copy into Current Note.

Locate the Current Encounter tab at the bottom of the pane and click on it.

## Step 6

In the previous exercise you worked with and removed problems in the patient's problem list located in the upper-right corner, under the patient's name. Problems are added to this list by dragging and dropping them.

Locate the finding **systemic HTN**, click on it, and hold the left mouse button down as you drag it upward toward the patient's name (as shown by the arrow in Figure 7-19).

**Figure 7-19** Add systemic HTN to the problem list by dragging and dropping it on the patient's name.

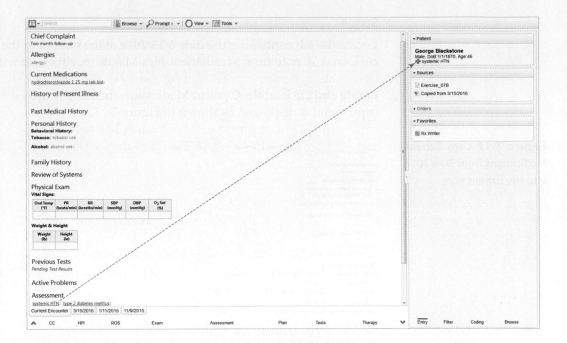

When the finding is over the pane containing the patient name, release the mouse button to drop it.

Unlike other drag-and-drop procedures you have done in previous exercises, this does not move the diagnosis from its previous location; it simply adds it to the problem list.

### Step 7

Locate the diagnosis **type 2 diabetes mellitus** in the Assessment section, and then using the same procedure as the previous step, drag-and-drop it onto the patient's problem list name (as shown by the arrow in Figure 7-20). When you have successfully added both diagnoses, the patient's problem list should resemble Figure 7-20.

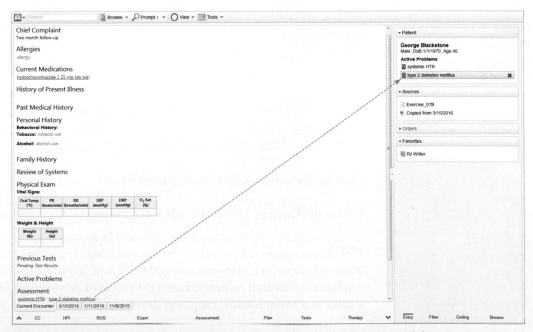

**Figure 7-20** Add type 2 diabetes mellitus to the problem list by dragging and dropping it on the Active Problems list.

## Step 8

Locate the Current Medications section. Mr. Blackstone is currently taking hydrochlorothiazide tablets to control his blood pressure. The clinician will renew the prescription, however, and wants to also keep the finding in current medications. This is done by duplicating the finding and then moving the duplicate.

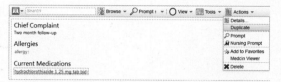

**Figure 7-21** Creating a duplicate finding using the Actions drop-down menu option.

*Right-click* on the finding **hydrochlorothiazide** to invoke the Actions drop-down menu, and then select the Duplicate option (as shown in Figure 7-21).

## Step 9

A duplicate finding will be added and have focus.

Click the Actions button on the toolbar, and select Details from the drop-down menu. In the Details pop-up window, click in the Prefix field and select **renew** from the drop-down list, as shown in Figure 7-22.

**Figure 7-22** Selecting the "renew" prefix for hydrochlorothiazide.

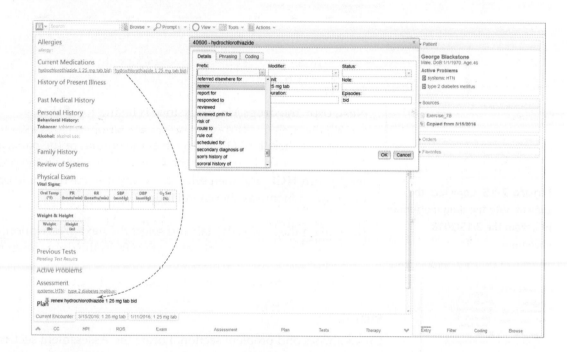

Click the OK button to close the pop-up window, and then drag "renew hydrochlorothiazide 1 25 mg tab bid" downward, and drop it on the Plan section, as illustrated by the arrow in Figure 7-22.

## Step 10

As you learned earlier in the chapter, problem-oriented charts group plan, orders, and therapy into problem sections related to a diagnosis or condition. In the previous exercise the problem sections had already been created and were simply copied into the current encounter. In this step, you will learn how problem sections are created.

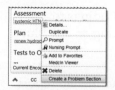

**Figure 7-23** Create a problem section for systemic HTN using the Actions drop-down menu option.

Locate the Assessment section and *right-click* on **systemic HTN** to invoke the Actions drop-down menu, and then select Create a Problem Section as shown in Figure 7-23.

This will move the diagnosis and the plan into a new section labeled "Problem 1." Compare your screen to Figure 7-24.

**Figure 7-24** Current encounter note after creating the Problem 1 section.

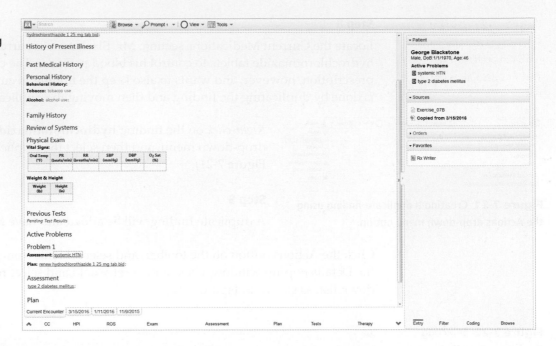

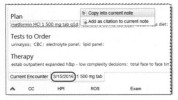

**Figure 7-25** Copy into the current note the drug metformin HCL from the 3/15/2016 encounter.

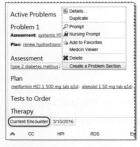

**Figure 7-26** Create a problem section for type 2 diabetes mellitus using the Actions drop-down menu option.

### Step 11

Next, copy the drugs Mr. Blackstone is taking for diabetes.

Locate and click the 3/15/2016 tab at the bottom of the pane, and when the previous encounter is displayed, locate the Plan section, click on the prescription for **metformin HCL**, and then select the Copy into current note option from the drop-down menu, as shown in Figure 7-25.

Remain on the 3/15/2016 tab and select the next prescription, **atenolol**, and then select the Copy into current note option from the drop-down menu.

Return to the current encounter by clicking on the Current Encounter tab.

### Step 12

Create the second problem section. Locate the Assessment section of the current encounter and *right-click* on **type 2 diabetes mellitus** to invoke the Actions drop-down menu, and then select Create a Problem Section as shown in Figure 7-26.

### Step 13

Compare your screen to Figure 7-27. Your encounter note should have two problem sections.

At this step, verify that all entered findings are red. If, while selecting findings to highlight them, you accidently changed their state, correct this by clicking on any blue finding until it turns red.

Prior to his appointment Mr. Blackstone had some lab work done and the lab report is ready, as indicated by the link under the Previous Tests section heading. To retrieve the results locate and *single-click* on the Pending Test Results link (circled in Figure 7-27).

**Figure 7-27** Current encounter with the second problem section. The Pending Test Results link is circled in red.

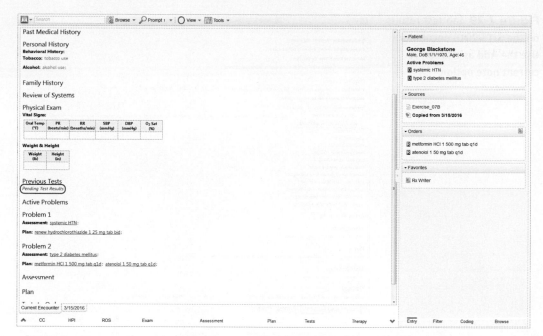

The lab test results will be merged into the current encounter as shown in Figure 7-28.

**Figure 7-28** Test Results retrieved from the lab for George Blackstone.

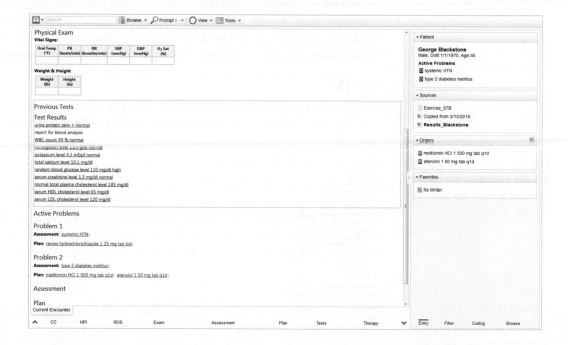

## Step 14

Similar tests were performed on the patient's previous visit, and the clinician wishes to compare the two reports, but does not wish to mingle the previous results with the new report. Therefore, we will *cite* them instead of copying them.

Click on any white space that does not highlight a finding or heading so that the date tabs reappear. Click on the **3/15/2015** tab to display the previous note.

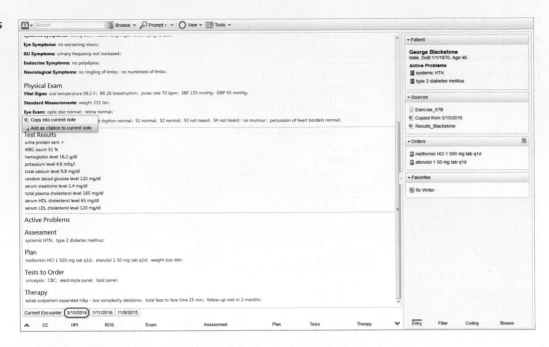

**Figure 7-29** Lab test results on the 3/15/2016 encounter. Use the Add as citation to current note option.

In the 3/15/2016 note, click on the Test Results heading to highlight the section, and display the drop-down menu. This time, however, select the Add as citation to current note option, as shown in Figure 7-29.

The difference between the two options is that copy merges the findings into the current encounter note, where they may be modified or moved as would any current finding. Citation places the cited data as a footnote at the bottom of the note, and the only valid action permitted on a cited item is that the citation may be deleted.

**Step 15**

Click on the Current Encounter tab and compare your screen to Figure 7-30. You should now be able to compare the current test results findings with the results at the bottom of

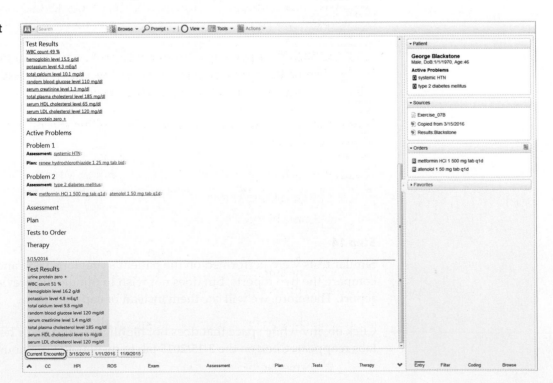

**Figure 7-30** 3/15/2016 Test Results added to the current encounter as a citation.

the encounter cited from his March 15, 2016 lab report. For example, Mr. Blackstone's white blood count (WBC) has gone down, while his hemoglobin level has gone up.

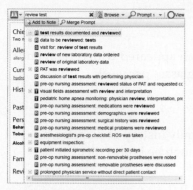

**Figure 7-31** The test results documented and reviewed finding highlighted in the search list.

Document that the clinician has reviewed the lab reports. Locate the Search box on the toolbar and click in it. Type **review test** and press the Enter key. Locate the test results documented and reviewed concept in the drop-down list, click on it to highlight it, and then click the Add to note button shown in Figure 7-31.

Scroll to the bottom of the encounter pane (if necessary) to locate and click on **test results documented and reviewed** until the finding turns red.

### Step 16

Scroll the encounter pane to the top. Proceed to the Physical Exam section and record Mr. Blackstone's vital signs in the corresponding fields of the encounter as follows:

| | |
|---|---|
| Temperature: | **98.6** |
| Pulse: | **78** |
| Respiration: | **26** |
| SBP: | **138** |
| DBP: | **90** |
| O$_2$ Sat: | **96** |
| Weight: | **235** |
| Height: | **68.5** |

### Step 17

As you learned in the previous exercise, the Active Problems in the upper corner of the Content pane can also be used to invoke the Merge Prompt function. Locate and *double-click* on the active problem **Type 2 Diabetes Mellitus**.

Related clinical concepts will be added to the encounter. Remember, underlined concepts indicate findings documented in previous encounters.

Scroll the encounter pane upward (if necessary) to document Past Medical History. Mr. Blackstone has not been to the podiatrist recently, opting to examine his feet himself. He is compliant with checking his blood sugar at home.

Locate and click on **recent examination by podiatrist** until it turns blue and the description changes.

Locate and click on the following findings until they turn red.

- foot self-exam recently
- home blood sugar check

### Step 18

Mr. Blackstone smoked a pack of cigarettes a day for 20 years, but quit last year. He continues to drink a glass of wine every night with supper.

Locate and click on the following findings until they turn red.

- tobacco use
- former smoker

- cigarettes
- recently stopped smoking
- alcohol use
- wine

Type the following numbers in the data detail fields, which appeared with certain findings: **20** pack-years, stopped smoking **1** year ago, wine **7** glasses per week.

**Step 19**

Mr. Blackstone has seen an eye doctor regularly, has a family history of diabetes, an increased appetite, and continues to gain weight even though he is on a diet.

Locate and click on the following findings until they turn red.

- seeing an eye doctor regularly
- diabetes mellitus (under Family History)
- recent change in weight
- recent weight gain
- increased appetite

The clinician reviews the rest of the symptoms and finds they are normal.

Click on the Review of Systems heading to highlight the section. Click the Actions button on the toolbar and select Otherwise Normal from the drop-down menu.

Compare your History, Review of Systems, and Vital Signs sections to Figure 7-32, scrolling as necessary.

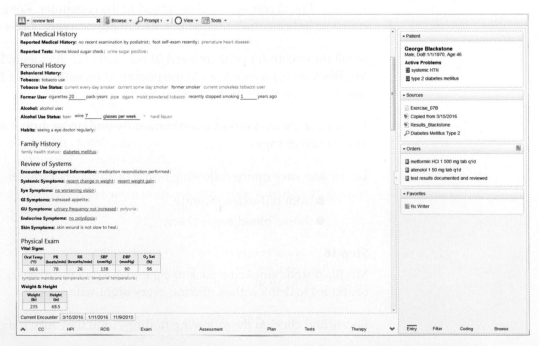

**Figure 7-32** Correctly completed findings for History, Review of Systems, and Vital signs sections.

Family History

family health status: systemic HTN; diabetes mellitus;

Review of Systems

**Encounter Background Information:** medication reconciliation performed;

**Systemic Symptoms:** recent change in weight; recent weight gain;

**Head Symptoms:** no headache;

**Eye Symptoms:** no worsening vision;

**Cardiovascular Symptoms:** no chest pain;

**GI Symptoms:** increased appetite;

**GU Symptoms:** urinary frequency not increased; polyuria;

**Endocrine Symptoms:** no polydipsia;

**Neurological Symptoms:** no dizziness;

**Skin Symptoms:** skin wound is not slow to heal;

Physical Exam

**Vital Signs:**

| Oral Temp (°F) | PR (beats/min) | RR (breaths/min) | SBP (mmHg) | DBP (mmHg) | $O_2$ Sat (%) |
|---|---|---|---|---|---|
| 98.6 | 78 | 26 | 138 | 90 | 96 |

tympanic membrane temperature; temporal temperature; blood pressure:combine

**Weight & Height**

| Weight (lb) | Height (in) |
|---|---|
| 235 | 68.5 |

**Standard Measurements:** patient obese; body mass index;

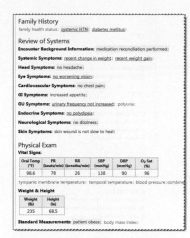

**Figure 7-33 Findings and additional concepts related to Hypertension highlighted in yellow.**

## Step 20

Locate and *double-click* on the active problem **Hypertension (systemic HTN)** in the upper-right corner of the Content pane.

Return to the Family History section to locate the **systemic HTN** finding and click on it until it turns red.

The clinician reviews additional symptoms added by the hypertension prompt and finds that they are negative. Click on the Review of Systems heading to highlight the section. Click the Actions button on the toolbar and select Otherwise Normal from the drop-down menu.

Proceed to the Physical Exam section. Locate the Standard Measurements group, and click on **patient obese** until it turns red.

Findings recorded in step 20 are highlighted yellow in Figure 7-33.

## Step 21

Scroll downward to the Therapy section. Locate and click on the following findings until they turn red.

- weight loss diet
- institute prescribed exercise plan
- patient education about proper diet
- patient education about diabetes

Compare your Therapy section to Figure 7-34.

Therapy

**Physician's Services:** test results documented and reviewed;

**Basic Management Procedures and Services:** diet; low sodium diet; weight loss diet; diabetic diet; institute prescribed exercise program; abstinence from smoking; patient education about a proper diet; patient education about diabetes; patient education about a blood glucose monitor; patient education about a home blood glucose monitor; patient education about diabetes home insulin administration; inquiry and counseling about medication administration and compliance; discussed concerns about properly fitting shoes; the patient's goal is to begin regular exercise; [illegible]

**Rehabilitation:** psychotherapeutic rehabilitation: behavior modification; lifestyle change;

**Medical Supplies and Equipment:** diabetic supplies glucose monitoring strips;

referral to diabetologist; referral to endocrinologist; referral to pediatric endocrinologist; consultation with an endocrinologist; consultation with a podiatrist; consultation with a nephrologist; consultation with an ophthalmologist; consultation with a nutritionist;

**Figure 7-34 Therapy section showing correctly recorded findings.**

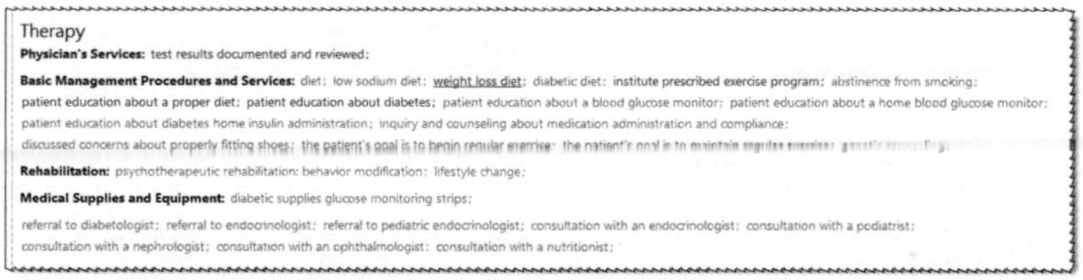

## Step 22

Click the View button on the toolbar and select Concise from the drop-down menu. Because there are so many findings, the completed encounter is shown in two figures. Compare your screen to Figure 7-35a and Figure 7-35b, scrolling your screen as necessary until you have compared all of it. If everything on your screen matches the figures, proceed to step 23. If there are any differences, review the preceding steps and correct your work.

## Step 23

If wish to print a copy of your completed encounter notes for yourself or because your instructor requires you to turn them in, use the Create PDF option, and then print or download the PDF at this time.

The final step in every exercise is to submit your completed work for a grade.

Locate and click the blue Quippe icon button on the toolbar, and then select the Submit for Grade option from the drop-down menu. This will complete Exercise 7B.

**Figure 7-35a** Concise view of upper portion of correctly completed encounter.

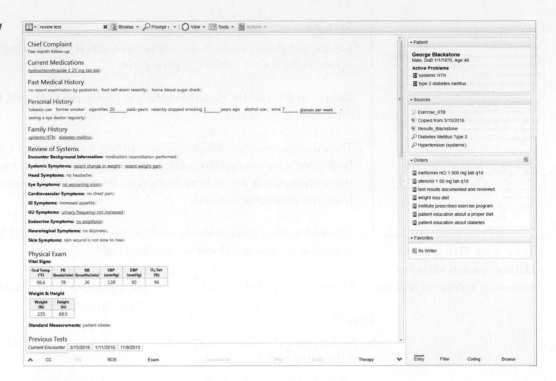

**Figure 7-35b** Concise view of remaining portion of correctly completed encounter.

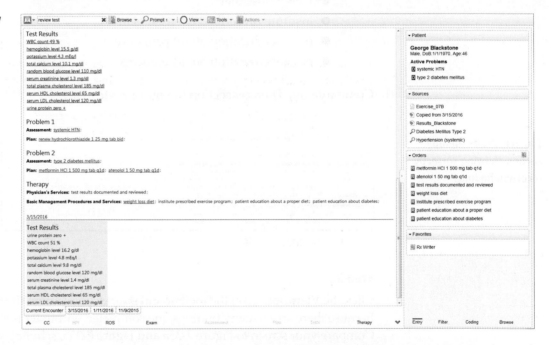

## Orders and Results Management

You will recall from Chapter 1 that Results Management was one of the eight criteria for an EHR in the IOM report. Orders are tracked in an EHR from the moment they are entered in the system. In Chapter 6 we mentioned that one of the benefits of CPOE systems is that they keep track of what has been ordered for each patient. Benefits of CPOE order tracking include:

◆ Preventing lost orders.

◆ Preventing duplicate orders.

◆ Detecting when a patient sent to an outside lab has failed to show up.

Benefits of results tracking include:

◆ Notifying the provider as soon as preliminary results are available.

◆ Notifying the provider anytime results status are updated to "final" or "corrected."

◆ Keeping track of which results need to be reviewed by the clinician.

Exercises in this chapter demonstrate the benefits of having test results available to the provider during the patient encounter. The ability to review results online improves the clinician's ability to make timely clinical decisions or to order subsequent additional tests when warranted. Another benefit is the ability to compare or "trend" the results of several iterations of the same test.

The Student Edition software does not contain a live electronic laboratory interface, as it would not be appropriate to order tests from a classroom. Consequently, lab order and result exercises merge data into the encounter without making an actual connection to a laboratory system. The purpose of the exercises is to demonstrate how useful it is to have lab data at hand while seeing the patient and to allow you to work with test result data.

## Guided Exercise 7C: Retrieving Pending Lab Results

In this exercise you will learn about lab data and retrieve some results for a patient.

### Case Study

In the previous chapter, this patient's mother reported that the family had possibly been exposed to lead-based paints while remodeling an older home. You will recall the treatment plan recommended screening other family members for lead poisoning. Accordingly, Alena Zabroski's 16-year-old son, Stanley, has had lab work done in preparation for his upcoming appointment. Today some of the results are ready.

### Step 1

Start a supported web browser program and follow the steps listed inside the cover of this text to log in to the MyHealthProfessionsLab for this course.

Locate and click on the link Exercise 7C.

### Step 2

In the New Encounter window, locate and click on **Zabroski, Stanley**.

Set the date to **05/22/2016** and the time to **3:00 PM**.

Compare your New Encounter window to Figure 7-36 to verify that the date and time are set *correctly*, and then click the OK button.

### Step 3

Locate the Previous Tests section heading and *single-click* on the Pending Test Results link, as you did in Exercise 7B. A pop-up window will display the pending lab report as shown in Figure 7-37.

As explained earlier, it would be inappropriate for student EHR software to have a live connection to a laboratory system. The purpose of this window is to illustrate the workflow of retrieving results and to help you to visualize the components of a lab

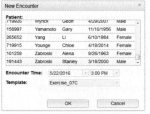

**Figure 7-36** Stanley Zabroski selected and date set to 5/22/2016 3:00 PM in the New Encounter window.

**Figure 7-37** Lab Results window showing the lab report to download.

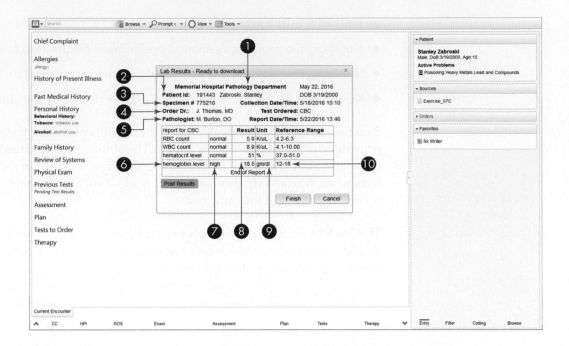

report. In an actual medical office it is unlikely you would see this screen. In practice, lab results are merged into the EHR without pausing unless there is a mismatch between the order and the report. In such a case, the report would be displayed for purposes of verifying that the requisition is correctly matched to the order.

**Step 4**

Since the report is displayed, study the sections that make up the report.

❶ At the top of the lab report is the name of the facility that performed the test(s) and the date of the report.

❷ The second line contains patient information to help identify the patient in the EHR. This information comes from the original order requisition sent by the EHR, so it should match the ordering physician's system exactly.

❸ The third line identifies the order to the lab by a unique specimen number. Sometimes this number is alternatively called the accession number or requisition number. The same line provides the date and time the specimen was taken from the patient. In inpatient settings where the patient may have blood drawn several times a day this is particularly useful for comparing changes over time. For an example of repeated tests results over time, refer to the Cumulative Summary Report shown in Figure 2-19 in Chapter 2.

❹ The fourth line identifies the ordering doctor and lists the tests ordered. Sometimes there is another doctor, such as the patient's primary care physician, to be copied on the report, in which case that doctor is also listed.

❺ The fifth line identifies the pathologist at the laboratory who has reviewed and is responsible for the report. Even when tests are performed by automated equipment, a pathologist reviews and approves the report before it is sent.

❻ The first column of the grid contains the test name and lists components of the test under it.

❼ The second column notes whether the result value is considered low, high, or normal. Results below the first number of the reference range (shown in the last column) are considered Low, while results above the second number of the reference range are considered High. If results are extremely far outside either end of the reference range, they are designated as Low-Low or High-High. These are also called critical or panic values because they are outside the normal range to a degree that may constitute an immediate health risk to the patient or require urgent action on the part of the ordering clinician.

**8** The third column is the actual result value.

**9** The fourth column is the unit of measure by which the result is reported. For example, locate hemoglobin. The value reported in column three is measured in grams (*gm*) (of oxygen carrying cells) per deciliter (*dl*) of whole blood. A deciliter is 100 milliliters.

**10** The last column lists a reference range within which the result is considered normal.

### Step 5

Once you have reviewed the report, locate and click the Post Results button. The report will be added to Stanley's chart. Locate and click the Finish button to close the pop-up window.

### Step 6

Compare your screen to Figure 7-38. If everything on your screen matches the figure, proceed to step 7. If there are any differences, click the Quippe icon button on the toolbar, select New Encounter from the drop-down menu, and restart the exercise at step 2.

**Figure 7-38** Test Results downloaded and merged into the current encounter.

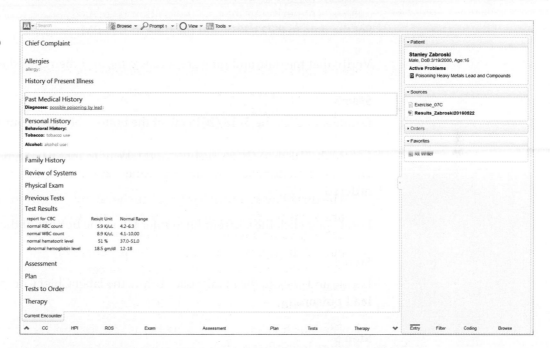

### Step 7

If wish to print a copy of your completed encounter notes for yourself or because your instructor requires you to turn them in, use the Create PDF option, and then print or download the PDF at this time.

The final step in every exercise is to submit your completed work for a grade.

Locate and click the blue Quippe icon button on the toolbar, and then select the Submit for Grade option from the drop-down menu. This will complete Exercise 7C.

## Critical Thinking Exercise 7D: Using Lab Results to Rule Out Lead Poisoning

In the previous exercise you retrieved lab results for one of several tests that had been ordered in preparation for a patient's appointment. In this exercise you will use what you have learned so far to retrieve the remaining test results, cite the earlier results, and clear an active problem.

### Case Study

Stanley Zabroski is a 16-year-old who was possibly exposed to peeling lead-based paint while living in his mother's childhood home. He has had lab work done in preparation for his appointment. The test results are ready. Today his office visit is for examination and to review the test results.

### Step 1

Start a supported web browser program and follow the steps listed inside the cover of this textbook to log in to the MyHealthProfessionsLab for this course.

Locate and click on the link Exercise 7D.

### Step 2

In the New Encounter window, locate and click on **Zabroski, Stanley**.

Set the date to **05/23/2016** and the time to **1:00 PM**.

Verify that the date and time are set *correctly*, and then click the OK button.

### Step 3

Locate and click the 5/18/2016 tab at the bottom of the encounter pane.

Locate the Tests to Order section, and take note that a CBC, basic metabolic panel with total calcium, hepatic function panel, serum lead, and urine lead tests were ordered.

Locate and click the Current Encounter tab at the bottom of the encounter pane.

### Step 4

Locate and click in the blank space below the label Chief Complaint, and type **Rule out lead poisoning**.

### Step 5

Locate the problem list in the upper-right corner of the Content Pane, and *double-click* on **Poisoning Heavy Metals Lead and Compounds.** This will merge relevant clinical concepts into the encounter pane.

Stanley denies having allergies, and doesn't have a history of abdominal tenderness. Locate and click on the following findings until they turn blue. The descriptions will change.

- allergy
- direct abdominal tenderness

**Step 6**

As his mother reported previously, there is a probable exposure to lead from remodeling work on their home. Locate and click on the following finding until it turns red.

- exposure to lead

*Right-click* on the finding and select Details from the Actions drop-down menu. Click in the Prefix field and select **probable** from the drop-down list. Click OK to close the pop-up window. The finding description should read "probable exposure to lead."

Locate and click on the following finding until it turns red.

- house has peeling lead-based paint

**Step 7**

Stanley denies smoking or using alcohol. Locate and click on the following findings until they turn blue. The descriptions will change.

- tobacco use
- alcohol use

**Step 8**

Proceed to Review of Systems. A medication reconciliation was not performed. Stanley has not been having headaches, nausea, or abdominal pain. His concentration is good and his school performance is not suffering.

Locate and click on the following finding until it turns red.

- medication reconciliation was not performed

Click on the Review of Systems heading to highlight the section. Click the Actions button on the toolbar and select Otherwise normal from the drop-down menu.

**Step 9**

Proceed to the Physical Exam section and enter the patient's Vital Signs using the following information:

| | |
|---|---|
| Temperature: | 98.6 |
| Pulse: | 70 |
| Respiration: | 20 |
| SBP: | 120 |
| DBP: | 80 |
| O$_2$ Sat. | 100 |
| Weight: | 155 |
| Height: | 73 |

**Step 10**

Locate and click on the following findings until they turn blue and their descriptions change.

- papilledema
- gums showed gingival line
- direct abdominal tenderness

**Step 11**

As discussed at the beginning of the exercise, the patient has had several lab tests performed prior to the office visit. The clinician will review results of the tests and document them in the encounter note.

Locate the Previous Tests section and *single-click* the Pending Test Results link.

The urine lead, serum lead, hepatic function panel, and basic metabolic panel with total calcium lab reports are retrieved and merged into the note. However, the CBC results were retrieved on the previous day. Bring them into the current encounter by citing them.

To restore the date tabs, click in any white space that does not highlight a heading or finding. Locate and click the **5/22/2016** tab at the bottom of the encounter pane.

Locate and click on the Tests Results heading to highlight the section. Select the Add as citation to current note option from the drop-down menu.

Locate and click the Current Encounter tab at the bottom of the encounter pane.

**Step 12**

Scroll the encounter pane to the bottom to confirm that the report for CBC was added.

Locate and click in the Search box on the toolbar. Type **review test** and press the Enter key.

Locate "test results documented and reviewed" in the search results list; click on it to highlight it, and then click the Add to Note button.

Locate the finding you have just added and click on it until it turns red.

- test results documented and reviewed

**Step 13**

The clinician has reviewed the test results and concludes that Stanley does not present any signs of lead poisoning.

Locate the Assessment section and note there are duplicate instances of poisoning by lead.

*Right-click* on the finding possible poisoning by lead to invoke the Actions drop-down menu, and then click on Delete.

There should now be only one instance remaining. Click on it until it turns blue and the description changes.

- poisoning by lead

**Step 14**

Since lead poisoning is no longer a concern, remove the item from Stanley's problem list.

Locate Active Problems in the upper-right corner of the content pane, under Stanley's name. *Single-click* Poisoning Heavy Metals Lead and Compounds to highlight it, and then click the X on the right end of the description to delete it.

## Step 15

Locate and click the blue Quippe icon button on the toolbar, and select Create PDF from the drop-down menu. This will produce a two-page PDF.

Compare your PDF to Figure 7-39a and Figure 7-39b, scrolling your screen as necessary until you have compared all of it. If everything on your screen matches the figures, proceed to step 16. If there are any differences, review the preceding steps and correct your work.

**Figure 7-39a** PDF encounter note for Stanley Zabroski (page 1 of 2). See overleaf for page 2.

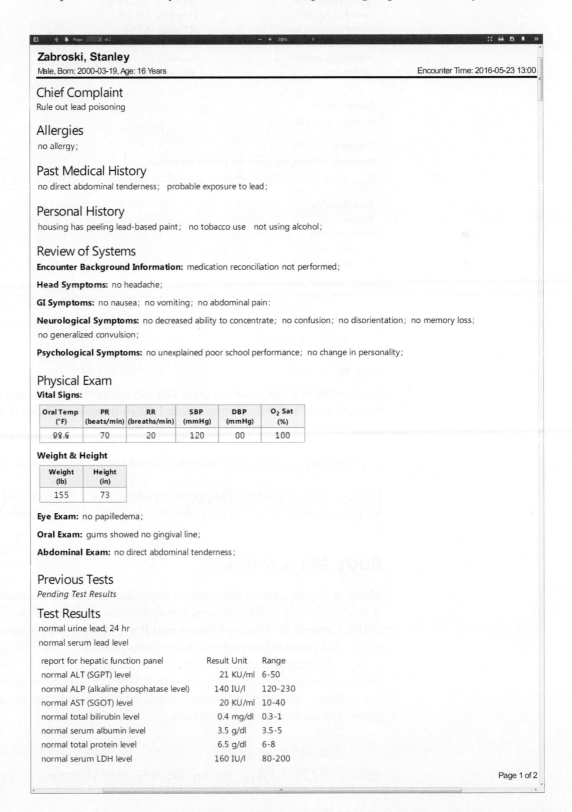

**Zabroski, Stanley**
Male, Born: 2000-03-19, Age: 16 Years                                          Encounter Time: 2016-05-23 13:00

### Chief Complaint
Rule out lead poisoning

### Allergies
no allergy;

### Past Medical History
no direct abdominal tenderness;   probable exposure to lead;

### Personal History
housing has peeling lead-based paint;   no tobacco use   not using alcohol;

### Review of Systems
**Encounter Background Information:** medication reconciliation not performed;

**Head Symptoms:** no headache;

**GI Symptoms:** no nausea;  no vomiting;  no abdominal pain;

**Neurological Symptoms:** no decreased ability to concentrate;  no confusion;  no disorientation;  no memory loss; no generalized convulsion;

**Psychological Symptoms:** no unexplained poor school performance;  no change in personality;

### Physical Exam
**Vital Signs:**

| Oral Temp (°F) | PR (beats/min) | RR (breaths/min) | SBP (mmHg) | DBP (mmHg) | O₂ Sat (%) |
|---|---|---|---|---|---|
| 98.6 | 70 | 20 | 120 | 00 | 100 |

**Weight & Height**

| Weight (lb) | Height (in) |
|---|---|
| 155 | 73 |

**Eye Exam:** no papilledema;

**Oral Exam:** gums showed no gingival line;

**Abdominal Exam:** no direct abdominal tenderness;

### Previous Tests
*Pending Test Results*

### Test Results
normal urine lead, 24 hr
normal serum lead level

| report for hepatic function panel | Result Unit | Range |
|---|---|---|
| normal ALT (SGPT) level | 21 KU/ml | 6-50 |
| normal ALP (alkaline phosphatase level) | 140 IU/l | 120-230 |
| normal AST (SGOT) level | 20 KU/ml | 10-40 |
| normal total bilirubin level | 0.4 mg/dl | 0.3-1 |
| normal serum albumin level | 3.5 g/dl | 3.5-5 |
| normal total protein level | 6.5 g/dl | 6-8 |
| normal serum LDH level | 160 IU/l | 80-200 |

Page 1 of 2

**Figure 7-39b** PDF encounter note for Stanley Zabroski (page 2 of 2).

**Zabroski, Stanley**
Male, Born: 2000-03-19, Age: 16 Years | Encounter Time: 2016-05-23 13:00

| report for basic metabolic panel with total calcium | Result Unit | Range |
|---|---|---|
| normal fasting glucose | 94 mg/dl | 60-99 |
| normal BUN level | 12 mg/dl | 7-25 |
| normal serum creatinine level | 0.9 mg/dl | 0.4-1.5 |
| BUN/Creatinine ratio | 13.3 % | 7.2-21.5 % |
| normal sodium level | 142 mEq/L | 135-145 |
| normal potassium level | 3.7 mEq/L | 3.5-5.1 |
| normal chloride level | 103 mEq/L | 96-112 |
| normal CO2 content | 26.5 mEq/L | 19.0-35.0 |
| calcium level | 9.6 mg/dl | 8.5-10.5 |

### Assessment
no poisoning by lead;

### Therapy
**Physician's Services:** test results documented and reviewed;

5/22/2016

### Test Results
RBC count 5.9
WBC count 8900
hematocrit level 51
hemoglobin level 17

Page 2 of 2

## Step 16

If you wish to print or save a copy of your completed encounter notes for yourself or because your instructor requires you to turn them in, print or download the PDF at this time.

The final step in every exercise is to submit your completed work for a grade.

Locate and click the blue Quippe icon button on the toolbar, and then select the Submit for Grade option from the drop-down menu. This will complete Exercise 7D.

# Body Mass Index

Many of the patients in the exercise data who have chronic conditions such as hypertension, diabetes, or heart problems are also overweight. The National Institute of Health (NIH), Centers for Disease Control and Prevention (CDC), American Medical Association (AMA), and other authorities are concerned about the rising percentage of obesity in both children and adults in America. A study published in *The Journal of the American Medical Association (JAMA)* reported that 34.9% of American adults and 17% of children were obese.[1] There are also many people who are below the threshold for the obese category, but are seriously overweight.

---

[1]Ogden, Carroll, Kit, and Flegal, "Prevalence of Childhood and Adult Obesity in the United States," *JAMA*, Vol. 311, No. 8, February 26, 2014.

# Real-Life Story

## Experiencing the Functional Benefits of an EHR

**by Henry Palmer, MD**

*Henry Palmer, MD, specializes in internal medicine and is affiliated with Rush University Medical Center.*

I am a physician practicing at two locations, neither of which is where my EHR computer is located. I have computers in the exam rooms and I am documenting with the patients, but the data is going over the Internet into the servers in real time.

Rush University Medical Center, like other large institutions, had many different computer systems in its departments. Trying to unite all these legacy systems was very difficult, but the center wanted to be able to access all the information relatively easily from one system. Rush has a CDR, or clinical data repository, which stores the data from various legacy systems. For example, the clinical notes section includes all of the radiology, ultrasound, stress testing, cardiology, and operative reports; these are transcribed reports, all text based.

Lab results, however, come in as fielded data. The results are imported automatically. You can set how far back in time you want to default your view of them. This is very handy because you are able to see the trends. You can also graph it. You can rearrange the view to see your results horizontally or vertically.

The CDR has demographic information for the patient, of course, and helpful information about admission and discharge. Let us say I want to look at the admission from two months ago. I can highlight it and find out who the providers were for that admission, the insurance information for that admission, as well as the diagnosis.

Rush also has an order entry system. When I sign in, it automatically shows if I have a patient who is in the hospital. This is handy, particularly in the case of primary care physicians, because sometimes your patients get admitted without your knowledge. A patient may get admitted into the surgical service and you might never be called.

The order entry screen first shows if there are any orders approaching expiration. It also asks me to authenticate any verbal orders I had given over the phone, but had not yet countersigned.

I can pull up a patient and view results through the order system. I can look at results in different ways—results for the last five days, all the results since admission, or just the ones that were critical. I can see details about particular results, the normal ranges, and some additional information about how to interpret those results.

When I write a medication order, it goes electronically to the pharmacy. The order system will also provide alerts to drug interactions or areas of concern the hospital has identified with the drug. When ordering potassium, for example, the system would advise me that it should only be given in a certain quantity if the patient is on certain medications that tend to increase potassium levels anyway.

It is easy to order labs by just clicking one box. I can also order a consult. CPOE works. It is not perfect, but in a large institution like this it has to work or it would not be used.

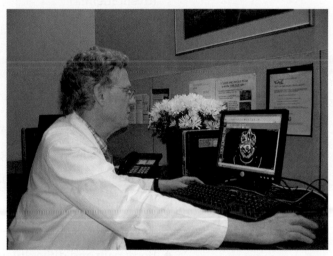

**Photo by Richard Gartee**
**Dr. Palmer reviews a CAT scan.**

Our PAC system eliminates the need to have to go down to radiology to see x-rays. On the average workstation I can view the images of the patients' x-rays with reasonable definition. If I want really fine detail, I can go to any of the high-definition monitors that are scattered around the hospital. I can also display the radiologist's report. Reading the report will guide me toward the areas of concern.

Additionally, we use an electronic signature program for signing off on charts. Basically this brings up the document, allowing me to edit it and finalize my signature. I can also indicate which doctors I want to receive copies of my document. The system will then automatically fax them to the doctors involved with the patient care.

Decision support includes access to the Rush medical library from inside our system. I enter my search term and it will

*(continued)*

retrieve an index of the article. I can go directly to what I want to read, for example, the treatment or the diagnostic approach to the disease.

One of the challenges as a primary care physician is that my patients search the Internet. They will often come in with research in hand and ask some very cogent questions. I think the downside can be that people assume because they have read it on the Internet that it applies to them or that they know what to do with the information—and that is not always the case.

The biggest problem I see in health information technology today is the segregation of records, particularly between inpatient and outpatient systems. When patients are admitted, their outpatient records are not there. Synchronizing those, I think, would be a big step forward and also eliminate redundancy in testing.

According to the CDC, people who are obese, compared to those with a normal or healthy weight, are at increased risk for many serious diseases and health conditions, including the following:[2]

◆ All-causes of death (mortality)

◆ High blood pressure (hypertension)

◆ High LDL cholesterol, low HDL cholesterol, or high levels of triglycerides (dyslipidemia)

◆ Type 2 diabetes

◆ Coronary heart disease

◆ Stroke

◆ Gallbladder disease

◆ Osteoarthritis (a breakdown of cartilage and bone within a joint)

◆ Sleep apnea and breathing problems

◆ Some cancers (endometrial, breast, colon, kidney, gallbladder, and liver)

◆ Low quality of life

◆ Mental illness such as clinical depression, anxiety, and other mental disorders

◆ Body pain and difficulty with physical functioning

How much body fat is too much? Traditionally, doctors used tables of height and weight to determine if patients were over- or underweight. However, Body Mass Index (BMI) has been identified as a better measuring method. BMI is a measure of body fat based on height and weight calculated using a simple formula that yields the same results with English or metric measurements.

The metric formula is $kg/m^2$ where weight is kilograms and height is meters. Metric height is more commonly measured in centimeters, in which case centimeters are converted to meters in the formula by multiplying the final product by $100^2$ (or 10,000).

When using pounds and inches, the formula is the same except the final product is multiplied by 703.

---

[2]Source: U.S. Department of Health and Human Services, Center for Disease Control web site http://www.cdc.gov.

The BMI number, as an indicator of body fat, determines which of four categories the patient falls in: underweight, normal, overweight, or obese.

**Adult BMI Categories**

| BMI | Category |
|---|---|
| 18.5 or less | Underweight |
| 18.5–24.9 | Normal weight |
| 25–29.9 | Overweight |
| 30 or greater | Obese |

For example, Briana Allen, a patient who drank too much coffee, is 5'4" (64 inches) and weighs 100 pounds. Her weight divided by her height squared, times 703 equals her BMI.

$$(100/(64 \times 64)) \times 703 = 17.2$$

Comparing the result of this calculation to the Adult BMI categories table, we can see that Briana is in the BMI category underweight.

For Adults age 20 years or older both genders share the same BMI chart. However, because BMI changes substantially as children get older, BMI categories are gender-specific and age-specific for children and teens ages 2 to 20 years.

The CDC encourages pediatricians to replace use of the older weight-for-stature charts with the new BMI-for-age charts.[3] There are several advantages to using BMI-for-age as a screening tool for overweight and underweight children. BMI-for-age provides a reference for adolescents, which was not available previously. Another advantage is that the BMI-for-age measure is consistent with the adult index, so BMI can be used continuously from two years of age into adulthood. This is important, as BMI in childhood is a determinant of adult BMI.

**Waist Circumference and BMI**   Some clinicians include measuring the circumference of their patients' waists as part of their standard measurements because changes in waist circumference over time can indicate an increase or decrease in abdominal fat. Increased abdominal fat is associated with an increased risk of heart disease. Although waist circumference is not part of the BMI Clinical Quality Measure, waist circumference and BMI are interrelated. Waist circumference provides an independent prediction of risk over and above that of BMI. However, according to the National Institutes of Health, it is not necessary to measure waist circumference in individuals with BMIs greater than or equal to 35, as waist circumference beyond that level of BMI has little added predictive power of disease risk over that of BMI.[4]

Conversely, BMI may not be a good predictor for patients with increased muscle mass such as athletes whose BMI may exceed 25, but who, in fact, are not overweight. For these patients waist circumference overrules BMI.

---

[3]Source: U.S. Department of Health and Human Services, Center for Disease Control web site http://www.cdc.gov.
[4]NIH National Heart, Lung, and Blood Institute. *Guidelines on Overweight and Obesity: Electonic Textbook.* http://www.nhlbi.nih.gov/health-pro/guidelines/current/obesity-guidelines/e_textbook/txgd/4142.htm (February 1, 2016).

## Critical Thinking Exercise 7E: Determining BMI Category for a Patient

BMI can be easily calculated for adults using the EHR. In this exercise you are going to see how BMI is calculated for a patient and determine the patient's BMI category. Do not worry if you do not have a calculator; the EHR software is going to calculate the BMI for you and display the math.

### Case Study

Rosa Garcia is a 27-year-old female with borderline diabetes. A nurse takes Rosa's height and weight measurements using the metric system (kilograms and centimeters). The medical assistant takes her height and weight measurements in pounds and inches. We are going to see if they both get the same BMI result.

### Step 1

Start a supported web browser program and follow the steps listed inside the cover of this textbook to log in to the MyHealthProfessionsLab for this course.

Locate and click on the link Exercise 7E.

### Step 2

In the New Encounter window, locate and click on **Garcia, Rosa**, and then click the OK button.

You do not need to set the date or time for this exercise.

### Step 3

The nurse weighs Rosa and her weight is **58.74** kilograms.

Locate the Weight (kg) field and enter her weight.

Next, she measures Rosa's height. She is **152.4** centimeters tall.

Locate the Height (cm) field and enter her height.

Click on the BMI field; the value will be calculated and the formula displayed.

### Step 4

The medical assistant weighs Rosa and her weight is **129.5** pounds.

Locate the Weight (lb) field and enter her weight.

Next, she measures Rosa's height. She is **60** inches tall.

Locate the Height (in) field and enter her height.

Click on the BMI field; the value will be calculated and the formula displayed.

### Step 5

Compare the BMI results from both metric and English units of measure. If they are not the same, recheck the numbers you typed in steps 3 and 4, and correct your error.

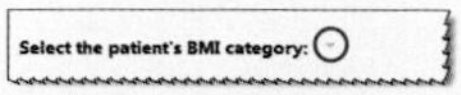

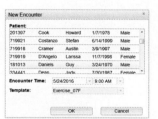

**Figure 7-40** Down-arrow to select BMI category is circled in red.

Locate the table of Adult BMI Categories in your textbook and compare the BMI ranges shown for each category to Rosa's BMI to determine her category.

### Step 6

Locate the field labeled **Select the patient's BMI category** and click the down-arrow button next to it (circled in red in Figure 7-40). A drop-down list will appear; click on the category that you determined was correct for Ms. Garcia in step 5.

### Step 7

A reference figure is not provided for this exercise.

If you wish to print a copy of your completed encounter notes for yourself or because your instructor requires you to turn them in, use the Create PDF option, and then print or download the PDF at this time.

The final step in every exercise is to submit your completed work for a grade.

Locate and click the blue Quippe icon button on the toolbar, and then select the Submit for Grade option from the drop-down menu. This will complete Exercise 7E.

## Guided Exercise 7F: Calculating BMI and Trending Weight for a Diabetic Patient

In the previous exercise, you learned how BMI is calculated and how the BMI number correlates to BMI categories in adults. Since BMI is one of the Clinical Quality Measures for Meaningful Use listed in Chapter 1 it will be included in most exercises in remaining chapters. However, as you will see in this exercise, the EHR can not only perform the calculations for BMI but also determine the BMI category.

In addition to BMI you will also cite past measures of the patient's weight into the encounter to document the patient's weights from his longitudinal record for comparison. This is called trending and is similar in purpose to cumulative summary analysis of lab results, discussed earlier.

### Case Study

Guy Daniels has been seen at the clinic quarterly for several visits. He has hypertension and Type 2 diabetes. Both conditions are exacerbated by his weight problem.

### Step 1

Start a supported web browser program and follow the steps listed inside the cover of this textbook to log in to the MyHealthProfessionsLab for this course.

Locate and click on the link Exercise 7F.

### Step 2

In the New Encounter window, locate and click on **Daniels, Guy**.

Set the date to **05/24/2016** and the time to **9:00 AM** as shown in Figure 7-41.

Verify that the date and time are set correctly, and then click the OK button.

**Figure 7-41** Select Guy Daniels and set the date to May 24, 2016 9:00 AM in the New Encounter window.

### Step 3

Locate and click in the blank space below Chief Complaint, and type **3 month checkup**.

### Step 4

Proceed to the Physical Exam section and record Mr. Daniels's vital signs in the corresponding fields of the encounter as follows:

| | |
|---|---|
| Temperature: | **98.2** |
| Pulse: | **68** |
| Respiration: | **20** |
| SBP: | **125** |
| DBP: | **85** |
| Weight: | **239** |
| Height: | **68.5** |

Once you have entered the weight and height, click on the label "BMI." Notice that the BMI was calculated by the EHR and Mr. Daniels's BMI category was automatically determined from the results.

### Step 5

Next, you are going to cite a list of his previous weight measurements.

Click on any white space in the encounter pane that does not highlight a heading or a finding. This will cause the date tabs at the bottom to reappear.

Locate and click on the **8/19/2015** tab, and the encounter note shown in Figure 7-42 will display.

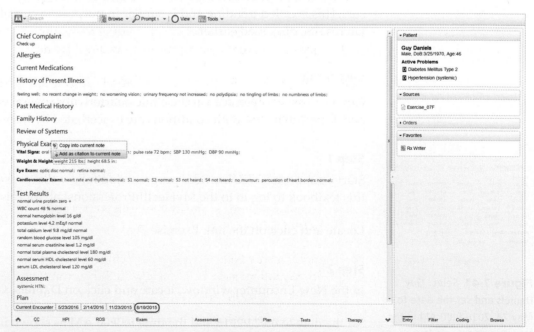

**Figure 7-42** Add as citation to current note the patient's weight from the 8/19/2015 encounter.

Locate the finding **weight 215 lbs;** click on it to highlight it, and then select Add as citation to current note from the drop-down menu.

Repeat this procedure, citing the weight findings from the **11/20/2015** and **2/14/2016** tabs as well. When you have finished, click on the Current Encounter tab.

### Step 6

Scroll to the bottom of the current encounter and observe the trend of weight increase for Mr. Daniels as shown in Figure 7-43. This figure can also be used to verify that the Vital Signs were entered correctly in step 4.

**Figure 7-43** Vital Signs and BMI category, and Weight from previous encounters added as citation to the current note.

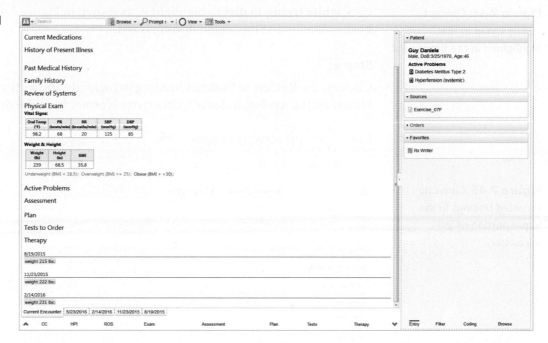

Results for Mr. Daniels's lab tests have been received. Locate and click on the **5/23/2016** tab.

Locate and click on the **Test Results** heading to highlight the entire section, and then click Copy into current note from the drop-down menu.

Also, copy Mr. Daniels's current medications. Locate and click on the heading **Current Medications** to highlight the entire section, and then click Copy into current note from the drop-down menu.

### Step 7

Return to the current encounter by clicking on the Current Encounter tab.

Locate Active Problems in the upper-right corner of the content pane, and *double-click* on **Diabetes Mellitus Type 2**.

Mr. Daniels has not been compliant with his diabetes care. However, the clinician has reviewed the patient's medications. Scroll the encounter pane to the top, and then locate and click the following findings until they turn blue and their descriptions change.

- recent examination by podiatrist
- home blood sugar check

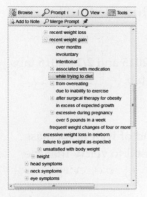

**Figure 7-44** Concept "while trying to diet" highlighted in the Browse list.

- seeing an eye doctor regularly
- medication reconciliation not performed

### Step 8

Proceed to Review of Systems. Locate and click on the following findings until they turn red.

- recent change in weight
- recent weight gain

Click the Browse button on the toolbar and in the Concepts drop-down list, locate and click **while trying to diet** to highlight it, as shown in Figure 7-44. Click the Add to Note button. Verify that the added finding is red.

### Step 9

Click on the Review of Systems heading to highlight the section. Click the Actions button on the toolbar and select Otherwise Normal from the drop-down menu.

Compare your screen to Figure 7-45.

**Figure 7-45** Correctly recorded findings in the upper portion of the encounter.

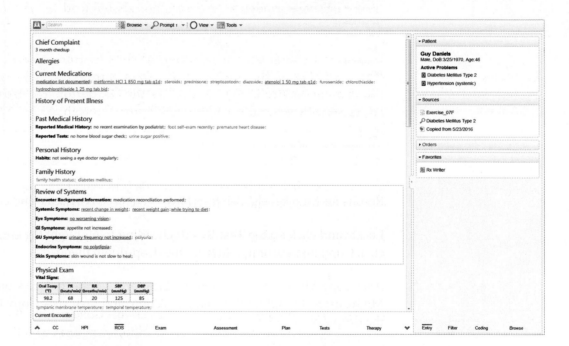

### Step 10

Scroll the encounter pane downward to the Plan section.

Locate and click **metformin HCL** until it turns red.

*Right-click* on the finding and select Details from the Actions drop-down menu. In the Details pop-up window click the down-arrow on the Prefix field, and change the prefix by selecting **renew** from the drop-down list. Click the OK button to close the Details window. The description should read "renew metformin HCL" and the finding should be red.

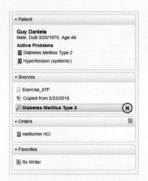

**Figure 7-46** Sources section of the content pane; click X (circled in red) to delete unentered concepts.

**Step 11**

Locate and *right-click* on **type 2 diabetes mellitus** in the Assessment section to invoke the Actions drop-down menu. Click on the Create a problem section option.

After the problem section is created, verify that the type 2 diabetes mellitus finding is red. If it is not, click on it until it turns red.

Next, clean up unentered concepts for diabetes. Locate the Sources section in the content pane and click on the prompt instance labeled "Diabetes Mellitus Type 2" as shown in Figure 7-46. Locate and click the X at the right end of the item. Unused concepts related to diabetes will be removed from the encounter pane.

**Step 12**

Locate Active Problems in the upper-right corner of the content pane, and *double-click* on **Hypertension (systemic)**.

Return to the Plan section. Locate and click **atenolol** until it turns red.

*Right-click* on the finding and select Details from the Actions drop-down menu. Change the prefix by selecting **renew** from the drop-down list, and then click the OK button to close the Details window. The description should read "renew atenolol" and the finding should be red.

Remain in the Plan section. Locate and click **hydrochlorothiazide** until it turns red. *Right-click* on the finding, select Details from the Actions drop-down menu, and change the prefix to renew. Click the OK button to close the Details window. The description should read "renew hydrochlorothiazide" and the finding should be red.

**Step 13**

Locate **systemic HTN** in the Assessment section and *right-click* on it to invoke the Actions drop-down menu. Click on the Create problem section option.

After the problem section is created, verify that the finding systemic HTN is red. If it is not, click on it until it turns red.

**Step 14**

Click the View button on the toolbar and select Concise from the drop-down menu. Compare your screen to Figure 7-47, scrolling as necessary until you have verified the entire encounter. If everything on your screen matches the figure, proceed to step 15. If there are any differences, review the preceding steps and correct your work.

**Step 15**

If wish to print a copy of your completed encounter notes for yourself or because your instructor requires you to turn them in, use the Create PDF option, and then print or download the PDF at this time.

The final step in every exercise is to submit your completed work for a grade.

Locate and click the blue Quippe icon button on the toolbar, and then select the Submit for Grade option from the drop-down menu. This will complete Exercise 7F.

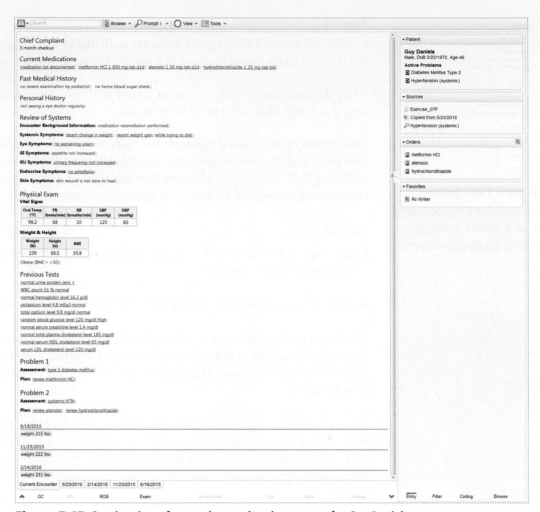

**Figure 7-47** Concise view of correctly completed encounter for Guy Daniels.

## Critical Thinking Exercise 7G: Discovering Your BMI and Category

Because BMI is a useful healthcare screening tool, the CDC provides a free online BMI calculator and is a source of information about diet and health. You may have an interest in seeing how you measure up. You will need to know your accurate height and weight for this exercise. If you have not recently weighed yourself, postpone the exercise until you have an opportunity to take your own measurements.

### Privacy Information About Exercise 7G

In this exercise you will enter personal information about your height, weight, and possibly date of birth. This data is used only for calculating BMI during the exercise. None of the data you enter will be shared with your instructor or reported to any entity. Your grade for this exercise is based solely on performing the exercise.

### Step 1

Start a supported web browser program and follow the steps listed inside the cover of this textbook to log in to the MyHealthProfessionsLab for this course.

Locate and click on the link Exercise 7G.

The web page shown in Figure 7-48 will be displayed.

**Figure 7-48** CDC BMI Calculators page.

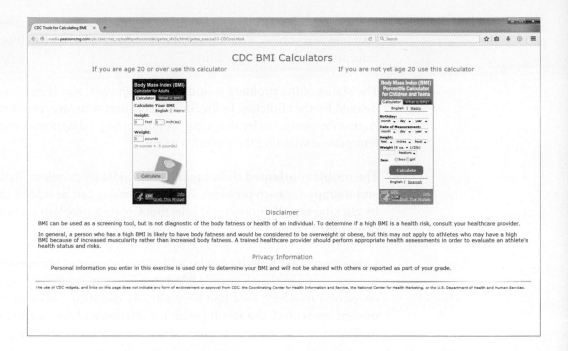

## Step 2

On the displayed page you will see two BMI calculators created by the CDC. As explained earlier, BMI categories are adjusted by age and gender for persons under age 20. Adult BMI categories are the same for either gender.

If you are at least 20 years old, use the Adult BMI Calculator.

If you are not yet age 20, use the Children and Teen BMI Calculator.

## Step 3

Once you have determined the appropriate BMI calculator to use, enter your data, following the on-screen instructions. As stated above, no one but you will see your personal information. Be honest about your weight, as the purpose of this exercise is for your own benefit.

When you have entered data in the calculator fields, click the Calculate button and your BMI category will be displayed. If your BMI category is outside the normal limits, you may find helpful information at the CDC website by clicking the links provided in the calculator.

This completes Exercise 7G.

## Chapter Seven Summary

This chapter explored Patient Lists and the problem-oriented chart as well as laboratory test results and body mass index. In this chapter you learned how to copy and cite findings from previous encounter notes into the current note, to calculate BMI, and to identify the BMI categories.

**Problem Lists** provide an up-to-date list of the diagnoses and conditions that affect that particular patient's care. Problem lists track both acute and chronic conditions.

Problems are removed from the list or set inactive once the patient is cured or the problem is resolved. Problems that normally resolve themselves over a short period of time are called *acute self-limiting*.

The status of the problem is updated at each visit, and if resolved, may be set inactive or deleted by the clinician. In the Student Edition software, problems can be added to the Active Problems list by dragging and dropping a diagnosis onto the section of the content pane containing the patient's name.

The **problem-oriented** chart organizes the data by problem, listing the diagnosis, plan, and therapy for each problem. Problem sections can be added to the current encounter by clicking on a diagnosis and selecting Create a problem section from the Actions drop-down menu.

**Laboratory Test Results** can be added to the current encounter note by retrieving the results from the electronic laboratory system, or by copying them from a previous encounter in which they had been already received. Laboratory reports list the component measured, the result (value), a reference of the normal value range, and an indicator of whether the result is considered normal, low, high, low-low, or high-high.

**Copy into current note** allows you to copy one or more findings from a previous encounter into the current note where they become findings that can be modified or acted upon like any finding in the note.

**Add as citation to current note** is used to cite one or more findings from a previous encounter into the current note. Cited findings are placed at the bottom of the note as reference data. Cited data does not behave as findings in the current note and cannot be edited, but the citation can be deleted.

**Body Mass Index (BMI)** is a useful screening tool for measuring body fat using body weight adjusted for height. The BMI formula $(wt/ht^2)$ works with either metric or English units by using a conversion multiplier. The calculated BMI number correlates to one of four BMI categories: underweight, normal, overweight, or obese.

CDC recommends using BMI for both children and adults. A single BMI chart is used to determine BMI categories of adults of either gender. However, BMI thresholds to determine categories for children and teens differ by gender and age.

As you continue through the course, you can refer to the Guided Exercises in this chapter when you need to remember how to perform a particular task.

| Task | Exercise | Page # |
|---|---|---|
| How to use problem lists and create problem sections | 7A | 257 |
| How to copy findings from a previous encounter | 7A | 257 |
| How to cite findings | 7B | 266 |
| How to duplicate findings in the current note | 7B | 266 |
| Retrieve pending lab results | 7B | 266 |
| How to calculate BMI | 7E | 288 |

## Testing Your Knowledge of Chapter 7

### Step 1

Log in to MyHealthProfessionsLab following the directions printed inside the cover of this textbook.

Locate and click on Chapter 7 Test.

### Step 2

Answer the test questions. When you have finished, click the Submit Test button to close the window.

## Testing Your Skill Exercise 7H: Patient with Upper Abdominal Chest Pain

Now that you have performed all the exercises in Chapter 7 this exercise will help you and your instructor evaluate your acquired skills. Use the information in the case study and the features of the software you already know to document the patient's encounter.

### Case Study

Linda Lewis is a 51-year-old female with a history of systolic hypertension who was recently hospitalized for congestive heart failure (CHF). She discharged from the hospital 10 days ago. On May 24, 2016, she presents with a chief complaint of upper abdominal pain.

After entering the chief complaint, the clinician copies current medications from her 5/14/2016 discharge record into the current note.

Linda says she has no allergies, and does not use tobacco, but enjoys two martinis before dinner every night and also has a glass of wine with her meal.

Here are Linda's vital signs:

| | |
|---|---|
| Temperature: | 97.8 |
| Pulse: | 68 |
| Respiration: | 18 |
| SBP: | 120 |
| DBP: | 88 |
| Weight: | 152 |
| Height: | 65 |

The clinician enters the chief complaint into the search box, and when the search results are displayed, expands the symptom, selects epigastric, and clicks Merge Prompt.

While discussing her past medical history Linda says she has had a peptic ulcer before, but her symptoms this time included chest pain as well as abdominal pain and epigastric pain. Because she recently had CHF she thought she better come right in. The clinician documents her symptoms and reconciles her medications.

The clinician performs the physical exam and finds her bowel sounds normal, with no abdominal mass, but there is direct abdominal tenderness.

The clinician notices Ms. Lewis has pending test results and retrieves them.

After reviewing the results, the clinician returns to the Past Medical History, locates peptic ulcer, and right-clicks on it, and selects Prompt from the Actions drop-down menu.

Revisiting Review of Systems, the clinician asks when the chest pains start. Linda says right after meals.

The clinician believes her peptic ulcer has returned, records the assessment, and writes a prescription for amoxicillin, one 250 milligram capsule three times a day for 7 days, by mouth, with food; zero refills, generic.

The clinician also orders antacids and counsels her about drinking.

### Step 1

Start a supported web browser program and follow the steps listed inside the cover of this textbook to log in to the MyHealthProfessionsLab for this course.

Locate and click on the link **Exercise 7H**. This will open the Quippe software window with the New Encounter window displayed in the center.

### Step 2

Locate and click on the patient name, and click the OK button. In this exercise, you **must** set the date as stated in the case study. You do not need to set the time of the encounter.

### Step 3

Read the case study *carefully*.

*Hint*: Copy her Current Medication into the note from her 5/14/2016 visit.

*Hint*: Remember to expand the search result and select epigastric before clicking merge prompt.

*Hint*: If you use the Actions button instead of right-click to prompt for peptic ulcer, verify that the finding state didn't change.

### Step 4

After recording the test results, primary diagnosis, and orders, the clinician will create a problem section based on the diagnosis.

Clinicians always document active problems every visit, even when they are not the primary reason for the visit.

*Hint*: *Double-click* on each diagnosis in her Active Problems list, and create a Problem section for each of them as well.

*Hint:* When you double-click active problems, additional related clinical concepts will load. You may need to scroll back down to the Assessment section to locate the diagnosis.

**Step 5**

After creating the problem sections, the clinician provides patient education about alcohol use.

*Hint*: Scroll to the therapy section and record the patient education finding.

**Step 6**

If you wish to print a copy of your completed encounter notes for yourself or because your instructor requires you to turn them in, use the Create PDF option, and then print or download the PDF at this time.

Submit your completed work for a grade. This will complete Exercise 7H.

# Chapter Eight

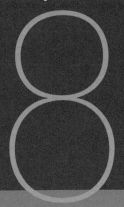

# Flow Sheets, Annotated Drawings, and Graphs

## Learning Outcomes

*After completing this chapter, you should be able to:*

◆ Describe flow sheets

◆ Work with a flow sheet

◆ Use an EHR drawing tool to annotate drawings in an encounter

◆ Graph weight and BMI, and annotate the graphs

## Learning to Use Flow Sheets

**Flow sheets** present data from multiple encounters in column form. This format allows for a side-by-side comparison of findings over a period of time. Some clinicians prefer to review patient records this way because it is easier to spot trends in the patient's health conditions. It is ideal for chronic disease management such as diabetes or long-term conditions such as pregnancy. OB offices use flow sheets to monitor pregnancy because they afford a view of previous visits when documenting the current one. Paper flow sheets were in use long before flow sheets were developed for EHR systems, but the flow sheet had to be updated by manually copying data from the paper chart, which created the risk of transposition errors. EHR systems have the ability to create flow sheets dynamically, involving no extra work for the practice.

Not all EHR systems implement flow sheets in the same manner, so flow sheets in your workplace may vary from these exercises. Some EHR systems limit flow sheets to lab results or vital signs. Whether the vendor implements it or not, any EHR using a codified nomenclature has the data structure necessary to create clinical flow sheets that present findings from entire encounters.

Another advantage of the flow sheet is that you do not have to click on the different date tabs to see previous instances of a finding, as the flow sheet row displays all previous instances of the finding. As you will see in the first exercise, you can switch easily between working in the encounter pane and the flow sheet.

### ALERT

Make certain you set the date and time correctly when instructed to do so, for all exercises in this chapter.

## Guided Exercise 8A: Working with a Flow Sheet

In previous exercises, you worked with patients who had multiple chronic conditions. You learned to view findings in previous encounters by clicking the tabs at the bottom of the encounter pane and to copy findings from previous encounters into the current note. This exercise will use what you learned previously and add a new concept, the flow sheet. In this exercise you will learn to use a flow sheet to compare previous findings and to document a patient encounter.

### Case Study

Guy Daniels is a patient with hypertension and borderline diabetes who has been seen quarterly at the outpatient clinic to better manage his health. Mr. Daniels returns for a 3-month checkup. Lab tests have been ordered and performed before his visit. The results were reviewed by the clinician when they arrived electronically yesterday.

### Step 1

Start a supported web browser program and follow the steps listed inside the cover of this textbook to log in to the MyHealthProfessionsLab for this course.

Locate and click on the link Exercise 8A.

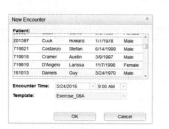

### Step 2

In the New Encounter window, locate and click on **Daniels, Guy**.

Set the date to **05/24/2016** and time to **9:00 AM** as shown in Figure 8-1.

Verify the date and time are set correctly, and then click the OK button.

**Figure 8-1** Select Guy Daniels and set the date to May 24, 2016 9:00 AM in the New Encounter window.

### Step 3

Locate and click in the blank space below the label "Chief Complaint," and type **3 month checkup**.

### Step 4

Click any white space in the encounter pane that does not highlight a heading or finding.

Locate and click the View button on the toolbar, and then select Flowsheet from the drop-down menu shown in Figure 8-2. The encounter pane workspace will divide and the flow sheet will display in the bottom portion (also shown in Figure 8-2).

## About the Flow Sheet View

The flow sheet view resembles a spreadsheet similar to Microsoft Excel®; that is, it is made up of rows and columns of cells.

The first column displays headings with clinical concepts or findings in the *current* encounter note. Section and Group headings are bolded, concepts and findings are displayed in normal text.

The second column, labeled "Current," shows findings in the current encounter. The remaining columns to the right are labeled with dates of previous encounter notes.

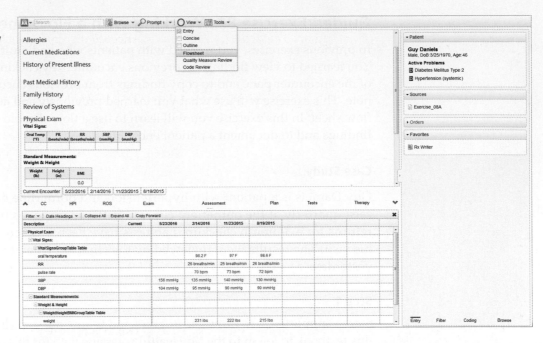

**Figure 8-2** Flow sheet invoked by selecting the View button, Flowsheet option.

The flow sheet rows horizontally display encounter data from previous visits for easy comparison. For example, locate the row labeled "oral temperature." Reading from left to right, you can easily compare the patient's temperature from three previous visits.

A scroll bar on the right of the flow sheet allows the flow sheet rows to be scrolled independently of the encounter note pane. If you cannot see the row of the flow sheet with Mr. Daniels's weight, scroll the flow sheet downward as necessary.

Flow sheets offer an improved method of trending results. Notice how much easier it is to compare changes in Mr. Daniels's weight than to cite the weight from each tab into the current note as you did in the previous chapter.

The rows of the flow sheet are limited to sections that have corresponding clinical concepts or findings in the current encounter. Even if a finding exists in a previous encounter, a row for it does not appear in the flow sheet unless the current encounter contains the same concept, or finding. At this point the encounter has only the Chief Complaint, Physical Exam Vital Signs, and weight and height sections, so those are the findings in the flow sheet.

**Step 5**

To increase the quantity of data displayed, add clinical concepts relevant to Mr. Daniels's condition.

Locate Active Problems at the top of the content pane on the right, and *double-click* on **Hypertension (systemic)**. The concepts related to hypertension are added to the encounter and corresponding rows appear in the flow sheet.

Rows displayed in the flow sheet can be restricted to a given section by giving that section focus. Initally, when the hypertension problem concepts were merged, the diagnosis was highlighted, thereby limiting the flow sheet rows to the Assessment section. To display rows for all concepts in the encounter, locate and click on any white space in the current encounter that does not highlight a heading, concept, or finding, and then click the View button on the toolbar and select Flowsheet from the drop-down menu, again. This will refresh the flow sheet to display all sections containing concepts.

**Step 6**

Scroll the flow sheet downward until Eye Exam is positioned in the top row as shown in Figure 8-3).

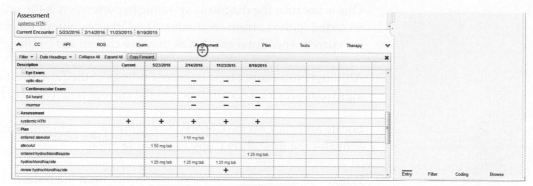

**Figure 8-3** Drag the division line (circled in red) to increase or decrease the vertical size of the flow sheet. Also the button to activate Copy Forward is highlighted blue.

The proportion of the encounter pane workspace allotted for the flow sheet can be resized at any time.

Locate the short horizontal line indicating the dividing point between the top of the flow sheet and the navigation bar at the bottom of the workspace. Position your mouse pointer over it and the mouse pointer will change to two vertical arrows as shown circled in red in Figure 8-3). Hold the left mouse button down as you drag the dividing line upward. This will vertically expand the flow sheet area. Continue dragging upward until you can at least see the previously ordered prescriptions in the plan section as shown in Figure 8-3).

In the future, if you wish to make the flow sheet take up less of the workspace pane, click on the dividing line and drag downward.

In previous chapters you learned that underlined concepts in the encounter note informed the clinician that findings for the concept were documented on previous visits. However, the clinician still had to click the previous encounter tabs to determine if the finding was normal or abnormal. Flow sheets display the state of the finding, saving the clinician time and effort.

Compare your screen to Figure 8-3. You will notice that most findings from previous encounters are represented by blue minus symbols and red plus symbols, except where a finding has a value. Red plus symbols represent positive or abnormal findings. Blue minus symbols represent negative or normal findings. If a finding has a value in the Details value field, the value and unit are displayed in red or blue (color related to the state of the finding). For example, the vital signs findings in Figure 8-2 and the prescription orders in Figure 8-3 have value/units that display, whereas the eye exam optic disc and assessment systemic HTN in Figure 8-3) do not have numerical values, so they merely display the blue minus symbol for "normal" and the red plus symbol for "positive." Cells that are blank do not have findings recorded in the encounter for the column date. For example, atenolol was only ordered on 2/14/2016, so the cells in the atenolol row are blank for other dates.

You may also notice that heading descriptions in the first column are preceded by small minus symbol icons. Clicking these plus or minus symbols allows you to collapse or expand the concepts displayed below them similar to the way you expand and collapse trees in the Browse drop-down lists.

### Step 7

You will notice there is only one row with a recorded finding in the Current column. This is because the diagnosis systemic hypertension is the only finding we have recorded in the current encounter. The Current column reflects findings documented in the current encounter as soon as they are clicked red or blue.

Although you cannot type or enter findings in the flow sheet cells, you can copy findings from previous encounters into the current note while in the Flowsheet view.

Locate and click on the Copy Forward button. It is highlighted blue in Figure 8-3. This activates the flow sheet Copy Forward feature.

When you move your mouse pointer away from the button, it will cease to be highlighted, but the Copy Forward function remains activated until you manually turn the function off by clicking the button a second time.

### Step 8

The clinician examines Mr. Daniels's eyes and reorders two prescriptions.

With the Copy Forward function active, locate the row for **optic disc** and the column labeled **2/14/2016**. Click the cell with the blue minus symbol at the junction of that row and column. A blue minus symbol should appear in the Current column for the optic disc row.

In the same column, move your mouse pointer downward to the row labeled "ordered atenolol" and click on the cell: **1 50 mg tab**. A copy of the order should appear in the row under the current column.

Locate the row labeled "ordered hydrochlorothiazide" and the column labeled **8/19/20015**. Click on the cell containing **1 25 mg tab**. A copy of the order should appear in the row under the current column.

Scroll the *encounter note* portion of the workspace pane until Eye Exam is at the top of the pane. This should allow you to see the recorded findings in both the encounter and flow sheet, as shown in Figure 8-4.

Locate and click the Copy Forward button to turn the copy function off. Figure 8-4 shows what the button looks like with the Copy Forward function still activated. When it is truly off, the button should resume the appearance it had in Figure 8-2, before you clicked it the first time.

The Flowsheet view can be closed by clicking the red X in the right corner of the flow sheet. The flow sheet can be redisplayed by selecting it from the View button drop-down menu.

Locate and click the X in the right corner of the flow sheet. The flow sheet will close and the encounter note will fill the workspace pane.

**Figure 8-4** Findings in the encounter note (above) added by clicking cells in the flow sheet with Copy Forward activated.

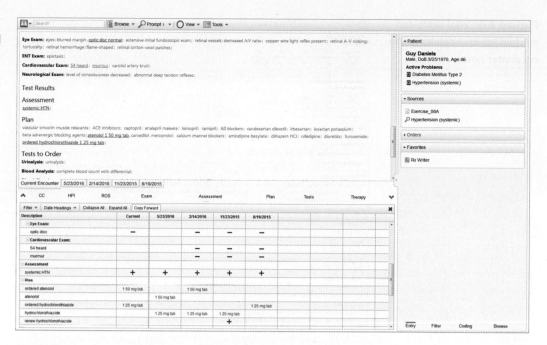

### Step 9

Scroll the encounter pane (if necessary) to the Physical Exam section and record Mr. Daniels's vital signs in the corresponding fields of the encounter as follows:

| | |
|---|---|
| Temperature: | **98.2** |
| Pulse: | **68** |
| Respiration: | **20** |
| SBP: | **125** |
| DBP: | **85** |
| Weight: | **239** |
| Height: | **68.5** |

### Step 10

Lab test results were received on May 23, 2016. Copy them into the current encounter.

Click any white space in the encounter pane that does not highlight a heading or finding. When the date tabs at the bottom of the encounter pane reappear, locate and click on the **5/23/2016** tab.

Locate and click on the heading Lab Results to highlight the lab results, and then select Copy into Current note from the drop-down menu, as you have done in previous exercises.

Click on the Current Encounter tab and compare your screen to Figure 8-5. You can also use this figure to verify you entered the vital signs correctly in step 9.

### Step 11

Click the View button on the toolbar and select Flowsheet from the drop-down menu, as you did in step 4. Scroll the flow sheet as necessary until you can see the Previous

**Figure 8-5** Vital signs and merged lab test results in the encounter note.

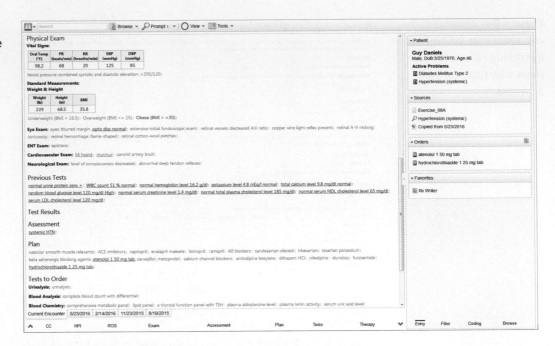

Tests section as shown in Figure 8-6. Compare the result values of various instances of test results components This example demonstrates how useful a flow sheet is in comparing result trends.

**Figure 8-6** Using the Flowsheet view to trend lab test results.

| Description | Current | 5/23/2016 | 2/14/2016 | 11/23/2015 | 8/19/2015 | | | |
|---|---|---|---|---|---|---|---|---|
| **Previous Tests** | | | | | | | | |
| urine protein | zero + | zero + | zero + | zero + | zero + | | | |
| WBC count | 51 % | 51 % | 51 % | 49 % | 48 % | | | |
| hemoglobin level | 16.2 g/dl | 16.2 g/dl | 16.2 g/dl | 15.5 g/dl | 16 g/dl | | | |
| potassium level | 4.8 mEq/l | 4.8 mEq/l | 4.8 mEq/l | 4.3 mEq/l | 4.2 mEq/l | | | |
| total calcium level | 9.8 mg/dl | 9.8 mg/dl | 9.8 mg/dl | 10.1 mg/dl | 9.8 mg/dl | | | |
| random blood glucose level 120 mg/dl High | 120 mg/dl | 120 mg/dl | 120 mg/dl | 110 mg/dl | 105 mg/dl | | | |
| serum creatinine level | 1.4 mg/dl | 1.4 mg/dl | 1.4 mg/dl | 1.3 mg/dl | 1.2 mg/dl | | | |
| total plasma cholesterol level | 185 mg/dl | 185 mg/dl | 185 mg/dl | 185 mg/dl | 180 mg/dl | | | |
| serum HDL cholesterol level | 65 mg/dl | 65 mg/dl | 65 mg/dl | 65 mg/dl | 60 mg/dl | | | |
| serum LDL cholesterol level | 120 mg/dl | 120 mg/dl | 120 mg/dl | 120 mg/dl | 120 mg/dl | | | |
| **Assessment** | | | | | | | | |
| systemic HTN | + | + | + | + | + | | | |

## Step 12

As stated earlier, although there are numerous findings in the previous encounters, the flow sheet rows display only headings and findings that correlate with those in the current encounter. Because the patient has two active problems, add the concepts for his second problem at this time.

Locate Active Problems at the top of the content pane on the right, and *double-click* on **Diabetes Mellitus Type 2**. The concepts related to the patient's type 2 diabetes are added to the encounter and a corresponding row is added to the flow sheet. Click on any white space in the encounter pane that does not highlight a heading or concept to see all rows for the added concepts.

Figure 8-7 shows the additional flow sheet rows; however, the figure includes data copied forward later in this step.

Locate and click the Copy Forward button at the top of the flow sheet to activate the function.

With the Copy Forward function active, locate the **while trying to diet** row and click the cell for that row in the **2/14/2016** column. A red plus symbol should appear in the row under the Current column.

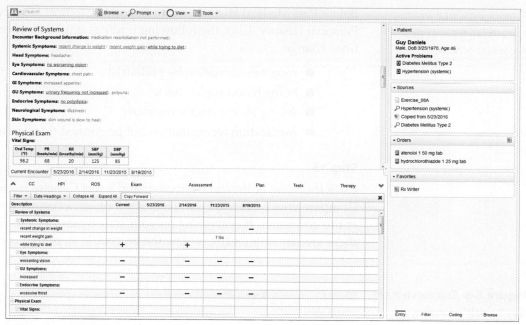

**Figure 8-7** Additional flow sheet rows added by diabetes problem. Current column symptoms were copied forward using the flow sheet.

Because the finding "while trying to diet" was not previously in the current note, it now has focus in the encounter, causing rows for other symptoms in the flow sheet not to display. Restore the display of all rows in the flow sheet by clicking on any white space in the encounter pane that does not highlight a heading or concept.

Locate the 2/14/2016 column in the flow sheet and click cells with blue minus symbols for the following symptoms:

- worsening vision
- increased (GI symptoms)
- excessive thirst

Scroll the encounter note portion of the workspace until you can see Review of Systems. Compare your screen to Figure 8-7.

Locate and click the Copy Forward button to turn off the copy function. Locate and click the X in the right corner of the flow sheet to close it. The encounter note will fill the workspace pane.

### Step 13

Copy Mr. Daniels's current medications from the previous encounter. Locate and click on the **5/23/2016** tab.

Locate and click on the heading **Current Medications** to highlight entire section, and then click Copy into current note from the drop-down menu.

Return to the current encounter by clicking on the Current Encounter tab.

### Step 14

If necessary, scroll the encounter pane until you can see the several history sections and Review of Systems.

Below Past Medical History, locate Reported Medical History and Reported Tests and Personal History. Click the following findings until they turn blue and their descriptions change.

- recent examination by podiatrist
- home blood sugar check
- seeing an eye doctor regularly
- medication reconciliation not performed (located in Review of Systems)

**Step 15**

Click the View button on the toolbar and select Concise from the drop-down menu. Compare your screen to Figure 8-8, scrolling as necessary until you have verified the entire encounter. If everything on your screen matches the figure, proceed to step 16. If there are any differences, review the preceding steps and correct your work.

**Figure 8-8** Concise view of Guy Daniels's correctly completed encounter note.

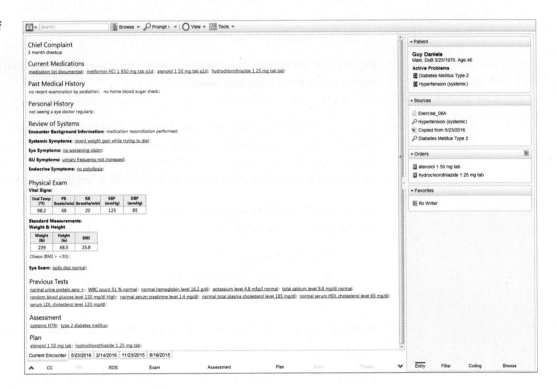

**Step 16**

If wish to print a copy of your completed encounter notes for yourself or because your instructor requires you to turn them in, use the Create PDF option, and then print or download the PDF at this time.

The final step in every exercise is to submit your completed work for a grade.

Locate and click the blue Quippe icon button on the toolbar, and then select the option Submit for Grade from the drop-down menu. This will complete Exercise 8A.

## Guided Exercise 8B: Obstetric Patient's Flow Sheet

Flow sheets are frequently used in obstetric offices because they assist the clinician and nurses in monitoring the course of the pregnancy over all three trimesters.

## Case Study

Gloria Natell is a 33-year-old in her third trimester of pregnancy. Ms. Natell was last seen 10 days ago, but as her expected delivery date is near, her visits are being scheduled more frequently.

### Step 1

Start a supported web browser program and follow the steps listed inside the cover of this textbook to log in to the MyHealthProfessionsLab for this course.

Locate and click on the link Exercise 8B.

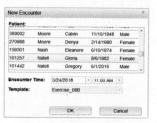

**Figure 8-9** Select Gloria Natell and set the date to May 24, 2016 11:00 AM in the New Encounter window.

### Step 2

In the New Encounter window, locate and click on **Natell, Gloria**.

Set the date to **05/24/2016** and the time to **11:00 AM** as shown in Figure 8-9.

Verify the date and time are set correctly, and then click the OK button.

### Step 3

Locate and click in the blank space below the label "Chief Complaint," and type **prenatal checkup**.

### Step 4

The nurse or medical assistant begins the visit by recording Ms. Natell's vital signs.

Scroll the encounter pane to the Physical Exam section and record Gloria's vital signs in the corresponding fields of the encounter as follows:

| | |
|---|---|
| Temperature: | **98.8** |
| Pulse: | **74** |
| Respiration: | **26** |
| SBP: | **145** |
| DBP: | **95** |
| Weight: | **152** |
| Height: | **65** |

### Step 5

Click any white space in the encounter pane that does not highlight a heading or finding to restore the date tabs.

Locate the **5/14/2016** tab at the bottom of the encounter pane and click on it.

When the 5/14/2016 encounter note is displayed, click on the heading **Allergies** to highlight it, and then select Copy into Current note from the drop-down menu. Repeat the procedure for the headings **Current Medications** and **Personal History**. Arrows in Figure 8-10 help identify the sections you are to copy into the current note.

After you have copied all three sections, click the tab at the bottom of the encounter pane labeled **Current Encounter**.

**Figure 8-10** Arrows indicate three sections of the 5/14/2016 encounter to copy into the current note.

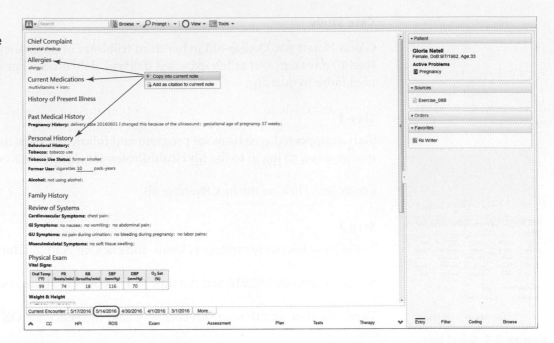

## Step 6

Locate and click the View button on the toolbar, and then select Flowsheet from the drop-down menu. When the flow sheet is displayed, increase the number of rows you can see by changing its proportion of the workspace.

Locate the short horizontal line indicating the dividing point between the top of the flow sheet and the navigation bar at the bottom of the workspace. Position your mouse pointer over it and the mouse pointer will change to two vertical arrows as shown circled in Figure 8-11. Hold the left mouse button down as you drag the dividing line upward. Continue dragging upward until you can at least see the Behavioral History, tobacco use section of the flow sheet as shown in Figure 8-11.

Notice the red plus and blue minus symbols in the Current column. These are findings copied from the 5/14/2016 encounter in step 5.

**Figure 8-11** Flow sheet resized by dragging the line circled in red. Red pluses, blue minus in the Current column are findings from the previous step.

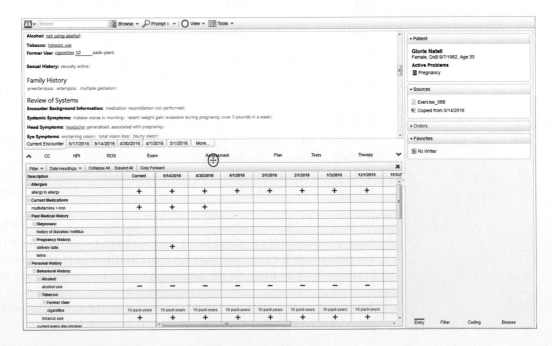

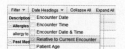

**Figure 8-12** Flow sheet drop-down menu for changing the date column heading labels.

**Figure 8-13** Flow sheet of Gloria Natell's vital signs.

### Step 7

In addition to the Copy Forward button with which you are familiar from the previous exercise, there are four other buttons on the flow sheet. These buttons change the information displayed in the flow sheet columns and rows.

Locate and click on the Date Headings button and the drop-down menu shown in Figure 8-12 will be displayed. Select the option **Relative to Current Encounter**. This will change the labels of the columns from calendar dates to intervals of days, weeks, and months prior to the current encounter, as shown in Figure 8-13.

| Description | Current | 10 days ago | 3 weeks ago | 6 weeks ago | 3 months ago | 4 months ago | 5 months ago | 6 months ago | 7 month |
|---|---|---|---|---|---|---|---|---|---|
| Physical Exam | | | | | | | | | |
| Vital Signs: | | | | | | | | | |
| VitalSignsGroupTable Table | | | | | | | | | |
| oral temperature | 98.8 | 99 F | 98 F | 99 F | 99 F | 98 F | 99 F | 99 F | 9 |
| RR | 26 | 18 breaths/min | 16 breaths/min | 18 breaths/min | 18 breaths/min | 18 breaths/min | 16 breaths/min | 18 breaths/min | 16 bre |
| pulse rate | 74 | 74 bpm | 68 bpm | 70 bpm | 72 bpm | 68 bpm | 68 bpm | 70 bpm | 7C |
| SBP | 145 | 116 mmHg | 110 mmHg | 112 mmHg | 114 mmHg | 114 mmHg | 110 mmHg | 110 mmHg | 114 |
| DBP | 95 | 70 mmHg | 58 mmHg | 72 mmHg | 78 mmHg | 78 mmHg | 70 mmHg | 70 mmHg | 72 |
| Weight & Height | | | | | | | | | |
| WeightHeightGroupTable Table | | | | | | | | | |
| weight | 152 | 147 lbs | 144 lbs | 142 lbs | 141 lbs | 140 lbs | 139 lbs | 138 lbs | 1: |
| height | 65 | 65 in | 65 in | 65 in | 65 in | 65 in | 65 in | 65 in | 6 |
| Cardiovascular Exam: | | | | | | | | | |
| edema | | | − | | − | + | − | − | |
| Female Genital Exam: | | | | | | | | | |
| fundal height abnormal | | | 29 cm | 25 cm | | 17 cm | | | |
| fetal movement | | | | | | − | | | |
| Assessment | | | | | | | | | |
| pregnancy | | | | | | | | | |

This alternate way of looking at the date is helpful to the obstetrician in monitoring the progression of Ms. Natell's pregnancy, although it could also be used by any specialty.

Following is information about the other buttons on the flow sheet, although it is not necessary to click them:

◆ **Filter** button contains options that control which findings in the current and previous encounters are displayed in the description column.

◆ **Collapse All** causes the flow sheet to display only section headings.

◆ **Expand All** simultaneously expands all heading rows to display all findings in the flow sheet.

As you learned in the previous exercise, the plus symbols next to headings in the description column expand individual sections. Using the Collapse All button, the clinician can quickly locate a section without scrolling, and then, by clicking the plus symbol next to the section heading, can better focus on the findings and group headings in that section.

### Step 8

The flow sheet and the encounter note can be scrolled independently. Scroll the flow sheet downward until you can see the Physical Exam, Vital Signs section as shown in Figure 8-13.

You can also document in the encounter pane without closing the flow sheet view. Actions taken in either the encounter note or the flow sheet instantly update the other portion of the workspace.

Reviewing vital signs in the flow sheet, the nurse notices that the patient's weight has increased from 147 lb to 152 lb in the last 10 days. Ms. Natell says the increase was sudden, occurring over the last few days. She also says she is having headaches, blurry vision, and pains in her upper right abdomen.

Locate Review of Systems, Systemic Symptoms group *in the encounter note*, and click the following findings until they turn red.

- recent weight gain
- over 5 pounds in a week
- headache
- blurry vision
- abdominal pain
- right upper quadrant abdominal pain

Click a white space so the last finding does not have focus and the Review of Systems section of the flow sheet is displayed. Compare your screen to Figure 8-14, scrolling either portion of the workspace as necessary.

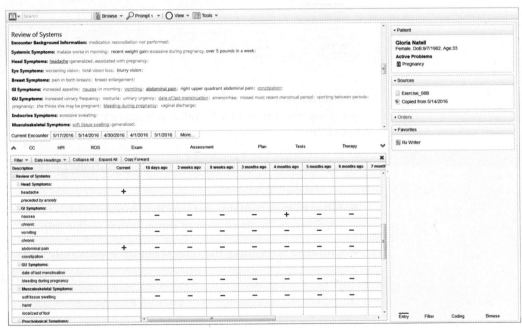

**Figure 8-14** Review of Systems findings recorded in the encounter note (above) are reflected in the flow sheet (below).

### Step 9

Scroll the encounter portion of the workspace to the Physical Exam section.

Locate and click on the following findings until they turn red.

- enlargement of breast
- edema
- fetal movement
- fetal heart sounds

Click any white space and then scroll the flow sheet portion of the workspace (if necessary) to see all of the newly added Physical Exam findings. Compare your screen to Figure 8-15.

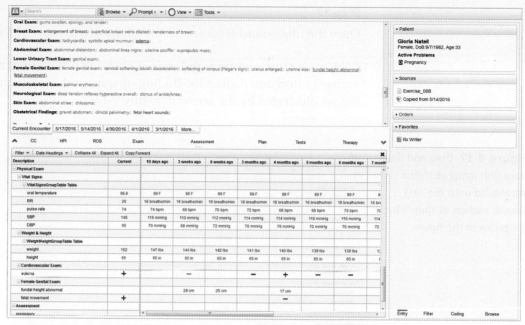

**Figure 8-15** Physical Exam findings in the encounter note and the flow sheet.

## Step 10

The clinician wants a urinalysis performed, stat.

Scroll the encounter pane to the Tests to Order section, and locate and click on the test until it turns red.

- urinalysis

*Right-click* on urinalysis to invoke the Actions drop-down menu and select Details. In the Details pop-up window, click in the note field and type **stat**. Click the OK button to close the Details window.

## Step 11

While waiting for the results of the urinalysis the clinician performs an ultrasound. Locate Imaging Studies and click on the following finding until it turns red.

- transabdominal obstetric ultrasound

Close the Flowsheet view by clicking the X in the right corner of the flow sheet. Compare your screen to Figure 8-16.

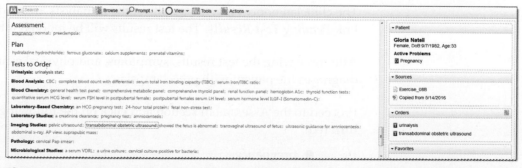

**Figure 8-16** Orders urinalysis stat and transabdominal obstetric ultrasound in the encounter note.

## Step 12

Once the ultrasound is complete, the clinician will move the finding to Test Results.

Click your mouse on **transabdominal obstetric ultrasound**, and while holding the left mouse button down, drag the finding upward and drop it on the Previous Tests heading, as illustrated by the arrow in Figure 8-17.

**Figure 8-17** Drag and drop transabdominal obstetric ultrasound onto the Test Results section as shown by the arrow in the figure.

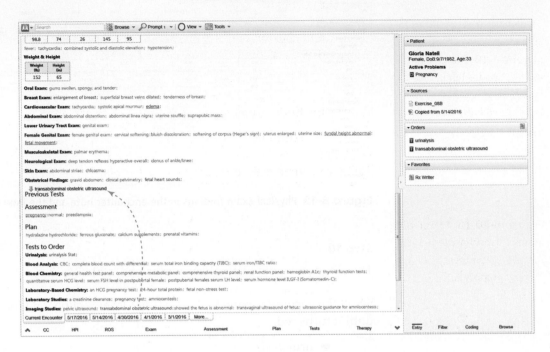

## Step 13

Next, change the finding prefix and state.

*Right-click* on **transabdominal obstetric ultrasound** to invoke the Actions drop-down menu, and select Details. In the Details pop-up window, click in the Prefix field and select the blank (first item) in the drop-down list as shown in Figure 8-18. Click the OK button to close the Details window.

Click on transabdominal obstetric ultrasound until the finding turns blue and the description changes to "transabdominal obstetric ultrasound normal."

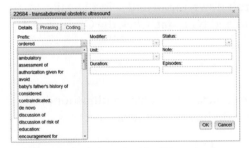

**Figure 8-18** Select the blank item in the Prefix drop-down list to clear ordered prefix.

## Step 14

The clinician notices that the results of the urinalysis are ready. Locate and click on the link *Pending Test Results*. The test results will be merged into the note.

After reviewing the test results, symptoms, and physical exam findings, the clinician diagnoses the patient with preeclampsia.

Proceed to the Assessment section and click on the following two diagnoses until they turn red.

- pregnancy
- preeclampsia

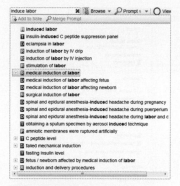

**Figure 8-19** Search results list for "induce labor." Medical induction of labor is highlighted light blue in the figure.

## Step 15

The clinician explains preeclampsia to Ms. Natell and discusses her options. The only cure for preeclampsia is delivering the baby. From the fetal ultrasound measurements and data in her records, the clinician calculates the gestational age of the baby to be 38½ weeks, and recommends inducing labor.

Click in the search box on the toolbar and type **induce labor**, and press the Enter key on your keyboard.

Locate and click on **medical induction of labor** in the search results list (highlighted in Figure 8-19), and then click on the Add to Note button.

## Step 16

Locate the finding you just added and click on it until it turns red.

- medical induction of labor

Compare your screen to Figure 8-20.

**Figure 8-20** Encounter with urinalysis results merged, and diagnoses and therapy findings recorded.

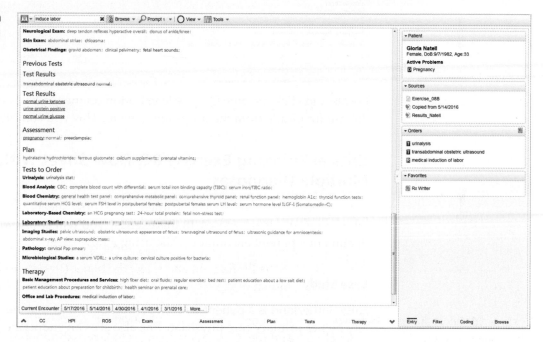

## Step 17

Click the View button on the toolbar and select Concise from the drop-down menu. Compare your screen to Figure 8-21, scrolling as necessary until you have verified the entire encounter. If everything on your screen matches the figure, proceed to step 18. If there are any differences, review the preceding steps and correct your work.

## Step 18

If you wish to print a copy of your completed encounter notes for yourself or because your instructor requires you to turn them in, use the Create PDF option, and then print or download the PDF at this time.

The final step in every exercise is to submit your completed work for a grade.

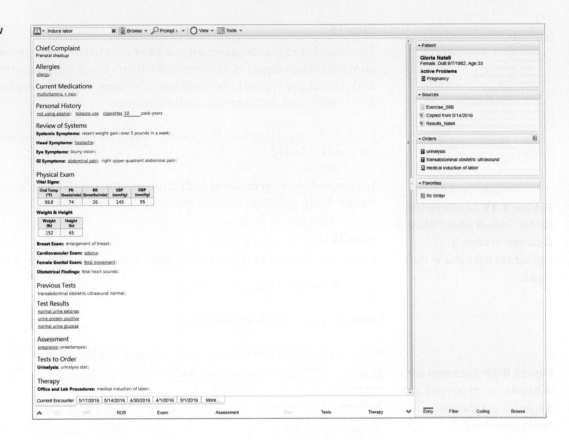

**Figure 8-21** Concise view of Gloria Natell's correctly completed encounter.

Locate and click the blue Quippe icon button on the toolbar, and then select the option Submit for Grade from the drop-down menu. This will complete Exercise 8B.

## Critical Thinking Exercise 8C: Flow Sheet with Multiple Diagnoses

In the preceding exercises, you learned to use flow sheets as you worked with patients who had multiple diagnoses. In this exercise you will apply what you have learned to document a patient encounter while using a flow sheet.

### Case Study

Sally Sutherland is a patient with hyperlipidemia and diabetes who has been seen annually by her primary care physician. She also sees an endocrinologist, who manages her diabetes, and an ob/gyn for her regular pelvic exams.

### Step 1

Start a supported web browser program and follow the steps listed inside the cover of this textbook to log in to the MyHealthProfessionsLab for this course.

Locate and click on the link Exercise 8C.

### Step 2

In the New Encounter window, locate and click on **Sutherland, Sally**.

Set the date to **05/24/2016** and the time to **1:00 PM**.

Verify that the date and time are set correctly, and then click the OK button.

**Step 3**

Locate and click in the blank space below the label "Chief Complaint," and type **Annual checkup**.

**Step 4**

Scroll the encounter pane to the Physical Exam section and record Sally's vital signs in the corresponding fields of the encounter as follows:

| | |
|---|---|
| Temperature: | **98.6** |
| Pulse: | **78** |
| Respiration: | **28** |
| SBP: | **134** |
| DBP: | **90** |
| Weight: | **153** |
| Height: | **60** |

Click on the label **BMI**, which will calculate her BMI and category.

**Step 5**

Locate Active Problems at the top of the content pane on the right, and *double-click* on **Diabetes Mellitus Type 2**. The concepts related to the patient's type 2 diabetes are added to the encounter.

Click any white space in the encounter pane that does not highlight a heading or finding.

Locate and click the View button on the toolbar, and then select Flowsheet from the drop-down-menu. The encounter pane workspace will divide and the flow sheet will display.

**Step 6**

Locate the Copy Forward button at the top of the flow sheet, and click on it.

In the flow sheet **5/15/2015** column, locate and click on cells with red plus, blue minus symbols, or value data, for the following findings; scroll the flow sheet as necessary.

- home blood sugar check
- never smoked
- 1 drinks/day
- drug use
- family history of diabetes mellitus

**Step 7**

Scroll flow sheet downward and compare vitals across all columns. Notice the change in her BMI status. In the **6/18/2013** column, locate and click the blue minus symbol in the patient obese row:

- patient obese

Close the flow sheet by clicking the X in the right corner of the flow sheet.

### Step 8

Copy Sally's current medications and several history items from the previous encounter. Locate and click on the **5/15/2015** tab.

Locate and click on the heading **Current Medications** to highlight the entire section, and then click Copy into current note from the drop-down menu.

Locate and click on the group heading **Pregnancy History** to highlight just that group, and then click Copy into current note from the drop-down menu.

Locate and click on the heading **Family History** to highlight the entire section, and then click Copy into current note from the drop-down menu.

Return to the current encounter by clicking on the **Current Encounter** tab.

### Step 9

Although it is true that Sally is not currently nursing, the fact is outdated and no longer relevant.

Locate Pregnancy History and *right-click* on **not currently nursing** to invoke the Actions menu, and then select **Delete** from the drop-down menu.

### Step 10

Because Sally has lost weight, scroll the encounter pane downward to Review of Systems. Locate **recent change in weight** and click on it until it turns red.

Click on the Review of Systems heading. Click the Actions button on the toolbar and select otherwise normal from the drop-down menu.

### Step 11

The clinician examines Sally, rechecking underlined clinical concepts that indicate corresponding findings in previous encounters, and finds everything normal.

Click on the Physical Exam heading. Click the Actions button on the toolbar and select otherwise normal from the drop-down menu.

### Step 12

The clinician proceeds to the Previous Tests section and notices that lab results are ready. Click on the *Pending Test Results* link. Several lab test results are added to the encounter note.

Click any white space outside the Test Results section to restore the date tabs at the bottom of the encounter note.

Click the View button on the toolbar, and select Flowsheet from the drop-down menu.

Scroll the flow sheet downward through the Test Results section, comparing lab results across the columns. Notice that total plasma cholesterol level has gone down, and the values have changed from red (abnormal–high) in the previous two columns to blue (normal) in the current column.

Scroll the flow sheet further downward to the plan section. Locate the row for "ordered metformin HCL" and click the cell containing **1 500 mg tab po.** This will Copy Forward the order.

Close the flow sheet by clicking the X in the right corner of the flow sheet.

### Step 13

The clinician has completed the diabetes-related portion of the exam. Clear unentered findings related to diabetes.

Locate the Sources section in the content pane and click on the prompt instance labeled "Diabetes Mellitus Type 2" (with the magnifying glass icon). Locate and click the X at the right end of the item.

The clinician next reviews Sally's hyperlipidemia condition. Locate the Active Problems section in the content pane and *double-click* on **Hyperlipidemia**.

The clinician finds that the concepts related to hyperlipidemia have improved. Click on the Physical Exam heading. Click the Actions button on the toolbar and select otherwise normal from the drop-down menu.

### Step 14

Based on the test results and physical exam findings, the clinician believes Sally's hyperlipidemia has resolved.

Proceed to the Assessments section. *Right-click* on **hyperlipidemia** to invoke the Actions drop-down menu and select Details. In the Details pop-up window, click in the Status field and select **resolved** from the drop-down list. Click the OK button to close the Details window. The description should read "hyperlipidemia – resolved."

### Step 15

Click the View button on the toolbar and select Concise from the drop-down menu. Because of the quantity of data added by the lab test results, the comparison of Concise view is shown in two figures. Compare your screen to Figure 8-22a and Figure 8-22b,

**Figure 8-22a** Upper portion of Sally Sutherland's correctly completed encounter (1 of 2 screen captures).

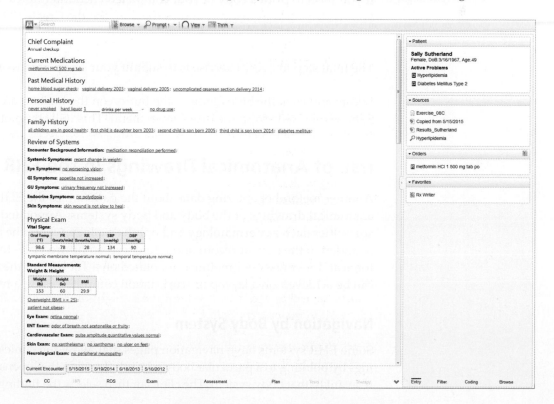

**Figure 8-22b** Bottom portion of Sally Sutherland's correctly completed encounter (2 of 2 screen captures).

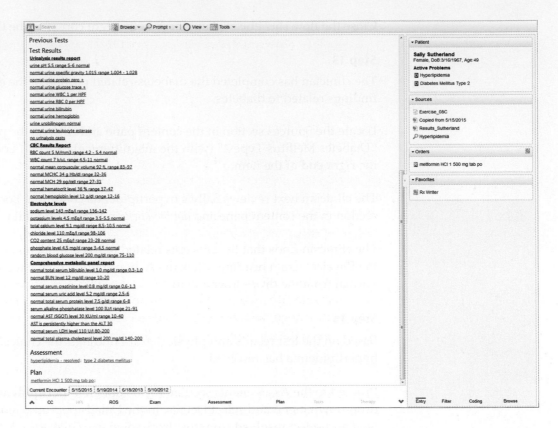

scrolling as necessary until you have verified the entire encounter. If everything on your screen matches the figure, proceed to step 16. If there are any differences, review the preceding steps and correct your work.

### Step 16

If you wish to print a copy of your completed encounter notes for yourself or because your instructor requires you to turn them in, use the Create PDF option, and then print or download the PDF at this time.

The final step in every exercise is to submit your completed work for a grade.

Locate and click the blue Quippe icon button on the toolbar, and then select the option Submit for Grade from the drop-down menu. This will complete Exercise 8C.

## Use of Anatomical Drawings in the EHR

Another method of entering data about the patient into the EHR involves the use of anatomical drawings of the body and body systems. Annotated drawings are used in specialties such as dermatology and ophthalmology where the annotated drawing is included in the patient record and referenced on future visits to compare changes. Anatomical drawings are sometimes annotated on a Tablet, but the same or a similar result can be achieved on a laptop or workstation computer using a mouse.

### Navigation by Body System

Some EHR systems have navigation pages that allow the clinician to quickly locate findings by pointing to a particular body part in a drawing that opens a list of clinical concepts relevant to that body system. The clinician then selects the findings appropriate to the visit.

In navigation usage, the pictures do not become part of the patient note; they are just a visual tool for browsing concepts. Think of this as searching with pictures rather than words.

## Annotated Drawings as EHR Data

Certain specialties routinely add information to the physical exam in the form of drawings or sketches. Two examples are dermatologists, who sometimes note the location of nevi (moles) on an outline of the body, and ophthalmologists, who frequently document changes to the retina on a drawing of the eye. These annotated drawings have long been a part of the patient's paper chart, and most EHR systems today include a tool to annotate drawings in the computer. The images created using the tools in the EHR become part of the electronic encounter. Annotated drawings are also useful for patient education, as we shall see in a later exercise.

Although annotated images in an EHR can become part of the encounter note, text or measurements added to the images are not codified data. This means that for the purpose of subsequent analysis of the EHR records, the clinician needs to document them as findings in the encounter note as well as on the image.

## Guided Exercise 8D: Annotated Dermatology Exam

This exercise will give you an opportunity to practice the annotation of a drawing using a simplified tool in the Student Edition software. As with previous exercises, the purpose here is to let you experience a function that is often available in commercial EHR systems. The drawing tools you will use here will be similar in principle but not identical to those you might use in a medical office. The method of invoking the annotation tool and the manner in which a drawing is subsequently merged into the patient note will vary by EHR vendor.

### Case Study

Arnie Greensher is a 66-year-old male who has a large number of moles on his back, the result of years of working in the sun without a shirt. His doctor has been monitoring them through regular follow-up visits. In addition to the encounter notes created at those visits, the clinician finds it useful to save annotated drawings, which show the placement of the moles. In subsequent visits, the doctor will compare the drawings from past encounters to the current state of the patient's skin to quickly identify new moles or changes from a previous visit.

### Step 1

Start a supported web browser program and follow the steps listed inside the cover of this textbook to log in to the MyHealthProfessionsLab for this course.

Locate and click on the link Exercise 8D.

### Step 2

In the New Encounter window, locate and click on **Greensher, Arnie**.

Set the date to **05/24/2016** and the time to **5:00 PM**, as shown in Figure 8-23.

Verify that the date and time are set correctly, and then click the OK button.

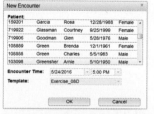

**Figure 8-23** Select Arnie Greensher and set the date to May 24, 2016 5:00 PM in the New Encounter window.

### Step 3

Locate and click in the blank space below the label "Chief Complaint," and type **Follow up visit for routine lesion recheck**.

**Step 4**

Mr. Greensher has no allergies, but is a former smoker who smoked two packs a day for 20 years. He enjoys a glass of wine with dinner every night.

Locate and click on the clinical concept **allergy** until the finding turns blue and the description changes to "no allergy."

Proceed to Personal History, Behavioral History, and click on the following findings until they turn red.

- tobacco use
- former smoker
- cigarettes

Type **40** in the pack-years field.

- alcohol use
- wine

Type **1** in the quantity field. Click the drop-down menu for the units field and change it to **glasses per day**.

**Step 5**

Mr. Greensher reports no change to his skin, but is concerned that there might be changes to moles on his back that he can feel but not see.

Proceed to Review of Systems and click on **skin changes** until the finding turns blue and the description reads "no skin changes."

Locate and click on **change in mole** until it turns red.

**Step 6**

The patient removes his clothes and the clinician examines Mr. Greensher's skin.

Click on the following findings until they turn blue and their descriptions change.

- occipital lesions on scalp
- lesions on face
- lesions on chest
- lesions on upper extremities in front
- lesions on lower extremities in front

Click on the following findings until they turn red.

- the skin was normal except as noted
- lesions on back

**Step 7**

Proceed to the Assessment section and click on the diagnosis until it turns red.

- dysplastic nevus

Compare your screen to Figure 8-24.

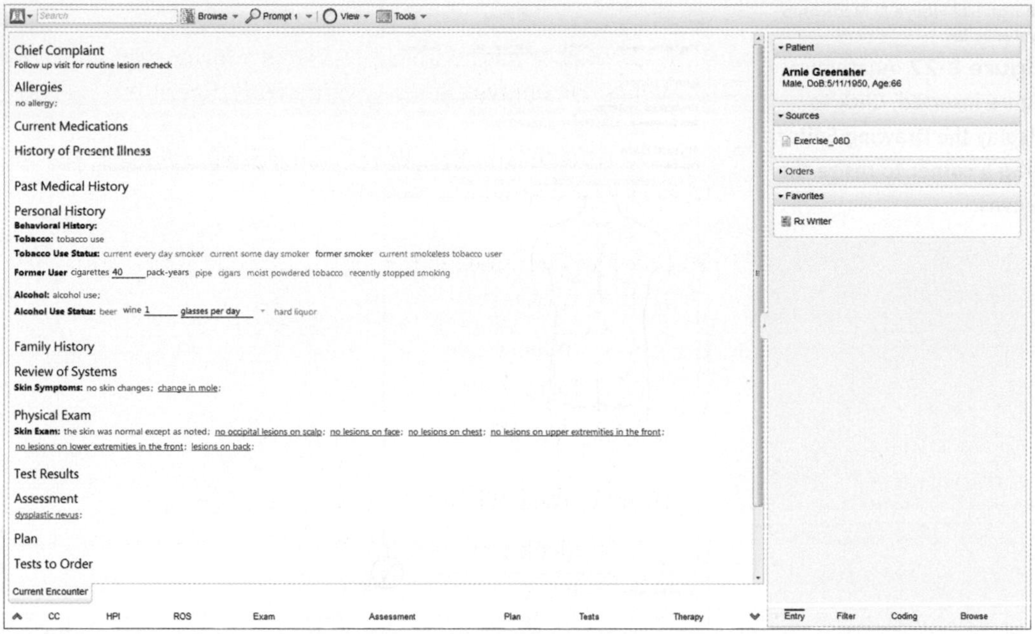

**Figure 8-24** Encounter note, Allergies through Assessment sections, for Arnie Greensher.

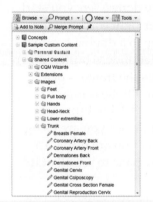

**Figure 8-25** Browse the drop-down list for Images with expanded folder for Trunk.

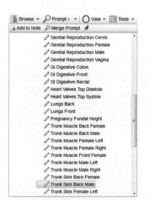

**Figure 8-26** Browse the drop-down list for Trunk scrolled further. Trunk Skin Back Male is highlighted light blue in the figure.

## Step 8

The clinician observes fifteen moles on the patient's back and wishes to document their locations for future reference. This will be done with an annotated drawing. The Student Edition software contains various anatomical illustrations, which may be used as the background for annotated drawings.

Click any white space in the encounter pane, so that neither the diagnosis nor any other finding is selected.

Locate and click the Browse button on the toolbar as you have in previous exercises. When the drop-down menu is displayed, click the plus symbol next to the Sample Custom Content icon. When the tree is expanded, locate and click on the plus symbol next to Shared Content and Images. Drawing images in the drop-down list are preceded by a pencil icon.

The drop-down list organizes images available for annotated drawings by body part. Locate and click on the plus symbol next to Trunk, as shown in Figure 8-25, to expand the tree.

The available drawings in the expanded Trunk portion of the tree are numerous. Scroll the list of images downward until you locate **Trunk Skin Back Male**, click on it to highlight it (as shown in Figure 8-26) and then click on the Add to Note button.

The anatomical drawing shown in Figure 8-27 will be inserted into the Physical Exam section of the encounter note.

## Step 9

Initially the drawing canvas will be smaller than the one shown in Figure 8-27. The drawing canvas and image can be resized larger to make it easier to draw on.

Click anywhere on the drawing canvas (the image or white space within it). Two things will happen: The drawing canvas will be outlined, and the content pane will display the Drawing Editor set of annotation tools.

**Figure 8-27** Anatomical figure inserted. Click to display the Drawing Editor. Drag a corner to resize the canvas.

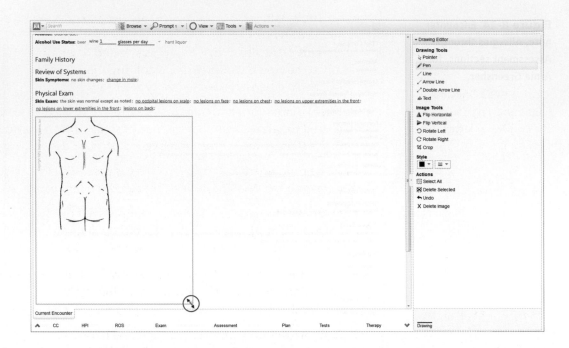

If you would like to size your drawing canvas larger, this must be done *before* you start annotating the image. Position your mouse pointer over the lower right corner of the canvas. When correctly positioned, the mouse pointer will change to a double-headed arrow as shown circled in red in Figure 8-27. Click and hold the left mouse button down as you drag the border of the canvas diagonally downward. When the frame is of a desired size, release the mouse button and the image will resize to fill the frame.

The ideal size of the canvas for you will depend on the computer device you are using for your exercises, the screen size and orientation, and the browser you are using. Do not make the canvas so large that you have to scroll the encounter pane to see all of it.

When you released the mouse, the image dynamically resized to fill the canvas. If you have sized your image too large, you can make it smaller by again clicking on the lower right corner and then dragging the corner diagonally upward.

When the drawing image is of a size you can work with comfortably, proceed to the next steps.

**WARNING**

Do not resize the drawing canvas once you begin adding annotations, as the annotated items will not resize or reposition. If you find you cannot work in the size canvas you have created, restart the exercise by clicking the Quippe menu icon on the toolbar and selecting New Encounter from the drop-down list.

### Step 10

This step will familiarize you with the Drawing Editor features. If at any point you click in the encounter note, outside the drawing canvas, the Drawing Editor will close. Simply click on the drawing again to redisplay the Drawing Editor in the content pane.

The Drawing Editor, located in the content pane, consists of four groups of features: Drawing Tools, Image Tools, Style, and Actions.

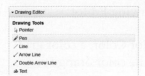

**Figure 8-28** Drawing Editor, Drawing Tools, showing Pen selected.

**Drawing Tools** (shown in Figure 8-28) are used to select the type of annotation to be added to the drawing canvas. Clicking the left mouse button on a tool selects the tool, and it remains on until a different tool is selected. Positioning the mouse pointer on the canvas, then moving the mouse while holding the left mouse button down creates the type of mark or action dictated by the type of tool currently selected.

**Pointer** Annotations added to the drawing canvas are discrete elements. The pointer is used to select annotations already on the drawing. Once an element is selected with the pointer tool, it can be moved, edited, or deleted.

**Pen** The fundamental drawing tool is the pen. With Pen selected you can make any free-form shape. Moving the pen repeatedly over an area will fill it in.

**Line** Draws straight lines between two points. Position the mouse pointer where you want to start the line, click and hold the left button as you move the mouse, and release the button where you want the line to end.

**Arrow Line** Draws a straight single arrow. Position the mouse pointer where you want to start the line, and click and hold the left button as you move the mouse. The arrow head will be on the end where you release the button.

**Double Arrow Line** Draws a straight line between two points with an arrow head at both the starting and ending points of the line you have drawn.

**ab Text** This tool opens a textbox on the drawing where you can type. This is useful for labeling the elements you have added to your drawing.

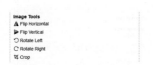

**Figure 8-29** Drawing Editor, Image Tools (not used in the exercise).

**Image Tools** (shown in Figure 8-29) allow you to flip an image, or to change the orientation of the image by rotating it. A crop tool allows a small portion of the image to be used. If you have worked with drawing or photo editing software, you may be familiar with these functions. The image tools will not be used in these exercises.

**Style** Consists of two buttons used to set the color and weight of the drawing tools (except text). Figure 8-30 shows the buttons as if their respective down-arrows had been clicked. In the Drawing Editor the buttons are situated closer together than show in the figure.

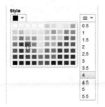

**Figure 8-30** Drawing Editor, Style buttons, Color and Weight. The figure illustrates selecting color orange-red and line thickness 4.

**Color** Clicking the down-arrow of the first button displays a grid of colors. Selecting a color in the grid sets the color in which pen, line, arrow, or text elements are created. The Square block icon of the button displays the color currently in effect.

**Weight** The second button whose icon is three horizontal lines of increasing thickness sets the weight or thickness of the marks made with the pen, line, or arrow tools. Smaller numbers make a narrower line, larger numbers make a thicker line.

**Actions** (shown in Figure 8-31) affect elements added to the image with drawing tools or undo the last action by the user.

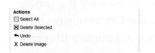

**Figure 8-31** Drawing Editor, Actions used to delete or undo drawing elements.

**Select All** selects all elements on the drawing canvas.

**Delete Selected** Deletes elements from the drawing canvas that are currently selected using the pointer tool or the Select All action option.

**Undo** Undoes the last activity related to the drawing canvas; for example, restoring a line deleted by mistake, or correcting an accidentally resized canvas.

**Delete Image** Removes the entire drawing canvas, anatomical image, and related annotations from the encounter note.

### Step 11

The best way to understand the tools is to use them. The doctor has noted fifteen small moles on Mr. Greensher's back.

If the Pen is not the tool currently selected, click on **Pen** in the Drawing Editor.

Locate the Style buttons and click the down-arrow on the button for Color; a color grid will appear as shown in Figure 8-30. Locate the grid square with the color orange-red and click on it. The grid will close, and the icon button should have an orange-red square.

Set the weight of the drawing tool (line thickness). Click the Style button whose icon is three horizontal lines and select **4** from the drop-down list of numbers.

### Step 12

Now you are ready to draw on the anatomical image. You are annotating the location of moles. Make your circles small.

Position the mouse pointer on the drawing canvas, over the patient's left shoulder at the place shown in Figure 8-32. Click and hold down the left mouse button while making a small circular motion, and then release the button. The size of the circle is controlled by how far you move the mouse before releasing the mouse button.

**Figure 8-32** Draw a small circle on the left shoulder to represent the position of a mole.

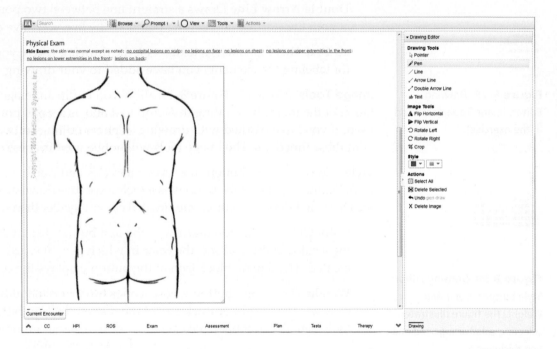

Compare the mole you have drawn Figure 8-32. It doesn't have to be exactly the same, but if yours is too small, too large, or in the wrong position, click the Undo button in the Actions section of the Drawing Editor and try again. When you are satisfied with your first drawing, proceed to the next step.

### Step 13

Before adding the rest of Arnie's moles you are going to learn how to remove an element added in error.

With the pen tool still selected, draw a small circle on the neck, well away from the mole you added in step 12.

After you have added it, locate Drawing Tools in the content pane, and click on the Pointer tool.

Position your mouse pointer over the spot you want to remove and click the left mouse button. The item will be selected as shown in Figure 8-33.

**Figure 8-33** Selecting an object to delete (hand-shaped pointer on neck).

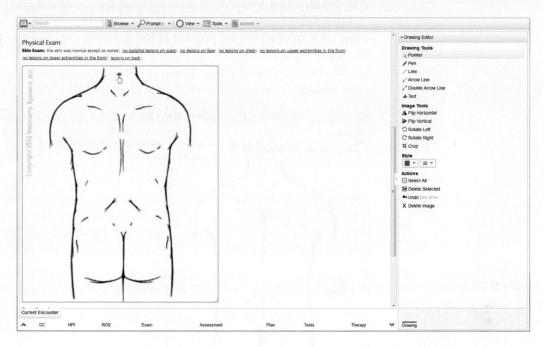

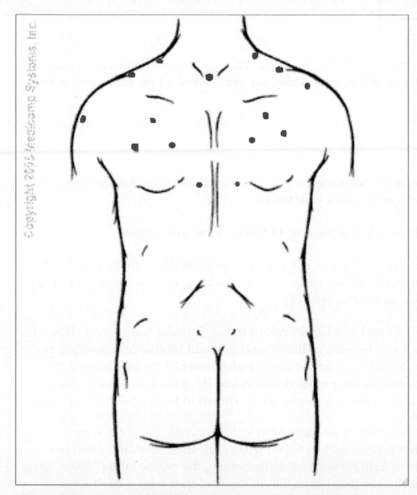

**Figure 8-34** Draw 14 additional small moles on the back (15 total).

Locate Drawing Editor, Actions section, and click on Delete Selected. The item will be removed, and your drawing should once again look like Figure 8-32.

### Step 14

Using what you have learned in step 12, you will now illustrate the location of moles on Mr. Greensher's back using the pen.

Restore pen function by locating and clicking on Pen in the Drawing Tools.

Draw **14** additional small moles on the patient's back, in the locations shown in Figure 8-34. You do not have to place them precisely where they are in the figure; just get reasonably close. When you are done, you should have 15 moles, total.

### Step 15

Clinicians can annotate the images by adding text directly on the drawing canvas with the Text tool. The clinician also can select a different color for the text. It is wise to make text a different color, as it will help the text stand out from the background figure and elements drawn on the image.

Locate and click on **ab Text** in the Drawing Tools.

Locate Styles in the Drawing Editor and click on the Color button. When the Color palette window is displayed, click on the blue square of the grid.

Now click over an empty portion of the drawing canvas and a text box will appear, as shown in Figure 8-35.

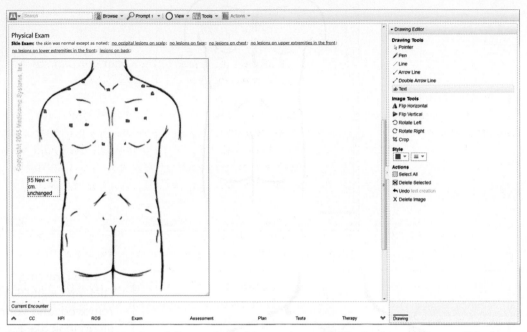

**Figure 8-35** Change tool to ab Text, color to blue, and type "15 Nevi < 1 cm. Unchanged" in the text box.

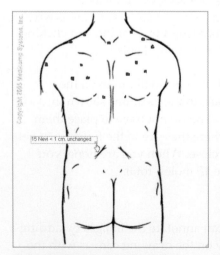

**Figure 8-36** Change the tool to Pointer, click the lower right corner of the text box, and drag horizontally.

If the text box is not positioned where you would like it, click elsewhere. It will move to wherever you click your mouse.

Type the following text in the box: **15 Nevi < 1 cm. unchanged**

While you are typing, the box will expand automatically to fit the text, but the text will wrap oddly. When you are finished adding the text, locate Drawing Tools and click on the Pointer tool.

After the pointer tool is selected, return to the drawing canvas and click on the text box. It will become outlined, and you will be able to reposition and resize it. Locate and click on the lower right corner of the highlighted text box. Hold the left mouse button down as you drag the frame horizontally until the entire text fits in a single line as shown in Figure 8-36, then release the mouse button.

If the box is not positioned where you wish, click anywhere on the text box except the lower right corner, and while holding the mouse button down, drag the box to the desired location on the canvas, and then release the button.

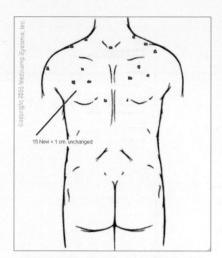

Figure 8-37 Change the tool to Line and draw a blue line from the text to the region of the moles.

### Step 16

Another useful drawing tool is the Line, which can be used to connect text to the drawing points.

Locate and click Line in the Drawing Tools.

Draw a line similar the one in Figure 8-37. Position your mouse on the canvas just above the text "15 Nevi." Hold down the left mouse button as you drag the mouse upward toward the moles on the left shoulder blade. Release the button when the line reaches the position shown in Figure 8-37.

### Step 17

Click any white space in the encounter pane that is outside the drawing canvas to close the canvas and Drawing Editor.

Annotated drawings provide an excellent means of recording the location and size of certain observed findings in a physical exam. However, as we have discussed several times, the contents of the image are not codified, searchable records. In this example, the text added to the drawing became part of the image and as such can only be read by a person, not the computer.

Therefore, the clinician also will record the text of the findings in the encounter note. This will result in the best of both worlds; codified data for the computer, and a visual record of the location of moles for use in future exams.

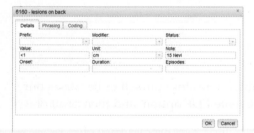

Figure 8-38 Add details in the pop-up window for the Physical Exam finding "lesions on back."

Locate the Physical Exam section, Skin Exam and *right-click* on the finding Lesions on the back. When the Actions button menu is displayed, select Details from the drop-down menu.

In the Details pop-up window Value field type **<1** and then select **cm** from the drop-down list in the Units field.

Click in the Note field and type **15 Nevi**.

Compare your pop-up window to Figure 8-38. When everything is entered correctly, click the OK button to close the window.

### Step 18

The clinician advises the patient to avoid sun exposure and to return for a follow-up in three months.

Scroll the encounter pane to the bottom. Locate and click the following findings until they turn red.

- follow-up visit in 3 months
- discussed avoiding sun exposure

### Step 19

Click the View button on the toolbar and select Concise from the drop-down menu. Compare your screen to Figure 8-39, scrolling as necessary until you have verified the entire encounter. If everything on your screen matches the figure, proceed to step 20. If there are any differences, review the preceding steps and correct your work.

**Figure 8-39** Concise view of correctly completed encounter with annotated drawing for Arnie Greensher.

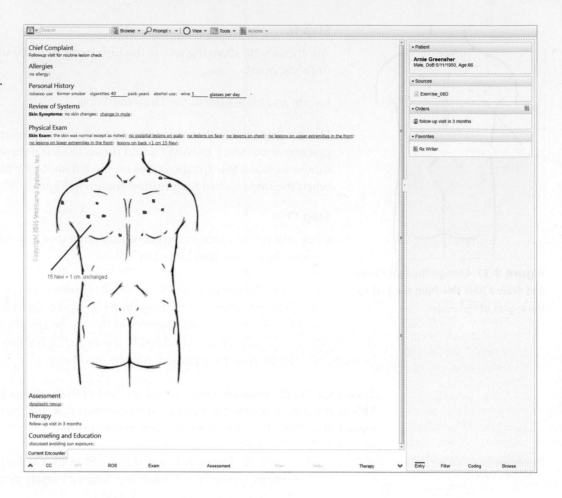

## Step 20

If wish to print a copy of your completed encounter notes for yourself or because your instructor requires you to turn them in, use the Create PDF option, and then print or download the PDF at this time.

The final step in every exercise is to submit your completed work for a grade.

Locate and click the blue Quippe icon button on the toolbar, and then select the option "Submit for Grade" from the drop-down menu. This will complete Exercise 8D.

## Critical Thinking Exercise 8E: Examination of a Patient with Pressure Sores

In this exercise, you will use the skills you have acquired in the previous exercise to document a patient with pressure sores.

### Case Study

Raj Patel is an 80-year-old male, who presents complaining of sores on his back and buttocks. Four years ago he had surgery to repair cervical and thoracic spinal fractures that were the result of an automobile accident. He was recently seen at the ER for shortness of breath caused by severe asthma. He has become sedentary over the last two weeks and has developed pressure sores on his shoulder blades and buttocks. Because he cannot see his sores, he mistakenly believes his pain is at the sites of his spinal and iliac incisions.

# Real-Life Story

## First Patient Whose Life Was Saved by Expert System Software He Operated Himself

*Courtesy of Primetime Medical Software and Instant Medical History, used by permission.*

Jack Gould of Columbia, South Carolina, became the first person in medical history to save his own life with software he operated himself.

One day Mr. Gould came to his physician's office to pick up a prescription renewal for his wife, who was also a patient there. In the waiting room was a computer kiosk running Instant Medical History, a patient-operated medical expert system. A sign posted near the system read, "Stay Healthy: Take our Prevention Questionnaire." While waiting for the prescription refill to be authorized, he decided to try it out.

In addition to eating and exercise recommendations, the software suggested that he needed the standard procedure to check for colon cancer because he could not recall having been checked within the timeframe suggested by standard guidelines. Normally, after the patient completes the questionnaire, the physician reviews the information with the patient. Because in this case he was not there to see the physician, he spoke with the triage nurse, who confirmed it was a wise preventive action to take and scheduled an appointment.

A few weeks later, the patient returned for his appointment. The doctor was surprised that the patient was there for such a specific preventative procedure months before his annual physical examination. The doctor asked who scheduled the procedure. In

a tone reflecting his expectation that it was common for patients to schedule proctosigmoidoscopies on their own volition, he replied, "Well, your computer did."

No physician can be expected to remember the thousands of recommended interventions for each patient. The preventive health screening software queried the patient for the appropriate items based on his sex, age, and risk factors and compared them to the preventive guidelines of the U.S. Preventive Services Task Force. In the case of Mr. Gould, a flexible sigmoidoscopy was scheduled and a resectable severely dysplasic polyp was removed easily from his colon.

The large precancerous polyp that was discovered might have gone completely undetected without the intelligent prompting of the Instant Medical History program. Mr. Gould knew the importance of his decision to take the interview after his physician explained that he would not have thought to do this test until his routine annual complete medical examination. The polyps were removed without complication, before they could develop into colon cancer.

He was totally unaware of his risk for other conditions until he took the preventive interview. Now he strongly believes that Instant Medical History saved his life.

### Step 1

Start a supported web browser program and follow the steps listed inside the cover of this textbook to log in to the MyHealthProfessionsLab for this course.

Locate and click on the link Exercise 8E.

### Step 2

In the New Encounter window, locate and click on **Patel, Raj**.

Set the date to **05/24/2016** and the time to **5:15 PM**.

Verify that the date and time are set correctly, and then click the OK button.

**Step 3**

Locate and click in the blank space below the label "Chief Complaint," and type **Post-surgical sores on back and buttocks**.

**Step 4**

Begin the visit by taking Mr. Patel's Vital Signs and history.

Enter Mr. Patel's vital signs in the corresponding fields on the form as follows:

| | |
|---|---|
| Temperature: | **98.6** |
| Pulse: | **78** |
| Respiration: | **28** |
| SBP: | **150** |
| DBP: | **90** |
| $O_2$ Sat | **99** |
| Weight: | **141** |
| Height: | **66** |

When you have finished, click on the cell labeled BMI to display his BMI category.

**Step 5**

Mr. Patel informs the nurse that he is not allergic to drugs, but has pollen allergies. He says he does not use tobacco, alcohol, or drugs.

Scroll the encounter pane to the top of the encounter. Begin in the Allergy section and then continue into the Personal History section. Locate and click on the following findings until they turn red.

- allergy
- allergy to pollens

Locate and click on the following findings until they turn blue. Their descriptions will change.

- allergy to drugs
- tobacco use
- alcohol use
- drug use

**Step 6**

Mr. Patel admits he is not exercising, has decreased his activity, and has become sedentary, lying in bed most of the time.

Locate the Habits group heading and click on the following findings until they turn red.

- poor exercise habits
- not exercising regularly
- sedentary
- a decrease in physical activity

### Step 7

Because Mr. Patel believes his surgical wounds are "acting up," the nurse views scanned documents of his surgical records and adds his surgical history.

Click in the Search box on the toolbar, type **prior surgery**, and press the Enter key on your keyboard.

Locate **Prior Surgery** preceded by the block letter H in the search results, click on it to highlight it, and then click the button labeled Add to Note.

Locate the concept you have just added to the Past Medical History section, and click on it until it turns red.

- prior surgery

### Step 8

Locate and click the Browse button on the toolbar. A list of history concepts will likely be displayed. Collapse the history tree by clicking the small minus symbol next to the domain History. Click the small plus symbol next to the block letter D to expand the Diagnoses, syndromes and conditions tree.

Scroll the drop-down list until you locate **orthopedic disorder**, and then click the small plus symbol next to it. (Hint: orthopedic disorder is between rheumatologic disorder and neurologic disorder.)

In the expanded tree of orthopedic disorders, locate **fracture** and click the small plus symbol to expand it. Locate and click on the clinical concept **vertebral column** to highlight it, and then click the Add to Note button.

Locate and *right-click* on the added finding

- fracture of vertebral column

When the Actions button menu is displayed, select Details from the drop-down menu. In the Details pop-up window click in the Onset field and type **3/25/2012**.

Click in the Note field and type **C7, T1, T2, T3**. These are the vertebrae of the spine listed on his surgery report.

When you have finished, click the OK button to close the pop-up window. The finding should be red and the description should read "fracture of vertebral column 3/25/2012 C7, T1, T2, T2."

### Step 9

The patient reports red sores, which his daughter says turn white when she presses on them.

Click the X in the Search box on the toolbar to clear it. Type **red sore** and press the Enter key on your keyboard.

When the search list is displayed, click the small plus symbol next to the symptom "a red sore" to expand the tree. Click the concept **blanching with pressure** to highlight it, and then click the button labeled Add to Note.

Locate the added finding in the Review of Symptoms section, and click it until it turns red.

● a red sore which blanches with pressure

**Step 10**

The clinician observes three pressure sores on the patient's back and examines them.

Click the X in the Search box on the toolbar to clear it. Type **lesions tender** and press the Enter key on your keyboard.

Locate "lesions tender" (about two-thirds of the way down the list) and click the small plus symbol to expand the tree. Click the concept **to direct pressure** to highlight it, and then click the Add to Note button.

Locate the added finding in the Physical Exam, Skin Exam section, and click it until it turns red.

● lesion tender to direct pressure

**Step 11**

Click the Browse button on the toolbar, which should cause the drop-down list to open with the Physical Examination tree expanded at lesion. Click the red pushpin at the top of the drop-down list, so you can add multiple concepts to your note.

Scroll the list downward to locate "Ulcer." Click the small plus symbol next to Ulcer to expand the tree further.

Locate and click the concept **on shoulders** to highlight it, and then click the Add to Note button.

Locate the concept **on buttocks** (scrolling the list, if necessary). Click on it to highlight it, and then click the Add to Note button.

Click the Browse button on the toolbar to close the drop-down list.

Verify that the added Skin Exam findings are red. If they are not, click them until they turn red.

● ulcer on shoulders
● buttocks

**Step 12**

Add the clinician's assessment.

Click again on the X in the Search box to clear it, and then type **pressure ulcer** and press the Enter key. In the search results list, locate and click on **stage I pressure ulcer of the buttock** (which is preceded by a block letter D for diagnosis). Click the Add to Note button.

Click in the Search box, but do not clear it. Simply add shoulder to your search criteria (i.e., **pressure ulcer shoulder**), and then press the Enter key. Locate **pressure ulcer of the upper left back** and click the plus symbol to expand the tree. In the expanded tree, click on **Stage I** and then click the Add to Note button.

Repeat the same search (**pressure ulcer shoulder**) by clicking in the Search box and pressing the Enter key. Locate **pressure ulcer of the upper right back** and click the plus symbol to expand the tree. In the expanded tree, click on **Stage I** and then click the Add to Note button.

**Step 13**

Locate the newly added diagnoses in the Assessment section and click on them until they turn red.

- stage I pressure ulcer of left upper back
- stage I pressure ulcer of right upper back
- stage I pressure ulcer of the buttock

**Step 14**

Using what you have learned in the previous exercise, create an annotated drawing to illustrate the position of Mr. Patel's incision scars and pressure sores.

Click on a white space in the encounter pane, so neither the diagnosis nor any heading or finding has focus.

Add the anatomical image **Trunk Skin Back Male** to the encounter note as you did in the previous exercise. (Hint: Click the Browse button on the toolbar, and expand the trees "Sample Custom Content," "Shared Content," and "Images." Scroll the list of images to locate and expand "Trunk" by clicking the plus symbol next to it. Scroll the expanded list of Trunk images downward until you locate **Trunk Skin Back Male**. Click on it and click the Add to Note button. Click the Browse button to close the drop-down list.)

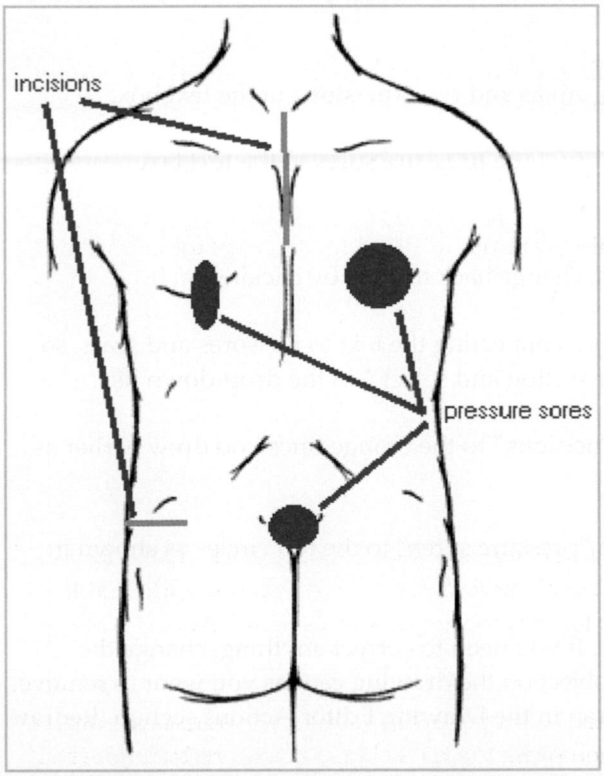

The anatomical drawing shown in Figure 8-40 will be inserted into the Physical Exam section of the encounter note.

**Step 15**

Click on the drawing to display the Drawing Editor in the content pane.

If desired, you can resize the drawing canvas larger. Click on the lower right corner of the drawing canvas and hold the mouse button down while dragging diagonally downward, until the canvas reaches a comfortable size for you to work in.

Locate the Style section of the Drawing Editor and click on the button that sets the color. The palette window shown previously in Figure 8-30 will be invoked. Locate and click on the grid cell containing the color **red**.

Next, click on the Weight (button with three lines). As you can see from Figure 8-40 you will need to draw large circles, so select **5.5** from the drop-down list to get the thickest line.

**Figure 8-40** Drawing of incisions and pressure sores to reproduce in the encounter.

Verify that **Pen** is the selected Drawing Tool.

### Step 16

As closely as possible, replicate the drawing in Figure 8-40. Depending on the mouse you are using, drawing large even circles can be difficult. Again, your drawing doesn't have to be as evenly drawn as the figure; just get the size and placement of the pressure sores as close as you can.

Draw a large red circle over the right shoulder blade, a red circle over the coccyx, and a vertical ellipse over the left shoulder blade (at locations shown in Figure 8-40). Fill in each circle before proceeding to the next. Do this by moving the mouse within the circle while continuing to hold the left button until the entire circle is red.

In the Drawing Editor, Drawing Tools, change to **Line** by clicking on it.

In the Style section of the Drawing Editor click on the Color button. When the palette is displayed, select the **orange** grid cell.

Draw a short horizontal line from the edge of the left hip toward the coccyx as shown in Figure 8-40.

Draw a long vertical line from the base of the neck to the center of the shoulder blades as shown in Figure 8-40.

### Step 17

Next, label the drawing parts with text.

In the Drawing Editor, Drawing Tools section, click on **ab Text**.

In the Style section of the Drawing Editor click on the Color button. When the palette is displayed, select the **blue** grid cell.

Click in the upper left of the drawing canvas and type **incisions** in the text box.

Click on the right side of the drawing and type **pressure sores** in the text box.

### Step 18

In the Drawing Editor, Drawing Tools, change back to **Line** by clicking on it.

You will need less thickness for the lines connecting the text to the sores and scars, so click on the Weight button in the Style section and select **3** in the drop-down list.

Draw two blue lines from the word "incisions" to the orange lines you drew earlier as shown in Figure 8-40.

Draw three blue lines from the phrase "pressure sores" to the red circles as shown in Figure 8-40.

Compare your drawing to Figure 8-40. If you need to correct anything, change the Drawing Tool to "Pointer." Click the object on the drawing canvas you want to remove, and then click the Delete Selected button in the Drawing Editor Actions section. Redraw the element correctly.

## Step 19

Click the View button on the toolbar and select Concise from the drop-down menu. Compare your screen to Figure 8-41, scrolling as necessary until you have verified the entire encounter. If everything on your screen matches the figure, proceed to step 15. If there are any differences, review the preceding steps and correct your work.

**Figure 8-41** Concise view of correctly completed encounter with annotated drawing for Raj Patel.

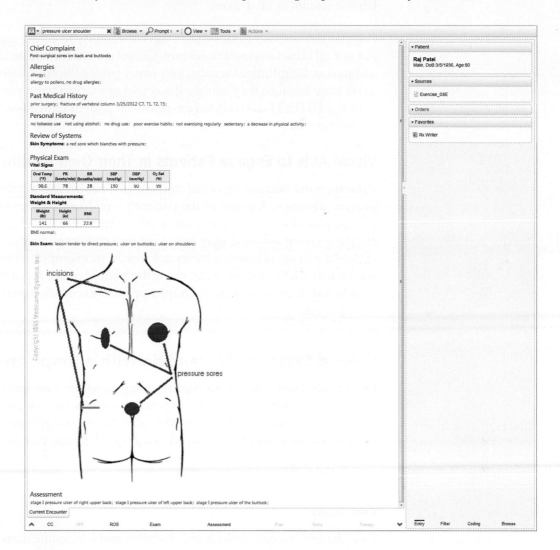

## Step 20

If wish to print a copy of your completed encounter notes for yourself or because your instructor requires you to turn them in, use the Create PDF option, and then print or download the PDF at this time.

The final step in every exercise is to submit your completed work for a grade.

Locate and click the blue Quippe icon button on the toolbar, and then select the option Submit for Grade from the drop-down menu. This will complete Exercise 8E.

## Using Graphs to View Trends

In Chapter 1 the IOM identified trending as one of the functional benefits derived from an EHR. Earlier in this chapter you have learned to use flow sheets as a means of "trending," which is comparing the change of certain findings or measurements over a period of time.

Another approach to trending is to view the data as a graph. Chapter 2 discussed the advantages of EHR records with codified results as opposed to EHR records that are scanned images of printed reports. Nowhere is that benefit more evident than with graphs. An EHR system with graphing capability can create a graph from longitudinal data of any finding that has numerical values recorded over multiple encounters, be it lab test results or vital signs.

Popular commercial EHR systems have the ability to create graphs from EHR data, but not all clinicians use the feature. Clinicians are trained to identify trends when comparing longitudinal results, and many prefer the cumulative summary or flow sheet view because they can see the actual numerical values in the report. However, with the HITECH Act's added emphasis on patient education, graphs can play an important role.

## Visual Aids to Engage Patients in Their Own Healthcare

Patients must become involved in their own healthcare to effectively manage and prevent diseases. A graph of the patient's weight measurements or body-mass index and graphs of key indicators such as cholesterol and blood glucose levels can be effective visual aids and may help to stimulate compliance with health regimens. The cliché "a picture is worth a thousand words" is exemplified when the clinician can, with a few clicks of the mouse, show the patient a graph portraying changes in relevant health factors over time. Graphs provide excellent visual aids for patient counseling or education.

## Guided Exercise 8F: Trending with a Graph and Flow Sheet

In previous exercises, you worked on citing previous measurements of a patient's weight to see trends. Subsequently you learned a better way, to view trends by using flow sheets. In this exercise, using the same patient, weight, and height data, you will see how the data may be portrayed as a graph. Because you are already familiar with the case after performing Exercise 8A, all findings except weight and height have been omitted to keep this exercise short.

### Case Study

Guy Daniels is a patient with hypertension and borderline diabetes who has been failing to follow his diet and irregular in his exercise habits. You are going to create a graph and annotate it to help him visualize his problem.

### Step 1

Start a supported web browser program and follow the steps listed inside the cover of this textbook to log in to the MyHealthProfessionsLab for this course.

Locate and click on the link Exercise 8F.

### Step 2

In the New Encounter window, locate and click on **Daniels, Guy**.

Set the date to **05/24/2016** and the time to **9:00 AM** as shown previously in Figure 8-1.

Verify that the date and the time are set correctly, and then click the OK button.

## Step 3

Record Mr. Daniels's weight and height in the corresponding fields of the encounter pane as you did in the first exercise.

Weight: **239**

Height: **68.5**

Verify that you have entered both fields correctly and then locate and click on the Graph Weight button.

A graph of Mr. Daniels's weight over three previous visits will appear, as shown in Figure 8-42.

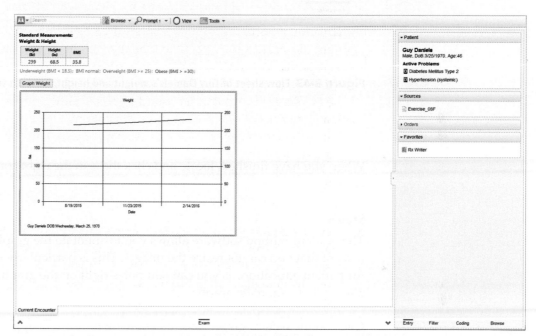

**Figure 8-42** Guy Daniels's weight, height, BMI, and graph of body weight.

## Step 4

You are probably familiar with graphs from other courses you have taken. The graph has labels at two axes. Numbers along the left edge label the horizontal lines demarking 10 lb increments. Vertical lines separate the graph into columns. The columns are labeled with dates at which the weight was measured. The blue graph line connects the points on the graph denoting the patient's weight on each date.

Now, let us compare the graph to the flow sheet.

Click on any white space below the graph to restore date tabs at the bottom of the encounter pane.

Click the View button on the toolbar and select Flowsheet from the drop-down menu. The flow sheet will display as shown in Figure 8-43.

Compare the graph and flow sheet simultaneously.

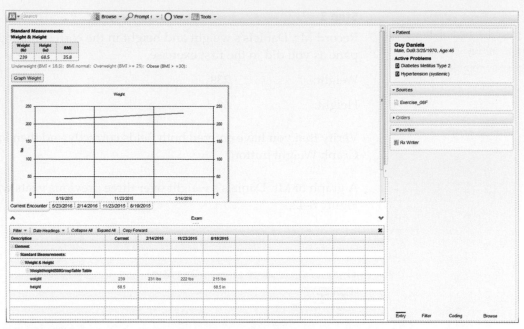

**Figure 8-43** Flow sheet of Guy Daniels's weight and height, beneath the graph of his weight.

When you have finished, locate and click the X in the right corner of the flow sheet to close it.

### Step 5

The Student Edition software allows you to annotate the graph as you would a drawing (except that you cannot resize the image). This is particularly useful when the graph is for patient education, as you can add notes right on the graph. Not all EHR systems allow you to annotate graphs.

Click on the weight graph, and the Drawing Editor will appear in the content pane on the right.

In the Drawing Tools section, click on the **ab Text** tool.

In the Styles section, click on the Color button, and select **blue** from the drop-down palette.

Locate the **11/23/2015** column of the graph, and click in that column in the space below the horizontal line labeled **200**. If the textbox appears it is too high or low, simply click in another location to reposition it before you start typing. In the text box, type **wt. gain while trying to diet**.

Locate the **2/14/2016** column, and click in that column at or near the horizontal line labeled **200**. In the text box, type **not exercising**.

Click on any white space below the graph to close the Drawing Editor.

Compare your screen to Figure 8-44. If everything on your screen matches the figure, proceed to step 6. If there are any differences, review the preceding steps and correct your work.

**Figure 8-44** Added annotation text on the weight graph in Guy Daniels's correctly completed encounter.

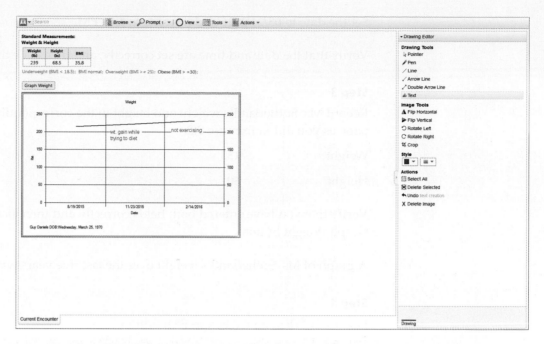

### Step 6

If wish to print a copy of your completed encounter notes for yourself or because your instructor requires you to turn them in, use the Create PDF option, and then print or download the PDF at this time.

The final step in every exercise is to submit your completed work for a grade.

Locate and click the blue Quippe icon button on the toolbar, and then select the option Submit for Grade from the drop-down menu. This will complete Exercise 8F.

## Critical Thinking Exercise 8G: Graphing Weight and BMI

Other numerical values can also be graphed. In the previous chapter, you learned how BMI is calculated and how the BMI number correlates to BMI categories in adults. Because BMI is one of the Clinical Quality Measures listed in Chapter 1, it might be useful to graph it for the patient. In this exercise, in addition to graphing the patient's weight you will also graph her BMI.

### Case Study

Sally Sutherland is a patient with hyperlipidemia and diabetes who has been seen annually by her primary care physician, so several years of data are available for graphing.

### Step 1

Start a supported web browser program and follow the steps listed inside the cover of this textbook to log in to the MyHealthProfessionsLab for this course.

Locate and click on the link Exercise 8G.

### Step 2

In the New Encounter window, locate and click on **Sutherland, Sally**.

Set the date to **05/24/2016** and the time to **1:00 PM**.

Verify that the date and time are set correctly, and then click the OK button.

**Step 3**

Record Ms. Sutherland's weight and height in the corresponding fields of the encounter pane as you did in Exercise 8C.

Weight:                153

Height:                60

Verify that you have entered both fields correctly and then locate and click on the Graph Weight button.

A graph of Ms. Sutherland's weight over the last five years will appear,

**Step 4**

Locate and click on the Graph BMI button.

A graph of Ms. Sutherland's BMI over the same five years will appear, below the weight graph.

**Step 5**

The clinician knows that Sally had a baby in 2014, and that the increase in her weight due to pregnancy caused her BMI to appear elevated. Add a note to her graph.

Click on the **BMI** graph, and the Drawing Editor will appear in the content pane on the right.

In the Drawing Tools section, click on the **ab Text** tool.

In the Styles section, click on the Color button, and select the cell for **blue** in the palette grid.

Locate the column labeled **5/19/2014** and click in that column at the line labeled **30**. In the textbox type **Disregard – pregnancy wt.**

Click any white space outside the graph to close the Drawing Editor.

**Step 6**

Compare your screen to Figure 8-45, scrolling as necessary until you have verified the entire encounter. If everything on your screen matches the figure, proceed to step 7. If there are any differences, review the preceding steps and correct your work.

**Step 7**

If wish to print a copy of your completed encounter notes for yourself or because your instructor requires you to turn them in, use the Create PDF option, and then print or download the PDF at this time.

The final step in every exercise is to submit your completed work for a grade.

Locate and click the blue Quippe icon button on the toolbar, and then select the option Submit for Grade from the drop-down menu. This will complete Exercise 8G.

**Figure 8-45** Sally Sutherland's correctly completed encounter with two graphs and added annotation text.

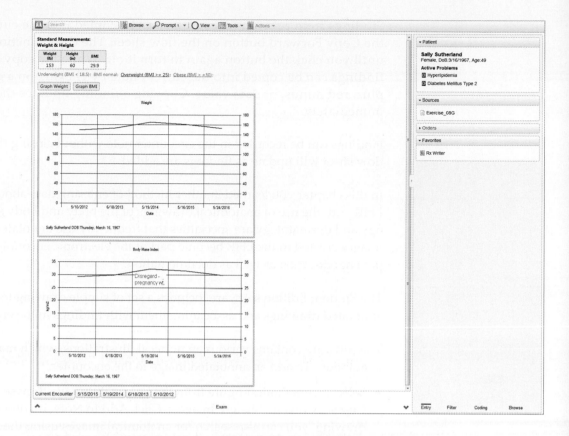

## Chapter Eight Summary

This chapter showed how codified data in the EHR can be displayed in a flow sheet and how findings with numerical values can be graphed.

Flow sheets present longitudinal data from multiple encounters for a side-by-side comparison of findings over a period of time. Flow sheets are displayed by clicking the View button and selecting Flowsheet from the drop-down menu. The Flowsheet view is closed by clicking an X in the upper right corner of the flow sheet.

The flow sheet view resembles a spreadsheet made up of rows and columns of cells. The first column displays descriptions of section and group headings as well as concepts and findings in the current encounter. The second column shows findings recorded in the current encounter. The remaining columns to the right are labeled with dates of previous encounters, and the column displays findings from that encounter note. A button on the flow sheet allows you to change the date labels to days, weeks, months, or years from the date of the current encounter.

The flow sheet rows are grouped vertically into logical sections and groups that match the sections in the current encounter. Quippe flow sheets do not display rows for findings from previous encounters unless there is a corresponding clinical concept in the current encounter.

Flow sheet rows can be collapsed or expanded by clicking the plus or minus symbols next to the headings. Buttons at the top of the flow sheet can expand or collapse all rows. When an individual heading or finding in the encounter note has focus, only rows for that section are displayed. Click on any white space in the encounter pane to redisplay all rows.

Findings from previous encounters can be copied into the current note by clicking the Copy Forward button on the flow sheet. The copy function remains active until you click the button again to turn it off. While the copy function is activated, findings can be copied into the current note by clicking on a cell containing a blue plus, red minus, or data value. Copying a finding updates the encounter note immediately.

Findings can be recorded in the encounter note without closing the flow sheet, and the flow sheet will update as findings are added.

In this chapter you learned another method of entering data about the patient into the EHR with the use of anatomical drawings of the body and body systems. Ophthalmology and dermatology are specialties that frequently use annotated drawings. Annotated images created in the EHR become part of the electronic encounter and are useful for patient education as well as documentation.

The Student Edition software includes a set of simple drawing tools for creating annotated drawings and associating them with findings in the encounter notes.

The software contains various anatomical illustrations, which may be selected for annotation. To add an annotated image to the encounter:

◆ Select an anatomical figure from the image library via Browse (Expand, Sample Custom Content, Shared, Images). Click Add to Note. If you know the name of the drawing, you can also search for anatomical images using the search box.

◆ Left-click on the image to enter drawing mode, which also opens the Drawing Editor in the content pane.

◆ Left-click on drawing tools to select them.

◆ Annotate the drawing by clicking and holding the left mouse button down as you move over the image (with "pen" selected for example).

◆ Change the color and line thickness of tools with the Color and Weight buttons located in the Style section of the Drawing Editor.

◆ Use Drawing Editor Action buttons to select, delete, or undo elements of the drawing.

◆ Exit out of drawing mode and close the Drawing Editor by clicking anywhere in the encounter pane outside the drawing canvas.

EHR software can also display trends using graphs of numerical data recorded in previous encounters. Graphs provide excellent visual aids for patient counseling or education.

| Task | Exercise | Page # |
|---|---|---|
| How to view a flow sheet | 8A | 301 |
| How to copy findings in flow sheet view into the current note using Copy Forward | 8A | 301 |
| How to insert drawing images in an encounter note | 8D | 321 |
| How to annotate drawings using the Drawing Editor | 8D | 321 |
| How to insert a graph into an encounter note and annotate it | 8F | 338 |

# Testing Your Knowledge of Chapter 8

### Step 1

Log in to MyHealthProfessionsLab following the directions printed inside the cover of this textbook.

Locate and click on Chapter 8 Test.

### Step 2

Answer the test questions. When you have finished, click the Submit Test button to close the window.

## Testing Your Skill Exercise 8H: Diabetic with High Blood Pressure

Now that you have performed all the exercises in Chapter 8 this exercise will help you and your instructor evaluate your acquired skills. Use the information in the case study and the features of the software you already know to document the patient's encounter.

### Case Study

The patient is George Blackstone, whom you used in a previous exercise, but in this exercise you will utilize a flow sheet and annotate a drawing. Mr. Blackstone has high blood pressure and diabetes. He comes in on **May 24, 2016** for a two-month follow-up visit.

George says he has no allergies. After entering the chief complaint and allergies, the clinician reviews the 3/15/2016 encounter and copies the Current Medications and Assessment sections into the current note.

Returning to the current encounter tab, the clinician notices there are pending test results and retrieves them.

The clinician records George's vital signs and performs a quick screening exam in which he finds everything normal. George's current medications indicated he was taking hydrochlorothiazide. The clinician orders it again.

Here are Mr. Blackstone's vital signs:

| | |
|---|---|
| Temperature: | **98.6** |
| Pulse: | **78** |
| Respiration: | **26** |
| SBP: | **138** |
| DBP: | **90** |
| Weight: | **235** |
| Height: | **68.5** |

Using flow sheet view the clinician compares lab test results from multiple visits. In the assessment section of the encounter he right-clicks on diabetes mellitus and selects Prompt from the drop-down menu. This adds rows to the flow sheet. He copies forward the family history of diabetes, and in the plan section of the flow sheet he copies medication orders for metformin HCL and atenolol and the weight loss diet.

Because it is important for diabetics to perform regular self-examination of their feet, the clinician annotates a drawing to remind George what areas to check.

### Step 1

Start a supported web browser program and follow the steps listed inside the cover of this textbook to log in to the MyHealthProfessionsLab for this course.

Locate and click on the link **Exercise 8H**. This will open the Quippe software window with the New Encounter window displayed in the center.

### Step 2

Locate and click on the patient name, and click the OK button. In this exercise, you **must** set the date as stated in the case study. You do not need to set the time of the encounter.

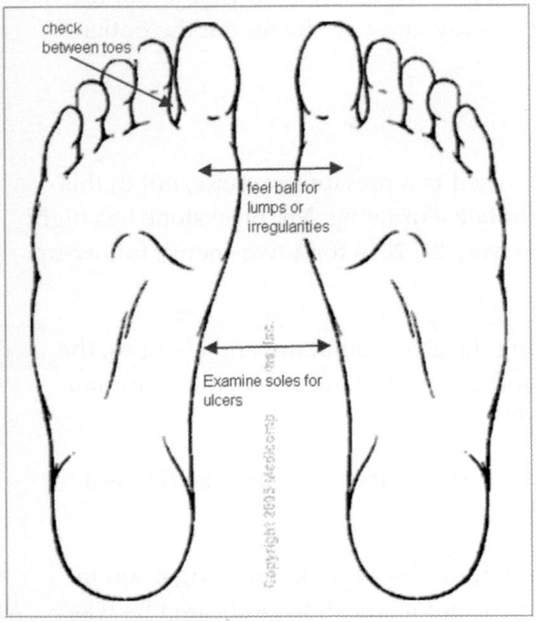

check
between toes

feel ball for
lumps or
irregularities

Examine soles for
ulcers

Copyright 2005 Medicomp

**Anatomical Figure © Medicomp Systems, Inc.**

**Figure 8-46** Replicate this annotated drawing as part of Exercise 8H.

### Step 3

Read the case study *carefully*.

*Hint*: Copy the Current Medication and Assessment sections while reviewing the 3/15/2016 note.

*Hint*: Use the Hypertension wizard to enter vital signs, document the quick exam, and order a renewal of George's current medication.

*Hint*: Prompt on the assessment diabetes mellitus to add rows to the flow sheet view so you can document copy forward family history and three remaining orders.

### Step 4

After closing the flow sheet view, add the image feet skin bottom to the note. As closely as possible, match Figure 8-46.

### Step 5

If you wish to print a copy of your completed encounter notes for yourself or because your instructor requires you to turn them in, use the Create PDF option, and then print or download the PDF at this time.

Submit your completed work for a grade. This will complete Exercise 8H.

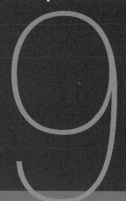

# Using the EHR to Improve Patient Health

## Learning Outcomes

*After completing this chapter, you should be able to:*

- ◆ Document a well-baby checkup
- ◆ Explain the relationship between vital signs and growth charts
- ◆ Create a pediatric growth chart
- ◆ Understand immunization schedules
- ◆ Order immunizations for a child
- ◆ Discuss preventive care guidelines
- ◆ Understand how EHR preventive care systems work
- ◆ Review and document Clinical Quality Measures
- ◆ Describe the concept of Patient-Centered Medical Home

## Prevention and Early Detection

The value of an EHR increases as a practice uses it. As more of the patient's health record is stored in a codified EHR, more can be done with it. As we have seen in previous chapters, longitudinal data from past encounters can be used to improve patient care through disease management, trending, and creating graphs for patient education and counseling.

Still, it is always better to prevent a disease than to treat it. Thus far, you have learned how to use an EHR to document patient visits. In this chapter, we will discuss various ways in which preventive care, immunization, preventive screening, education, and counseling can help people live longer, healthier lives.

# Pediatric Wellness Visits

Whereas those of us who are adults may have an electronic health record, we may never have a completely codified health record, because too much of our medical history is isolated in paper records at medical offices that we no longer visit. Those who are just being born, however, have an excellent chance that their health records are being created and stored electronically today and will be for the whole of their lives.

The care we receive in the early years is fundamental to lifelong health. Early screening, detection, education, and immunizations have all contributed to increased life spans of the population as a whole. Nowhere does this have more support than in the pediatric practice, where regular examinations are recommended for wellness visits, not just when the child is ill.

In the next three exercises, you will use the Student Edition software to record a pediatric visit, create a different kind of graph called a *growth chart*, and learn about childhood immunizations. This is a lot of material to cover, and for that reason the pediatric visit will span several exercises.

## Guided Exercise 9A: Well-Baby Checkup

### Case Study

Tyrell Williams is a 6-month-old male who is brought by his mother to the pediatric clinic where he has always been seen. As a result, the clinic has a lifelong history of his care and growth.

### Step 1

Start a supported web browser program and follow the steps listed inside the cover of this textbook to log in to the MyHealthProfessionsLab for this course.

Locate and click on the link Exercise 9A.

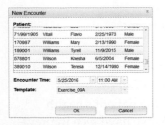

**Figure 9-1** Select Tyrell Williams and set the date to May 25, 2016 11:00 in the New Encounter window.

### Step 2

In the New Encounter window, locate and click on **Williams, Tyrell**.

Set the date to **05/25/2016** and the time to **11:00 AM** as shown in Figure 9-1.

Verify the date and time are set correctly, and then click the OK button.

### Step 3

The pediatric template will be displayed. Take a moment to orient yourself. You will notice that there are quite a few clinical concepts on the encounter note.

Whereas medical practices seeing adult patients with chronic illnesses might use a general template and rely on lists or forms to add concepts for specific conditions, pediatric practices have to document numerous age-specific growth and development milestones during well-baby checkups. For this reason pediatric practices typically create multiple templates or forms, with each template or form containing concepts appropriate to an age group. For example, newborn to two weeks, two months, four months, six months to one year, one to two years, and another for age two and beyond.

This pediatric template uses checkboxes to record findings as you did in Chapter 3. This type of design allows the medical assistants or nurses and pediatricians to move through the exam quickly, ensuring that nothing is forgotten or overlooked.

Well-baby checkups are usually quite extensive and involve the social history of the parents as well as of the baby. This template contains the items a practice might cover during a checkup for a 6-month-old baby. In the interest of time, you will not enter data for every question, although you would during an actual pediatric wellness visit.

Tyrell is brought here by his mother for his 6-month checkup. Begin at the top of the encounter note and click in the appropriate checkboxes. A check mark will appear.

✓ 6-month visit

✓ mother

In this template, the reason for visit finding suffices for the Chief Complaint, unless there is an illness or additional condition to be covered during the visit. In this case there is not.

The remainder of the template uses checkboxes. Most contain the letters "Y" and "N," which you click to record a finding as positive or negative, similar to forms and templates you worked with previously. In this template, some but not all findings change color and description when Y or N is clicked. This provides a visual clue to the clinician, but the state of the finding is determined by the box checked regardless of whether or not the finding changes color.

## Step 4

The Growth and Development section, as mentioned earlier, is used to document developmental milestones (of a 6-month-old in this case). These are observations either the nurse or pediatrician makes while watching and interacting with the baby or from answers supplied by the adult who brought the baby to the clinic.

Tyrell is not shy. Locate **shy with strangers** and click the checkbox:

✓ **N** shy with strangers

The description will change to "Is not shy with strangers."

Tyrell sits independently, babbles, rolls over from back to front, and passes an object from hand to hand. His mother says he pulls himself to standing position.

Click on the heading Growth and Development to highlight the section. Click the Actions button on the toolbar and select Otherwise Normal from the drop-down menu. This will set all unentered findings in this section to **Y**.

Compare the upper portion of your screen to Figure 9-2.

**Figure 9-2** Portion of the encounter with the correctly completed Growth and Development findings.

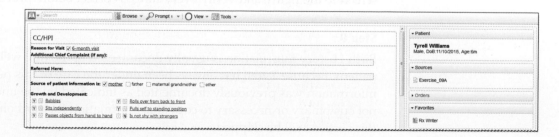

**Step 5**

Proceed to GI Symptoms. Tyrell's mother says he is going through six to eight diapers a day and usually one of them is a bowel movement. He is nursing and hasn't been constipated.

Type the numeric information into the fields at the end of each line and click the N checkbox for constipated.

Bowel movements per day: **1**

Bowel movements per week: **7**

Wet diapers per day: **6-8**

✓ **N** constipation

**Step 6**

Tyrell's mother says he is sleeping normally and has no difficulty breast feeding; usually about every four hours.

Click on the checkboxes corresponding to her response and enter the hours and number of feedings where indicated.

✓ **N** an abnormal sleep pattern

✓ **Y** Infant is breastfeeding

✓ **N** difficulty breast feeding

Number of hours between feedings: **4**

Number of feedings in 24 hours: **6**

Compare the GI Symptoms through Breast Feeding sections of your screen with Figure 9-3.

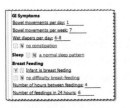

**Figure 9-3** Portion of the encounter showing GI Symptoms, Sleep patterns, and Breast Feeding.

**Step 7**

The remaining findings in this section concern his diet. Tyrell is not bottle fed and has been eating rice cereal since he was 4 months old. His mother has just started giving him pureed fruits and vegetables, and estimates he is eating about two ounces of each per day. As you have in previous steps, click on the checkboxes corresponding to her response and enter the numeric information where indicated.

✓ **N** Infant is bottle feeding

✓ **Y** Is rice cereal introduced (type **4** when prompted for months)

✓ **Y** Vegetables oz/day (type **2** in oz/day field)

✓ **Y** Fruits oz/day (type **2** in oz/day field)

Figure 9-4 shows all of the findings completed in this and previous steps. Compare your screen to the figure and verify everything is correct before proceeding.

**Step 8**

Birth History information is usually documented at the first well-baby visit of a new patient. Because Tyrell has always been under the care of this pediatric practice, the information was previously documented as indicated by the underlined findings. It is not customary or necessary to copy this information forward on subsequent visits, so this section will be skipped.

**Figure 9-4** Correctly completed CC/HPI and developmental portion of Tyrell Williams' note.

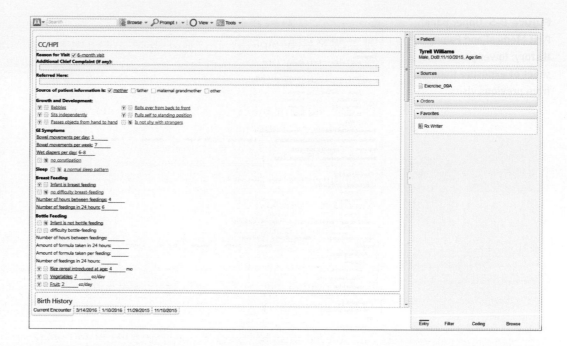

Scroll the encounter pane so the Past Medical History section is positioned at the top. There are no new conditions in the interval since his previous visit, he has never had surgery, and there are no changes to the family history, which was documented on an earlier visit. Therefore locate and click the following checkboxes:

✓ No significant past medical history

✓ No significant surgical history

✓ No significant family history

### Step 9

The clinician notices that two findings at the bottom of the Past Medical History section are underlined, indicating they were documented on an earlier visit. The clinician would like to quickly see the previous findings and document them again.

Click any white space in the encounter pane that does not highlight a heading or finding so that the date tabs at the bottom of the encounter pane reappear.

Click the View button on the toolbar and select Flowsheet from the drop-down menu.

A Flowsheet similar to Figure 9-5 will be displayed. If necessary scroll the flow sheet until you can see the rows labeled Exposure and Environmental Exposure.

Locate the Copy Forward button at the top of the flow sheet and click it on.

Locate the column dated **11/29/2015** and click the cells containing blue minus symbols for the following rows:

- exposure to tuberculosis
- exposure to lead

The findings will be recorded in the encounter note above.

Close the flow sheet view by clicking the X in the right corner of the flow sheet.

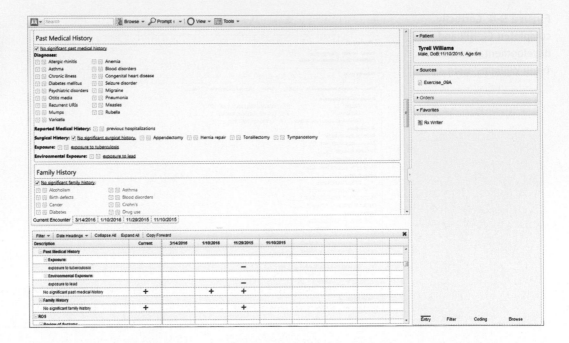

**Figure 9-5** Upper pane: Past Medical and Family History; lower pane: flow sheet of exposure findings from previous visits.

## Step 10

Scroll the encounter pane until the section labeled Family Social History is positioned at the top of the encounter pane.

In pediatric visits, the parent's or other caregiver's social habits and environment are health factors that can affect the child. This section is used to record findings about the infant's family environment and the behavioral habits of adults living there. Whereas with adult and teen patients, behavioral history is about the patient's habits, in well-baby visits, the behavioral history is not about if the baby uses tobacco, alcohol, or drugs, but if the adults around him or her do.

Ms. Williams says she is not smoking or drinking because she is nursing, but her husband smokes cigarettes and drinks moderately. She denies that either of them uses drugs.

Locate and click on the checkboxes indicated for the following Family Social History findings:

✓ **Y** lives with parents

✓ **Y** tobacco use

✓ **Y** alcohol use

✓ **N** drug use

✓ **Y** secondhand tobacco smoke in home

## Step 11

The nurse or pediatrician discusses with Ms. Williams if Tyrell is having any symptoms. He has none.

Click on the ROS heading to highlight the section. Click the Actions button on the toolbar and select Otherwise Normal from the drop-down menu.

Compare the top portion of your screen to Figure 9-6. Verify that your Family Social History and ROS symptom findings match the figure.

**Figure 9-6** Family Social History and ROS sections of encounter note.

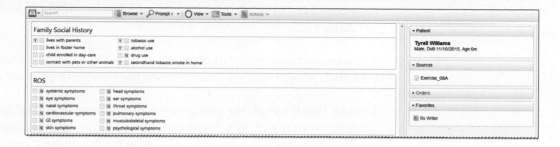

## Step 12

Scroll the encounter pane until the section labeled Physical Exam is positioned at the top of the encounter pane. Although you would normally enter Tyrell's vital signs at this section, we are going to defer that to the next exercise. As mentioned earlier, Tyrell's well-baby visit will be documented over the course of three exercises.

Locate and click the following checkboxes as indicated.

✓ Y alert

✓ Y well hydrated

✓ Y active

✓ Y normal growth and development

The pediatrician examines the remaining body systems and finds that Tyrell is normal and healthy.

Click on the Physical Exam heading to highlight the section. Click the Actions button on the toolbar and select Otherwise Normal from the drop-down menu.

Compare your screen to Figure 9-7.

**Figure 9-7** Physical Exam section of encounter note with vital signs entry omitted.

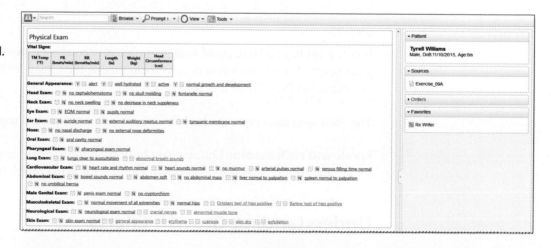

## Step 13

Completion of the Immunizations section will be deferred to a subsequent exercise. Scroll the encounter pane all the way to the bottom so you can see the Assessment and Education sections. Two characteristics of well-baby visits are seen here.

First, unless the child is ill, the diagnosis for a well-baby checkup is the same for every child: one of a special group of diagnosis codes that, instead of indicating an ailment or condition, indicate a state of wellness. Codes for well-baby (age: birth to two years) correlate to ICD-10CM codes Z00.121 and Z00.129. ICD-10CM codes will be discussed in Chapter 12.

The second characteristic of pediatric visits is the focus on providing counseling and education about health-related issues to the parents or primary caregivers.

During Tyrell's visit, the pediatrician provides educational information to his mother about the child's development, nutrition, immunizations, and safety. The pediatrician, having noticed Tyrell's first tooth is nearly ready to push through his gum, also discusses teething and subsequent dental hygiene for when he does have teeth.

Locate and click on the checkbox for the Assessment:

✓   normal routine history and physical well-baby (birth–2 yr)

Locate and click the indicated checkboxes for the following to indicate that these topics were covered during the visit:

✓   **Y** Nutrition

✓   **Y** Teething

✓   **Y** Stranger Safety

✓   **Y** Safety Guidelines

✓   **Y** Dental Hygiene

### Step 14

Click the View button on the toolbar and select Concise from the drop-down menu. Compare your screen to Figure 9-8, scrolling as necessary until you have verified the entire encounter. If everything on your screen matches the figure, proceed to step 15. If there are any differences, review the preceding steps and correct your work.

### Step 15

If you wish to print a copy of your completed encounter notes for yourself or because your instructor requires you to turn them in, use the Create PDF option, and then print or download the PDF at this time.

The final step in every exercise is to submit your completed work for a grade.

Locate and click the blue Quippe icon button on the toolbar, and then select the Submit for Grade option from the drop-down menu. This will complete Exercise 9A.

## Understanding Growth Charts

Childhood growth depends on nutritional, health, and environmental conditions. Changes in any of these factors influence how well a child grows and develops. A child's measurements can be compared against a graph of statistical information gathered from studies of the growth rate of well-babies in a reference population. These graphs are called **growth charts**.

**Figure 9-8** Elongated image of correctly completed encounter note in Concise view.

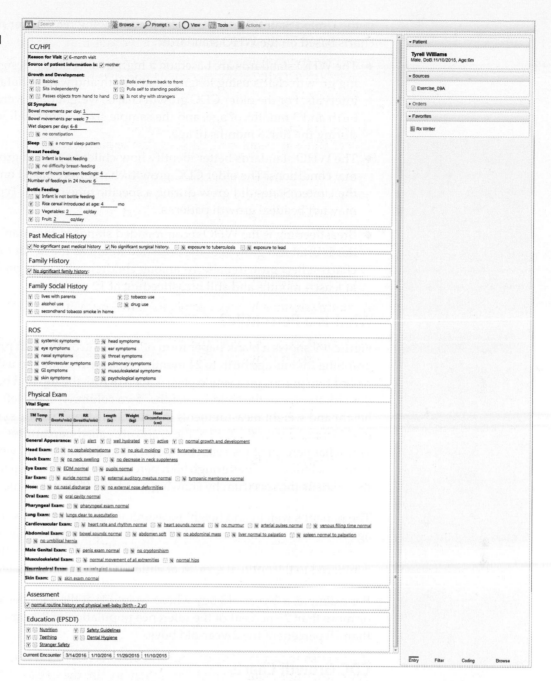

Pediatric growth charts have been used to track the growth of infants, children, and adolescents in the United States since 1977, when the National Center for Health Statistics (NCHS) created a set of graphs as a clinical tool for health professionals to determine if the growth of a child was adequate. In 2006 the World Health Organization (WHO) released a new international growth standard statistical distribution, which describes the growth of children ages 0 to 59 months living in environments believed to support what WHO researchers view as optimal growth of children in six countries throughout the world, including the United States. The distribution shows how infants and young children grow under these conditions, rather than how they grow in environments that may not support optimal growth.

Although the CDC encourages pediatricians to replace use of weight-for-stature charts with the new BMI-for-age charts for patients age two and up, CDC recommends use of the WHO growth charts to monitor growth for infants and children 0 to 2 years of age in the United States. The CDC offers the following reasons for recommending growth charts based on the WHO standards:

◆ The WHO standards are based on a high-quality study designed explicitly for creating growth charts using longitudinal length and weight data measured at frequent intervals. For the older CDC growth charts, weight data were not available between birth and 3 months of age, and the sample sizes were small for sex and age groups during the first 6 months of age.

◆ The WHO standards better identify how children should grow when provided optimal conditions. The older CDC growth charts were based on how typical children in the United States did grow during a specific time period. Typical growth patterns may not be ideal growth patterns.

◆ Breastfeeding is the WHO recommended standard for infant feeding. The WHO standards establish growth of the breastfed infant as the norm for growth. The WHO charts reflect growth patterns among children who were predominantly breastfed for at least 4 months and still breastfeeding at 12 months.

## What Is a Percentile?

Figure 9-9 shows a blank paper form of a WHO growth chart provided by the CDC for graphing infants age birth to 24 months. This form would be used by a clinic to manually record two graphs on a single page. Labels across the top and bottom of the graph demark the age of the child in months. Two columns on the left axis serve as a legend of height and weight measurements in both English and metric systems. The curved blue lines printed across the face of the graph are called percentiles. The curved lines represent what percent of the reference population the individual would equal or exceed. This graph includes the 5th through 95th percentiles; the CDC also has a version available that widens the spectrum by showing a 3rd and 97th percentile.

The patient's weight and height measurements can be marked on the chart under each age for which readings are available. By finding the percentile line closest to the patient's measurements, the clinician can assess the size and growth patterns of the individual as compared to the optimal growth of children in the United States and five other countries.

For example, a 2-year-old boy whose weight is at the 25th percentile weighs the same as or more than 25 percent of the reference population of 2-year-old boys but weighs less than 75 percent of the 2-year-old boys.

## CDC Growth Charts

Two sets of 10 pediatric growth charts are maintained and distributed by the Centers for Disease Control and Prevention (CDC), five for boys and five for girls in each set. Set 1 has the outer limits of the curves at the 5th and 95th percentiles. Most pediatricians in the United States use set 1 for the majority of routine clinical assessments. Set 2 has the outer limits of the curves at the 3rd and 97th percentiles for selected applications. For example, pediatric endocrinologists and others who assess the growth of children with special health care requirements may choose to use set 2 for certain patients.

In addition to the WHO growth charts recommended for age birth to 24 months, the CDC provides two gender-specific versions of the following pediatric growth charts:

Infants, birth to 36 months

◆ Length-for-age and Weight-for-age

◆ Head circumference-for-age and Weight-for-length

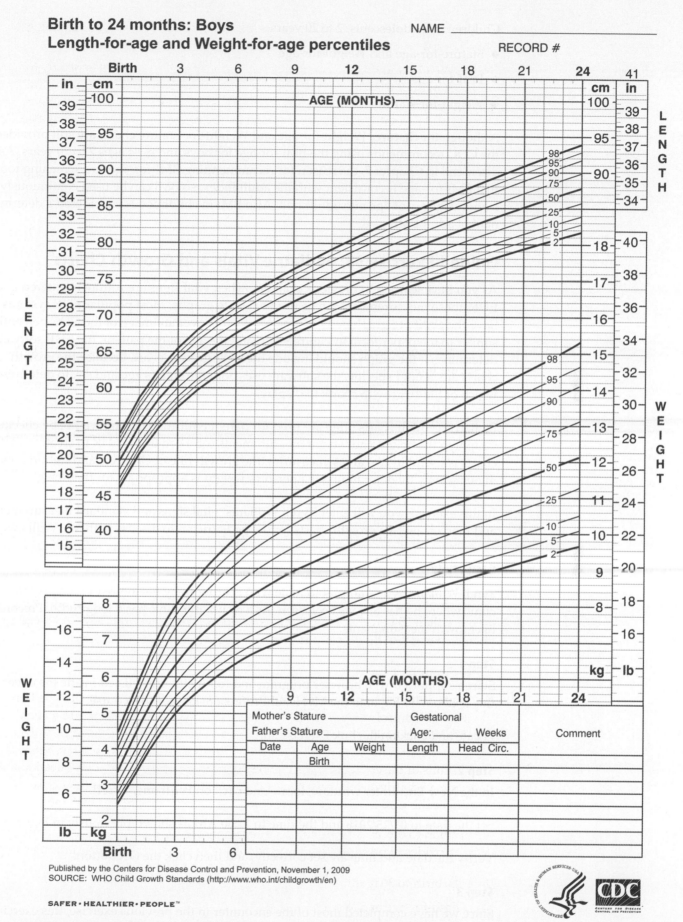

## Birth to 24 months: Boys
### Length-for-age and Weight-for-age percentiles

NAME _____

RECORD # _____

Published by the Centers for Disease Control and Prevention, November 1, 2009
SOURCE: WHO Child Growth Standards (http://www.who.int/childgrowth/en)

SAFER · HEALTHIER · PEOPLE™

**Figure 9-9** Boys birth to 24 months Length-for-age/Weight-for-age growth chart.

Children and adolescents, 2 to 20 years

◆ Stature-for-age and Weight-for-age

◆ BMI-for-age

◆ Weight-for-stature

Although the Stature/Weight-for-age and Weight-for-stature charts are still provided, the CDC recommends using the BMI-for-age for boys and girls ages 2 to 20 years. As discussed in Chapter 7, the reason for recommending BMI-for-age as a screening tool is that BMI-for-age is consistent with the adult index, so BMI can be used continuously from two years of age into adulthood. Also BMI in childhood is considered a determinant of adult BMI.

## Guided Exercise 9B: Pediatric Vitals and Growth Charts

As you have learned in previous chapters, when vital signs are routinely entered in an EHR, those measurements can be used to create graphs. Most popular EHR systems have the ability to graph pediatric measurements over an image of the CDC percentiles, similar to the paper form in Figure 9-9. Using the age of the patient, the EHR software determines if the graph should include the CDC growth chart. Because the growth charts are gender specific, the software uses both the child's age and sex to determine which of the 16 growth charts to display.

Pediatric growth charts often are used for parent education during well-baby checkups. Graphing the height and weight measurements recorded in the EHR to create growth charts is useful in two areas: measuring the growth rate of children, and fighting obesity in our society by determining if a person's weight is appropriate for their height.

In this exercise, you will enter Tyrell Williams' vital signs and standard measurements, and then create two growth charts for the pediatrician to discuss with Ms. Williams.

### Case Study

Tyrell Williams is a 6-month-old male who is brought by his mother to the pediatric clinic where he has always been seen. As a result, the clinic has a longitudinal record of his growth measurements.

### Step 1

Start a supported web browser program and follow the steps listed inside the cover of this textbook to log in to the MyHealthProfessionsLab for this course.

Locate and click on the link Exercise 9B.

### Step 2

In the New Encounter window, locate and click on **Williams, Tyrell**.

Set the date to **05/25/2016** and the time to **11:00 AM** as shown previously in Figure 9-1.

Verify the date and time are set correctly, and then click the OK button.

### Step 3

Since we have completed most of the encounter in the previous exercise, this exercise focuses on the vital signs portion of the encounter.

Notice that there are several differences between pediatric and adult vital signs:

◆ Infant growth is referred to as length not stature or height.

◆ The temperature is measured in the ear (tympanic).

◆ The circumference of the head is also recorded.

◆ Blood pressure readings are not typically taken in healthy children under the age of three.

Enter the following measurements for Tyrell in the corresponding Vital Signs fields:

| | |
|---|---|
| Temperature: | **99** |
| Pulse: | **128** |
| Respiration Rate: | **40** |
| Length (in): | **27.5** |
| Weight (kg): | **8.7** |
| Head Circumference (cm): | **43.9** |

Compare your screen with Figure 9-10. If there are any differences, review the above information and correct your work. When you have verified the vital signs are entered correctly, proceed to step 4.

**Figure 9-10** Correctly completed entry of Tyrell Williams' vital signs.

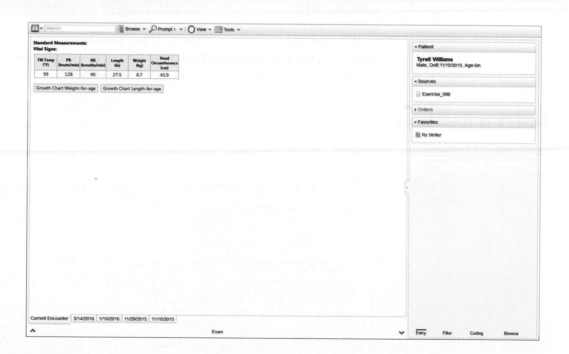

**Step 4**

Click on the Growth Chart Weight-for-age button.

Compare your screen to Figure 9-11. Review the growth chart for Tyrell Williams displayed on your screen. The blue X marks the patient's weight at the various months, listed across the bottom of the graph. The curved lines represent the comparable growth rate as a percentage of the general population. This is the percentile described previously. Similar growth charts also can be generated for a child's length and head circumference.

**Figure 9-11** Tyrell Williams'
weight-for-age growth chart.

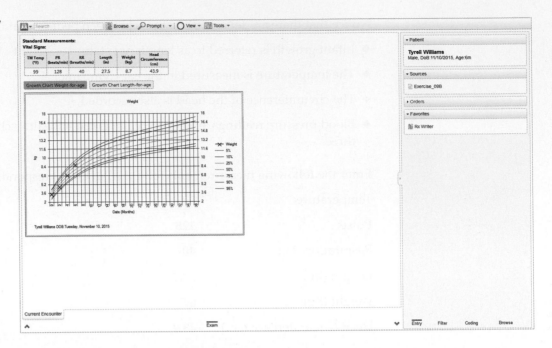

### Step 5

Compare the graph to the EHR data by invoking the flow sheet view.

Click any white space in the encounter pane, so the graph does not have focus and the date tabs again appear at the bottom of the pane.

Click the View button on the toolbar and select Flowsheet from the drop-down menu. The flow sheet will display, as shown in Figure 9-12.

**Figure 9-12** Weight-for-age
growth chart compared with
flow sheet of vital signs.

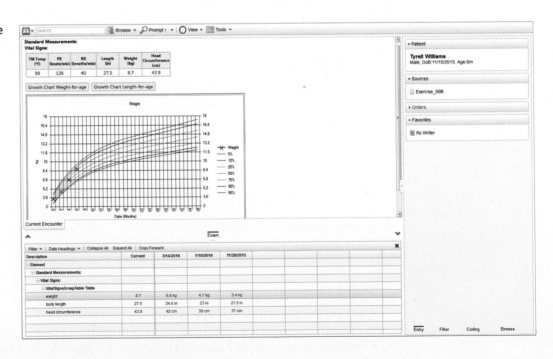

### Step 6

Change the column headings of the flow sheet to show Tyrell's age instead of the dates of his previous visits.

**Figure 9-13** Date Headings drop-down menu with Patient Age selected.

Locate and click the down-arrow on the Date Headings button at the top of the flow sheet. The drop-down menu shown in Figure 9-13 will be displayed.

Locate and click on the option **Patient Age**. The headings of the columns will change to Current, 4 Months old, 8 Weeks old, 19 Days old, and 1 Day old, Tyrell's ages on the dates of the previous visits.

Locate the weight row of the flow sheet (highlighted in Figure 9-12) and compare his weight at each age to the location of the X in the graph. The curved line that each X intersects is his percentile at that age. Notice that as Tyrell grows older he is moving into a higher percentile. This may be because he is breast fed, and the WHO data is standardized for breast-fed infants.

### Step 7

Close the flow sheet before adding the second graph by clicking the X in the right corner of the Flowsheet section of the pane.

Click on the Growth Chart Length-for-age button. A pediatric growth chart for length will be added to the encounter, as shown in Figure 9-14. Scroll the encounter pane if necessary to see the entire length-for-age graph. Notice that Quippe has automatically converted the length unit of measure, inches, to centimeters for purposes of the graph, but the unit of measure in the encounter is not changed.

**Figure 9-14** Tyrell Williams' length-for-age growth chart added to the encounter note.

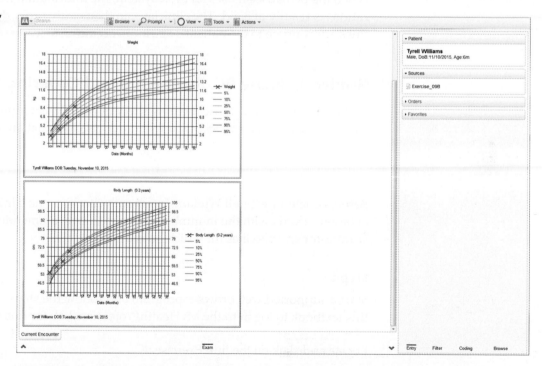

### Step 8

If you wish to print a copy of your completed encounter notes for yourself or because your instructor requires you to turn them in, use the Create PDF option, and then print or download the PDF at this time.

The final step in every exercise is to submit your completed work for a grade.

Locate and click the blue Quippe icon button on the toolbar, and then select the Submit for Grade option from the drop-down menu. This will complete Exercise 9B.

# The Importance of Childhood Immunizations

Immunization slows down or stops disease outbreaks. Vaccines prevent disease in the people who receive them and protect those who come into contact with unvaccinated individuals.

Although it is true that newborn babies are immune to many diseases because they have antibodies they obtained from their mothers, the duration of this immunity may only last as little as a month, and not more than a year. If a child is not vaccinated and is exposed to a disease germ, the child's body may not be strong enough to fight the disease. Before vaccines, many children died from diseases that vaccines now prevent. For example, through childhood immunization, we are now able to control many infectious diseases that were once common in this country, including polio, measles, diphtheria, pertussis (whooping cough), rubella (German measles), mumps, tetanus, and Haemophilus influenzae type b (Hib).[1]

One of the things a pediatrician does during the first two years of well-baby checkups is to compare the child's immunization history against a recommended schedule of immunizations. At regular intervals, the well-baby will receive one or more vaccines. By the age of 2 years, the child is then protected against numerous diseases that once caused the death of many children.

When the pediatrician uses an EHR system, the information from all previous immunizations is readily at hand. The clinician can then easily order the next scheduled vaccines appropriate to the patient's age and vaccine history.

## Guided Exercise 9C: Reviewing and Ordering Vaccines

In this exercise, you will use the flow sheet to verify what immunizations the child has had, and in a subsequent step you will order vaccines that are required.

### Case Study

Before concluding Tyrell Williams's 6-month checkup, the clinic will compare his immunization records with the immunization schedule recommended by the CDC and administer any vaccines for which he is due.

### Step 1

Start a supported web browser program and follow the steps listed inside the cover of this textbook to log in to the MyHealthProfessionsLab for this course.

Locate and click on the link Exercise 9C.

### Step 2

In the New Encounter window, locate and click on **Williams, Tyrell**.

Set the date to **05/25/2016** and the time to **11:00 AM** as shown previously in Figure 9-1.

Verify the date and time are set correctly, and then click the OK button.

---

[1]Source: U.S. Department of Health and Human Services, Centers for Disease Control website http://www.cdc.gov.

## Step 3

Because this exercise is a continuation of Tyrell's well-baby checkup on 5/25/2016, the encounter note documented in the previous two exercises will be displayed as shown in Figure 9-15.

**Figure 9-15** Existing encounter for Tyrell Williams for May 25, 2016 11:00 AM.

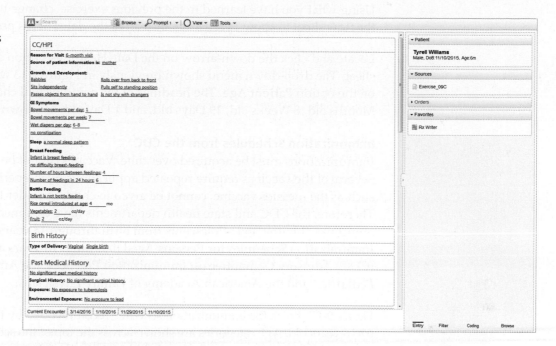

To prepare for the next step, where you will use the flow sheet to compare immunizations Tyrell has already received against the CDC-recommended immunization schedule, turn on the flow sheet view.

Click the View button on the toolbar and select Flowsheet from the drop-down menu.

Remember that the encounter note and the flow sheet can be scrolled separately. Scroll the flow sheet downward until you can see the immunizations section, as shown in Figure 9-16. Also scroll the encounter note portion of the pane to the bottom of the note

**Figure 9-16** Immunizations section of encounter (above) and flow sheet showing vaccines scheduled for 6-month visit.

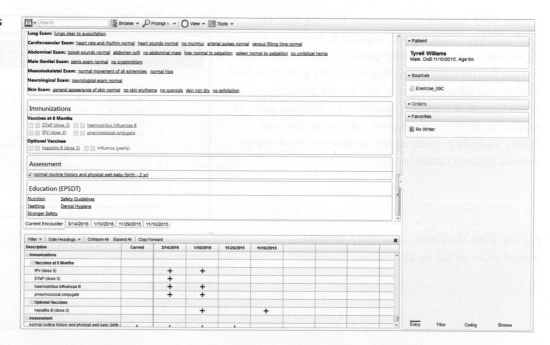

where you will find the Immunizations section. Position the two sections on your screen to resemble Figure 9-16.

### Step 4

Using what you have learned in the previous exercise, change the column headings of the flow sheet to show Tyrell's age instead of the dates of his previous visits.

Locate and click the down-arrow on the Date Headings button at the top of the flow sheet. The drop-down menu shown previously in Figure 9-13 will be displayed. Click on the option **Patient Age**. The headings of the columns will change to Current, 4 Months old, 8 Weeks old, 19 Days old, and 1 Day old, as shown in Figure 9-18.

### Immunization Schedules from the CDC

Immunizations must be acquired over time. Vaccines cannot be given all at once. Several of the vaccines require repeated applications over a period of time, and some, such as the measles vaccine, cannot be given to children under the age of 1 year. Therefore, the CDC and state health departments have designed a schedule to immunize children and adolescents from birth through 18 years. The Recommended Immunization Schedules for Persons Aged 0 through 18 Years are approved by the (CDC) Advisory Committee on Immunization Practices, the American Academy of Pediatrics, and the American Academy of Family Physicians.

Figure 9-17 shows the immunization schedule recommended by the CDC for children age 0 to 6 years old. Age categories are shown across the top of the schedule. The standard abbreviation for each vaccine is shown within the grid under the ages at which it should be administered. A key in the caption provides full names of the vaccine abbreviations.

Yellow bars within the grid indicate the ideal range of ages at which a particular series should be completed. The fact that yellow bars extend over multiple age categories indicates the flexibility that is built into the recommended schedule.

For example, the chart shows that the CDC recommends that infants should receive the first dose of Hepatitis B vaccine (HepB) soon after birth and ideally before hospital

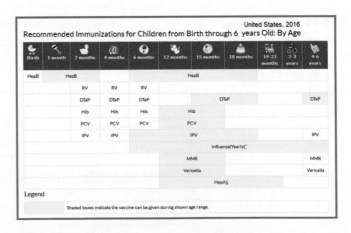

**Figure 9-17** Immunization schedule from the CDC. Key: *HepB* vaccine protects against hepatitis B. *RV* vaccine protects against rotavirus. *DTaP* vaccine protects against diphtheria, tetanus, and pertussis (whooping cough). *Hib* protects against Haemophilus influenzae type b. *PCV* vaccine protects against pneumococcus. *IPV* protects against polio. *Influenza* protects against flu. *MMR* protects against measles, mumps, and rubella. *Varicella* protects against chickenpox. *HepA* vaccine protects against hepatitis A.

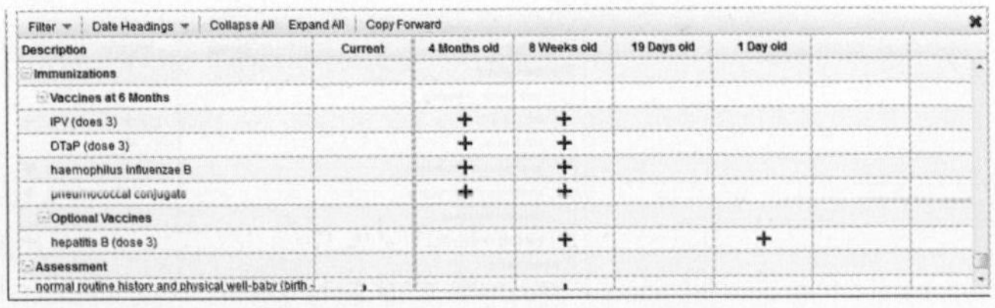

**Figure 9-18** Flow sheet showing Tyrell Williams' immunization history by age.

discharge. The second dose would be administered at least 4 weeks after the first dose. The third dose should be given at least 16 weeks after the first dose and at least 8 weeks after the second dose. The last dose in the vaccination series (third or fourth dose) should not be administered before the age of 24 weeks.

**Step 5**

Compare the CDC schedule shown in Figure 9-17 to the vaccine list in your flow sheet shown in Figure 9-18. Also, the patient date of birth is displayed in the right content pane of your screen. Notice the following:

Compare Tyrell's HepB (Hepatitis B) vaccine to the CDC schedule.

> Tyrell was born November 10, 2015. He had his first dose of Hepatitis B (HepB) before leaving the hospital on 11/11/2015 when he was 1 day old.

> He had his second dose during his 2-month checkup, when he was 8 weeks old.

> Because the yellow bar for HepB in Figure 9-17 spans several columns, he could receive his third dose during this visit (six months) or at his 12-month visit.

Compare his DTaP (Diphtheria, Tetanus, and Pertussis) vaccines to the CDC schedule.

> He had his first dose of DTaP at 8 weeks during his 2-month checkup.

> He had his second dose during his 4-month checkup as noted in the 4-month column.

> He is due for his third dose during this visit.

Compare his Haemophilus influenzae type B (Hib) doses to the CDC schedule.

> He had his first dose of Hib during his 2-month checkup, when he was 8 weeks old.

> He had his second dose during his 4-month checkup.

> He is due for his third dose during this visit.

Compare his IPV (Inactivated Polio Virus) doses to the CDC schedule.

> He had his first dose of IPV during his 2-month checkup, when he was 8 weeks old.

> He had his second dose during his 4-month checkup.

> He is due for his third dose during this visit.

Compare his Pneumococcal Conjugate Vaccine (PCV) doses to the CDC schedule.

> He had his first dose of PCV during his 2-month checkup, when he was 8 weeks old.

> He had his second dose during his 4-month checkup.

> He is due for his third dose during this visit.

Of the vaccines remaining on the CDC schedule, he is too young for the Varicella vaccine as well as the Measles, Mumps, Rubella (MMR) vaccine, which is not administered before 12 months.

He is old enough for a flu shot, but the office visit occurs in May, which historically is not flu season, so the pediatrician decides to wait until his 9-month visit.

**Step 6**

Now that the clinician has a clear picture of the patient's immunization needs, the vaccine can be ordered and administered.

Although the Rx code for a vaccine is the same regardless of when it is administered, EHR systems differentiate which dose is being given (first dose, second dose, third dose) in order to facilitate tracking and comparison of patient immunizations with the CDC schedule, which, as you can see in Figure 9-17, allows for variance in the ages at which doses are given. Therefore, the clinician cannot merely copy forward the flow sheet cells of previous immunizations, as those finding descriptions include the dose number. Instead the clinician will order the immunizations in the encounter portion of the pane.

Close the flow sheet view by clicking the X in the right corner of the Flowsheet view.

### Step 7

Locate the Immunizations, Vaccines at 6 Months section of the encounter note and then click the checkbox for each of the following:

✓  **Y** DTaP (dose 3)

✓  **Y** Haemophilus influ B (dose 3)

✓  **Y** IPV (dose 3)

✓  **Y** Pneumococcal Conjugate (dose 3)

Proceed to the Optional Vaccines group, and then click the checkbox for each of the following:

✓  **Y** hepatitis B (dose 3)

✓  **N** influenza vaccine (yearly)

Compare your screen to Figure 9-19.

**Figure 9-19** Encounter for May 25, 2016 11:00 AM with the correctly completed immunization section.

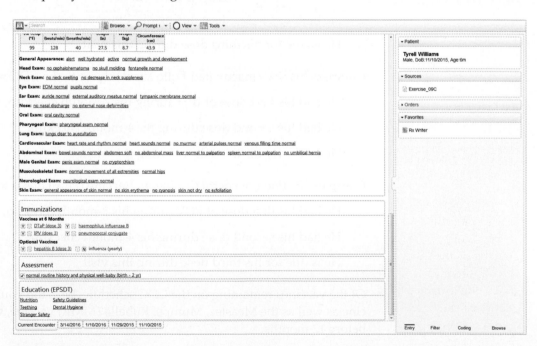

### Step 8

If you wish to print a copy of your completed encounter notes for yourself or because your instructor requires you to turn them in, use the Create PDF option, and then print or download the PDF at this time.

The final step in every exercise is to submit your completed work for a grade.

Locate and click the blue Quippe icon button on the toolbar, and then select the Submit for Grade option from the drop-down menu. This will complete Exercise 9C.

## Critical Thinking Exercise 9D: Determine Your Adult Immunizations

The CDC also publishes a recommended immunization schedule for adults. Because adult immunizations are different from those you had as a child, you may have an interest in seeing what you need as an adult. The CDC provides free online information about immunizations. This exercise accesses portions of the CDC website.

### Privacy Information About Exercise 9D

In step 4 of this exercise you will enter personal information about yourself. This data is used only for generating a personalized list of recommended immunizations, specific to you. None of the data you enter will be shared with your instructor or reported to any entity. Your grade for this exercise is based solely on performing the exercise.

### Step 1

Start a supported web browser program and follow the steps listed inside the cover of this textbook to log in to the MyHealthProfessionsLab for this course.

Locate and click on the link Exercise 9D.

### Step 2

A page similar to Figure 9-20 will display the CDC Recommended Immunizations for Adults: By Age.[2] Links at the top will take you to a second adult immunization schedule, and a useful tool to determine your adult immunization needs.

**Figure 9-20** CDC Recommended Immunizations for Adults: By Age.

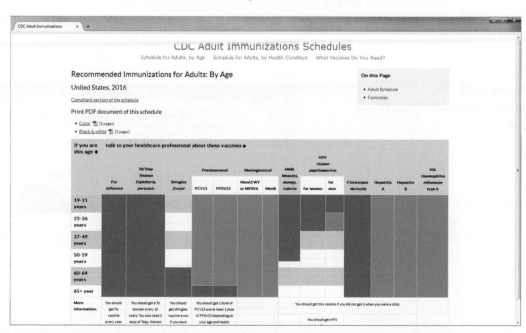

NOTE

The web pages used in this exercise are automatically updated by the CDC, and therefore your screen display may differ from the figures in these steps, which were accurate representations at the time of printing.

After you have reviewed the Recommended Immunizations for Adults: By Age page, click the Schedule for Adults by Health Condition link at the top of the page.

[2]Ibid.

### Step 3

The Recommended Immunizations for Adults: By Health Condition page similar to Figure 9-21 will be displayed. Some vaccines are not recommended for persons with certain health conditions or for women who are pregnant or trying to become pregnant. This page shows both the recommended vaccines and those that are contraindicated.

**Figure 9-21** CDC Recommended Immunizations for Adults: By Health Condition.

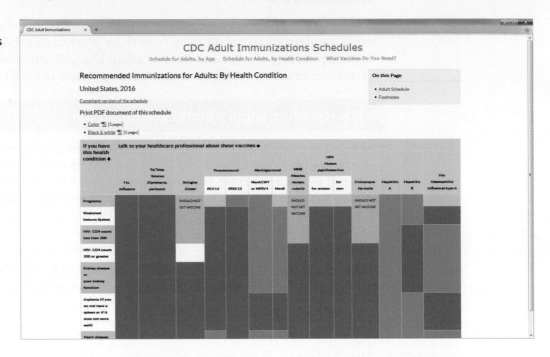

After you have reviewed the Recommended Immunizations for Adults: By Health Condition page, click the What Vaccines Do You Need? link at the top of the page.

### Step 4

The Adolescent and Adult Vaccine Quiz similar to Figure 9-22 will be displayed. Despite the word "Quiz" in its title, this is not a test. The information you enter into this page is private and is not saved or reported back to the grade book.

**Figure 9-22** CDC Adolescent and Adult Vaccine Quiz.

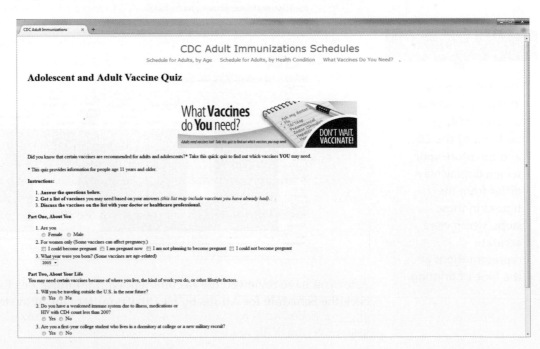

**Figure 9-23**

My Results

Follow the on-screen instructions. When you have completed all the questions, click the My Results button, shown in Figure 9-23. A personal report of immunizations you may need will be generated based on the information you provided. You may print out your immunization schedule and discuss any items listed with your healthcare provider.

### Step 5

When you are finished printing or reviewing your personal immunization schedule, you may close your browser. This completes Exercise 9D.

## Preventative Care Screening

The U.S. Preventive Services Task Force is an independent panel of experts in primary care and prevention that systematically reviews the evidence of effectiveness and develops recommendations for clinical preventive services. The task force recommendations about preventive services are based on age, sex, and risk factors for disease.

Research has shown that the best way to ensure that preventive services are delivered appropriately is to make evidence-based information readily available at the point of care. As far back as 1990 EHR systems were developed to compare patient information in a medical office computer with age, sex, and risk factors. The systems generated a list of preventive care measures individualized to the patient based on the U.S. Preventive Services Task Force guidelines at the point of care. The task force recommendations form the majority of the Clinical Quality Measures (CQM) introduced in Chapter 1.

### Clinical Quality Measures

U.S. Preventive Services Task Force guidelines and other measures selected by the Secretary of Health and Human Services as Clinical Quality Measures (CQMs) are evidence-based, meaning they were developed by analyzing scientific evidence from current research and studies to determine the effectiveness of preventive services. The guidelines recommend both for and against certain measures, including screening, counseling, and preventive medications. However, the guidelines are not set in stone. They vary not only by age and sex but change the recommended intervals for the screening or test based on the individual patient. For example, a blood test measuring total cholesterol and high-density lipoprotein (HDL-C) is recommended every five years for a male over 35, but the interval shortens to every two years if the patient has additional risk factors such as high blood pressure, abnormal lipid levels on previous tests, or a family history of cardiovascular disease before age 50.

Using data in the EHR, the computer is able to find the appropriate Clinical Care Measure based on the patient's age and sex, add to it based on the patient's problem list and history findings, and then reduce the intervals a screening needs to be repeated based on abnormal values of previous test results. The system then generates a list of CQMs unique to the patient and delivers it to the clinician's computer screen. Using this information, the clinician can order tests, discuss important health care options, and recommend lifestyle changes to the patient at the point of care.

Preventive care screening programs, such as the Patient Alert screenshown in Chapter 2, Figure 2-24, makes effective use of the EHR to present the provider with recommended screening tests for early detection, immunizations for prevention, and suggested areas for patient education and counseling.

# Real-Life Story

## Quality Care for Pediatric and Adult Patients

**By Alison Connelly, P.A. (edited by the author)**

*Alison Connelly is a physician assistant in a large multispecialty group in New York City. She was instrumental in setting up the preventative screening guidelines and designing many of the forms used in the EHR at her practice. Her group has eight clinics and 350 employees.*

Our practice implemented EHR and uses many of the options the system offers. These include the electronic prescription system, document imaging, a Medcin-based EHR, a referral system, and Quality Care Guidelines (the preventative screening component of our EHR).

The document imaging component is terrific! That was actually what got doctors who were resistant to adopting the EHR to start using the system, because they could access their results and reports instantly. Now that we are on the imaging system, any type of patient results that comes in is immediately scanned in so that doctors do not have to wait. This is especially useful in the off-site clinics. We have eight locations. Previously, a document would come in and it could float around for a couple of weeks before it got to the proper clinician, but now as soon as it arrives it is scanned and the clinicians have immediate access to the results on the report on the computer.

A little more than half our total providers enter their own exam notes in the EHR, but all of the pediatric clinicians use it. We created multiple forms for pediatrics based on age and what the milestones and programs for that visit are. We have forms for well-baby visits at 2 months, 4 months, 6 months, 1 year, 15 months, 2 years, and so on. We also created one comprehensive pediatric form for all types of sick visits.

The pediatricians use the growth charts to ensure the pattern of the child's growth is appropriate and follows a trend. The vitals are automatically plotted on the growth chart after they are entered.

We use the Quality Care Guidelines module for age, sex, and disease-specific clinical reminders, primarily in the adult population. I will explain more about that later. Although the guideline system can be used for child immunization scheduling, in New York City, we have to use the Citywide Immunization Registry (CIR) to report every vaccine we give to children between birth and 18 years old. So, in addition to putting it in the encounter, we have to send it into the city. If that were computerized, it would be much better; we could eliminate double entry by recording it in the EHR and then transmitting it to the city registry.

From a practical standpoint, the guideline system worked well for adults in our practice. An adult population has more things that have to be monitored and more of the patients have chronic diseases than do children. In addition to the preventive health measures recommended by age and sex, we have special guidelines for the following conditions:

▶ Diabetes

▶ HIV

▶ Hypertension

▶ Hyperlipidemia

▶ Renal failure

▶ Ischemic heart disease

▶ Anemia

▶ Asthma

Using the guideline system, we are able to make sure, for example, that a diabetes patient has a hemoglobin A1C done every three months.

The guideline system uses patient data that is updated either manually or automatically. Many of the items on the guidelines are tests, and it is possible to have the electronic lab system update them with orders and results. However, the interface to our local lab company never worked consistently, so most of our guideline data is updated via the encounter. These are entered by the clinician, and then our system automatically updates the guideline when the encounter is processed.

The other update process we use is related to our document image system, which updates the patient data when we scan images. For instance, we actually capture the mammogram referral and the mammogram result. When a mammogram result comes in, it is scanned and we update our system. This does three things: it stores an image of the results, it updates the patient data for the guideline, and it updates the managed care referral portion of the EMR.

We also run reports off the EHR data using the guideline system. In the case of the mammogram, this allows us to reconcile patients that are referred out with results we received back. We can then follow up with patients that just never went for their appointment.

I work in the HIV clinic and use both the guideline system and custom forms I designed for the EHR. While I write my notes in the EHR, I pull up the guidelines; it is a great monitor.

Because HIV has a lot of clinical guidelines to follow, clinicians can become very focused on HIV and overlook the normal orders that would be done based on age and sex, such as a mammogram or a fecal occult blood test. From that standpoint, the guideline system is very helpful, because it produces a complete list of recommendations for the patient's age and sex as well as any diseases the patient may have. I use it almost like a checklist that I go down to make sure I do not forget anything.

I also created forms in our EHR system specific for the HIV clinic that monitors certain clinical guidelines we have to follow and information such as the percentage of pills taken per week and the number of hours slept a night. I used an option in the form designer to make those fields required. The clinician cannot exit the form until those questions are answered.

The EHR system is great, but if it becomes more interconnected we could do so much more. I like the idea that it could automatically update guidelines when results are received or automatically send vaccine data to the immunization registry. Similarly, we have to report sexually transmitted diseases within a certain time frame. If we could do that electronically when we received the lab result as well, it would be great.

In relationship to the HITECH Act, reporting which Clinical Quality Measures have been met by eligible professionals, eligible hospitals, and critical access hospitals helps measure and track the quality of healthcare services provided and relates to strategic goals for ensuring that our healthcare system is delivering effective, safe, efficient, patient-centered, equitable, and timely care.

CQMs measure many aspects of patient care including:

◆ health outcomes

◆ clinical processes

◆ patient safety

◆ efficient use of healthcare resources

◆ care coordination

◆ patient engagements

◆ population and public health

◆ adherence to clinical guidelines

CQM reporting is derived directly from data entered into the EHR, as you will do in the next exercise. CMS maintains and provides specifications for each Clinical Quality Measure in both computer and human readable (HTML) format. These documents identify the CQM with a unique number, data criteria, population criteria, and supplemental data elements. The Rationale section of the CQM document describes the source and scientific evidence supporting the measure. Additionally, the CQM document includes a Clinical Recommendation Statement, which summarizes relevant guidelines. Quippe brings this information to the point of care, and you will have an opportunity to view the CQM documents during the following exercises.

### Guided Exercise 9E: Applying Quality Measures to Patient Care

In this exercise you will learn to use the Clinical Measure Review feature, which analyzes a patient's longitudinal record and presents Clinical Quality Measures uniquely tailored to a patient by age, gender, and health conditions. While doing so, you will have an opportunity to view the requirements and scientific reasoning behind the preventative care recommendations.

### Case Study

Guy Daniels is a patient with hypertension and borderline diabetes who has been the subject of several previous exercises. Imagine, if you will, this exercise occurring during that same visit. The clinician will review preventative care health screening recommendations and order or document findings as necessary.

### Step 1

Start a supported web browser program and follow the steps listed inside the cover of this textbook to log in to the MyHealthProfessionsLab for this course.

Locate and click on the link Exercise 9E.

### Step 2

In the New Encounter window, locate and click on **Daniels, Guy**.

Set the date to **05/24/2016** and time to **9:00 AM** as shown previously in Figure 9-1.

Verify the date and time are set correctly, and then click the OK button.

### Step 3

Locate and click in the blank space below the label Chief Complaint, and type **3 month checkup**.

### Step 4

Click any white space in the encounter pane that does not highlight a heading or finding to restore the date tabs at the bottom of the encounter pane.

Locate and click the **5/23/2016** tab.

When the encounter note is displayed, click on the Current Medications heading, and select **Copy into current note** from the drop-down menu.

Locate and click the **Current Encounter** tab.

### Step 5

Proceed to the Physical Exam section and record Mr. Daniels's vital signs in the corresponding fields of the encounter as follows:

| | |
|---|---|
| Temperature: | **98.2** |
| Pulse: | **68** |
| Respiration: | **20** |
| SBP: | **125** |
| DBP: | **85** |
| Weight: | **239** |
| Height: | **68.5** |

Verify that the CC and vitals in Figure 9-24 match yours.

**Figure 9-24** Encounter note with CC, Current Medications, and Vital signs. The View menu is also shown.

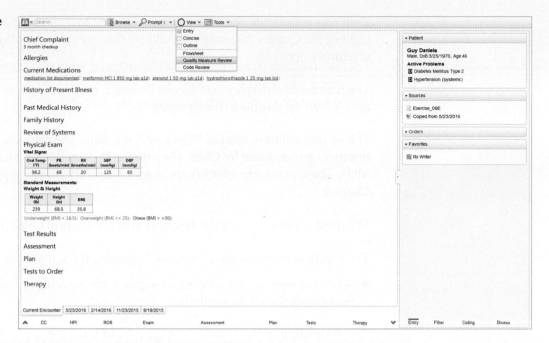

Locate and click the View button on the toolbar, and then select Quality Measures Review from the drop-down menu (also shown in Figure 9-24). The encounter pane workspace will divide and Quality Measures relevant to Mr. Daniels will display in the bottom portion as shown in Figure 9-25. In the figure it has already been sorted by measure.

**Figure 9-25** Quality Measure Review displays at the bottom of the pane.

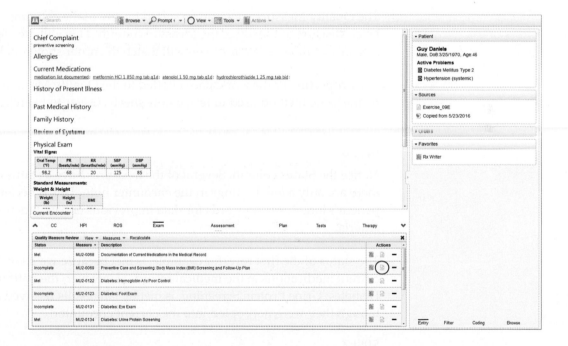

## About the Quality Measures Review

The quality measures view resembles the flow sheet in that it displays in the lower portion of the encounter pane workspace, is resizable, and is made up of rows and columns. As with flow sheet view, there is an X in the right corner that can be used to close the quality measure view.

Each row represents one of the Clinical Quality Measures (CQM). A scroll bar on the right of the Quality Measure view allows the rows to be scrolled independently of the encounter note pane.

The first column displays status of a measure: met, incomplete, pending, excluded, or n/a (not applicable to the patient).

The second column, labeled "Measure," identifies the measure by a number. The numbers are assigned by CMS. The number is preceded by an acronym: MU1, MU2, or MU3. These acronyms identify the stage of meaningful use reporting discussed in Chapter 1

The third column provides a description of the Clinical Quality Measure.

The fourth column, labeled "Actions," contains three icons for each row:

◆ A wizard icon, which invokes a Quippe form for adding findings to the encounter that satisfy the CQM's criteria.

◆ A **document** icon (circled in Figure 9-25) opens a separate tab of your browser to display detailed information about the medical reasoning behind the CQM and scientific authority responsible for the measure.

◆ A **minus symbol** icon, when clicked, hides a CQM from the list for the duration of the current session. The CQM will be restored to the list on the patient's next encounter, or if the list is refreshed.

The Quality Measure view can be sorted by any of the columns. Locate and click on the label **Measure** at the top of the Measure column. This will reorder the view, sorted by measure number, so your screen will match the order shown in Figure 9-25.

The proportion of the workspace allotted to the Quality Measure view can be changed by the same method used to resize flow sheets. (Refer to Exercise 8A, step 6 if you need to resize the Quality Measure portion of your screen.)

### Step 6

Notice the Status column. Several of the measures have a status of "Met" even though there are only a few findings in the encounter note. This is because Quippe searches the patient's longitudinal records for data in previous encounters that meet a CQM's criteria.

The status of the first row, for example, is met because we have "Documentation of current medications in the medical record." However, the bottom row (in Figure 9-25, Diabetes: Urine Protein Screening, is met by lab results received at an earlier date though they were not copied into the current encounter.

### Step 7

Locate the second row, Preventive Care and Screening Body Mass Index (BMI) Screening and Follow-up Plan. Locate the Actions column and click on the document icon (circled in Figure 9-25) for that row.

A new tab of your browser will open to display the CMS-provided documentation for this CQM as shown in Figure 9-26. Locate and read the Description section. Scroll if necessary until you locate and can read the Rationale section explanation regarding "BMI above upper parameters."

**Figure 9-26** CMS documentation for BMI CQM opens in a separate tab.

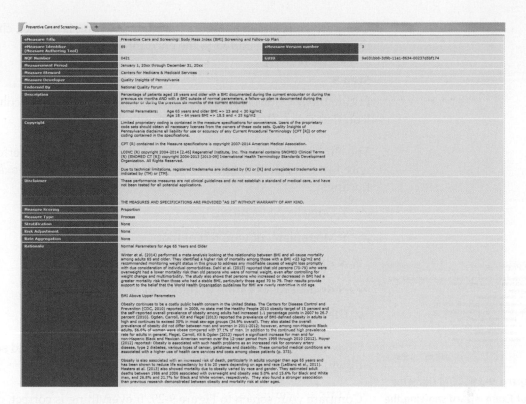

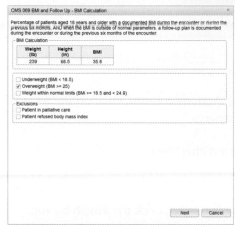

**Figure 9-27** BMI CQM wizard page 1. Next button located in the lower right corner.

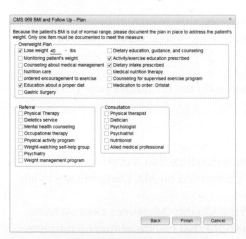

**Figure 9-28** BMI CQM wizard page 2 showing the correctly checked findings.

## Step 8

The Clinical Measure Review not only informs the clinician of what needs to be ordered or done for the patient, but the wizard icon allows the orders or findings to be added to the encounter note without closing the view.

Remain in the second row, Actions column, and click on the left icon to invoke the wizard shown in Figure 9-27. A wizard is a form similar to other forms you have used, except that it may have multiple pages and may require you to select certain findings before the Finish button is enabled.

The BMI wizard displays Mr. Daniels's weight, height, and BMI level from the current encounter. Had you not entered the vital signs in the encounter already, the fields in the wizard would allow you to enter the data here. Click on the Next button as shown in Figure 9-27.

The page containing the follow-up plan is displayed, as shown in Figure 9-28. Notice that the Finish button at the bottom of the wizard is grayed out, meaning it is disabled. Instructions at the top of the screen inform the clinician that at least one plan item must be selected to complete the measure. This is a minimum; as many of the items as the clinician wants to add to the plan can be checked. Locate and click checkboxes for the following findings:

✓ Lose weight

✓ Education about a proper diet

✓ Activity/exercise education prescribed

✓ Dietary intake prescribed

Click the down arrow for the Lose weight ___ lbs field and select **40** from the drop-down list.

Compare your screen to Figure 9-28. If everything is correct, click the Finish button and the findings will be added to the encounter note.

**Step 9**

Locate the row for Diabetes: Foot Exam, and in the Actions column, click on the wizard icon (left icon). The Diabetes Foot Exam wizard displays.

The clinician takes the patient's Dorsalis pedis pulses and performs a monofilament wire test on each foot. Locate and click the indicated checkboxes for the following findings:

✓ **Y** Dorsalis pedis pulses

✓ **Y** Monofilament wire test of foot

✓ **N** decreased sensation of left foot

✓ **N** decreased sensation of right foot

✓ Diabetic foot examination performed

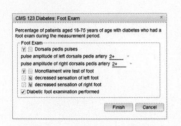

**Figure 9-29** CQM Diabetes Foot Exam wizard showing the correct checkboxes and values.

Click the down arrow for both of the pedis artery fields and select 2+ from the drop-down list.

Compare your screen to Figure 9-29. If everything is correct, click the Finish button. The findings will be added to your encounter note.

**Step 10**

The clinician examines the patient's retinas.

Locate the row for Diabetes: Eye Exam, and in the Actions column, click on the wizard icon (left icon). The Diabetes Eye Exam wizard displays.

Locate **Examination of retina** and click the indicated checkbox.

✓ **N** Results Neg

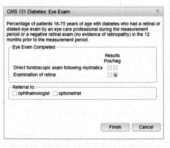

**Figure 9-30** CQM Diabetes Eye Exam wizard showing Examination of retina negative.

Compare your screen to Figure 9-30. If everything is correct, click the Finish button. The finding will be added to your encounter note.

**Step 11**

Scroll the encounter note portion of the workspace pane downward until you can see the bottom of the encounter note as shown in Figure 9-31. Notice that all rows of CQMs displayed in the figure have a status of "Met."

Compare the encounter note portion of your screen with the encounter note portion of Figure 9-31.

**Step 12**

Scroll the Quality Measures view downward. You will notice that some incomplete items remain. In the interest of time, they will be performed on Mr. Daniels's next visit.

Locate the minus symbol icon (rightmost icon) in the Quality Measures view Actions column and click the minus symbol icon for each CQM that has the status incomplete. The minus symbol icon hides the measure from view for the current session only and the clinician will see the CQMs again on Mr. Daniels's next visit.

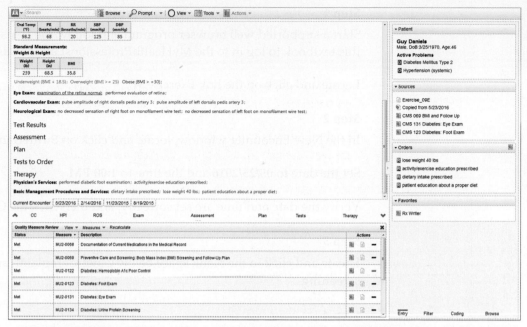

**Figure 9-31** Encounter note portion shows the correct findings. Quality Measure view shows the correct status of CQMs.

Close the Quality Measures Review by clicking the X in the right corner of the view.

### Step 13

Verify that the findings in your encounter note are correct. All correctly entered findings for the encounter can be seen by comparing your screen to Figures 9-25 and 9-31. If everything on your screen matches the figures, proceed. If there are any differences, review the preceding steps and correct your work.

If you wish to print a copy of your completed encounter notes for yourself or because your instructor requires you to turn them in, use the Create PDF option, and then print or download the PDF at this time.

The final step in every exercise is to submit your completed work for a grade.

Locate and click the blue Quippe icon button on the toolbar, and then select the Submit for Grade option from the drop-down menu. This will complete Exercise 9E.

## Critical Thinking Exercise 9F: Clinical Quality Measures for a Female Patient

In the previous exercise it was stated that the Quality Measures Review function created a list of recommended health measures, unique to a patient based on age, gender, and health conditions. In this exercise you will apply what you have learned to a patient of different gender with slightly different health conditions.

### Case Study

Sally Sutherland is a patient with hyperlipidemia and diabetes who was the subject of a previous exercise graphing her weight and BMI.

**Step 1**

Start a supported web browser program and follow the steps listed inside the cover of this textbook to log in to the MyHealthProfessionsLab for this course.

Locate and click on the link Exercise 9F.

**Step 2**

In the New Encounter window, locate and click on **Sutherland, Sally**.

Set the date to **05/25/2016** and the time to **1:00 PM**.

Verify the date and time are set correctly, and then click the OK button.

**Step 3**

Locate and click in the blank space below Chief Complaint, and type **preventive screening**.

**Step 4**

Click any white space in the encounter pane that does not highlight a heading or finding to restore the date tabs at the bottom of the encounter pane.

Locate and click the **5/15/2016** tab.

When the encounter note is displayed, click on the Current Medications heading, and select **Copy into current note** from the drop-down menu.

Locate and click on the **Tobacco Use Status** group heading, and then select **Copy into current note** from the drop-down menu.

Locate and click the **Current Encounter** tab.

**Step 5**

Record Ms. Sutherland's vital signs in the corresponding fields of the encounter as follows:

| | |
|---|---|
| Temperature: | **98.6** |
| Pulse: | **78** |
| Respiration: | **28** |
| SBP: | **134** |
| DBP: | **90** |
| Weight: | **153** |
| Height: | **60** |

Verify that you have entered her vital signs correctly and then locate and click on the BMI cell.

**Step 6**

Locate and click the View button on the toolbar, and then select Quality Measures Review from the drop-down menu. The encounter pane workspace will split into two portions, and Quality Measures relevant to Ms. Sutherland will display in the bottom portion of the pane.

The Quality Measure view will likely display, sorted by Status. Locate the heading of the second column and click on the label "Measure." This will rearrange the rows by CQM measure number. This is done to help you locate rows in the subsequent steps.

Locate the CQM "Documentation of Current Medications" in the first row, and click the wizard icon (leftmost icon in the Actions column). As you have just copied the medications into the current encounter, click the checkbox "medications listed in document," and click the Finish button. A finding will be added to the encounter and the CQM status will change to "Met."

### Step 7

The CQM in the second row, Preventive Care and Screening BMI Screening and Follow-up Plan, has a status of "Excluded." You will recall in a previous exercise that the clinician's comment to disregard the spike in her BMI due to pregnancy. In her case the CQM is excluded by rule.

Because the CQM in the third row has already been met, proceed to the fourth CQM row, Diabetes: Foot Exam.

Locate the Actions column, and click on the wizard for the fourth CQM. The Diabetes Foot Exam wizard displays.

The clinician takes the patient's Dorsalis pedis pulses and performs a monofilament wire test on each foot. Locate and click the indicated checkboxes for the following findings:

- ✓ **Y** Dorsalis pedis pulses
- ✓ **Y** Monofilament wire test of foot
- ✓ **N** decreased sensation of left foot
- ✓ **N** decreased sensation of right foot
- ✓ Diabetic foot examination performed

Click the down arrow for both of the pedis artery fields and select 2+ from the drop-down list.

Verify that everything is entered correctly, and then click the Finish button. The findings will be added to your encounter note and the status will change to "Met."

### Step 8

The next CQM is an example of a preventive screening recommendation based on age, gender, and health factors. The CQM Breast Cancer Screening did not appear in Mr. Daniels's review because it is gender specific to females over a certain age.

Locate the Actions column for the fifth row, Breast Cancer Screening, and click the **document** icon (center icon in the column). A new tab of your browser will open to display the CMS-provided documentation for this CQM. Locate and read the Description section to determine the gender and age range the CQM is recommended for.

Locate and click the wizard icon in the Actions column for the Breast Cancer Screening CQM.

The clinician orders a mammogram. Locate and click on the checkbox:

- ✓ Place order

Click the Finish button. The order will be added to your encounter note and the status will change to "Pending." In this example, the test has been ordered, but the CQM will not be met until the radiology report is received and reviewed by the ordering clinician.

### Step 9

The clinician examines the patient's retinas and the results are negative.

Locate the row for Diabetes: Eye Exam, and click on the wizard icon in the Actions column. The Diabetes Eye Exam wizard displays.

Locate **Examination of retina** and click the indicated checkbox.

✓ **N** Results Neg

Click the Finish button. The finding will be added to your encounter note and the status will change to "Met."

### Step 10

Use the scroll bar on the right of the Quality Measure view to scroll the list of CQMs downward, so you can complete the remaining CQMs.

Locate the row for Diabetes: Urine Protein Screening, and click on the wizard icon in the Actions column. The wizard displays. The doctor orders a urinalysis. Locate and click the checkbox for Urinalysis:

✓ Place Order

Click the Finish button. The finding will be added to your encounter note, but the CQM will have a status of "Pending" until the test results are received and reviewed.

### Step 11

Locate the row for Preventive Care and Screening Tobacco Use Screening and Cessation Intervention, and click on the wizard icon in the Actions column. The wizard displays. Ms. Sutherland has never smoked. Because we copied her tobacco use into the note in step 4, it is already checked in the wizard. Click the Finish button to add the fact that the assessment of tobacco use has been met.

### Step 12

Locate the row for Preventive Care Screening Influenza Immunization. Because Ms. Sutherland is not due for her annual flu shot, locate and click the minus symbol (rightmost icon) in the Actions column. The CQM will disappear from the list.

### Step 13

Locate the row for Diabetes: Low Density Lipoprotein (LDL) Management, and click on the wizard icon in the Actions column. The wizard displays. The doctor orders an LDL Cholesterol. Locate and click the checkbox:

✓ Order

Click the Finish button. The finding will be added to your encounter note, but the CQM will have a status of "Pending" until the test results are received and reviewed.

## Step 14

Compare your Quality Measures Review to Figure 9-32, scrolling as necessary. Verify that none of the CQMs have a status of incomplete. If there are any incomplete CQMs, review the previous steps and correct your error. When the statuses of all of your CQMs match Figure 9-32, close the Quality Measures Review by clicking the X in the right corner of the view.

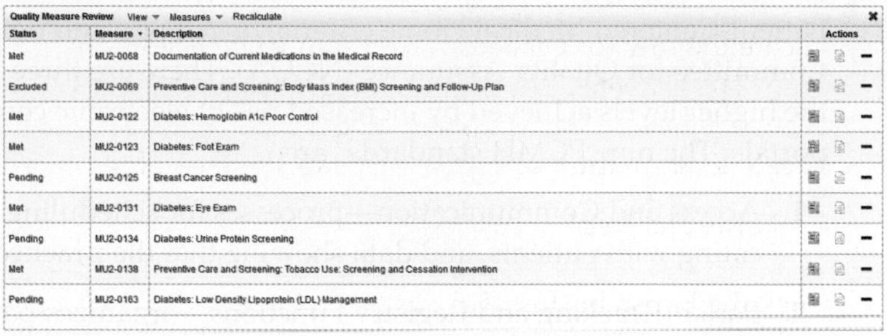

**Figure 9-32** Quality Measure view shows the correct status of Sally Sutherland's CQMs.

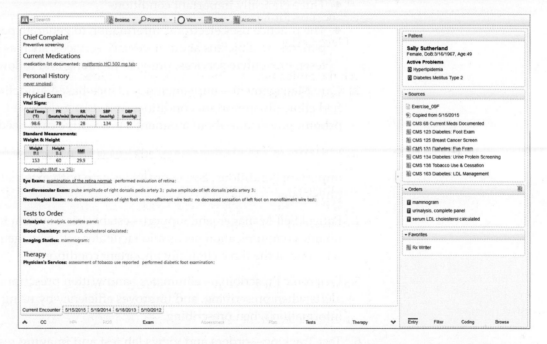

## Step 15

Click the View button on the toolbar and select Concise from the drop-down menu. Compare your screen to Figure 9-33, scrolling as necessary until you have verified the entire encounter. If everything on your screen matches the figure, proceed to step 16. If there are any differences, review the preceding steps and correct your work.

**Figure 9-33** Concise view of Sally Sutherland's correctly completed encounter note.

## Step 16

If wish to print a copy of your completed encounter notes for yourself or because your instructor requires you to turn them in, use the Create PDF option, and then print or download the PDF at this time.

The final step in every exercise is to submit your completed work for a grade.

Locate and click the blue Quippe icon button on the toolbar, and then select the Submit for Grade option from the drop-down menu. This will complete Exercise 9F.

# The Patient-Centered Medical Home

Another approach to providing comprehensive primary care for both children and adults is **Patient-Centered Medical Home (PCMH)**. The PCMH is a healthcare setting that facilitates partnerships between patients, and their primary care physicians, and when appropriate, the patient's family.

Practices qualify for PCMH status by meeting the Physicians Practice Connections Patient-Centered Medical Home criteria, developed and owned by the National Committee for Quality Assurance (NCQA). There are three levels of recognition, with the higher levels achieved by increased use of electronic communication and web portals. The nine PCMH standards[3] are:

1. Access and Communication—processes for scheduling appointments, communicating with patients, and data showing that the practice meets this standard.

2. Patient Tracking and Registry Functions—organizes patient-population data using an electronic system that includes searchable patient clinical information used to manage patient care. The practice applies electronic or paper-based charting tools to organize and document clinical information consistently using standard data fields and uses the system to identify the following:

   ◆ Most frequently seen diagnoses

   ◆ Most important risk factors

   ◆ Three clinically important conditions

   ◆ The practice uses electronic information to generate patient lists and remind patients or clinicians about necessary services, such as specific medications or tests, preventive services, pre-visit planning and follow-up visits.

3. Care Management—implements evidence-based guidelines for the three identified clinically important conditions and uses guideline-based reminders to prompt physicians about a patient's preventive care needs at the time of the patient's visit. Maintains a team approach to managing patient care, uses various components of care management for patients with one or more of the clinically important conditions, and coordinates care with external organizations and other physicians.

4. Patient Self-Management Support—establishes a system to identify patients with unique communication needs and facilitates self-management of care for patients with one of the three clinically important conditions.

5. Electronic Prescribing—eliminates handwritten prescriptions, uses drug safety alerts when prescribing, and improves efficiency by using cost (drug formulary) information when prescribing.

6. Test Tracking—orders and views lab test and imaging results electronically, with electronic alerts; manages the timely receipt of information on all tests and results.

7. Referral Tracking—coordination of care and following through critical consultations with other practitioners.

---

[3]Adapted from *PPC-PCMH Companion Guide* (Washington, DC: National Committee for Quality Assurance, 2010, www.ncqa.org/ppcpcmh.aspx).

8. Performance Reporting and Improvement—measures or receives performance data by physician or across the practice and reports on:

- ◆ Clinical process
- ◆ Clinical outcomes
- ◆ Service data
- ◆ Patient safety

Collects data on patient experience with, and reports on:

- ◆ Access to care
- ◆ Quality of physician communication
- ◆ Patient/family confidence in self-care
- ◆ Patient/family satisfaction with care

Uses performance data to set goals based on measurement results and, where necessary, acts to improve performance. Produces reports using nationally approved clinical measures and electronically transmits them to external entities.

9. Advanced Electronic Communication—maximizes electronic communication with patients via the web to support patient access and self-management. Sends patients e-mail about specific needs and clinical alerts. Uses electronic communication among the care management team for patients with one of the three identified clinically important conditions.

## Chapter Nine Summary

In this chapter you learned to create a pediatric growth chart. You also learned about pediatric vital signs, family social history, and other aspects unique to well-baby checkups.

The baby's length, weight, and head circumference are measured on each visit. These measurements can be plotted on a graph called a growth chart that compares the individual's growth to statistical information from a reference population. Lines on the chart called percentiles represent the percentage of the population that was the same size at the same age. A child who is at the 50th percentile weighs the same or more than 50% of the reference population at that age.

For children age 2 and up, the CDC now recommends using Body Mass Index (BMI) growth charts instead of the weight-for-age and weight-for-stature. BMI growth charts are gender specific and age specific for children, but a single BMI chart is used for adults of both genders.

Immunizations must be acquired over time. Vaccines cannot all be given at once. CDC-recommended immunizations are aligned with the well-baby visit intervals. You learned how to compare a child's immunization history to the schedule recommended by the CDC (or state health department) to determine what is required each visit.

Disease prevention through periodic screening and early detection also can save lives. Preventive guidelines that make up many of the Clinical Quality Measures were developed by the U.S. Preventive Services Task Force and others. CQMs are tools for helping providers deliver effective, safe, efficient, patient-centered care. A list of CQMs relevant to individual patients can be generated by an EHR system and tailored by the computer to suit the individual's risk factors, based on the patient's age and sex, and health conditions. Using the CQM wizard, the clinician can order tests, discuss important healthcare options, and recommend lifestyle changes to the patient at the point of care. Using the CQM document button, the clinician can view evidence-based documentation citing the research and rationale for performing the measure.

A Patient-Centered Medical Home (PCMH) is a model for providing primary care. PCMH standards encourage electronic orders, results, and communication with patients.

| Task | Exercise | Page # |
| --- | --- | --- |
| How to document a well-baby visit | 9A | 348 |
| How to create growth charts | 9B | 358 |
| How to interpret immunization schedules | 9C | 362 |
| How to use Quality Measures Review to document preventive care objectives | 9E | 371 |

## Testing Your Knowledge of Chapter 9

### Step 1

Log in to MyHealthProfessionsLab following the directions printed inside the cover of this textbook.

Locate and click on Chapter 9 Test.

### Step 2

Answer the test questions. When you have finished, click the Submit Test button to close the window.

## Testing Your Skill Exercise 9G: Baby's First Checkup

Now that you have performed all the exercises in Chapter 9 this exercise will help you and your instructor evaluate your acquired skills. Use the information in the case study and the features of the software you already know to document the patient's encounter.

### Case Study

Chloe Younge is a 2-month-old female infant who is having her first visit for a well-baby checkup on May 25, 2016. She is brought by both of her parents. She has not had any of her immunizations, but her growth and development milestones are normal.

She is being breast-fed every 4 hours and nurses without difficulty. Her parents do not give her formula and have not started her on cereal or solid food. She is using 8–10 diapers a day, and though she only has bowel movements about 3 times a week, she is not constipated. She sleeps normally.

There is no significant past medical, surgical, or family history. She lives with her parents, who do not drink or use drugs and do not smoke or allow it in their home. They do have a dog, who loves Chloe.

The pediatrician reviews symptoms and performs a physical exam. Everything is normal. Chloe weighs 5 kilograms, is 57 centimeters long, and has a head circumference of 38.5 centimeters. The clinician provides parent education about basic baby care and immunizations. Chloe receives all the vaccinations she is due at her age.

### Step 1

Start a supported web browser program and follow the steps listed inside the cover of this textbook to log in to the MyHealthProfessionsLab for this course.

Locate and click on the link **Exercise 9G**. This will open the Quippe software window with the New Encounter window displayed in the center.

### Step 2

Locate and click on the patient name, and click the OK button. In this exercise, you **must** set the date as stated in the case study. You do not need to set the time of the encounter.

### Step 3

Read the case study *carefully*. Use the case study information above to identify Chloe's measurements and other findings.

*Hint*: Use Otherwise Normal where appropriate.

Once you have documented all the information provided in the case study, proceed to step 4.

### Step 4

If you wish to print a copy of your completed encounter notes for yourself or because your instructor requires you to turn them in, use the Create PDF option, and then print or download the PDF at this time.

Submit your completed work for a grade. This will complete Exercise 9G.

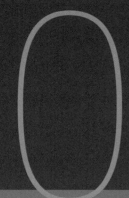

# Decision Support and Patient Involvement

## Learning Outcomes

*After completing this chapter, you should be able to:*

◆ Discuss the effect of the impact of Internet technology on healthcare

◆ Describe decision support available on the web

◆ Explain integrated decision support

◆ Discuss how patients can be engaged in their own care

◆ Access and review patient education documents

◆ Discuss secure methods of remotely accessing the EHR

◆ Compare different types of telemedicine

◆ Describe the advantages and workflow of patient-entered data

◆ Understand the workflow of an E-visit

◆ Discuss patient access to electronic health records

## Enriching the EHR Through Connectivity

This chapter will address two more of the eight core functions of an EHR defined by the IOM, decision support and patient support or engagement. Decision support means giving clinicians access to evidence-based information at the point of care. Patient support means getting patients involved in their own care and educating them on how to stay healthy. Both of these core functions have been enriched by the Internet.

Chapter 1 named the Internet as one of the social forces driving EHR adoption. The flexibility of the Internet and its ability to get information to and from almost any point in a worldwide network enables providers to access their patients' charts, communicate with patients, transmit medical images, and work from anywhere. Thanks to the Internet the clinician has instant access to a worldwide body of medical knowledge. No longer is it necessary for a physician to make a trip to the medical library or maintain a vast library in the office.

The Internet is one of the key technologies impacting our society in general. It has changed the way that people communicate, research, shop, and conduct business. It has also fostered changes in healthcare.

People shop for doctors online, insurance companies provide online participating provider lists, and physician specialty associations and state and local medical societies all offer web sites that help patients locate a provider near them.

Later in this chapter we are going to discuss how the Internet and related technologies are changing patients' expectations of the healthcare system and changing the way healthcare is delivered. Patient portals help medical practices meet HITECH Act objectives and HIPAA compliance by providing patients online access to their health records and patient education information. In some practices, they also expedite patients' access to care through E-visits.

## Decision Support

The rapidly expanding body of medical information challenges the clinician to continuously keep current with all the changes in healthcare practices. Regardless of the clinical setting where providers work, the need for up-to-date clinical support information is necessary. Sometimes a provider may treat a patient who presents with a health problem with which the provider has little or no care experience or who requires new and unfamiliar medications. In other situations a provider may be called upon to share his or her expertise with committees to develop new care protocols to support developing best practice guidelines. Providers may also be involved in new program development to meet needs in their community or to be involved in research to improve patient outcomes.

The quantity of information available to clinicians regarding conditions, disease management, protocols, case studies, and treatments far exceeds their available time to read it.

Although the Internet offers easy access to myriad web sites that can quickly provide information to help support any knowledge deficit, it is important to obtain information from sites that can be depended on for accurate and quality information to guide their care. Two such sites are the Centers for Disease Control and Prevention (shown in Figure 10-1) and Medscape®.

The official web site of the Centers for Disease Control and Prevention (CDC) is an online source for credible health information. Providers and patients may use its resources at no cost and without specific permission. The site provides direct access to important health and safety topics, scientific articles, data and statistics, tools and resources—and over 900 topics. Several decision support and patient education exercises in this chapter link to online CDC documents.

Medscape is the leading web site for providers as a source of objective, credible, relevant clinical information and educational tools. The site provides online continuing medical education (CME) as well as online coverage of medical conferences, access to over 100 medical journals, and specialty-specific daily medical news. Large numbers of research papers and nearly every medical journal is available on the site.

In addition to physician-oriented sites, professional organizations for other healthcare professionals are reliable sources of information on guidelines, practice standards,

**Figure 10-1** CDC web site used by patients and clinicians.

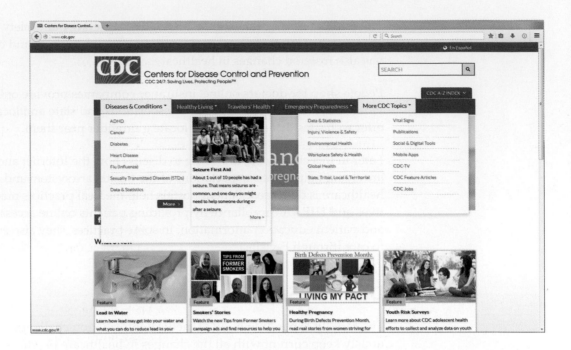

continuing education credits, upcoming conferences, and a variety of online networking opportunities. Here are three examples for allied healthcare professionals:

◆ Nursing professional organizations have many web sites offering information on professional practice and even include areas specifically designed for student nurses. Additionally, if the nurse is working within a particular clinical specialty, the professional nursing organization associated with the specialty will contain information that is clinically relevant and supportive of best practice standards.

◆ The American Association of Medical Assistants (AAMA) web site provides information on certification programs, online CME courses, and news useful to the medical assistant.

◆ The American Health Information Management Association (AHIMA) web site offers resources and tools to advance health information professional practice and standards for the delivery of quality healthcare.

## Integrated Decision Support

Although continuing education classes, medical journals, and web sites such as Medscape are available to a majority of clinicians, the information relevant to a particular case may not be easy to locate during the patient encounter when it is most needed. Incorporating decision support into the EHR can reduce the occurrence of medical errors and thus improve healthcare safety.

Two features you have used previously may also be considered forms of decision support:

1. For EHRs based on the Medcin nomenclature, the ability to prompt for clinical concepts based on a finding not only adds unentered concepts to speed documentation, but may also cause the clinician to consider additional causes or suggested treatments. For example, a patient with a cough who keeps pet birds may have parrot fever (psittacosis).

2. The Clinical Quality Measures Review feature also provides decision support, not only by recommending preventive care, but also with the ability to display CQM documentation containing specific details of the measure and additional reference material.

A third feature, introduced in this chapter, is the ability to integrate decision support links into the EHR, giving the clinician direct access to materials relevant to the findings of the current case without having to search the web.

Clinics can imbed links to external documents into templates or forms that, when clicked, display any type of helpful material. These might include defined protocols, results of case studies, or standard care guidelines prepared by specialists, medical societies, or government organizations.

In current EHR systems, external decision support documents are selected and links are set up in the system by someone at the facility. The selection of decision support items is generally the responsibility of the clinician or of a committee in a hospital or group practice. The author is not aware of any EHR vendor that automatically installs standard decision support documents or links, so decision support documents in your workplace will vary from the examples here.

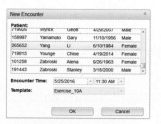

NOTE

### About Decision Support Scenarios

The intent of the decision support exercises in this chapter is to provide the student an opportunity to experience how clinical information about conditions or diseases can be accessed by a clinician at the point of care. The case study scenarios are not intended to imply that a trained clinician would not know the information the student is retrieving.

## Guided Exercise 10A: Patient with Dengue Fever

### Case Study

Li Yang is a 31-year-old female who after a relaxing Hawaiian vacation has developed a high fever, severe headache, and muscle and joint pain. She believes she contracted the flu from the close confines of the plane during the flight home and goes to her family physician.

### Step 1

Start a supported web browser program and follow the steps listed inside the cover of this textbook to log in to the MyHealthProfessionsLab for this course.

Locate and click on the link Exercise 10A.

### Step 2

In the New Encounter window, locate and click on **Yang, Li**, as shown in Figure 10-2. You do not need to set the date and time for this encounter. Click the OK button.

**Figure 10-2** Selecting Li Yang from the New Encounter window patient list.

### Step 3

Click in the blank space under the heading Chief Complaint, and type **Patient reports cold or flu**.

### Step 4

Li says she has had a high fever for two days, and a severe headache, so she has been taking Extra Strength Excedrin® to relieve the pain and reduce her fever, but it isn't working.

Click in the toolbar Search box and type Excedrin, and press the Enter key on your keyboard. When the list is displayed the clinician knows Excedrin is a combination of acetaminophen, aspirin, and caffeine. Click on **acetaminophen + aspirin + caffeine**, and then click the Add to Note button.

The finding will be added to the Plan section. Click on the finding, drag your mouse upward, and drop it onto the Current Medications heading.

*Right-click* on the finding and select Details from the Actions drop-down menu. Change the Prefix from ordered to blank (the first item in the prefix field drop-down list shown in Figure 10-3).

**Figure 10-3** Select blank row in the drop-down list to clear ordered from the Prefix field.

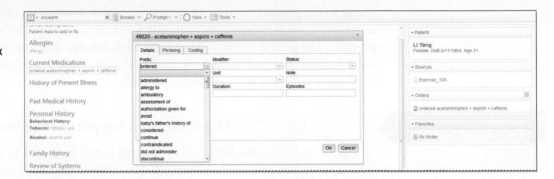

Click the OK button to close the Details pop-up window. The finding should be red and the description should be as it is in Figure 10-4, and no longer include the word ordered.

### Step 5

Next, document her personal history and vital signs. Li does not use tobacco, but does drink a glass of wine per week. She denies having any allergies.

Locate and click the following findings until they turn blue and their descriptions change.

- allergy
- tobacco use

Click on two alcohol findings until they turn red.

- alcohol use
- wine

Type **1** in the field "Glasses per week."

Enter Li's vital signs in the corresponding fields of the encounter as follows:

| | |
|---|---|
| Temperature: | 104 |
| Pulse: | 80 |
| Respiration: | 28 |
| SBP: | 140 |
| DBP: | 90 |
| O₂ Sat: | 99 |
| Weight: | 110 |
| Height: | 62 |

Compare your screen to Figure 10-4 to verify you have entered the Chief Complaint, Allergies, Current Medications, and Vital Signs correctly.

**Figure 10-4** Correct entries for the Chief Complaint, Allergies, Current Medications and Vital Signs sections.

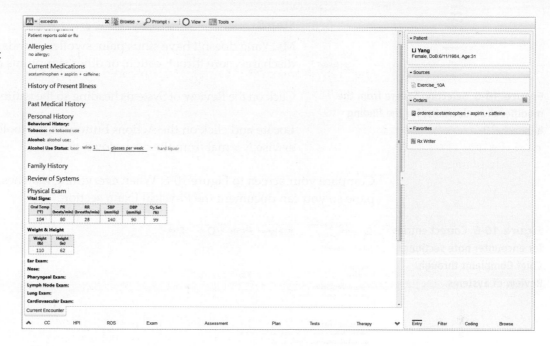

### Step 6

Click anywhere in the workspace pane that is not a finding or a heading, and then click the Browse button on the Toolbar at the top of the screen.

Locate and click the plus symbol to expand "Sample Custom Content," "Shared Content," and "Student Edition Lists." Locate and click on the list named **Adult URI** to highlight it and then click on the Add to Note button.

### Step 7

Begin in Past Medical History, then proceed to Review of Systems. Ms. Yang is not feeling well. She has had a fever for two days, a severe headache, and muscle aches. She denies any recent URI.

Locate and click on the following finding until it turns blue and the description changes.

- recent upper respiratory infection

Locate and click on the following findings until they turn red.

- taking medications
- not feeling well
- fever
- headache
- muscle aches

*Right-click* on **fever**, and select Details from the Actions drop-down menu. Click in the Duration field and type **2d** and then click OK to close the Details pop-up window.

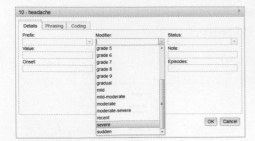

**Figure 10-5** Selecting Severe from the modifier drop-down list for the finding headache.

*Right-click* on **headache**, and select Details from the Actions drop-down menu. Click in the Modifier field and select **severe** from the drop-down list shown in Figure 10-5. Click the OK button to close the Details pop-up window.

### Step 8

Ms. Yang doesn't have sinus pain, swollen glands, earache, nasal discharge, sore throat, cough, or other symptoms of a cold.

Click on the Review of Systems heading so the entire section becomes outlined.

Locate and click on the Actions button on the toolbar, and then select Otherwise Normal from the drop-down menu.

Compare your screen to Figure 10-6. When everything matches, scroll the encounter pane so you can document the Physical Exam section.

**Figure 10-6** Correct entries for encounter note sections Chief Complaint through Review of Systems.

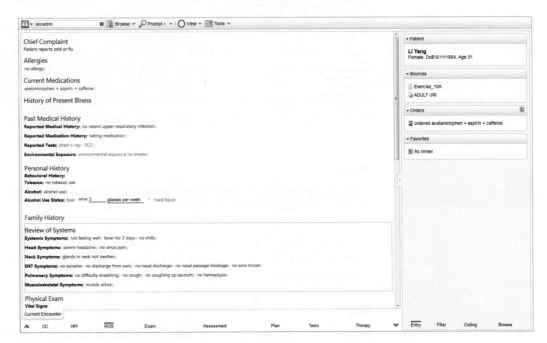

### Step 9

The clinician thoroughly examines the patient and cannot find any sign of a typical URI.

Click on the Physical Exam heading so the entire section becomes outlined, and then click the Actions button on the toolbar, and select Otherwise Normal from the drop-down menu.

Upon examination of her skin the clinician notices a lot of mosquito bites.

Locate and click on the X in the Search box on the toolbar to clear it, and then type **mosquito** and press the Enter key on your keyboard.

Locate mosquito bite (prefaced by the block letter H) in the search results list. Click on it to highlight it, and then click the Add to Note button. The finding will be added to the Past Medical History section.

Click on the **mosquito bite** finding until it turns red.

Ms. Yang says she got the mosquito bites on her trip to Hawaii.

Locate and click on the X in the Search box on the toolbar to clear it, and then type **travel hawaii** and press the Enter key on your keyboard.

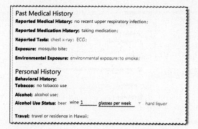

Locate "travel or residence in Hawaii" in the search results list, click on it to highlight it, and then click the Add to Note button. The finding will be added to the Personal History section.

Click on the travel finding until it turns red. Figure 10-7 shows the two new findings in the two history sections.

**Figure 10-7** History findings mosquito bite and travel added in step 9.

### Step 10

The clinician is aware that dengue virus can be transmitted by mosquitos in the tropics and recalls hearing about some cases in Hawaii, but has not seen a case of it before. However, since Ms. Yang does not have the symptoms of a typical respiratory infection, and does have a history of travel to the South Pacific and the presence of mosquito bites, it is worth considering.

Locate and click on the X in the Search box on the toolbar to clear it again, and then type **dengue** and press the Enter key on your keyboard.

Locate **dengue fever** in the search results list, click on it to highlight it, and then click the **Merge Prompt** button. Clinical concepts related to dengue fever will be added to the encounter note.

### Step 11

Since it is a condition the clinician has not treated before, the clinician accesses Decision Support.

Click anywhere in the workspace pane that is not a finding or a heading, and then click the Browse button on the toolbar, and then expand the Sample Custom Content, Shared Content, and Student Edition Forms trees. Locate the form **Decision Support**, click on it to highlight it, and then click the Add to Note button.

In the pop-up window locate **Dengue virus**, and click on the small button with three dots located to the left of it (circled in Figure 10-8). A separate tab or window will display decision support content from the CDC.

Review the document, scrolling as necessary. The clinician believes Ms. Yang's case is mild and notes the treatment plan (on page 2) for mild cases.

Return to the window or tab in which you are documenting your exercise encounter. In the pop-up window click the checkbox indicating that the clinician has reviewed the dengue virus document (as shown in Figure 10-8). Click the OK button to close the form window.

### Step 12

The clinician orders a test to confirm the diagnosis and orders oral fluids as the treatment. Locate and click the following findings in the Assessment, Test to Order, and Therapy sections until they turn red.

- dengue fever
- serum ELISA for dengue fever
- oral fluids

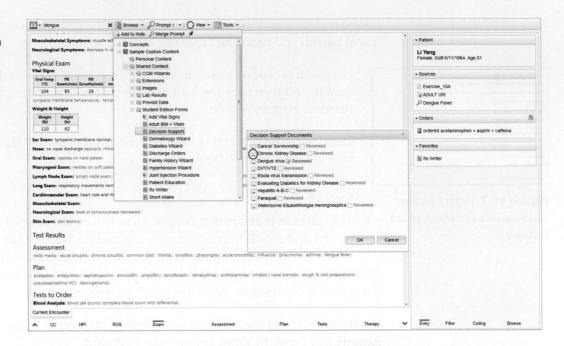

**Figure 10-8** Decision Support Documents form on the right invoked from the Student Editions Forms list on the left.

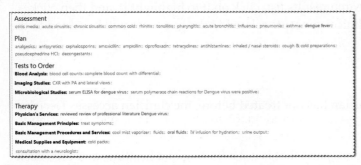

**Figure 10-9** Correctly completed Assessment and Plan sections of the encounter note.

Compare the Assessment and Plan portions of your screen to Figure 10-9.

### Step 13

Having reviewed the decision support material the clinician realizes that dengue fever increases risk of bleeding and therefore analgesics containing aspirin are contraindicated.

Scroll the encounter upward to Current Medications and click on the finding avoid aspirin until it turns red.

● avoid aspirin

*Right-click* on **acetaminophen + aspirin + caffeine**, and select Details from the Actions drop-down menu. Click on the prefix field and select **discontinue** from the drop-down list. Click on the OK button to close the Details pop-up window. The description should read "discontinue acetaminophen + aspirin + caffeine."

### Step 14

Click the View button on the toolbar and select Concise from the drop-down menu. Compare your screen to Figure 10-10, scrolling as necessary until you have verified the entire encounter. If everything on your screen matches the figure, proceed to step 15. If there are any differences, review the preceding steps and correct your work.

### Step 15

If wish to print a copy of your completed encounter notes for yourself or because your instructor requires you to turn them in, use the Create PDF option, and then print or download the PDF at this time.

The final step in every exercise is to submit your completed work for a grade.

**Figure 10-10** Concise view of the correctly completed encounter for Li Yang.

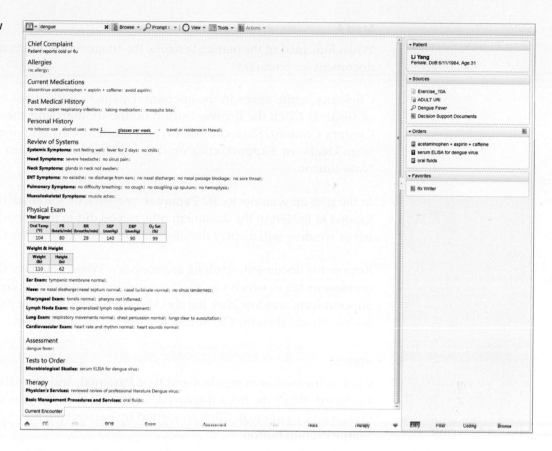

Locate and click the blue Quippe icon button on the toolbar, and then select the Submit for Grade option from the drop-down menu. This will complete Exercise 10A.

## Critical Thinking Exercise 10B: Accidental Exposure to Paraquat

### Case Study

Ethan is a student who has an afterschool job on a farm. He was messing around in the barn when he spilled a container of herbicide. He is having trouble breathing. His employer, who is trained and licensed to use paraquat, has Ethan immediately shower, and loans him some clean clothes. Ethan is having trouble breathing, so his employer calls Ethan's mother, telling her to meet them at the ER

### Step 1

Start a supported web browser program and follow the steps listed inside the cover of this textbook to log in to the MyHealthProfessionsLab for this course.

Locate and click on the link Exercise 10B.

### Step 2

In the New Encounter window, locate and click on **Farmer, Ethan**, and click the OK button. You do not need to set the date and time for this encounter.

### Step 3

Click in the blank space under the heading Chief Complaint, and type **accidental contact with herbicide**.

### Step 4

When informed of the herbicide name, the triage nurse brings up the decision support document for paraquat.

Click any white space in the encounter pane that does not highlight a heading or finding. Click the Browse button on the toolbar, and then expand the Sample Custom Content, Shared Content, and Student Edition Forms trees. Locate the form **Decision Support**, click on it to highlight it, and then click the Add to Note button.

In the pop-up window locate **Paraquat**, and click on the small button with three dots located to the left of the document title, as you did in the previous exercise. A separate tab or window will display decision support content from the CDC.

Review the document, scrolling as necessary. When you have finished, return to the window or tab in which you are documenting your exercise encounter. In the Decision Support form window click the checkbox indicating that the paraquat information was reviewed, and then the OK button to close the form window.

### Step 5

Click in the toolbar Search box and type **Paraquat**, and press the Enter key on your keyboard. When the list is displayed, locate and click the plus symbol to expand poisoning by paraquat. Click **accidental by paraquat** to highlight it, and then click the Merge Prompt button.

### Step 6

After confirming that Ethan has already showered and his contaminated clothes were properly disposed of, the nurse proceeds to document the encounter. Ethan has no allergies, but started smoking cigarettes a few months ago. He denies alcohol use, but admits smoking marijuana occasionally. He is not on any medications.

Locate and click the following findings until they turn blue and their descriptions change.

- allergy
- alcohol use
- medication reconciliation not performed

Locate and click the following findings until they turn red.

- tobacco use
- current some day smoker
- cigarettes
- using marijuana
- difficulty breathing

Click in the cigarettes pack-years field and type **<1**. This means less than one.

### Step 7

Ethan's breathing is rapid and shallow. Although the ER monitoring equipment electronically transfers vital signs data into the chart, *for purposes of this exercise* you will enter the data manually.

Enter Ethan's vital signs and standard measurements in the corresponding fields of the encounter as follows:

| | |
|---|---|
| Temperature: | 98.8 |
| Pulse: | 80 |
| Respiration: | 30 |
| SBP: | 100 |
| DBP: | 78 |
| O$_2$ Sat: | 90 |
| Weight: | 160 |
| Height: | 70 |

Locate and click the following finding until it turns red.

- tachypnea

## Step 8

Click in the Search box on the toolbar. Without erasing paraquat, press the Enter key on your keyboard to redisplay the search results for paraquat. Locate **urine paraquat** (prefaced by the block letter "T"). Click on it to highlight it, and then click the Add to Note button.

Locate the added finding in Tests to Order, and click it until it turns red.

- urine paraquat

## Step 9

When the lab results are ready, the ER doctor reviews the urine test results, confirms the diagnosis, orders two additional blood tests, oxygen, an IV, and admits Ethan to the hospital.

Locate and click the following findings until they turn red.

- accidental poisoning by paraquat
- comprehensive metabolic panel
- hepatic function panel

*Right-click* **urine paraquat** and select Details from the Actions drop-down menu. Click the down-arrow on the Prefix field and select **reviewed** from the drop-down list. Click the OK button to close the pop-up window. The description should read "reviewed urine paraquat."

## Step 10

Click any white space in the encounter that does not cause a heading or finding to have focus, and then click the Browse button on the toolbar. Expand the tree by clicking the small plus symbols next to Sample Custom Content, Shared Content, and Student Edition Lists.

Locate the list named "N Hospital Admission" by scrolling lists to the bottom. Click on the name to highlight it, and then click the Add to Note button.

Locate and click the following findings until they turn red.

- oxygen
- normal saline infusion ml/hr
- hospital admission

*Right-click* on **normal saline infusion ml/hr**, and select Details from the Actions drop-down menu. In the Details pop-up window type **1000** in the Value field and **4h** in the Duration field. Click the down-arrow on the Unit field and select **ml/hr**. Click the OK button. The finding description should read "normal saline infusion 1000 ml/hr for 4 hours."

## Step 11

Click the View button on the toolbar and select Concise from the drop-down menu. Compare your screen to Figure 10-11, scrolling as necessary until you have verified the entire encounter. If everything on your screen matches the figure, proceed to step 12. If there are any differences, review the preceding steps and correct your work.

**Figure 10-11** Concise view of the correctly completed encounter for Ethan Farmer.

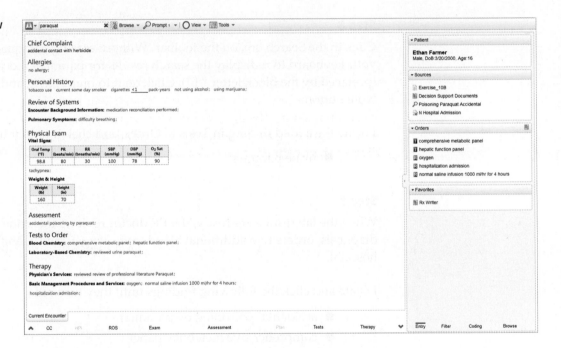

## Step 12

If you wish to print a copy of your completed encounter notes for yourself or because your instructor requires you to turn them in, use the Create PDF option, and then print or download the PDF at this time.

The final step in every exercise is to submit your completed work for a grade.

Locate and click the blue Quippe icon button on the toolbar, and then select the Submit for Grade option from the drop-down menu. This will complete Exercise 10B.

# Patient Involvement in Their Own Healthcare

Patients must become involved in their own healthcare to effectively manage and prevent diseases. One such example was the immunization quiz you completed in Exercise

9D. Other examples are the use of patient-specific graphs, growth charts, and BMI that were used for in-patient education and counseling in previous chapters.

Patients can also be engaged in their own healthcare by measuring their own blood pressure at home and keeping a log that they bring to the doctor's office when they have a checkup. Dr. Allen Wenner provides a spreadsheet template to patients who have Microsoft Excel on their home computers. The template is available to his patients on his web site. He encourages them to record their daily blood pressure in an Excel workbook instead of on paper, and to bring or e-mail a copy of the workbook file when they come to his office.

During the patient's office visit, Dr. Wenner and the patient discuss the graph of the daily blood pressure readings compared with the regimen of blood pressure medicine. The clinician tells the patient what are the parameters of control, for example, 140/90 for most patients and 130/80 for diabetics. The patient also can view the graph at home as he builds it with his own data. Following the graph on his home computer, the patient knows whether the therapy is working.

Figure 10-12 shows a graph created in Excel by Dr. Wenner and his patient. Notice that during the Hyzaar treatment the patient's blood pressure is trending higher than 140 over 90. The graph indicates the medication needs to be changed. After the doctor shows the patient how to read the graph during the office visit, the patient understands the normal and abnormal range. The patient knows when to call Dr. Wenner for advice rather than wait until the next appointment. This shared information results in shared decision making. The interaction is transformed from one of gathering information to one of managing the patient's problem. Patients can now look actively at issues of the illness, the treatment regime, and the desired outcome.

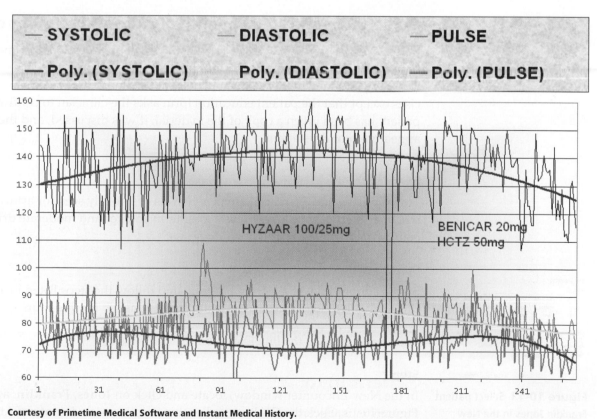

Courtesy of Primetime Medical Software and Instant Medical History.

**Figure 10-12** Graph of patient-entered blood pressure readings from February to May.

This is one example of patients using technology to improve blood pressure management. Research has shown that controlling blood pressure will reduce stroke, heart attack, and vascular disease. Nearly 200 medications are approved for controlling hypertension. There is a combination of drugs that will work for most patients without side effects. Currently in the United States, only about one-third of hypertensive patients have their illness under good control. A number of reasons contribute to this, but increased patient involvement can improve their health.

## Patient Education Material

Doctors Wenner and Bachman discussed, in Chapter 1, the concept of giving the patient a copy of the exam note at the conclusion of the visit. Their recommendation of this practice has become one of the meaningful use requirements (also introduced in Chapter 1). One effect of giving the patient written documentation of the diagnosis, therapy, and plan of care discussed during the visit is that it improves the patient's recollection of the clinician's advice. The other effect is that it stimulates compliance by the patient with the plan of care. Another standard practice is for a medical office to maintain a list of patient education documents about various conditions and provide copies to patients.

Patient education documents can be printed and given to the patient during the visit, e-mailed, or provided on the clinic's web portal (discussed later in this chapter). Patient education documents differ from the decision support documents accessed during the previous exercises in that the vocabulary is oriented to the layman and the material often contains colorful illustrations to help the patient understand the body part or medical concepts being discussed. Although easier to read, patient education materials provided by a medical office are generally evidence-based, and come from a reliable medical authority such as the CDC, or non-profit organizations such as the American Heart Association or American Cancer Society.

## Guided Exercise 10C: Patient Education About Risk of COPD

In this exercise you will access a form listing patient education documents that the practice has decided would be useful for patients. In most respects the process of accessing and viewing these documents will be similar to the decision support exercises except that the patient education form asks the clinician to confirm that the patient has been given a copy of the material, it was discussed, and the patient appeared to understand it.

### Case Study

Franklin Jones is a 77-year-old male who was previously seen for arthritic pain and seasonal allergy symptoms. He is a long-term smoker and moderate drinker. He is continuing to have difficulty breathing.

### Step 1

Start a supported web browser program and follow the steps listed inside the cover of this textbook to log in to the MyHealthProfessionsLab for this course.

Locate and click on the link Exercise 10C.

### Step 2

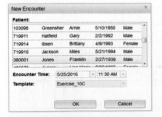

**Figure 10-13 Select patient Franklin Jones in the New Encounter window.**

In the New Encounter window, locate and click on **Jones, Franklin**, as shown in Figure 10-13. Click the OK button. For this exercise, you do not need to set the date and time of the encounter.

**Step 3**

Click in the blank space under the heading Chief Complaint as you have in previous exercises, and type **Difficulty breathing**.

**Step 4**

You take Mr. Jones' vital signs and enter them into the corresponding fields on the encounter note. They are as follows:

| | |
|---|---|
| Temperature: | **98.6** |
| Pulse: | **72** |
| Respiration: | **22** |
| SBP (systolic) | **125** |
| DBP (diastolic) | **80** |
| $O_2$ Sat: | **95** |
| Weight: | **147** |
| Height: | **67** |

Verify that you have entered the vital signs correctly.

**Step 5**

Locate and click on the following findings until they turn red.

- allergy
- allergy to pollens

Locate and click on the following finding until it turns blue and the description changes.

- allergy to drugs

**Step 6**

As you may recall from Chapter 4, Mr. Jones has been smoking for 50 years and drinks a six-pack of beer a week. Proceed to the Personal History section.

Locate and click on the following findings until they turn red.

- tobacco use
- current everyday smoker
- cigarettes
- alcohol use
- beer

Locate cigarettes and type **50** in the pack-years field.

Locate beer and type **6** in the bottles per week field.

Compare your Chief Complaint, Allergy, Personal History, and Vital Signs sections to Figure 10-14.

**Step 7**

Click any white space in the encounter pane that does not highlight a heading or finding.

**Figure 10-14** Correctly completed Chief Complaint, Allergy, Personal History, and Vital Signs sections.

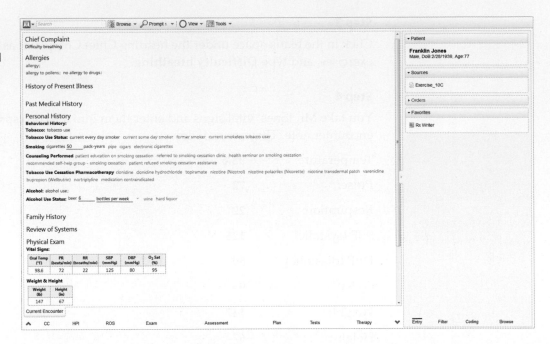

Click the Browse button on the toolbar, and then expand the Sample Custom Content, Shared Content, and Student Edition Forms trees. Locate the form **Short Intake**, click on it to highlight it, and then click the Add to Note button. The form will open on the Review of Systems tab.

Mr. Jones is having difficulty breathing and is awakening at night. The clinician discusses the other symptoms listed on the form, but Mr. Jones denies having them.

Locate and click the indicated checkboxes for the following findings.

✓  **Y** difficulty breathing

✓  **Y** sleep disturbance

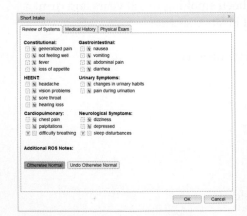

**Figure 10-15** Correctly completed Review of Systems page of the Short Intake form.

Locate and click the Otherwise Normal button (highlighted in Figure 10-15).

Compare your Short Intake Form, Review of Systems tab to Figure 10-15. If everything is correct, click on the Medical History tab.

**Step 8**

Notice that Personal History items on the form are already checked. These were set from findings already documented in the encounter. Click the checkboxes for only the Patient History and Family History items indicated in the following table:

| Diagnosis | Patient History | Family History |
|---|---|---|
| Angina | N | |
| Asthma | Y | |
| Cancer | N | Y |
| CHF (congestive heart failure) | N | Y |
| Hypertension | Y | |

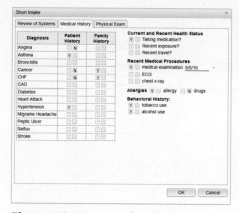

**Figure 10-16** Correctly completed Medical History page of the Short Intake form.

On the right side of the form page locate and click the indicated checkboxes for the following findings.

✓  Y Taking medications

✓  Y medical examination

A field will appear to enter the date of the recent medical examination. Mr. Jones was last seen on May 5, 2016. Click in the field and type 5/5/2016.

Compare your Short Intake Form, Medical History tab to Figure 10-16. If everything is correct, click the OK button to close the form and record the findings.

### Step 9

Noting that Mr. Jones has a history of asthma, the clinician uses the asthma list for the remainder of the exam.

Click any white space in the encounter pane that does not highlight a heading or finding.

Click the Browse button on the toolbar, and then expand the Sample Custom Content, Shared Content, and Student Edition Lists trees. Locate and click on the list **Asthma** to highlight it, and then click the Add to Note button.

For ease of entry, scroll the encounter pane until Review of Systems is at the top. Locate Pulmonary Symptoms and click on the following findings until they turn red.

- awakening at night short of breath
- wheezing
- recurs intermittently

### Step 10

Proceed to the Physical Exam section, Lung exam, and click on the following findings until they turn red.

- accessory muscles used during expiration
- wheezing
- prolonged expiratory time

Compare your screen to Figure 10-17.

### Step 11

The clinician's diagnosis is that Mr. Jones' asthma is the cause of his difficulty and orders albuterol. He also recognizes this visit is an excellent opportunity to provide patient education on chronic obstructive pulmonary disease (COPD) and counseling to stop smoking.

Locate the following findings in the Assessment and Plan sections and click on them until they turn red.

- asthma
- albuterol

**Figure 10-17** Correctly completed Review of Systems and Physical Exam sections of the encounter note.

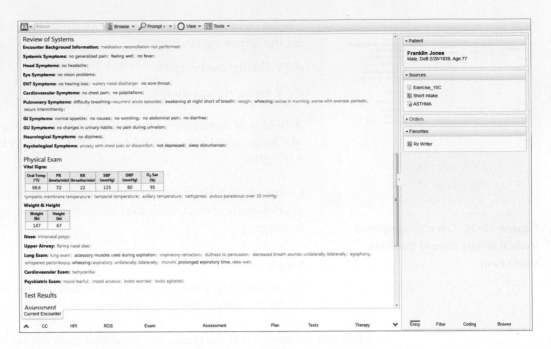

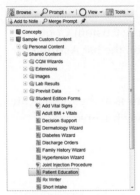

**Figure 10-18** Expanded tree of Forms with Patient Education form highlighted.

**Figure 10-19** Patient Education Documents selection form with checked boxes for COPD.

### Step 12

Click any white space in the encounter pane that does not highlight a heading or finding.

Click the Browse button on the toolbar, and then expand the Sample Custom Content, Shared Content, and Student Edition Forms trees. Locate the form **Patient Education**, click on it to highlight it as shown in Figure 10-18, and then click the Add to Note button. The pop-up window shown in Figure 10-19 displays a list of patient education materials the clinic prefers to use.

Locate the row for COPD and click on the underlined title "CDC: COPD, Are You at Risk?" The document will open as a PDF in a separate tab. Review the document.

The clinician discusses the risk of continuing to smoke. Mr. Jones says he understands, and will try to quit, but says he has had the habit a long time. The clinician refers him to a smoking cessation clinic and gives Mr. Jones a printed copy of the patient education material to take home.

Return to the tab or window with your encounter note and click three checkboxes in the COPD row under the following column headings:

✓ **Information Shared with Patient**

✓ **Education Sheet Given**

✓ **Patient Indicated Understanding**

Click the OK button to close the Patient Education window.

### Step 13

Scroll the encounter pane upward to the Personal History. Locate the Tobacco section, Counseling Performed group, and click on the following findings until they turn red.

- patient education on smoking cessation
- referred to a smoking cessation clinic

## Step 14

Click the View button on the toolbar and select Concise from the drop-down menu. Compare your screen to Figure 10-20, scrolling as necessary until you have verified the entire encounter. If everything on your screen matches the figure, proceed to step 15. If there are any differences, review the preceding steps and correct your work.

**Figure 10-20** Concise view of the correctly completed encounter for Franklin Jones.

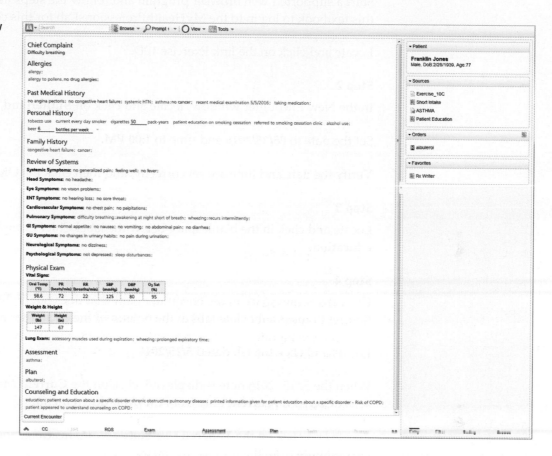

## Step 15

If wish to print a copy of your completed encounter notes for yourself or because your instructor requires you to turn them in, use the Create PDF option, and then print or download the PDF at this time.

The final step in every exercise is to submit your completed work for a grade.

Locate and click the blue Quippe icon button on the toolbar, and then select the Submit for Grade option from the drop-down menu. This will complete Exercise 10C.

## Critical Thinking Exercise 10D: Patient Education About Diabetes

In this exercise you will review patient education materials and document that they have been understood. The patient has been the subject of several previous exercises, and this exercise portrays the conclusion of a single encounter that has spanned several chapters. In the interest of time, this exercise omits reentry of many findings added for this encounter in previous chapters.

### Case Study

Sally Sutherland is a patient with hyperlipidemia and diabetes who is at the conclusion of her May 25 visit to the clinic. Her clinician will review patient education materials with Sally and give her patient education documents to take home.

### Step 1

Start a supported web browser program and follow the steps listed inside the cover of this textbook to log in to the MyHealthProfessionsLab for this course.

Locate and click on the link Exercise 10D.

### Step 2

In the New Encounter window, locate and click on **Sutherland, Sally**.

Set the date to **05/25/2016** and time to **1:00 PM**.

Verify the date and time are set correctly, and then click the OK button.

### Step 3

Locate and click in the blank space below the label Chief Complaint, and type **patient education**.

### Step 4

Click any white space in the encounter pane that does not highlight a heading or finding to restore the date tabs at the bottom of the encounter pane.

Locate and click the tab dated **5/15/2016**.

When the 5/15/2016 note is displayed, click on the **Current Medications** heading, and select **Copy into current note** from the drop-down menu.

Locate and click on the **Tobacco Use Status** group heading, and then select **Copy into current note** from the drop-down menu.

Locate and click on the **Previous Tests** heading, and select **Copy into current note** from the drop-down menu.

Locate and click the **Current Encounter** tab.

### Step 5

Record Ms. Sutherland's vital signs in the corresponding fields of the encounter as follows:

| | |
|---|---|
| Temperature: | 98.6 |
| Pulse: | 78 |
| Respiration: | 28 |
| SBP: | 134 |
| DBP: | 90 |
| Weight: | 153 |
| Height: | 60 |

Verify that you have entered her vital signs correctly and then locate and click on the cell labeled "BMI."

**Step 6**

Click any white space in the encounter pane that does not highlight a heading or finding.

Click the Browse button on the toolbar, and then expand the Sample Custom Content, Shared Content, and Student Edition Forms trees. Locate the form **Diabetes Wizard**, click on it to highlight it, and then click the Add to Note button.

When the pop-up window opens, you will notice that many of the fields already have data from findings in the current encounter. Locate Diabetes Diagnosis at the bottom of the form and click the checkbox for Type II.

✓ type II

Locate and click the Next button. The second page will be displayed.

Locate Dietary Orders and click the following checkboxes:

✓ weight loss diet

✓ diabetic diet

Locate and click the Finish button. The form window will close and the findings will be added to the encounter note.

**Step 7**

Click any white space in the encounter pane that does not highlight a heading or finding.

Click the Browse button on the toolbar, and then expand the Sample Custom Content, Shared Content, and Student Edition Forms trees. Locate the form **Patient Education**, click on it to highlight it, and then click the Add to Note button. The pop-up window previously shown in Figure 10-19 displays a list of patient education materials the clinic uses.

Locate the row for Diabetes and click on the underlined title "NIDDK: Guide to Diabetes Type I and Type II." The document will open as a PDF in a separate tab. Review the document.

The clinician discusses diabetes with the patient, and warns that her diabetes presents a danger to her heart as well. Locate the second document in the Diabetes row and click on the underlined title "NDEP: Take Care of Your Heart Manage Your Diabetes." The document will open as a PDF in a separate tab (this may replace the first document you opened). Review the document.

Return to the tab or window with your encounter note and form. Click four checkboxes in the Diabetes row under the following column headings:

✓ **Information Shared with Patient**

✓ **Education Sheet Given** (Guide to Diabetes Type I and Type II)

✓ **Education Sheet Given** (Take Care of Your Heart Manage Your Diabetes)

✓ **Patient Indicated Understanding**

Click the OK button to close the Patient Education window.

## Step 8

Click the View button on the toolbar and select Concise from the drop-down menu. Compare your screen to Figure 10-21, scrolling as necessary until you have verified the entire encounter. If everything on your screen matches the figure, proceed to step 9. If there are any differences, review the preceding steps and correct your work.

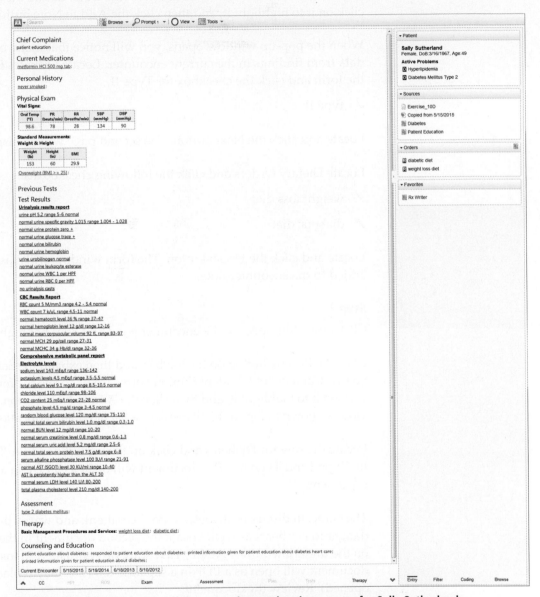

**Figure 10-21** Concise view of the correctly completed encounter for Sally Sutherland.

## Step 9

If wish to print a copy of your completed encounter notes for yourself or because your instructor requires you to turn them in, use the Create PDF option, and then print or download the PDF at this time.

The final step in every exercise is to submit your completed work for a grade.

Locate and click the blue Quippe icon button on the toolbar, and then select the Submit for Grade option from the drop-down menu. This will complete Exercise 10D.

## Using the Internet

Patients also become involved in their own care by using the Internet for research. Many clinicians are finding their patients are coming to visits armed with printouts about their conditions gathered from web sites. Some of these web sites provide reliable information; some do not. Social media and web sites trying to sell the patient something are not what is meant by evidence-based, credible sources of patient education information.

There are trustworthy sources of health information on the Internet. For example, one of the most trusted sources of consumer information on the web is WebMD® (www.webmd.com). On the WebMD consumer portal, patients can access health and wellness news, support communities, interactive health management tools, and more. Online communities and special events allow individuals to participate in real-time discussions with experts and with other people who share similar health conditions or concerns. Other web sites offering evidence-based patient education are those sponsored by notable healthcare organizations such as Johns Hopkins, Mayo Clinic, and others, as well as government-sponsored sites including CDC, National Institute of Health, and state health departments. By using sites such as these, patients can play an active role in managing their own health.

## Critical Thinking Exercise 10E: Internet Medical Research

In this exercise you will need access to the Internet. You will visit the WebMD web site to obtain factual information for a patient and then record your answers to the exercise questions.

### Case Study

Brenda Green is a 54-year-old established patient with a history of hypertension and possible peripheral arterial disease of the legs. She has been prescribed Coumadin, a drug that has specific dangers. Follow the steps listed here to locate the answers to the questions in step 4.

### Step 1

Start a supported web browser program and follow the steps listed inside the cover of this textbook to log in to the MyHealthProfessionsLab for this course.

Locate and click on the link Exercise 10E.

### Step 2

Without closing the exercise window, open an additional browser window or tab of the current browser.

Type the following URL in the address field of the new window: www.webmd.com.

**Step 3**

When the web page is displayed, locate the search field, type **Coumadin**, and press the Enter key on your keyboard or click on the search icon.

A page of search results will be displayed. Locate and click on the link "Drug Results for Coumadin."

**Step 4**

From the information displayed on the page answer the following questions:

What is the generic drug name for Coumadin?

What is a very serious (possibly fatal) effect of this drug?

What lab test must be performed periodically to monitor the effect of this drug?

Name a food that affects how the drug works in the body.

**Step 5**

Click on the window or tab of the browser that has Exercise 10E displayed. Enter your answers to the questions posed in step 4 and then click the Submit Quiz button.

You may close your browser windows. This completes Exercise 10E.

One way clinicians help patients find reliable information is for hospitals and medical practices to set up their own web sites. These are called Patient Portals. Patient educational information on a clinic's web site has the advantage of being consistent with the medical philosophy of the practice. A sample web site is shown in Figure 10-22. Beyond providing information about the medical practice, clinicians, and office hours, the site shown in Figure 10-22 includes online information about preventative health measures, diseases, and conditions that the practice treats.

The ONC strategies discussed in Chapter 1 call for the use of technology to make health information available to the patient. "Consumer-centric information helps individuals manage their own wellness and assists with their personal health care decisions."[1] The HITECH Act, also discussed in Chapter 1, established objectives for providers to engage patients and families through the use of web portals for their patients:

◆ Provide patients the ability to view online, download and transmit their health information

◆ Provide clinical summaries for patients for each office visit

◆ Use secure electronic messaging to communicate with patients on relevant health information

Modern patient portals allow patients secure access to their lab results and medical records as well as other features we will discuss later.

---

[1] *The Decade of Health Information Technology: Delivering Consumer-centric and Information-rich Health Care* (Washington, DC: U.S. Department of Health and Human Services Office of National Coordinator, July 21, 2004).

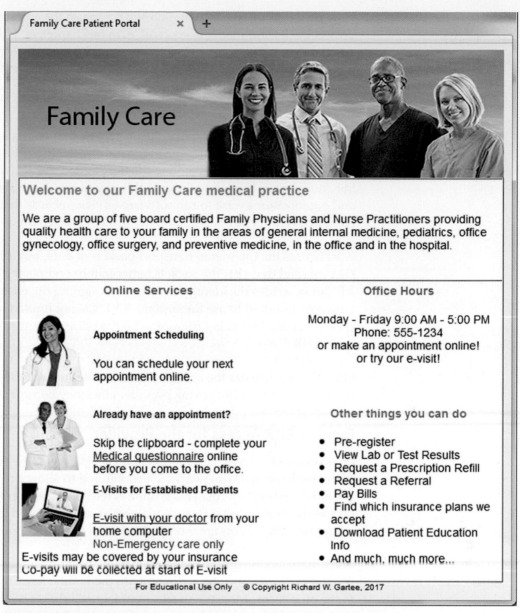

For Educational Use Only   © Copyright Richard W. Gartee, 2017

**Figure 10-22** Simulated provider web portal used for exercises in Chapter 10.

## Secure Internet Data

Most people know the Internet because of the services they use on it such as e-mail, games, and social media. However, before proceeding further it may be helpful to understand how it works.

The Internet is a worldwide public network that can be accessed by any computer device or smart phone anywhere there is connectivity. The Internet was created by interconnecting millions of smaller business-, academic-, and government-run networks. It is really a very large network of networks. The Internet Protocol encloses data in packets that are sent through the various networks making up the Internet until they arrive at your browser or email.

The problem is that the Internet is not secure. The packets of data pass through many computers and networks on their way to their destination. They can be copied, opened, and read by anyone with enough technical savvy.

How do we secure the information so we can use the accessibility of the Internet, but protect the information? As you will learn in Chapter 11, HIPAA requires encryption when transmitting personal health information over the Internet. Secure transmission of data over the Internet usually relies on either of two methods. These are secured socket layer (SSL) or a virtual private network (VPN). There are additional secure transmission schemes not covered here.

SSL adds security by encrypting the content of web pages, and the receiving browser that initiated the SSL connection automatically decrypts the page content to display it. This prevents anyone intercepting the transmitted packets from making sense of them. SSL, however, is limited to the only things you can do on a web page. Some providers and organizations want to run software or view records that are on their office network computers from elsewhere. To do this, a VPN may be used.

A VPN uses the Internet to transport packets of data, but it has its own software that encrypts and decrypts the packets between the sending and receiving systems. The VPN also verifies the identity of the person signing on, ensuring access only to those who are permitted to use the system. A VPN is not limited to web pages and may be used to secure data being transmitted by application software other than browsers, such as an EHR.

Once the practice has the ability to operate software securely over the Internet, numerous possibilities for improving provider efficiency become available.

## Remote EHR Access for the Provider

Providers increasingly want access to their EHR when they are away from the office. Many medical facility networks are configured to allow providers to access their patients' medical records. This is often is referred to as "remote access." Clinicians connect to their office network and sign on just as they would in the office, except the sign in and resulting access are wrapped securely in a VPN connection.

The benefits to the provider and the patient are tremendous. Instead of staying late, the provider can go home, have dinner with the family, relax for a few hours, then sign on to the office computer system and complete any chart reviews or other work that previously would have meant staying late. Additionally, if the clinician receives an emergency call from or about a patient, the patient's records can be accessed from home, helping the clinician make better decisions.

## Practicing Medicine Online

Beyond allowing the clinician to work from home and allowing patients to access their records, the Internet has enabled the delivery of actual medical services online. Principally this takes two forms, telemedicine and E-visits (which we will discuss later).

Telemedicine uses communication technology to deliver care to a patient in another location. A consulting health professional studies the patient's case and offers advice or instructions to the referring physician or directly to the patient, neither of whom are at the consultant's location.

Telemedicine can take many forms, ranging from a simple phone call between two doctors to a videoconference between a nurse and a client, as shown in Figure 10-23. Even examinations or surgical procedures have been conducted remotely.

Telemedicine can be practiced in real time or asynchronously (independent sessions not occurring at the same time). Before the Internet, early pioneers of telemedicine conceived of it in terms of the technology of their time, television. They imagined a scenario in which the doctor and patient could see each other on television sets at each end. Satellites that carry television signals would securely transmit the bidirectional video sessions. There were several drawbacks to this approach.

- Synchronous telemedicine requires the presence of all parties at the same time. When participants are located in different time zones, real-time telemedicine sessions can be difficult to schedule.

- Television could not transmit or display at a sufficient resolution for diagnostic images such as x-rays or CAT scans. Although modern computers can do this, large digital files of CAT scans or MRI can be time consuming to load remotely.

- Some states' laws prohibit treatment of patients by providers not licensed in that state.

## Asynchronous Telemedicine at Mayo Clinic

Known worldwide for their medical expertise, specialists at Mayo Clinic in Rochester, Minnesota, are in great demand. However, doctors and clients seeking consultations are frequently in other time zones or even other countries. In those cases, real-time telemedicine is impractical.

Rather than trying to get participants in different time zones to be available at the same time, the doctors at Mayo decided to conduct **telemedicine asynchronously**. Marvin Mitchell, division chair of Media Support Services at Mayo Clinic, calls this **store-and-forward telemedicine**. It allows a doctor requesting a consult to send case information that is saved and then reviewed and responded to later by a specialist at Mayo.

If a video conference is an example of real-time telemedicine, voice mail would be a simple analogy of store-and-forward telemedicine. One doctor sends a message stating the facts of the case and supporting documents; the other doctor reviews the message and then responds with a detailed analysis and conclusion for the original doctor.

In Mayo Clinic's practice, the patient's physician in a remote location does the necessary examinations and diagnostic tests he or she would normally do. Then the doctor creates an electronic package including high-resolution images, scanned paper documents, motion image capture, angiography, and anything else that the specialist at Mayo might need to review. The information is then transmitted with a consultation request to the Mayo telemedicine office via a secure Internet connection.

The Mayo telemedicine system follows the same workflow as if the patient were at the clinic. When the Mayo Clinic telemedicine office receives the electronic package, the patient is registered and given a Mayo Clinic patient number, and an electronic medical record is created. The diagnostic images from the package are stored in the Mayo PAC system and orders to the radiologist are created. Other records are imported into the EHR.

The principal advantage of this workflow is that it is as transparent to the Mayo physicians as possible. Specialists at Mayo see the remote patient's records in the same system they use every day. A Mayo radiologist views the diagnostic images, interprets them, and dictates a report. Similarly, other specialties look at the imported EHR data and enter their second opinion into Mayo's clinical notes system.

When all the subspecialists' reports have been completed, a comprehensive second-opinion document is compiled and sent back to the remote physician. That physician can use the second opinion to work up the diagnosis and treatment plan for the patient. In Mayo Clinic's case, real-time interactions between remote physicians are not necessary.

Although store-and-forward telemedicine works well for consults, it can involve delays when additional information or tests are needed and one must wait for the response to arrive. Other forms of telemedicine conducted in real time include remote, robotic, or even guided surgery. Using telemedicine, it is possible for a local physician to get advice from a distant expert and guidance in treating the patient.

## Teleradiology

Another form of telemedicine, specifically concerned with the transmission of diagnostic images from one location to another, is teleradiology. Usually this is for the purpose of having the images "read" by a radiologist at the receiving end. This may be to obtain a second opinion or consult, or because the sending facility does not have enough radiologists on staff and has contracted to have radiology interpretations done by another facility. In the latter case, state laws may require the radiologist to be licensed by the state from which the images are sent.

Currently, most states require a physician to be licensed by that state to treat patients in that state. Mayo Clinic's method of telemedicine solves the problem of licensure that has hindered telemedicine in the United States. At Mayo, the telemedicine consultation is physician to physician as a resource for the patient's doctor. Because they are not giving advice directly to a patient in another state, no laws are broken. This method also has the additional advantage of keeping the patient's local physician in control of the patient care at all times.

The benefit of telemedicine is that it makes high-level medical expertise available to remote and rural areas. Many communities do not have medical specialists. Even fewer places in the world have subspecialists, or sub-subspecialists who can recognize and treat rare or complex medical problems.

## Telemedicine in Nursing

One area where real-time telemedicine seems to work well is home health nursing. Home health agencies and their clients are typically in the same time zone and always licensed in the same state as their clients. Although home care nurses have been monitoring clients using the telephone for a long time, the availability of faster Internet speeds has made video conferencing via computer possible as shown in Figure 10-23. It has been reported that the older generation is among the fastest growing segment of computer users. Because this group is the larger portion of home health clients, the field is ready for telemedicine nursing.

There are many advantages for the client. Home nurses do not see clients as frequently as they would in other healthcare settings. Using Internet video conferencing, the client can not only talk to but also see the nurse between visits. Questions can be answered and issues addressed sooner. Nurses can download data from home

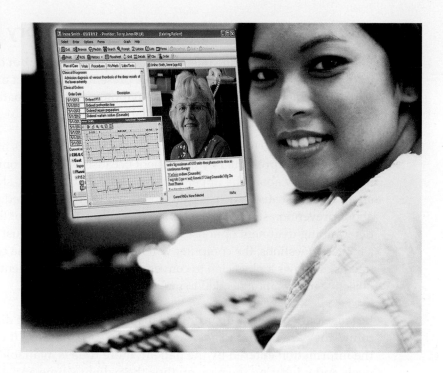

**Figure 10-23** Home health nurse video conferences with the client, while monitoring her heart rate.

medical devices that monitor the client's heart rate, blood pressure, glucose, and other measures.

Using the downloaded data and the nurse's impressions from face-to-face video communication, the nurse can determine the client's progress. In addition to the elderly, telemedicine works well for home care nursing for clients with AIDS and for monitoring women at risk for preterm labor. Telemedicine does not replace, but supplements, home visits, and thereby home care is improved.

## Telemedicine via E-Visits

It is less common for physicians to practice a video chat type of telemedicine without first having the patient's signs and symptoms documented. Clinicians have concerns about the potential for medical liability, the lack of structured documentation, and the difficulty of accurately documenting what was discussed in the teleconference as part of the patient's medical record. Also, the clinician's medical decision making is based in part on the symptoms, history of present illness, and physical exam of the patient. Who inputs that into the record? One solution is to use the patient portal as a mechanism for patients to describe their condition in a structured question format whose answers can be imported into the encounter note.

An E-visit allows the patient to be treated by a clinician for nonurgent health problems without the patient having to come into the office. Using the patient portal for an E-visit, patients enter their own symptom and HPI information, creating a documented medical encounter. When the E-visit data is imported into the EHR it becomes a part of the patient's chart, just like any other visit, and the clinician has a documented starting point for medical decision making. As we shall see in later exercises, using the patient portal for E-visits enhances the efficiency of providers and improves the accessibility of healthcare for the patients.

Long before the concepts of Meaningful Use, or E-visits, or even the Internet existed, several leading physicians recognized the value of having patients document their symptoms and history.

## Patient Entry of Symptoms and History

EHR systems facilitate documentation at the point of care, but only the patient has the information about what symptoms were present at the outset of the illness and what the outcome of medical treatment of those symptoms was. The patient is also typically the source of past medical, family, and social history.

Allen Wenner, MD has found the use of computer interviews improves the quality of the information presented by the patient because it is more complete. For example, an ideal interview about the upper respiratory tract and sinuses should include questions about unusual causes such as psittacosis, an infection acquired from raising birds, query about prevention such as use of tobacco, and consideration of the risk for pregnancy in determining treatment options. The clinician may forget or just not have enough time to ask these questions; the computer will not forget. Because the computer never forgets details, it allows a physician to converse casually with a patient while clarifying the objective information needed to make a confident diagnosis.

Because patients want their physicians to arrive at the best diagnosis, Dr. Wenner found they are willing to answer questions. Also, because the physician can review the information entered by the patient, more time is available for explaining the diagnosis and educating the patient; thus the patient's time and effort to enter the data are rewarded.

### Workflow Using Patient-Entered Data

Instant Medical History can be administered on a kiosk or on a Tablet in the waiting room, in a subwaiting area, in the exam room, or at home via the web. Figure 10-24

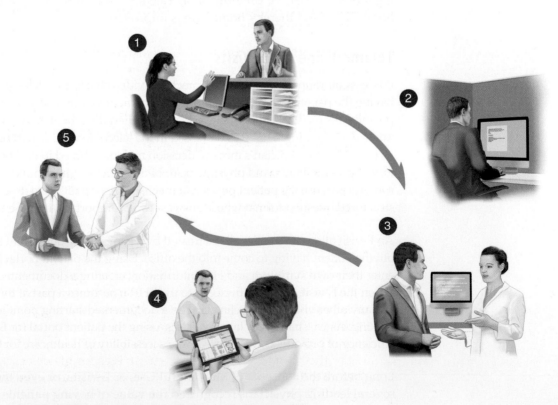

**Figure 10-24** Workflow of patient entering his own data.

illustrates one workflow of an office using Instant Medical History. As you will see in Exercise 10F, it is also easily administered over the Internet.

❶ When the patient arrives, a receptionist, nurse, or medical assistant asks the patient to complete a medical history and reason for today's visit using a computer in a private area of the waiting room.

❷ The patient is given access to a kiosk or other computing device to enter his or her own history and symptom information using a computer-guided questionnaire. The questions are asked one at a time and can dynamically branch to other question sets based on the answers provided by the patient.

The patient completes the questions at his or her own pace and has an opportunity to change answers. Patients can review their histories and are better prepared to interact with the physician.

❸ When the patient has completed the questionnaire, the system alerts the nurse or medical assistant that the patient is ready to move to an exam room. The nurse and patient review the patient-entered symptoms and history together. Where necessary, the nurse edits the record if there is additional information.

The computer organizes the patient-entered information for the provider in a succinct and easy-to-read format that becomes the starting point for the encounter. After review of the data, the nurse or clinician can merge it into the EHR encounter note.

❹ The physician examines the patient and discusses the reason for the visit and reviews with the patient the HPI information now in the chart. Having a complete history in the EHR in advance of the exam provides the clinician with a great deal of useful information to begin making the proper diagnosis and considering appropriate treatment. It also allows the physician to spend less time documenting and more time with the patient discussing the effects of the illness on the patient. It also allows the clinician time to discuss the treatment plan with the patient.

Because interview software records subjective information from the patient, the data represents a more complete and accurate reflection of a patient's complaints.

After asking a few confirmatory questions, physicians can complete the physical exam, assessment, and plan portions of the encounter note in the examination room while the patient is still present.

❺ The encounter note has been completed at the point of care. As the patient leaves, the patient is given a copy of the encounter note along with any patient education materials or prescriptions.

## Internet Workflow

Providers and patients soon realized that it was possible to complete the symptom and history interview before the visit by using the Internet. Today many medical practices enable the patient to complete the Instant Medical History questionnaire online before the visit. This saves time during the office visit and allows the patient to give more thought to their answers when completing the interview from the comfort of their home. When the patient arrives for his or her appointment, the data will already be available to the clinician. Imagine the same workflow scenario as Figure 10-24 except step ❷ is performed on the patient's home computer before coming to the office.

## Improved Patient Information

Data from patient screening is useful for providing pertinent information that allows an immediate diagnosis. Not only does the physician have a reasonable idea of the patient's problems before any examination begins, but the data are also instantly ready to become part of the medical record.

Patient-entered data transforms the visit from a data-gathering session into an opportunity to concentrate on the most important task at hand: caring for the patient.

The increased efficiency that computer screening allows makes office visits more enjoyable because the physician has more time to explain the diagnosis and educate the patient.

Dr. Wenner and his peers have found most patients willing and eager to answer a computer interview about their reason for the visit. The patient benefits because the time the doctor has saved from having to input the symptoms and history can be focused fully on the patient and used for counseling and education.

When the exam room is configured as shown in step ❸ of Figure 10-24, so that the patient and clinician can both see the screen, the patient is able to engage in the mutual process of documenting the visit. The patient benefits from this arrangement because when the patient and provider share information, the patient feels a part of the decisions and has a vested interest in following the plan of care.

John Mayne at the Mayo Clinic observed, "If the time physicians spend collecting, organizing, recording, and retrieving data could be reduced, at least in part, by information technology, more time would be available for actual delivery of medical care (and, thus, in effect increase the number of physicians) and at the same time the physician's capabilities for collecting information from patients would be extended."[2]

## Guided Exercise 10F: Experiencing Patient-Entered HPI

In this exercise you will have an opportunity to experience what we have been discussing by taking on the role of a patient who is completing his "paperwork" for an upcoming appointment online. Note, in step 5 you will enter your own name or student ID, which will be used to identify your work to your instructor.

### Case Study

Tomas Martiniz is a 24-year-old male who injured his knee when he jumped off a loading dock at work. He has an appointment at the Family Care medical clinic on May 26, 2016. He is going online to complete his medical questionnaire in advance.

### Step 1

Start a supported web browser program and follow the steps listed inside the cover of this textbook to log in to the MyHealthProfessionsLab for this course.

Locate and click on the link Exercise 10F.

> **NOTE**
>
> It is important to understand that a patient entering medical history either at a kiosk in the doctor's office or via the Internet is not accessing the actual EHR, but rather a separate application. Using a separate application protects the security and integrity of the EHR.

---

[2]J. G. Mayne, W. Weksel, and P. N. Sholtz, "Toward Automating the Medical History," *Mayo Clinic Proceedings*, 43 (1968): 1–25.

### Step 2

The sample provider web portal shown previously in Figure 10-22 will be displayed.

### Step 3

Locate the section of the web page labeled "Already have an appointment?" and click on the link "Medical Questionnaire."

The interview web page, "Get started preparing for your next doctor's visit," will be displayed.

### Step 4

Locate and click on the Start Interview button.

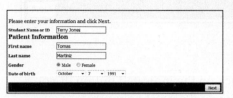

**Figure 10-25** Student ID and patient information portion of interview.

### Step 5

The center portion of the web page will display the Interview dialog as shown in Figure 10-25.

Enter the following:

Student Name or ID: Enter either your name or student ID as directed by your instructor. Do not enter the student name shown in the figure.

Patient Information:

First Name: **Tomas**

Last Name: **Martiniz**

Click on the circle next to **Male**.

Click on the down arrow buttons in each of the Date of Birth fields and select from the drop-down lists: **October, 7**, and **1991**.

Compare your screen to Figure 10-25. When everything has been entered correctly, locate and click on the Next button.

### Step 6

The reason for visit screen will be displayed.

The interview on web page is functionally identical to online questionnaires on web sites such as the one Karen Smith, MD described in the Real-Life Story and portals of other forward-thinking doctors.

Locate the free text field (circled in red in Figure 10-26) and type **Knee pain**.

Compare your screen to Figure 10-26. When you have finished typing, locate and click on the Next button.

### Step 7

The software at the web site will conduct the interview by asking Mr. Martiniz the questions listed below, one question at a time. For each question there will be buttons labeled with various answers to the question. Additional buttons allow you to skip a question or go back to the previous question.

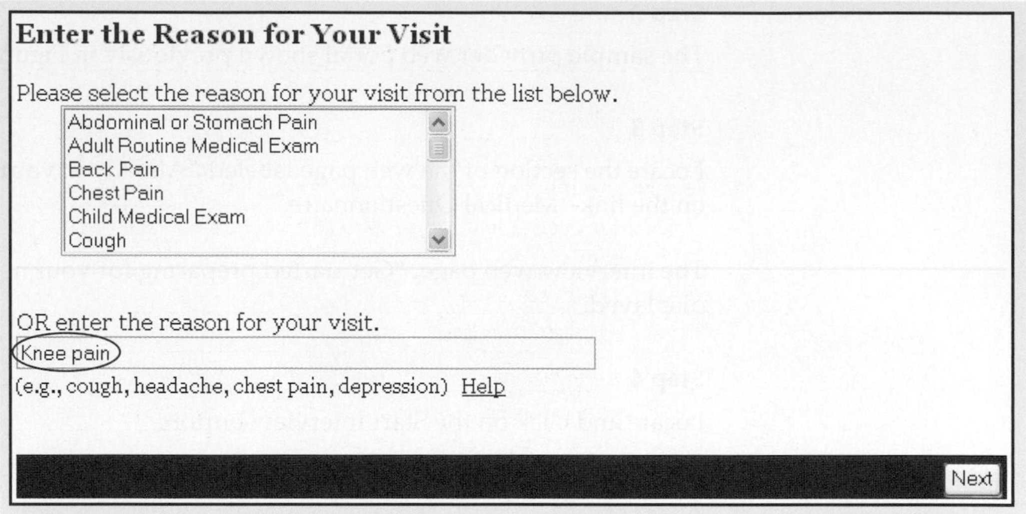

**Figure 10-26** Type reason for visit: Knee pain.

**Enter the Reason for Your Visit**

Please select the reason for your visit from the list below.

```
Abdominal or Stomach Pain
Adult Routine Medical Exam
Back Pain
Chest Pain
Child Medical Exam
Cough
```

OR enter the reason for your visit.

Knee pain

(e.g., cough, headache, chest pain, depression)  Help

Next

ALERT

The interview software dynamically changes questions based on the patient's input. If the order of questions deviates from the sequence listed in the table, click on the Previous Question button until you find your mistake and then resume.

For each question in the table below, locate and click on the indicated button. If you make an error, click on the Previous Question button and correct your error.

| Interview Question | Click on the button labeled: |
|---|---|
| What kind of problem are you having with your knee (or knees)? | Pain |
| What were you doing when the problem or pain began? | Fell |
| How long ago did your knee symptoms begin? | 3 to 4 days |
| How did your knee symptoms begin? | Suddenly or quickly |
| Please select the best answer which most closely describes the pace of your knee problem. | My symptoms seem to be getting better but improvement is slow |
| Has your knee symptoms caused you to stop or reduce work, exercise, or other activities? | Yes |
| On a scale of 0 (no pain) to 10 (severe), how severe is your knee problems? | 5 to 6 moderate |
| What time of day does your knee problem occur? | No specific time of day |
| Do your knee problems improve with activity? | No |
| Are your knee problems made worse by walking, running or other movement? | Yes |
| Are your knee problems worse when at rest or not moved? | No |
| Does your knee swell? | Yes |
| Is your painful knee joint red? | No |
| Is the painful knee joint warm? | No |
| Is the painful knee joint tender when you touch it? | Yes |
| Is the skin of the knee draining or open? | No |
| Which best describes where your knee is tender? | On the outside of the knee |
| How long have you had knee pain? | 1 to 3 days |
| Which knee is painful? | Left knee |
| Which part of your knee hurts? | The part towards the outside |
| Does your painful knee joint creak or make a grating noise when you move it? | No |
| Does your painful knee joint lock when it is moved in certain ways? | No |
| Does your knee give way? | No |

| Interview Question | Click on the button labeled: |
|---|---|
| Are you able to completely bend and extend your knee? | Yes |
| Is the skin around your knee red, warm, swollen, tender, or draining fluid? | No |
| Have you noticed any lumps under the skin around your knee along with the pain? | No |
| Does your knee(s) seem to be enlarged or larger on one or both sides? | Yes |
| When do you have knee pain? | Only during activity |
| Does your knee pain become worse when climbing up stairs? | Yes |
| Does your knee pain become worse when going down stairs? | No |
| Is your knee pain worse when you are bearing weight on your legs? | Yes |
| Is your knee pain worse when you are kneeling? | Yes |
| Is your knee pain worse when you turn or twist on your leg with your foot planted? | Yes |
| What happens to your painful knee joint when you are active? | Joint pain become worse during use |
| Does your knee pain become worse if you actively move the knee joint (that is if you make the knee joint move as you would during activity but without any stress or pressure on the knee joint)? | No |
| Does your knee pain become worse if you move the knee joint passively (that is if you make the knee joint move by having someone else move it for you)? | No |
| Have you ever injured the knee joint that is now painful? | Yes |
| Have you ever had the knee joint that is now painful immobilized (motionless) for 3 days or more? | No |
| Did this episode of knee pain start at the same time as an injury to the knee? | Yes |
| Which best describes the way that you injured your knee? | I jumped or fell from a high place |
| Which best describes how quickly your knee pain has come on? | Suddenly and worsened quickly over hours |
| What time of day does your knee pain occur? | No specific time of day |
| How would you describe the pain you usually have in your knee? | Moderate |
| On a scale of 0 (no pain) to 10 (severe), how is your knee pain with walking on flat surfaces? | 5 to 6 (moderate) |
| On a scale of 0 (no pain) to 10 (severe), how is your knee pain with walking up stairs? | 7 to 8 (severe) |
| On a scale of 0 (no pain) to 10 (severe), how is your knee pain with walking up hills? | Skip this question |
| On a scale of 0 (no pain) to 10 (severe), how is your knee pain with walking down stairs? | 5 to 6 (moderate) |
| On a scale of 0 (no pain) to 10 (severe), how is your knee pain with walking down hills? | Skip this question |
| On a scale of 0 (no pain) to 10 (severe), how is your knee pain while running? | Skip this question |
| On a scale of 0 (no pain) to 10 (severe), how is your knee pain while kneeling? | 9 to 10 (unbearable) |
| On a scale of 0 (no pain) to 10 (severe), how is your knee pain sitting with knee straight? | 3 to 4 (mild) |

*(continued)*

| Interview Question | Click on the button labeled: |
|---|---|
| On a scale of 0 (no pain) to 10 (severe), how is your knee pain at night? | 3 to 4 (mild) |
| Do you have a skin rash? | No |
| Have you had any fever in the past 4 weeks? | No |
| Do you have discolored blood vessels or varicose veins in your skin? | No |
| Do you have tenderness, swelling, redness, or pain anywhere on your leg in addition to around your knee? | No |
| Do you have a new hard lump or mass anywhere on your leg? | No |
| Do you have pain from your back shooting down your leg? | No |
| Have you tried any treatments for your knee problem? | No |
| Do you have rheumatoid arthritis? | No |
| Do you have osteoarthritis also known as degenerative arthritis? | No |
| Has a doctor ever diagnose you as having bursitis? | No |
| Has a doctor or other health professional ever told you that you had back problems? | No |
| Have you ever broken a bone of your lower extremity (thigh, knee, calf, ankle etc.)? | No |
| Have you ever dislocated a joint of your lower extremity (hip, knee, ankle, foot, etc.)? | No |
| Have you ever had a problem with phlebitis? | No |
| Have you had knee surgery? | No |
| Have you ever had an injury to your knee ligaments, knee tendons, or knee cartilage problem? | No |
| Have you ever had an infection in your knee? | No |

### Step 8

When you have reached the end of the interview, a free-text note box is displayed to allow the patient to enter additional comments in his or her own words.

Type **I jumped off a loading dock at work**.

Locate and click on the Next button.

### Step 9

The final screen of the interview allows you to review your work.

Compare your screen to Figure 10-27 by scrolling the window as necessary. If there are any differences (other than the patient's age), repeat the exercise, making certain you answer each of the questions in steps 6 and 7 correctly.

### Step 10

At the bottom of the interview report screen are two buttons labeled "Print" and "Save." The Save button will export the report to a file with the extension RTF, which you may save on your computer. RTF files can be opened with any word processor.

When everything in your report is correct, locate and click on the appropriate button to either print or save to a file, as directed by your instructor. Once you have your printout in hand or RTF saved, you have completed Exercise 10F.

Close your browser and, if sufficient class time remains, proceed to Exercise 10G.

**Figure 10-27** Completed interview for Tomas Martiniz.

**Chief Complaint**
Tomas Martiniz is a 24 year old male. His reason for visit is "Knee Pain".

**History of Present Illness**

#1. "Knee Pain"

Location
He reported: Left knee joint pain. Tenderness on the outside of the knee. Pain towards the outside of the knee.

Quality
He reported: Knee larger than normal.
He denied: Knee unstable when stressed. Painful knee joint locks in certain positions. Back pain moves down the leg. Knee joint movement associated with grating noise. Lumps under the skin. Leg redness, swelling, or tenderness. New lump on leg. He reported: No limitation of range of motion of the knee.

Severity
He reported: Knee pain moderate. Knee pain moderate (5-6/10) walking on flat surfaces and walking down stairs. Knee pain mild (3-4/10) sitting with knee straight and at night. Knee problem slowly improving and moderate (5-6/10). Knee pain severe (7-8/10) walking up stairs. Knee pain unbearable (9-10/10) while kneeling.

Duration
He reported: Knee pain 1 to 3 days. Knee problem 3 to 4 days.

Timing
He reported: Knee pain occurs at no specific time of day. Knee problem started with a fall, started suddenly or quickly, and at no specific time of day. Knee pain began with injury. Knee pain starting suddenly and quickly worsening over hours.

Context
He reported: Knee pain only with movement.
He denied: Previous immobilization of painful knee joint.

Modifying Factors
He reported: Knee pain becomes worse during use. Knee pain worse when climbing stairs, bearing weight, kneeling, and twisting.
He denied: Knee pain worse when descending stairs. Knee problem improved with activity. Knee problem worsened by activity. Knee pain worsened by active motion. Knee pain worsened by passive motion.

Associated Signs and Symptoms
He reported: Knee swells and tender.
He denied: Knee red and warm.

**Past, Family, and Social History**

Past Medical History
He denied: Bursitis. Rheumatoid arthritis. Back pain. Inflamed blood vessel. Internal derangement of knee. Knee infection.

Surgical History
He denied: Knee surgery.

Accidents and Injuries
History of: Previous injury to painful knee joint. Knee injured by jumping from a high place.
He denied: Broken hip or leg. Lower extremity dislocation.

Social History
History of: Treatment for knee problem.

Activities for Daily Living
History of: Knee problem reduced activity.

**Review of Systems**

Constitutional
He denied: Fever in the last month.

Cardiovascular
He denied: Varicose veins.

Skin
He denied: Knee draining. Rash.

**Additional Comments**
I jumped off a loading dock at work

Save   Print   Next

## Guided Exercise 10G: Reviewing Patient-Entered Data

In the previous exercise, you learned how Instant Medical History guides the patient through a series of questions to gather symptom and history data. Once the data is reviewed, the data can be imported or merged directly into the EHR to become part of the encounter note. In this exercise you will merge the data Mr. Martiniz has entered into the encounter note.

### Case Study

Tomas Martiniz is a 24-year-old male who has an appointment May 26, 2016, at 9:00 AM. Tomas is an established patient who has used the Internet to complete his medical questionnaire on the clinic's portal. His data is ready to import into the EHR to initiate the encounter note for his visit.

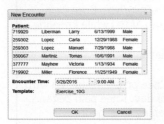

**Figure 10-28** Select patient Tomas Martiniz, set the date to 5/26/2016, and the time to 9:00 AM.

### Step 1

Start a supported web browser program and follow the steps listed inside the cover of this textbook to log in to the MyHealthProfessionsLab for this course.

Locate and click on the link Exercise 10G.

### Step 2

In the New Encounter window, locate and click on **Martiniz, Tomas**.

Set the date to **05/26/2016** and the time to **9:00 AM** as shown in Figure 10-28.

Verify the date and time are set correctly, and then click the OK button.

### Step 3

At check-in the patient informed the staff that last evening he completed the history and symptom questionnaire online using the patient portal. You will begin the encounter by retrieving the patient-entered data.

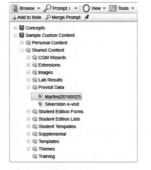

**Figure 10-29** Browse drop-down list with expanded trees, and Martiniz previsit interview selected.

Click the Browse button on the toolbar, and then expand the Sample Custom Content and Shared Content trees. Locate the folder **Previsit Data** and click the plus symbol to expand it. Locate and click on **Martiniz20160525** to highlight it (as shown in Figure 10-29) and then click the Add to Note button.

Compare the answers from the interview report you printed or saved in the previous exercise with the encounter note on your screen. Although the interview report contains the same data, its presentation is less verbose in the encounter note (exchanging "no" for "he denied" for example). Another difference is the organization of the data, which in the interview software places symptoms directly related to his problem in the History of Present Illness (HPI) section, while the Review of Systems section contains symptoms not related to his knee problem.

### Step 4

Notice that the online questionnaire did not ask about his personal habits. Locate and click the following Personal History findings until they turn blue and the descriptions change.

- tobacco use
- alcohol use

## Step 5

Enter the patient's vital signs in the corresponding fields of the encounter as follows:

Temperature:    **98.6**

Pulse:    **75**

Respiration:    **22**

SBP:    **117**

DBP:    **78**

Weight:    **154**

Height:    **68**

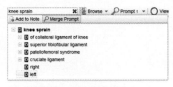

**Figure 10-30** Search results for knee sprain, "left" selected, and Merge Prompt button is highlighted.

## Step 6

Click in the Search box on the toolbar at the top of the screen.

Type **knee sprain** and press the Enter key on your keyboard.

The search function will return a drop-down list with the diagnosis knee sprain. Click the plus symbol next to it to expand the tree as shown in Figure 10-30.

In the expanded tree for knee sprain locate and click on **left** to highlight it and then click the Merge Prompt button at the top of the list.

Clinical concepts related to knee sprain will be added to your encounter pane.

## Step 7

Since the symptom findings for knee sprain merged from by the patient portal questionnaire are already in the HPI, you can proceed to the Physical Exam section. Scroll the encounter pane to locate the Physical Exam, Musculoskeletal Exam group. Locate and click on the following findings until they turn red:

- swelling of knee
- tenderness on palpitation of knee
- pain elicited by motion of knee

Proceed to the Assessment section and click on the following diagnosis until it turns red:

- sprained left knee

## Step 8

To be certain there is no further damage the clinician orders an x-ray. Proceed to the Tests to Order section. Locate and click on the following imaging study:

- x-ray of knee, oblique view, three or more views

Proceed to Therapy. Locate and click on the following findings:

- rest the extremity
- ice

Compare the Physical Exam, Assessment, Tests to Order, and Therapy sections of your encounter note to Figure 10-31. Also verify that you entered the vital signs correctly in step 5.

**Figure 10-31** Correctly completed Physical Exam, Assessment, Tests to Order, and Therapy sections.

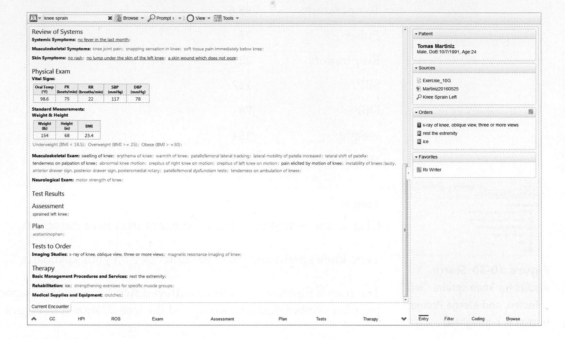

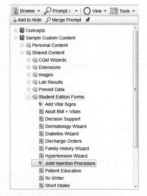

**Figure 10-32** Browse drop-down list with expanded trees and Joint Injection Procedure selected.

### Step 9

The clinician discusses the merits of a steroid and lidocaine injection and the patient consents. The clinician injects the left knee with 4 mL. Click in any white space of the encounter pane that does not highlight a heading or finding.

Click the Browse button on the toolbar, and then expand the Sample Custom Content, Shared Content, and Student Edition Forms trees. Locate the form **Joint Injection Procedure** (shown in Figure 10-32). Click on it to highlight it, and then click the Add to Note button.

Locate **Joint Injection Consent** in the Therapy section and click on the following finding until it turns red.

● Authorization given for joint injection

### Step 10

Locate the Summary block of text and click on the word **select**. A drop-down list will display. Click on **Left** in the drop-down list as shown in Figure 10-33.

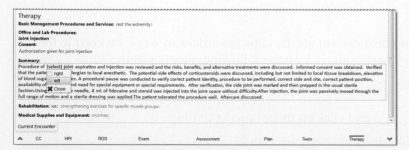

**Figure 10-33** Therapy section with Joint Injection Procedure and "select" drop-down list with "left" checked.

Next, click on the word "joint" and another drop-down list will display. Select **knee joint** from the drop-down list.

The summary text should now begin: "Procedure of left knee joint…"

### Step 11

Click the View button on the toolbar and select Concise from the drop-down menu. Compare your screen to Figure 10-34, scrolling as necessary until you have verified the entire encounter. If everything on your screen matches the figure, proceed to step 12. If there are any differences, review the preceding steps and correct your work.

**Figure 10-34** Concise view of correctly completed encounter for Tomas Martiniz.

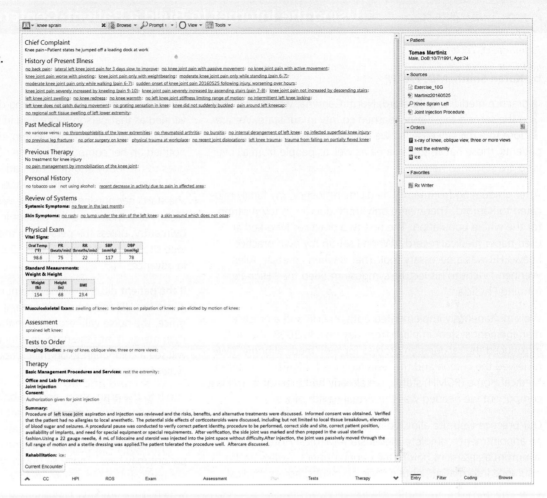

## Step 12

If wish to print a copy of your completed encounter notes for yourself or because your instructor requires you to turn them in, use the Create PDF option, and then print or download the PDF at this time.

The final step in every exercise is to submit your completed work for a grade.

Locate and click the blue Quippe icon button on the toolbar, and then select the Submit for Grade option from the drop-down menu. This will complete Exercise 10G.

## E-Visits

As we have seen from the previous exercises, patient data entered through a responsive and intelligent questionnaire provides a sound basis for gathering history and ROS needed for the encounter note. It also provides an excellent mechanism for E-visits. As described earlier, an E-visit allows the patient to be treated by a clinician for nonurgent health problems without the patient having to come into the office. E-visits may be conducted asynchronously or combined with a video teleconference.

by Karen Smith, MD, FAAFP

I practice medicine in Raeford, North Carolina, which is located in the second-most impoverished county in our state. We are close to a military base, so we have a culturally diverse mix of patients, those native to this area as well as people from all over who are stationed here.

After graduating from family medicine residency, my family relocated to Raeford. There were only three doctors in town caring for the whole population. The first two practices I worked at used paper medical records. When I set up my own practice I knew EHR was a necessary tool. That is when I met Dr. Allen Wenner. I went to his lecture symposium titled the "High-Performing Physician."

We simultaneously implemented both an EHR and a practice management system in place from day one. In 2008, the NCQA introduced the recognition process for the "medical home." We reviewed the criteria and the requirements for Patient-Centered Medical Home (PCMH) status; we already had most of it. The last component we needed was the virtual health office.

Our practice web site allows patients to register online, request an appointment, complete their Instant Medical History (IMH) symptom assessment before their appointment, review health insurance information, obtain their lab results, access medical information for common medical conditions, and have a virtual office visit with their doctor online.

Instant Medical History is readily accepted by our patients, especially military families. Because of a base realignment of the military, we have 30,000 new military personnel coming into our community and a lot of them have already registered online and completed their IMH before they come into the office.

## Workflow of Our Office

Our patients have several ways of contacting us; some call on the telephone and some just walk in. Our preferred first point of contact, however, is our web site. We automate a lot of our pre-visit activity. I have already mentioned they can complete the IMH symptom assessment over the Internet. We also have an automated system that telephones patients to remind them of their appointments. Once the Televox system has confirmed their appointment, one of my staff reviews their chart to see if their immunizations are up to date, if they have a balance due, or need anything else before their visit. In addition, we have now introduced a live operator system via the practice portal and Athena communicator, which is a very important combination of the web with a person who is familiar with the office systems.

When a patient shows up, existing demographic information is verified as that person is checked in on the computer. Once the patient is checked into the system, the nurse is automatically notified on her computer that the patient is checked in. She then goes to the lobby and gets the patient. She takes the patient's vital signs and then brings the patient into the exam room. There she starts her nursing intake. She will start the Instant Medical History and then leave the patient in the room to do his or her own entry, unless the person did the entry from home via our web site before coming. About 15 percent of our patients do it in advance.

If the patient did it at home, the nurse would extract it and bring it into the HPI section of the note. If the patient does it in the office, the nurse will return when that person is finished and then merge it into the note. In either case, when that is done I will see a color change on my computer and know that the patient is ready for me.

I go into the exam room and log on to the EHR. I have computers in every exam room, so I do not have to carry anything around. I have the patient elaborate a little more on the purpose of the visit. I perform the exam and go over any issues the patient may have. Then I sit down with that person so that we are both on the same level and can both see the computer screen. The computer is positioned where we can both see it at the same time and yet I can maintain eye-to-eye contact. My exam room computers are set up the way Dr. Wenner recommends (as shown in step ❸ of Figure 10-24) and it works well.

Many of my patients have hypertension or hyperlipidemia. By sharing the screen, the patient can actually see the objective information: "Here is your cholesterol and what you have been doing is working well." To get the patient to be compliant with the treatment plan, we put it in together. I am literally entering the orders in front of the patient as a way of emphasizing "I am putting this in the way we mutually agreed." When I have everything ordered, I look at the patient and ask, "Did we cover everything today, or is there anything else we need to take care of?" When the person answers no, then I close the encounter note. I stand up and we walk out the room together.

All of our office systems are interfaced. For example, if I had ordered labs when I wrote the order, the lab system automatically printed the labels and if an ABN (advanced beneficiary notice) is necessary, it printed out as well. Many times I will walk the patient to the lab and the phlebotomist already has the tubes ready. Because I use a bidirectional interface, the lab orders have already gone to the lab company.

When the patient is finished, he or she is taken to the front desk where my instructions to the patient, follow-up visit information, and a summary of today's visit are already prepared—all of this from the click of a button on the exam room computer. By the time the patient gets to the front desk to check out, he or she already has an appointment card ready for the next appointment, the billing information for the claim has gone into the billing system, the charges have been posted, and the patient due amount has been calculated and is ready for the front desk to collect, including any deductible that has not been met.

Even after the patient goes home, if he or she has a question about treatment, medication, or just forgot to ask something, the patient can go online to our web site and send me a secure message.

## Virtual Office Visits

We also offer patients the ability to use our web portal to have their office visit online instead of coming into the office. What we had to do was make it clear to the patient that "using the virtual office means the doctor is going to see and take care of your problems online; you do not need to physically present to the office." Our virtual office visit uses an interview question format similar to the IMH symptom assessment.

◆ The patient logs in and chooses Virtual Office Visit. The normal E-visit workflow is to collect the payment on the web site at the time of service.

◆ The patient confirms personal information and answers the health questions specific to the topic of the consultation, which normally takes about five minutes.

◆ Upon completion of their Virtual Office Visit, the system sends me a message.

◆ I log on and review the visit. I can see everything that the patient put in. I then create the response. I can reply with any further questions, but in most cases the online interview has gathered sufficient data. I also have access to my patient's medical history in the EHR. If I put in a prescription, it is sent to the pharmacy and adds information to the patient message that this is the patient's medication and the name of the drug store where it has been sent. Alternatively, I can say that the patient needs to come into the office in person.

◆ The patient then receives an e-mail notification from us. The confidential e-mail message does not disclose any information about the nature of the visit to our site. It simply asks the patient to return to our site for more information.

◆ Upon revisiting our site, the patient logs in and views the message from the physician. This message contains the treatment plan or a request for additional information. If the treatment plan involves prescription medications, the patient is given the pharmacy information.

In most cases, that completes the E-visit because very specific conditions and treatments can be done this way. Also, because these are my patients, I know what their health conditions are. I usually do not have to ask patients for further information and can close out the E-visit.

The utility of the E-visit occurring is very useful for our group. We promote the use of our web site everywhere, including our practice policies and patient care information sheets, but using the web portal and virtual office visits has been a learning curve in our community. I think in part this is because of the impoverishment in our county; only 30 percent of the households have Internet access within the home. I have noticed our military patients and their families use E-visits more than my other patients, but the Army has given the families computers and Internet access, so that may be a factor.

E-visits are conducted only for established patients, and only for routine conditions which are not likely to require an in-person physical examination. The American Academy of Family Physicians (AAFP) "defines an E-visit as an evaluation and management service provided by a physician or other qualified health professional to an established patient using a web-based or similar electronic-based communication network for a single patient encounter and offers the following guidelines for E-visits:

1. E-visits are available only to established patients who have previously received care from the physician's practice;

2. the patient initiates the process, and agrees to E-visit service terms, privacy policy, and charge for receiving asynchronous care from a physician or other qualified health professional;

3. electronic communication occurs over a HIPAA-compliant online connection;

4. an E-visit includes the total interchange of online inquiries and other communications associated with this single patient encounter;

5. the physician appropriately documents the E-visits, including all pertinent communication related to the encounter, in the patient's medical/health record;

6. the physician or other qualified health professional has a defined period of time within which responses to an E-visit request are completed; and

7. E-visits should be a payable physician service."[3]

Patients who are used to conducting banking, shopping, and bill paying transactions online embrace the speed and convenience of E-visits. In an independent study sponsored by Blue Shield of California, most patients and doctors in the study preferred a web visit to an office visit for nonurgent medical needs. Providers found that the E-visit gathered the important details and eliminated multiple messages back and forth that occur when trying to provide patient care via e-mail. The patients found that the time spent scheduling, driving, parking, and waiting was saved with an E-visit.[4]

Equally as important to the clinician, E-visits are reimbursed as a legitimate E&M visit. E-visits are covered by Blue Cross/Blue Shield™ plans, HMOs, and other private insurance carriers in numerous states. However, at the time that this book was published Medicare limited reimbursement for E-visits to patients living in areas designated as a Health Professional Shortage Area and required the E-visit include a face-to-face video session except in Alaska and Hawaii, where Medicare permits asynchronous E-visits.

## Mayo Clinic Study of E-visits

The largest study of Internet use for online care (E-visits) using a structured history was conducted in the Department of Family Medicine at Mayo Clinic in Rochester, Minnesota. Here are excerpts from the study.[5]

"Patients in the department preregistered for the service and then were able to use the online portal for consultations with their primary care providers.

"After completing (data entry for) the E-visit, the patients received an e-mail stating that their clinician would review their consultation within 24 hours. Another e-mail was forwarded to the clinician informing him or her of an E-visit waiting in the secure portal.

"The portal allowed the clinician to use templated encounter forms for many common illnesses so that information such as diagnostic codes, links to patient education, and treatment plans could be stored and reused. This standardization of treatment greatly speeded the process of reviewing an online visit. Medications were often prescribed during the process and faxed to the pharmacy. At the conclusion of the online visit, patients received an e-mail stating that the results of their encounter could be found on the portal. Patients would then log in and view the materials.

"Generally, online consultations were completed by clinicians within 24 hours of the E-visit submission; only 11 were not completed. E-visits were completed by the patient's primary provider 89% of the time; 11% of the consultations were provided by an on-call clinician for absent providers or if the patient selected 'first available doctor.'

"Because patients could enter any symptom or concern, ask questions, and add additional comments, the E-visits eliminated the need for clinicians to ask for further information in most instances. This was because the patient's history was organized and pertinent information including all medications, allergies, and vital signs such as weight

---

[3]http://aafp.org/about/policies/all/E-visits.html, January 1, 2016.

[4]Relay Health webVisit Study: Final Report, www.relayhealth.com © 2002–2003 RelayHealth Corporation.

[5]M. D. Adamson, C. Steven, M. D. Bachman, and W. John, *Pilot Study of Providing Online Care in a Primary Care Setting* (Rochester, MN: Department of Family Medicine, Mayo Clinic, 2010).

were always obtained. The volume of exchanges could be decreased further by emphasizing the need to send pictures of rashes. . . .

"Some consultations for patients with chronic disease seemed to show promise. Patients with diabetes mellitus first had laboratory tests and then were asked to complete an online visit regarding their diabetes. If all was well according to the interview and laboratory results, the patients did not need to visit the office. Hypertension was also managed online; patients sent in their blood pressure responses and clinicians managed their medications and laboratory studies online.

"During the 2-year study, 4,282 patients were registered for the service. Patients made 2,531 online visits, and billings were made for 1,159 patients. E-visits were made primarily by working-aged women who completed E-visits for themselves, their dependents, and their older parents during office hours and involved 294 different conditions. Two percent of the visits included uploaded photographs, and 16% of the E-visits replaced nonbillable telephone protocols with billable encounters. The E-visits made office visits unnecessary in 40% of cases; in 12.8% of cases, the patient was asked to schedule an appointment for a face-to-face encounter.

"The study showed the feasibility of online visits to educate, treat, and bill patients. The extent of conditions possible for treatment by online care was far ranging and was managed with a minimum of message exchanges by using structured histories."

## E-Visits in Practice

Two examples of other organizations with experience in E-visits are the University of Pittsburgh Medical Center (UPMC) and the University of Wisconsin (UW).

UPMC health system has been offering E-visits since 2009. The UMPC E-visit combines an online questionnaire in which patients enter data, followed up by an online video telehealth consultation.

UW Health and Unity Health Insurance, both affiliated with the University of Wisconsin, offer members asynchronous E-visits, some of which require patient prepay with a credit card at the start of the E-visit, depending on the patient's insurance plan. The patient completes the online questionnaire and a provider responds within two hours.

In either type of E-visit, the clinician may determine that the patient needs to be seen in person and will ask the patient to come in. When this occurs, generally there is no charge for the E-visit.

## Workflow of an E-Visit

The basic workflow of an E-visit begins with patient-entered symptom, history, and history of present illness information. Some E-visit web sites use Instant Medical History to gather HPI data from the patient. Other E-visit web sites use a combination of check boxes and free-text messages, similar to the secure messaging discussed earlier. Some E-visit web sites such as the one at the Mayo Clinic allow the patient to upload digital photos.

The workflow begins when a patient accesses his or her physician's web site and signs on. The patient must already be an established patient with the practice and have medical records on file. E-visits are not permitted for a new patient who has never been seen at the practice.

The patient's insurance plan information on file is accessed to determine if a copay is required and the amount (if any). If payment is required, credit card information is entered and processed.

The patient selects the reason for the visit from a list of the type of problems the practice will handle as E-visits. This allows the portal software to determine which question sets would be appropriate to ask.

The patient answers online interview questions related to his or her reported complaint, as shown later in Exercise 10H. Answers to certain medically significant questions could cause the software to ask different sets of medically related questions automatically. On some portals the patient can add free-text clarification at various points in the interview.

E-visits are only used for nonurgent visits. If the software detects that the condition seems urgent, the patient is advised to seek immediate medical care and the provider is notified. If the software determines that although the condition is not urgent, it is one for which the patient should be seen in person, the patient is given a message to that effect and automatically offered a choice of available appointments.

When the interview is complete, the data entered by the patient is stored and the clinician is notified that an E-visit is ready to review. Even if the clinician determines that the patient must come in person, the patient is better served because the symptom and history information is already complete.

The clinician reviews the patient-entered data, reviews any relevant patient medical records, and replies to the patient. The system allows the provider and patient to continue to exchange messages, much as a question-and-answer session in the exam room, except for the factor of time, which is sometimes delayed by one or both parties' responses.

The clinician also can prescribe electronically during the E-visit, just as he or she would during an office visit. When the patient receives the clinician's reply to the E-visit, that patient is prompted to select a preferred pharmacy from a list (if it is not already known to the EHR) and the prescription is electronically transmitted to the pharmacy by the doctor's system.

The doctor's response also can include patient education material and comments or care instructions from the doctor, all of which are recorded in the care plan. The doctor's practice management system can verify the patient eligibility for the E-visit, and submit the claim electronically.

## Guided Exercise 10H: Patient Requests an E-Visit

This exercise utilizes an IMH questionnaire, similar to Exercise 10F. Again in this exercise, you will first take on the role of a patient requesting an E-visit. Once you have finished, you will proceed to the next exercise where you will take on the role of the clinician who completes the E-visit.

Reminder: In step 5 you will enter your own name or student ID, which will be used to identify your work to your instructor.

### Case Study

Jacob Silverstein is a 46-year-old male with a history of hypertension and diabetes. He is on medication and has regular check-ups at his family practice. He has an issue with his medication and is going to try an online E-visit instead of coming to the office.

### Step 1

Start a supported web browser program and follow the steps listed inside the cover of this textbook to log in to the MyHealthProfessionsLab for this course.

Locate and click on the link Exercise 10H.

### Step 2

The sample provider web portal shown previously in Figure 10-22 will be displayed.

### Step 3

Locate the section labeled "E-visits for Established Patients" and click on the E-visit link.

### Step 4

The "Welcome to Family Care E-visit" web page shown in Figure 10-35 will be displayed. It includes simulated payment information in section 1 of the page. A key difference between an E-visit and a pre-visit questionnaire is that providers collect copay at the time of the E-visit. It is not necessary to collect the copay on the pre-visit questionnaire page, as the patient will be coming into the office, where the payment will be collected.

**Figure 10-35** Family Care portal E-visit page, with copay section and Start Interview button.

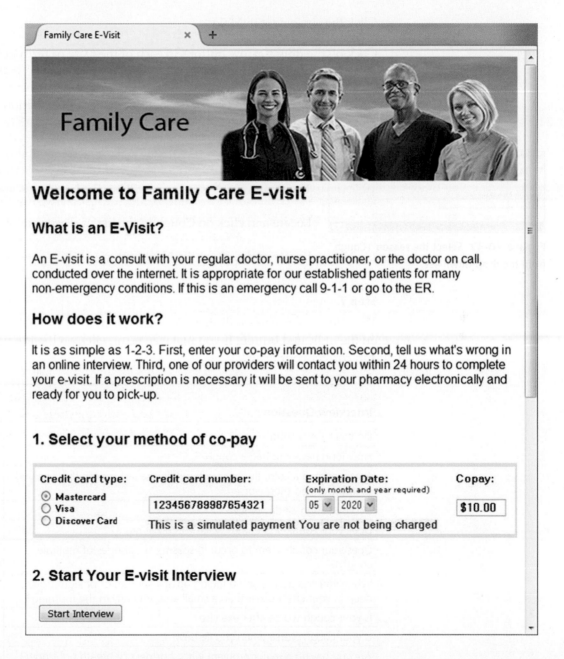

This is a student exercise; you will not be charged. Do not enter any personal credit card data; simply locate and click on the Start Interview button in section 2.

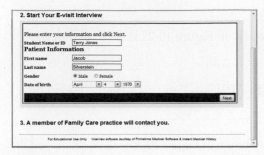

**Figure 10-36** Patient Interview screen for E-visit.

The center portion of your web page will open the student ID and patient information fields shown in Figure 10-36.

**Step 5**

Enter the following:

Enter your name or student ID as you did in the previous exercise.

Enter the following information about the patient:

First Name: **Jacob**

Last Name: **Silverstein**

Click the circle next to **Male**

Click on the down-arrow buttons in each of the Date of Birth fields and select **April, 4**, and **1970** from the drop-down lists.

Compare your screen to Figure 10-36. If the patient information has been entered correctly, locate and click on the Next button.

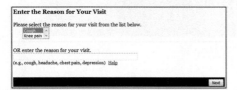

**Figure 10-37** Select the reason "Cough" from the drop-down list.

**Step 6**

The Reason for Visit screen will be displayed.

Locate and click on Cough in the list of reasons as shown in Figure 10-37.

Locate and click on the Next button.

**Step 7**

The interview process will start. For each question in the table below, locate and click on the indicated button. If you make an error, click on the Previous Question button and correct your error.

| Interview Question | Click on the following buttons |
|---|---|
| Do you have a cough? | Yes |
| How long have you had a cough? | 16 – 20 days |
| Have you had a cold, flu, or cough within the last month that seemed to improve and then worsen? | No |
| Do you cough all day long? | Yes |
| Does your cough sometimes wake you up at night? | No |
| Does your cough seem to occur in spasms or episodes of multiple coughs? | No |
| When you cough, are you bringing up any sputum or phlegm from deep in your chest other than a small amount early in the morning? | No |
| Is your cough worse after exercise? | No |
| Is your cough worse when you lie down? | No |
| Are you having a major problem with shortness of breath right now? | No |
| Do you have chest discomfort when you breathe? | No |

| Interview Question | Click on the following buttons |
|---|---|
| Do you have any wheezing when you breathe? | No |
| Do you sound hoarse? | No |
| Do you have post-nasal drip or are you always clearing the back of your throat? | No |
| Have you had a fever in the past week? | No |
| Do you sometimes wake up with soaking sweats at night? | No |
| Did your cough begin after any change in your medications? | Yes |
| Do you have a cough at certain seasons of the year? | No |
| Have you ever had pneumonia? | No |
| Have you ever kept or raised birds? | No |
| Describe your use of tobacco | Never used |

**Step 8**

When you have reached the end of the interview, a free-text note box is displayed to allow patients to enter messages in their own words. Leave the box empty. Locate and click on the Next button.

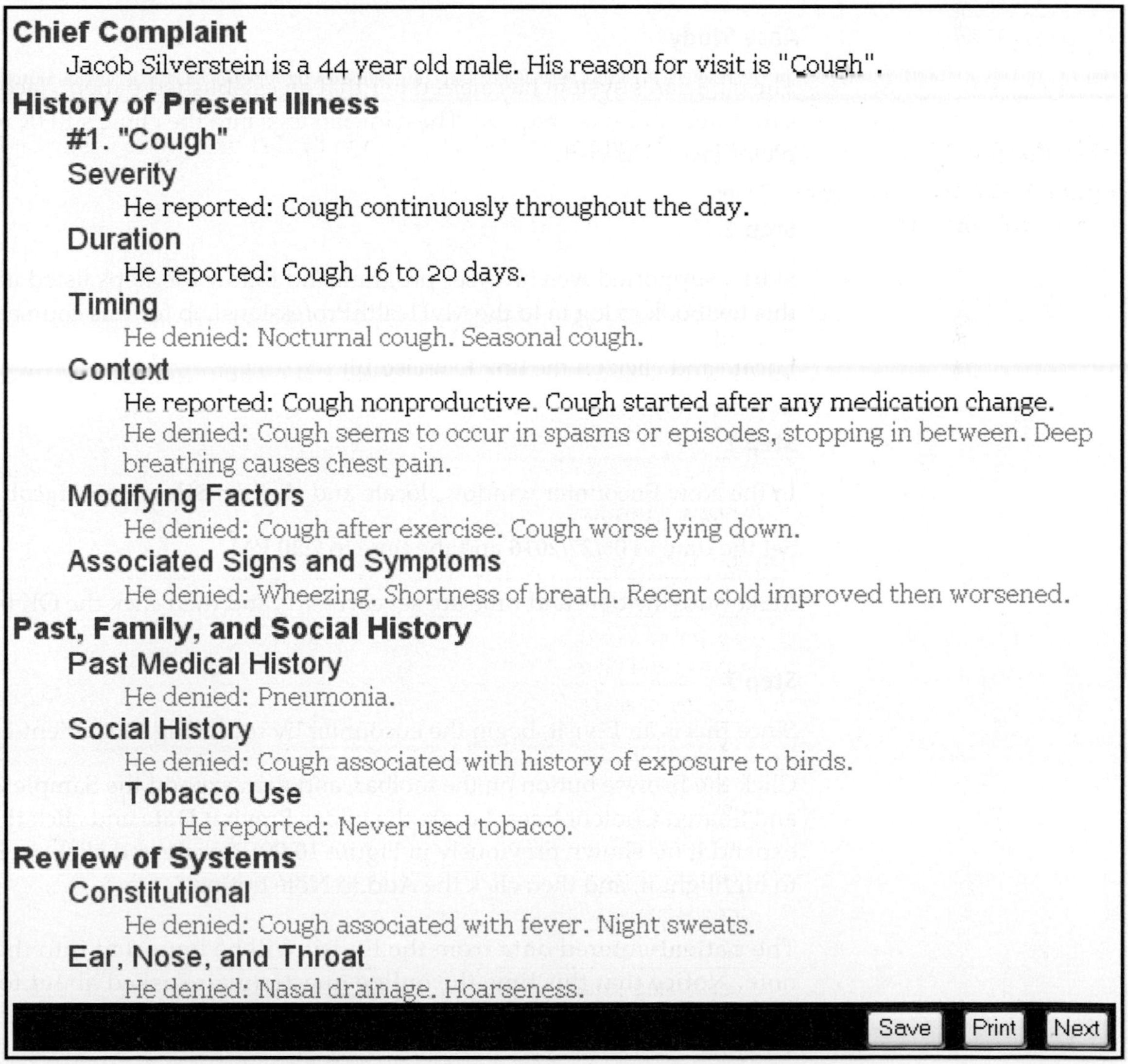

**Figure 10-38**
Correctly completed interview for E-visit.

## Chief Complaint
Jacob Silverstein is a 44 year old male. His reason for visit is "Cough".

## History of Present Illness
### #1. "Cough"
### Severity
He reported: Cough continuously throughout the day.
### Duration
He reported: Cough 16 to 20 days.
### Timing
He denied: Nocturnal cough. Seasonal cough.
### Context
He reported: Cough nonproductive. Cough started after any medication change.
He denied: Cough seems to occur in spasms or episodes, stopping in between. Deep breathing causes chest pain.
### Modifying Factors
He denied: Cough after exercise. Cough worse lying down.
### Associated Signs and Symptoms
He denied: Wheezing. Shortness of breath. Recent cold improved then worsened.

## Past, Family, and Social History
### Past Medical History
He denied: Pneumonia.
### Social History
He denied: Cough associated with history of exposure to birds.
### Tobacco Use
He reported: Never used tobacco.

## Review of Systems
### Constitutional
He denied: Cough associated with fever. Night sweats.
### Ear, Nose, and Throat
He denied: Nasal drainage. Hoarseness.

Save | Print | Next

### Step 9

The final screen of the interview allows you to review your work.

Compare your screen to Figure 10-38 by scrolling the window as necessary. If there are any differences (other than the patient's age), repeat the exercise, making certain you answer each of the questions in steps 6 through 8 correctly.

### Step 10

At the bottom of the Interview Report screen are two buttons labeled "Print" and "Save."

When everything in your report is correct, locate and click on the appropriate button to either print or save a RTF file, as directed by your instructor. Once you have your printout in hand or output file saved, close your browser and proceed to Exercise 10J.

## Critical Thinking Exercise 10J: Clinician Completes the E-Visit

In this exercise, you will take on the role of the clinician, reviewing and completing a patient's E-visit.

### Case Study

The clinician's system has alerted her that an established patient, Jacob Silverstein, has submitted an E-visit request. The clinician logs into the clinic's EHR remotely and completes Jacob's E-visit.

### Step 1

Start a supported web browser program and follow the steps listed inside the cover of this textbook to log in to the MyHealthProfessionsLab for this course.

Locate and click on the link Exercise 10J.

### Step 2

In the New Encounter window, locate and click on **Silverstein, Jacob**.

Set the date to **05/27/2016** and the time to **7:30 PM**.

Make sure the date and time are set correctly, and then click the OK button.

### Step 3

Since this is an E-visit, begin the encounter by retrieving the patient-entered data.

Click the Browse button on the toolbar, and then expand the Sample Custom Content and Shared Content trees. Locate the folder **Previsit Data** and click the plus symbol to expand it (as shown previously in Figure 10-29). Locate and click on **Silverstein E-visit** to highlight it, and then click the Add to Note button.

The patient-entered data from the E-visit will be imported into the encounter note. Notice that this time the online questionnaire asked about tobacco use and a change in medications, so these history items are included in the appropriate sections.

**Step 4**

The clinician wants to review Mr. Silverstein's medications. Locate the **5/11/2016** tab at the bottom of the encounter pane, and click on it.

When the 5/11/2016 note is displayed, click on the heading Current Medications and select **Copy into current note** from the drop-down menu.

Click on the **Current Encounter** tab.

**Step 5**

The clinician notes that Jacob is on lisinopril for his hypertension. Lisinopril is in a class of drugs called ACE inhibitors. ACE is an acronym for angiotensin converting-enzyme. A persistent dry cough is a well-known side-effect of ACE inhibitors.

The clinician decides to change Jacob's prescription.

Locate Current Medications and *right-click* on **lisinopril**. Select Details from the Actions drop-down menu. When the Details pop-up window opens, click the down-arrow on the prefix field and select **discontinue**. Click OK to close the Details window.

**Step 6**

Click in the Search box on the toolbar, type **adverse effect of ACE**, and press the Enter key on your keyboard.

In the search results list locate and click on **adverse effect of angiotensin-converting-enzyme** to highlight it. Click the Add to Note button.

Proceed to the Assessment section and click the finding until it turns red.

- adverse effect of angiotensin-converting-enzyme

**Step 7**

Locate Favorites in the content pane on the right, and *double-click* on the Rx Writer.

When the Rx Writer window opens, click on the Drug field, and select **Amlodipine maleate**.

Select the dosage 10 milligram tab from the drop-down list

Complete the prescription by entering the following information in the remaining fields:

| | |
|---|---|
| Quantity: | **1** |
| Unit: | **tab** |
| Interval: | **once a day** |
| Days: | **30** |
| Route: | **by mouth** |
| Dispense: | **30** |
| Refills: | **3** |
| Generic: | **Yes** |

Verify that everything is entered correctly, and then click the OK button.

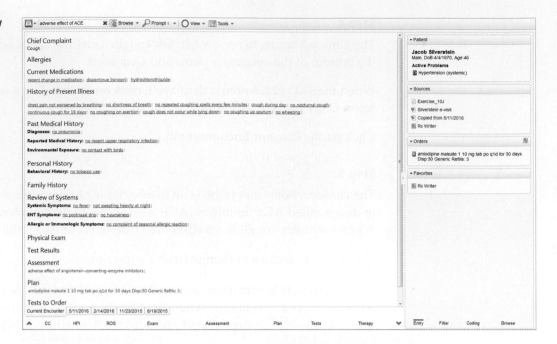

**Step 8**

Click the View button on the toolbar and select Concise from the drop-down menu. Compare your screen to Figure 10-39. If there are any differences, review the preceding steps and correct your work.

**Step 9**

At this point, the clinician's system will e-mail the patient to return to the portal for a message. Once he logs into the portal a message will inform Mr. Silverstein to discontinue his current medication and that a prescription for a new medication has been sent to his pharmacy. The patient, who has access to his records through the portal, will also be able to view a clinical summary of the E-visit.

**Step 10**

If you wish to print a copy of your completed encounter notes for yourself or because your instructor requires you to turn them in, use the Create PDF option, and then print or download the PDF at this time.

The final step in every exercise is to submit your completed work for a grade.

Locate and click the blue Quippe icon button on the toolbar, and then select the Submit for Grade option from the drop-down menu. This will complete Exercise 10J.

## Patient Access to Electronic Health Records

HIPAA (which we will cover in the next chapter) guarantees patients' rights to obtain copies of their health records. The HITECH Act goes further. As we discussed in Chapter 1, CMS criteria include:

◆ Providing patients with timely electronic access to their health information (including lab results, problem list, medication lists, allergies, and so on) within 96 hours of the information being available to the provider.

- Providing patients with an electronic copy of their health information upon request.

- Providing inpatients with an electronic copy of their discharge instructions and procedures at time of discharge, upon request.

- Sending reminders to patients per patient preference for preventive/follow-up care.

The number of medical offices with interactive web sites is growing. Practice portal web sites provide a secure means of communication, as demonstrated in this chapter's exercises. In addition, portal web sites allow the patient to request an appointment time, prescription renewals, and E-visits. Portals that provide secure access to results of recent lab tests, clinical visit summaries, and other information in the patient record help to further engage the patient in their own healthcare. A web site maintained by the patient's provider also provides a source of reliable patient education materials that promote health and well-being.

## Chapter Ten Summary

The Internet is one of the key technologies impacting healthcare. It not only gives the provider instant access to medical research and medical libraries for decision support, but allows the provider to engage the patient with web portals. Practice portals are secure web sites, where patients can see their medical information and consult with their doctor using secure messaging.

Patients research their conditions using the Internet and bring the information with them to their office visits. A medical practice web portal can provide links to reliable, credible patient education information.

The Internet is really a large network of networked computers, which is sometimes referred to as a "cloud." Personally identifiable health information that is sent over the Internet needs to be secured.

SSL is used to secure data exchanged via web pages such as the practice web portal. Remote provider access to the EHR via the Internet usually involves setting up a VPN.

Telemedicine provides specialist consultation to patients in remote locations and home care nurses to teleconference with their clients. Teleradiology allows a radiologist to interpret diagnostic images from another location.

One feature of practice portals is the ability for patients to use the Internet to enter information about their history and symptoms before arriving at a scheduled appointment.

Numerous studies have shown that patient data can become a significant contributor to the EHR, for some of the following reasons:

- Only the patient has the information about what symptoms were present at the outset of the illness.

- Only the patient knows the outcome of medical treatment of those symptoms.

- The patient is also the source of past medical, family, and social history.

- Patient-entered data is a more accurate reflection of a patient's complaints.

- Patients who can review their histories are better prepared for the visit.

- Up to 67 percent of the nurse or clinician's time with the patient is spent entering the patient's symptom into the visit documentation.

- A computer can be used by the patient over the Internet or in the waiting room to enter the same symptom and history information that the nurse or clinician would have entered.

- Patient-entered data is organized by the computer for the provider in a succinct and easy-to-read format that becomes the starting point for the encounter.

- Having a complete history in advance of the visit allows the clinician to ask fewer questions about the diagnosis and concentrate more on the effects of the illness on the patient. It also allows the clinician more time to discuss the treatment plan with the patient.

Other features found on practice web sites allow patients to request an appointment time or a prescription renewal, provide secure access to information from their medical record, and securely communicate with their doctor. HIPAA guarantees patients' right to obtain copies of their health records, and the HITECH Act criteria include providing patients with electronic access to their health information within 96 hours, and sending e-mail reminders about preventive and follow-up care.

Some practices offer E-visits, which allows patients to be treated online for nonurgent health problems without having to come into the office. The E-visit gathers symptom and history information and creates a documented encounter. It can be integrated into the EHR to become part of patients' charts, and, equally important to the clinician, E-visits are reimbursed as legitimate E&M visits by private payers (and by Medicare in areas with physician shortages).

## Testing Your Knowledge of Chapter 10

### Step 1

Login to MyHealthProfessionsLab following the directions printed inside the cover of this textbook.

Locate and click on Chapter 10 Test.

### Step 2

Answer the test questions. When you have finished, click the Submit Test button to close the window.

## Testing Your Skills Exercise 10K: A Patient with Hepatitis A

Now that you have performed all the exercises in Chapter 10 this exercise will help you and your instructor evaluate your acquired skills. Use the information in the case study and the features of the software you already know to document the patient's encounter.

### Case Study

Taylor Scott is a 20-year-old male who just returned from a trip to Africa. His chief complaint is abdominal pain, nausea, and jaundice. He tells the clinician he has lost his appetite and has been puking a lot. He thinks he might have eaten bad shellfish while he was there.

Taylor has no allergies, doesn't use tobacco or alcohol, but was never vaccinated for hepatitis, because his parents didn't believe in immunizations.

The clinician observers a generalized yellowish discoloration of skin, and asks Taylor if his abdominal symptoms are in the upper right quadrant. Taylor says yes. The clinician selects the Decision Support form and reviews the CDC document for Hepatitis.

Here are Taylor's vital signs:

| | |
|---|---|
| Temperature: | 102 |
| Pulse: | 70 |
| Respiration: | 20 |
| SBP: | 118 |
| DBP: | 76 |
| Weight: | 150 |
| Height: | 72 |

The clinician performs an abdominal exam and observes abdominal tenderness in the right upper quadrant, as well as an enlarged, tender, liver. He also documents Taylor's skin color.

The clinician refers back to the decision support document, and locates (in the column for Hepatitis A) the correct serum test to order. After ordering the test, the clinician records the assessment, and then locates and reviews patient education documents with the patient, who indicates that he understands.

### Step 1

Start a supported web browser program and follow the steps listed inside the cover of this textbook to log in to the MyHealthProfessionsLab for this course.

Locate and click on the link **Exercise 10K**. This will open the Quippe software window with the New Encounter window displayed in the center.

### Step 2

Locate and click on the patient name, and then click the OK button. In this exercise, you do not need to set the date or time of the encounter.

Read the case study *carefully*.

### Step 3

Hint: Open and read the decision support document before you add any findings. You can check the review box and close the form, but do not close the tab or window displaying the CDC document. The document gives the three-letter acronym for the virus that causes hepatitis A. Use the acronym to search in Quippe. When the search results display, click on the diagnosis description and Merge Prompt button.

Use the case study information above to record vital signs and other findings. Hint: After recording travel, click the Browse button to locate the country and add it to the note.

Once you have documented all the information provided in the case study, proceed to step 4.

### Step 4

If wish to print a copy of your completed encounter notes for yourself or because your instructor requires you to turn them in, use the Create PDF option, and then print or download the PDF at this time.

Submit your completed work for a grade. This will complete Exercise 10K.

# Privacy and Security of Health Records

## Learning Outcomes

*After completing this chapter, you should be able to:*

◆ List HIPAA transactions and uniform identifiers

◆ Understand HIPAA privacy and security concepts

◆ Apply HIPAA privacy policy in a medical facility

◆ Describe HIPAA security requirements and safeguards

◆ Discuss the importance of contingency plans

◆ Follow security policy guidelines in a medical facility

◆ Explain electronic signatures

## Understanding HIPAA

In Chapter 10 we discussed various ways the Internet is being used for healthcare, including patient access to their records through a web portal and remote access for providers using VPN or similar secure encryption. In Chapter 12 we will explore the relationship of the EHR data to the determination of codes required for medical billing. Between those topics it is prudent to understand HIPAA. HIPAA is an acronym for the Health Insurance Portability and Accountability Act, passed by Congress in 1996.

The HIPAA law was intended to:

◆ Improve portability and continuity of health insurance coverage

◆ Combat waste, fraud, and abuse in health insurance and healthcare delivery

◆ Promote use of medical savings accounts

◆ Improve access to long-term care

◆ Simplify administration of health insurance

HIPAA law regulates many things. However, a portion known as the Administrative Simplification Subsection[1] of HIPAA covers entities such as health plans, clearing-houses, and healthcare providers. HIPAA refers to these as *covered entities* or a *covered entity*. This means a healthcare facility or health plan and all of its employees. If you work in the healthcare field, these regulations likely govern your job and behavior. Therefore, it is not uncommon for healthcare workers to use the acronym HIPAA when they actually mean only the Administrative Simplification Subsection of HIPAA.

As someone who will work with patients' health records, it is especially important for you to understand the regulations regarding privacy and security. However, let us begin with a quick review of HIPAA, then study the privacy and security portions in more depth.

HIPAA implementation and enforcement is under the jurisdiction of several entities within the U.S. Department of Health and Human Services (HHS). This chapter will make extensive use of documents prepared by HHS.

## Administrative Simplification Subsection

The Administrative Simplification Subsection has four distinct components:

1. Transactions and code sets
2. Uniform identifiers
3. Privacy
4. Security

## HIPAA Transactions and Code Sets

The first section of the regulations to be implemented governed the electronic transfer of medical information for business purposes such as insurance claims, payments, and eligibility. When information is exchanged electronically, both sides of the transaction must agree to use the same format in order to make the information intelligible to the receiving system. Before HIPAA, transactions for nearly every insurance plan used a format that contained variations that made it different from another plan's format. This meant that plans could not easily exchange or forward claims to secondary payers and that most providers could only transmit electronically to a few plans.

### HIPAA Transactions

HIPAA standardized these formats by requiring specific transaction standards for nine types of EDI or Electronic Data Interchange. One additional transaction named in the rule has not been finalized. The Affordable Care Act (ACA), passed in 2010, also included Administrative Simplification provisions,[2] which expanded, or revised, several HIPAA provisions. The HIPAA transactions are:

1. Claims or Equivalent Encounters and Coordination of Benefits (COB)
2. Claim Payment and Remittance Advice

---

[1]Health Insurance Portability and Accountability Act, Title 2, subsection f.
[2]Administrative Simplification Provisions, Affordable Care Act of 2010, Sections 1104 and 10109.

3. Claims Status

4. Eligibility and Benefit Inquiry and Response

5. Referral Certification and Authorization

6. Premium Payments

7. Enrollment and De-enrollment in a Health Plan

8. Retail Drug Claims, Coordination of Drug Benefits, and Eligibility Inquiry

9. Health Claims Attachments

10. First Report of Injury (Not Implemented)

ACA added a requirement for electronic funds transfer (EFT) standards to be used in conjunction with claim payment/remittance advice transactions.

## Standard Code Sets

In an EDI transaction, certain portions of the information are sent as codes. For the receiving entity to understand the content of the transaction, both the sender and the receiver must use the same codes. In most cases, these are not the nomenclature codes discussed in Chapter 2, but rather standardized codes used to effectively communicate demographic and billing information.

For example, in an insurance claim, services and patient visits are identified by procedure codes instead of their long descriptions. The medical reasons for the procedure are sent in the claim as diagnosis codes. HIPAA requires the use of standard sets of codes. Two of those standards are:

◆ CPT-4 and HCPCS (Procedure codes)

◆ ICD10-CM (Diagnoses codes)

ICD10-CM, CPT-4, and HCPCS codes will be discussed in Chapter 12.

There are additional codes sets for demographic and payment information. Under HIPAA, any coded information within a transaction is also subject to standards. Just a few examples of the hundreds of other codes include codes for sex, race, type of provider, and relation of the policyholder to the patient.

## HIPAA Uniform Identifiers

You can see the importance of both the sending and receiving system using the same formats and code sets to report exactly what was done for the patient. Similarly, it is necessary for multiple systems to identify the providers and healthcare businesses sending the claim or receiving the payment. ID numbers are used in computer processing instead of names because, for example, there could be many providers named John Smith.

However, before HIPAA, all providers had multiple ID numbers assigned to them for use on insurance claims, prescriptions, and so on. A provider typically received a different ID from each plan and sometimes multiple numbers from the same plan. This created a problem for the billing office to get the right ID on the right claim and made electronic coordination of benefits all but impossible.

HIPAA established uniform identifier standards to be used on all claims and other data transmissions. These include the following:

◆ **National Provider Identifier** This type of identifier is assigned to doctors, nurse practitioners, and other healthcare providers.

◆ **Employer Identifier** This identifier is used to identify employer-sponsored health insurance. It is the same as the federal Employer Identification Number (EIN) that employers are assigned for their taxes by the Internal Revenue Service.

◆ **National Health Plan Identifier** This is a unique identification number assigned to each insurance plan. Implementation of the rule requiring its use in HIPAA transactions has been delayed.[3]

## HIPAA Privacy Rule

### NOTE

### PHI

HIPAA privacy rules frequently refer to PHI or Protected Health Information. PHI is the patient's individually identifiable health information.

The HIPAA Privacy Rule establishes standards for the protection of **personally identifiable health information**, called **PHI**, held by covered entities and their business associates and gives patients important rights with respect to their health information. Additionally, the Privacy Rule permits the use and disclosure of health information needed for patient care and other important purposes.

The Privacy Rule protects PHI held or transmitted by a covered entity or its business associate, in any form, whether electronic, paper, or verbal. PHI includes information that relates to the following:

◆ The individual's past, present, or future physical or mental health or condition;

◆ The provision of health care to the individual;

◆ The past, present, or future payment for the provision of health care to the individual.

PHI includes many common identifiers, such as name, address, birth date, and Social Security Number.[4]

When the HIPAA legislation was passed, "Congress recognized that advances in electronic technology could erode the privacy of health information. Consequently, Congress incorporated into HIPAA provisions that mandated the adoption of Federal privacy protections for individually identifiable health information."[5]

The Privacy Rule established, for the first time, a foundation of federal protections for the privacy of protected health information. "The Rule does not replace federal, state, or other law that grants individuals even greater privacy protections, and covered entities are free to retain or adopt more protective policies or practices."[6]

The 2013 Omnibus HIPAA final rule[7] enhanced patient privacy protections, provided patients new rights to their health information, and strengthened the government's ability to enforce the law. The 2013 HIPAA rule:

---

[3]https://www.cms.gov/regulations-and-guidance/hipaa-administrative-simplification/affordable-care-act/health-plan-identifier.html, December 17, 2015.
[4]HIPAA Basics for Providers: Privacy, Security, and Breach Notification Rules, publication ICN 909001, May 2015, The Medicare Learning Network®, U.S. Department of Health & Human Services.
[5]*Guidance on HIPAA Standards for Privacy of Individually Identifiable Health Information* (Washington, DC: U.S. Department of Health and Human Services Office for Civil Rights, December 3, 2002, and revised April 3, 2003).
[6]*Ibid.*
[7]Omnibus HIPAA final rule, 45 CFR Parts 160 and 164, Federal Register, January 25, 2013.

- Allows patients to ask for a copy of their electronic medical record in an electronic form;

- Allows patients to instruct their provider not to share information about their treatment with their health plan when they pay by cash;

- Reduces burden by streamlining individuals' abilities to authorize the use of their health information for research purposes;

- Clarifies that genetic information is protected under the HIPAA Privacy Rule and prohibits most health plans from using or disclosing genetic information for underwriting purposes.

To comply with HIPAA law, privacy activities in the average medical facility might include the following:

- Providing a copy of the office privacy policy informing patients about their privacy rights and how their information can be used.

- Asking the patient to acknowledge receiving a copy of the policy or signing a consent form.

- Obtaining signed authorization forms and in some cases tracking the disclosures of patient health information when it is to be given to a person or organization outside the practice for purposes other than treatment, billing, or payment purposes.

- Adopting clear privacy procedures for its practice.

- Training employees so that they understand the privacy procedures.

- Designating an individual to be responsible for seeing that the privacy procedures are adopted and followed.

- Securing patient records containing individually identifiable health information so that they are not readily available to those who do not need them.

Let us examine each of these points.

## Privacy Policy

"The HIPAA Privacy Rule gives individuals a fundamental new right to be informed of the privacy practices of their health plans and of most of their healthcare providers, as well as to be informed of their privacy rights with respect to their personal health information. Health plans and covered healthcare providers are required to develop and distribute a notice that provides a clear explanation of these rights and practices. The notice is intended to focus individuals on privacy issues and concerns, and to prompt them to have discussions with their health plans and healthcare providers and exercise their rights.

"Covered entities are required to provide a notice in *plain language* that describes:

- How the covered entity may use and disclose protected health information about an individual.

- The individual's rights with respect to the information and how the individual may exercise these rights, including how the individual may complain to the covered entity.

- The covered entity's legal duties with respect to the information, including a statement that the covered entity is required by law to maintain the privacy of protected health information.

- Whom individuals can contact for further information about the covered entity's privacy policies."[8]

---

[8]*Guidance on HIPAA Standards for Privacy of Individually Identifiable Health Information* (Washington, DC: U.S. Department of Health and Human Services Office for Civil Rights, December 3, 2002, and revised April 3, 2003).

The privacy policy must meet the requirements of HIPAA law, and the use or disclosure of PHI must be consistent with the privacy notice provided to the patient.

## Consent

The term **consent** has multiple meanings in a medical setting. **Informed consent** refers to the patient's agreement to receive medical treatment having been provided sufficient information to make an informed decision. Exercises 4B and 10G documented the patient's informed consent before administering the injection procedure. Consent for medical procedures must still be obtained by the practice.

Under the Privacy Rule the term *consent* is only concerned with use of the patient's information and *should not be confused with consent for the treatment itself*. The Privacy Rule originally required providers to obtain patient "consent" to use and disclose PHI except in emergencies. The rule was almost immediately revised to make it easier to use PHI for the purposes of treatment, payment, or operation of the healthcare practice.

Under the revised Privacy Rule, the patient gives consent to the use of their PHI for the purposes of treatment, payment, and operation of the healthcare practice. The patient does this by signing a consent form or signing an acknowledgment that he or she has received a copy of the office's privacy policy. Figure 11-1 shows a patient receiving a copy of the medical facility's privacy policy. The patient registration form shown in Chapter 1, Figure 1-11, contains a statement acknowledging receipt of the privacy policy. This approach to obtaining HIPAA "consent" by making it part of the routine demographic and insurance forms that patients sign is common in many healthcare facilities.

**Figure 11-1** The patient acknowledges receipt of the medical facility's privacy policy.

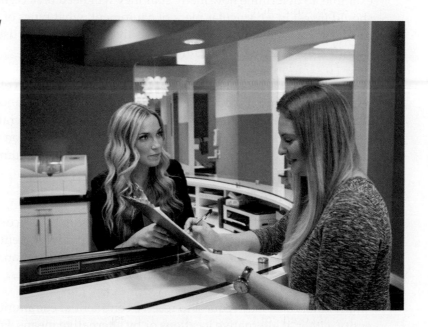

However, the rule permits healthcare providers some uses of PHI without the individual's authorization:

◆ A healthcare entity may use or disclose PHI for its own treatment, payment, and healthcare operations activities. For example, a hospital may use PHI to provide healthcare to the individual and may consult with other healthcare providers about the individual's treatment.

- A healthcare provider may disclose PHI about an individual as part of a claim for payment to a health plan.

- A healthcare provider may disclose PHI related to the treatment or payment activities of any healthcare provider (including providers not covered by the Privacy Rule). Consider these examples:

    A doctor may send a copy of an individual's medical record to a specialist who needs the information to treat the individual.

    A hospital may send a patient's healthcare instructions to a nursing home to which the patient is transferred.

    A physician may send an individual's health plan coverage information to a laboratory that needs the information to bill for tests ordered by the physician.

    A hospital emergency department may give a patient's payment information to an ambulance service that transported the patient to the hospital in order for the ambulance provider to bill for its treatment.

- A health plan may use protected health information to provide customer service to its enrollees.

Others within the office can use PHI also. For example, doctors and nurses can share the patient's chart to discuss what the best course of care might be. The doctor's administrative staff can access patient information to perform billing, transmit claims electronically, post payments, file the charts, type up the doctor's progress notes, and print and send out patient statements.

The office administrators can also use PHI for operation of the medical practice—for example, to determine how many staff they will need on a certain day, whether they should invest in a particular piece of equipment, what types of patients they are seeing the most of, where most of their patients live, and any other uses that will help make the office operate more efficiently.

The HHS *Guidance* document states: "A covered entity may voluntarily choose, but is not required, to obtain the individual's consent for it to use and disclose information about him or her for treatment, payment, and healthcare operations. A covered entity that chooses to have a consent process has complete discretion under the Privacy Rule to design a process that works best for its business and consumers."[9]

## Modifying HIPAA Consent

"Individuals have the right to request restrictions on how a covered entity will use and disclose protected health information about them for treatment, payment, and healthcare operations. A covered entity is not required to agree to an individual's request for a restriction, but is bound by any restrictions to which it agrees.

"Individuals also may request to receive confidential communications from the covered entity, either at alternative locations or by alternative means. For example, an individual may request that her healthcare provider call her at her office, rather than her home. A healthcare provider must accommodate an individual's reasonable request for such confidential communications."[10]

---

[9]Ibid.
[10]Ibid.

## Critical Thinking Exercise 11A: Creating a Privacy Policy

The purpose of this exercise is to let you apply what you have learned in this chapter to create a privacy policy that meets the minimum requirements to protect patient rights under the Privacy Rule.

### Case Study

You have been hired at a new clinic that is just opening and have been asked to create a compliant privacy policy notice.

### Step 1

Start a supported web browser program and follow the steps listed inside the cover of this textbook to log in to the MyHealthProfessionsLab for this course.

Locate and click on Exercise 11A.

### Step 2

Click the button labeled "I am ready to start".

An empty HIPAA Policy form will display along with a list of statements that *may* or *may not* belong in a privacy policy. The HIPAA form has four sections. Drag and drop only the correct statements into the sections of the form to which they belong.

### Step 3

When you are satisfied with your privacy policy click the Submit Quiz button and close the window.

## Authorization

"A *consent* document is not a valid permission to use or disclose protected health information for a purpose that requires an *authorization* under the Privacy Rule."[11]

**Authorization** differs from consent in that it *does* require the patient's permission to disclose PHI.

Some instances that would require an authorization include sending the results of an employment physical to an employer and sending immunization records or the results of an athletic physical to the school.

The appearance of an authorization form is up to the practice, but the Privacy Rule requires that it contain specific information. The required elements are:

◆ Date signed

◆ Expiration date

◆ To whom the information may be disclosed

◆ What is permitted to be disclosed

◆ For what purpose the information may be used

Unlike the Privacy Rule concept of consent, authorizations are not global. A new authorization is signed each time there is a different purpose or need for the patient's information to be disclosed.

---

[11]Ibid.

**Research**   Authorizations are usually required for researchers to use PHI. The only difference in a research authorization form is that it is not required to have an expiration date. The authorization may be combined with consent to participate in a clinical trial study for example.

**Research Exceptions**   To protect the patient's information while at the same time ensuring that researchers continue to have access to medical information necessary to conduct vital research, the Privacy Rule does allow some exceptions that permit researchers to access PHI without individual authorizations. Typically, these are cases where the patients are deceased; where the researcher is using PHI only to prepare a research protocol; or where a waiver has been issued by an internal review board, specifying that none of the information will be removed or used for any other purpose.

**Marketing**   The Privacy Rule specifically defines marketing and *requires* individual authorization for all uses or disclosures of PHI for *marketing purposes* with limited exceptions. These exceptions generally apply when information from the provider is sent to all patients in the practice about improvements or additions to the practice; or when the information is sent to the patient about their own treatments. For example, a reminder about an annual checkup is *not* marketing.

## Guided Exercise 11B: Authorization for Release of PHI

The purpose of this exercise is to let you apply what you have learned in this section to record an authorization.

### Case Study

Knesha Wilson wants to attend summer cheerleading camp at Champion Cheer and Dance Academy. The camp requires a health physical and Knesha's immunization records. She recently had a physical for her school's cheerleading program. As Knesha is a minor, her mother, Teresa Wilson, accompanies her to the Family Care medical practice to sign the release. Teresa informs the practice health information manager she wants to release only Knesha's cheerleading physical and immunization records. She says it is only to be used for camp admission and should expire in one month.

### Step 1

Start a supported web browser program and follow the steps listed inside the cover of this textbook to log in to the MyHealthProfessionsLab for this course.

Locate and click on Exercise 11B.

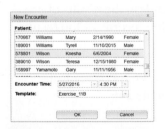

**Figure 11-2** New Encounter window with Knesha Wilson selected.

### Step 2

In the New Encounter window, locate and click on **Wilson, Knesha**, as shown in Figure 11-2. Click the OK button. You do not need to set the date in the New Encounter window for this exercise.

### Step 3

Locate the address lines below "Disclosure To" and type the following:

Champion Cheer and Dance Academy

Director of Admissions

1792 Forest Ridge Road

Anywhere, ID 83207

### Step 4

Locate and click in the blank line below "Information authorized to be disclosed" and type **cheerleading physical and immunization records**.

### Step 5

Locate and click in the blank line below "Purpose of release" and type **camp admission**.

### Step 6

Locate "This authorization is to remain in effect for" and type **1** in the value field. Click the down-arrow on the units field and select **month** from the drop-down list. This will set the expiration date to 1 month from the date you are doing the exercise.

### Step 7

Since Knesha is a minor, her mother Teresa will sign the form today. Proceed to the Signatures section and click the check box next to Legal Representative.

The current date will display in the date field for Legal Representative's signature.

Locate the Relationship to Patient field and click the down-arrow. Select Parent from the drop-down list as shown in Figure 11-3.

Note: The expiration date and the date signed on your form will be different from the dates in Figure 11-3.

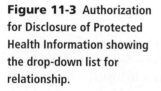

**Figure 11-3** Authorization for Disclosure of Protected Health Information showing the drop-down list for relationship.

### Step 8

Locate and click the blue Quippe icon button on the toolbar, and then select the option Create PDF. Review the PDF to verify you have entered all the information correctly.

Imagine Teresa Wilson signed it. You do not have to actually print it unless required to do so by your instructor. If your instructor requires you to turn in your completed work, then print or download the PDF as directed by your instructor.

The final step in every exercise is to submit your completed work for a grade.

Locate and click the blue Quippe icon button again, and select the Submit for Grade option from the drop-down menu. This will complete Exercise 11B.

## Government Agencies

One area that permits the disclosure of PHI without a patient's authorization or consent is when it is requested by an authorized government agency. Generally, such requests are for legal (law enforcement, subpoena, court orders, and so on) or public health purposes. A request by the FDA for information on patients who are having adverse reactions to a particular drug might be an example. Another example might be an audit of medical records by CMS to determine if sufficient documentation exists to justify Medicare claims.

The Privacy Rule also permits the disclosure of PHI, without authorization, to public health authorities for the purpose of preventing or controlling disease or injury as well as maintaining records of births and deaths. This would include, for example, the reporting of a contagious disease to the CDC or an adverse reaction to a regulated drug or product to the FDA.

Similarly, providers are also permitted to disclose PHI concerning on-the-job injuries to workers' compensation insurers, state administrators, and other entities to the extent required by state workers' compensation laws.

To ensure that covered entities protect patients' privacy as required, the Privacy Rule requires that health plans, hospitals, and other covered entities cooperate with efforts by the HHS Office for Civil Rights (OCR) to investigate complaints or otherwise ensure compliance.

## Minimum Necessary

The Privacy Rule **minimum necessary standard** is intended to limit unnecessary or inappropriate access to and disclosure of PHI beyond what is necessary. For example, if an insurance plan requests the value of a patient's hematocrit test to justify a claim for administering a drug, then the minimum necessary disclosure would be to send only the hematocrit result, not the patient's entire panel of tests.

> ### No Restrictions on PHI for Treatment of the Patient
>
> The minimum necessary standard does not apply to disclosures to or requests by a healthcare provider for PHI used for treatment purposes.

"The Privacy Rule generally requires covered entities to take reasonable steps to limit the use or disclosure of, and requests for, protected health information to the minimum necessary to accomplish the intended purpose. The minimum necessary standard does not apply to the following:

◆ Disclosures to or requests by a healthcare provider for treatment purposes.

◆ Disclosures to the individual who is the subject of the information.

◆ Uses or disclosures made pursuant to an individual's authorization.

◆ Uses or disclosures required for compliance with the Health Insurance Portability and Accountability Act (HIPAA) Administrative Simplification Rules.

◆ Disclosures to the Department of Health and Human Services (HHS) when disclosure of information is required under the Privacy Rule for enforcement purposes.

◆ Uses or disclosures that are required by other law.

The implementation specifications for this provision require a covered entity to develop and implement policies and procedures appropriate for its own organization, reflecting the entity's business practices and workforce."[12]

## Incidental Disclosures

"Many customary healthcare communications and practices play an important or even essential role in ensuring that individuals receive prompt and effective healthcare. Due to the nature of these communications, as well as the various environments in which individuals receive healthcare, the potential exists for an individual's health information to be disclosed incidentally.

For example, a hospital visitor may overhear a provider's confidential conversation with another provider or a patient, or may glimpse a patient's information on a sign-in sheet or nursing station whiteboard.

The HIPAA Privacy Rule is not intended to impede customary and essential communications and practices and, thus, does not require that *all* risk of incidental use or disclosure be eliminated to satisfy its standards. In fact the Privacy Rule permits certain incidental uses and disclosures of protected health information to occur where there is in place reasonable safeguards and minimum necessary policies and procedures that normally protect an individual's privacy."[13]

Incidental disclosure is one of the exceptions to the Breach Notification Requirements discussed later in the chapter.

## A Patient's Right to Know About Disclosures

Whether the practice has disclosed PHI based on a signed authorization or to comply with a government agency, the patient is entitled to know about it. Therefore, in most cases the medical office must track the disclosure.

The Privacy Rule gives individuals the right to receive a report of all disclosures made for purposes *other than* treatment, payment, or operation of the healthcare facility. The report must include the date of the disclosure, to whom the information was provided, a description of the information, and the stated purpose for the disclosure. The patient can request the report at any time and the practice must keep the records for at least six years.

Furthermore, Breach Notification Requirements, discussed later in the chapter, require the patient to be notified in writing when a breach of his or her PHI has occurred.

## Patient Access to Medical Records

In addition to protecting privacy, the law generally allows patients to be able to see and obtain copies of their medical records and request amendments to their records if they identify errors and mistakes. Health plans, doctors, hospitals, clinics, nursing homes, and other covered entities generally must provide access to these records within 30 days of a patient request, but may charge patients for the cost of copying and sending paper records.

---

[12]Ibid.
[13]Ibid.

The 2013 Omnibus HIPAA rule extended this provision by also giving patients the right to ask for their records in electronic form. However, if the provider is an eligible professional under the HITECH Act, then the provider must also provide patients with timely electronic access to their health records within 96 hours of the information being available to the provider. Meeting the HITECH Act requirement will more than satisfy the HIPAA requirement.

## Personal Representatives

"There may be times when individuals are legally or otherwise incapable of exercising their rights, or simply choose to designate another to act on their behalf with respect to these rights. Under the Rule, a person authorized to act on behalf of the individual in making healthcare related decisions is the individual's **personal representative**.

"The Privacy Rule requires covered entities to treat an individual's personal representative as the individual with respect to uses and disclosure of the individual's protected health information, as well as the individual's rights under the Rule.

"The personal representative stands in the shoes of the individual and has the ability to act for the individual and exercise the individual's rights. . . . In addition to exercising the individual's rights under the Rule, a personal representative may also authorize disclosures of the individual's protected health information."[14]

A personal representative is designated by signing a healthcare power of attorney or other form. In general, the personal representative's authority over privacy matters parallels his or her authority to act on other healthcare decisions.

◆ Where the personal representative has broad authority in making healthcare decisions, the personal representative is treated as the individual for all purposes under the Privacy Rule.

◆ Examples include a parent with respect to a minor child or a legal guardian of a mentally incompetent adult.

◆ Where the representative's authority is limited to particular healthcare decisions, his or her authority concerning PHI is limited to the same area.

◆ For example, a person with limited healthcare power of attorney about artificial life support could not sign an authorization for the disclosure of protected health information for marketing purposes.

◆ When the patient is deceased, a person who has authority to act on the behalf of the deceased or the deceased's estate is the personal representative for all purposes under the Privacy Rule.

Figure 11-4 provides a chart of who must be recognized as the personal representative for a category of individuals.

## Minor Children

In most cases, the parent, guardian, or other person acting as parent is the personal representative and acts on behalf of the minor child with respect to PHI. Even if a parent is not the child's personal representative, the Privacy Rule permits a parent access to a minor child's PHI when and to the extent it is permitted or required by state or other laws.

---

[14]Ibid.

**Figure 11-4** Persons automatically recognized as personal representatives for patients.

| If the Individual Is: | The Personal Representative Is: | Examples: |
|---|---|---|
| An Adult or an Emancipated Minor | A person with legal authority to make healthcare decisions on behalf of the individual | Healthcare power of attorney Court appointed legal guardian General power of attorney |
| A Minor (not emancipated) | A parent, guardian, or other person acting in loco parentis with legal authority to make healthcare decisions on behalf of the minor child | Parent, guardian, or other person (with exceptions in state law) |
| Deceased | A person with legal authority to act on behalf of the decedent or the estate (not restricted to healthcare decisions) | Executor of the estate Next of kin or other family member Durable power of attorney |

Conversely, regardless of the parent's status as personal representative, the Privacy Rule prohibits providing access to or disclosing the child's PHI to the parent, when and to the extent it is expressly prohibited under state or other laws.

However, the Privacy Rule specifies three circumstances in which the parent is not the personal representative with respect to certain health information about the minor child. "The three exceptional circumstances when a parent is not the minor's personal representative are:

◆ When State or other law does not require the consent of a parent or other person before a minor can obtain a particular healthcare service, and the minor consents to the healthcare service;

Example: A State law provides an adolescent the right to obtain mental health treatment without the consent of his or her parent, and the adolescent consents to such treatment without the parent's consent.

◆ When a court determines or other law authorizes someone other than the parent to make treatment decisions for a minor;

Example: A court may grant authority to make healthcare decisions for the minor to an adult other than the parent, to the minor, or the court may make the decision(s) itself.

◆ When a parent agrees to a confidential relationship between the minor and the physician.

Example: A physician asks the parent of a 16-year-old if the physician can talk with the child confidentially about a medical condition and the parent agrees.

If state or other laws are silent or unclear about parental access to the minor's PHI, the Privacy Rule grants healthcare professionals the discretion to allow or deny a parent access to a minor's PHI based on their professional judgment."[15]

## Critical Thinking Exercise 11C: What Is Required?

The purpose of this exercise is to let you see how you would apply what you have learned in this section.

---

[15]Ibid.

### Case Study

You are employed at a medical facility. One of your patients is being treated for injuries resulting from an accident. To meet state and federal regulations you will need the patient to sign several forms.

### Step 1

Start a supported web browser program and follow the steps listed inside the cover of this textbook to log in to the MyHealthProfessionsLab for this course.

Locate and click on Exercise 11C.

### Step 2

Read the four case studies and select the correct answer for each situation. When you have finished, click the Submit Quiz button and close the window.

## Business Associates

"The HIPAA Privacy Rule applies only to covered entities—healthcare providers, plans, and clearinghouses. However, most healthcare providers and health plans do not carry out all of their healthcare activities and functions by themselves. Instead, they often use the services of a variety of other persons or businesses. The Privacy Rule allows covered providers and health plans to disclose protected health information to these business associates if the providers or plans obtain written satisfactory assurances that the business associate will use the information only for the purposes for which it was engaged by the covered entity, will safeguard the information from misuse, and will help the covered entity comply with some of the covered entity's duties under the Privacy Rule.

"The covered entity's contract or other written arrangement with its business associate must contain the elements specified in the privacy rule. For example, the contract must:

◆ Describe the permitted and required uses of protected health information by the business associate;

◆ Provide that the business associate will not use or further disclose the protected health information other than as permitted or required by the contract or as required by law; and

◆ Require the business associate to use appropriate safeguards to prevent a use or disclosure of the protected health information other than as provided for by the contract."[16]

**Electronic Health Information Exchange**   Electronic health information exchange (HIE or eHIE) is an important part of the ONC Strategic Goals and Framework discussed in Chapter 1. The way most healthcare organizations implement HIE is to use a third party, called a health information exchange organization, to route information among various participating providers. The OCR recommends that participating providers execute Business Associate agreements with the HIE.

It will generally fall to the privacy officer (or in larger healthcare organizations, the legal department) to ensure that business associate agreements are on file for clearinghouses,

---

[16]Ibid.

# Real-Life Story

## The First HIPAA Privacy Case

*From the United States Attorney's Office, Western District of Washington[17]*

The first legal case under the privacy rule concerned the theft of patient demographic information (name, address, date of birth, Social Security number) by an employee in a medical office.

The former employee of a cancer care facility pled guilty in federal court in Seattle, Washington, to wrongful disclosure of individually identifiable health information for economic gain. This is the first criminal conviction in the United States under the health information privacy provisions of the Health Insurance Portability and Accountability Act (HIPAA), which became effective in April 2003. Those provisions made it illegal to wrongfully disclose personally identifiable health information.

The ex-employee admitted that he obtained a cancer patient's name, date of birth, and Social Security number while employed at the medical facility, and that he disclosed that information to get four credit cards in the patient's name. He also admitted that he used several of those cards to rack up more than $9,000 in debt in the patient's name. He used the cards to purchase various items, including video games, home improvement supplies, apparel, jewelry, porcelain figurines, groceries, and gasoline for his personal use. He was fired shortly after the identity theft was discovered.

"Too many Americans have experienced identity theft and the nightmare of dealing with bills they never incurred. To be a vulnerable cancer patient, fighting for your life, and having to cope with identity theft is just unconscionable," stated United States Attorney John McKay. "This case should serve as a reminder that misuse of patient information may result in criminal prosecution."

The case was investigated by the Federal Bureau of Investigation (FBI) and prosecuted by the United States Attorney's Office. The man was sentenced to a term of 10 to 16 months. He also has agreed to pay restitution to the credit card companies, and to the patient for expenses he incurred as a result of the misuse of his identity.

Although identity theft is serious, the consequences are much greater in a medical setting than if the same information had been stolen from an ordinary business. Why? Because even the patient's name and date of birth are part of the PHI. Additionally, the disclosure of medical information for financial gain could have resulted in a sentence of 10 years for each violation. The case serves as a reminder for everyone in the healthcare field of the personal responsibility for protecting PHI.

Although the patient privacy rule under HIPAA does not restrict the internal use of health information by the staff for treatment, payment, and office operations, you should make every effort to protect your patients' privacy and always follow the privacy policy of the practice.

---

> ### NOTE
>
> ### HIPAA Duties of OCR versus CMS
>
> OCR within HHS oversees and enforces the Privacy Rule, whereas CMS oversees and enforces all other Administrative Simplification requirements, including the Security Rule.

transcription services, HIE, and other businesses with whom your employer will exchange PHI.

## Civil and Criminal Penalties

Congress provided civil and criminal penalties for covered entities that misuse personal health information. For civil violations of the standards, OCR may impose monetary penalties from $100 to $50,000 per violation, up to $1,500,000 per year, for each requirement or prohibition violated. Criminal penalties apply for certain actions such as knowingly obtaining protected health information in violation of the law. Criminal penalties can range up to $50,000 and one year in prison for certain offenses; up to $100,000 and up to five years in prison if the offenses are committed under "false pretenses"; and up to $250,000 and up to 10 years in prison if the offenses are committed with the intent to sell, transfer, or use protected health information for commercial advantage, personal gain or malicious harm.

---

[17]Press release, United States Attorney's Office, Western District of Washington, August 19, 2004.

The HITECH Act also addressed privacy and security concerns associated with the electronic transmission of health information, in part through several provisions that strengthen the civil and criminal enforcement of the HIPAA rules. Subtitle D of the HITECH Act strengthens the civil and criminal enforcement of the HIPAA rules by establishing:

◆ Four categories of violations that reflect increasing levels of culpability

◆ Four corresponding tiers of penalty amounts that significantly increase the minimum penalty amount for each violation

◆ A maximum penalty amount of $1.5 million per calendar year for all violations of an identical provision

## HIPAA Security Rule

To fully comply with the Privacy Rule, it is necessary to understand and implement the requirements of the Security Rule. There are clearly areas in which the two rules supplement each other because both the HIPAA Privacy and Security rules are designed to protect identifiable health information. However, the Privacy Rule covers PHI in all forms of communications, whereas the Security Rule covers only electronic information. Because of this difference, security discussions are assumed to be about the protection of electronic health records, but the Security Rule actually covers all PHI that is stored electronically. This is called **EPHI**.

In this section, you will learn about the Security Rule. As with the previous section, much of the information provided is drawn directly from HHS documents. HHS regulates and enforces HIPAA using two different divisions for enforcement. OCR or Office of Civil Rights enforces the Privacy Rule whereas CMS enforces the Security Rule. As an employee of a covered entity, it is important that you participate in the security training and follow the security policy and procedures of your healthcare organization.

### Why a Security Rule?

Before HIPAA, no generally accepted set of security standards or general requirements for protecting health information existed in the healthcare industry. At the same time, new technologies were evolving, and the healthcare industry began to move away from paper processes and rely more heavily on the use of computers to pay claims, answer eligibility questions, provide health information, and conduct a host of other administrative and clinically based functions.

In order to provide more efficient access to critical health information, covered entities are using web-based applications, portals, and mobile devices that give medical staff and administrative employees more access to electronic health information. Although this means that the medical workforce can be more mobile and efficient (i.e., physicians can check patient records and test results from wherever they are), the rise in the adoption rate of these technologies creates an increase in potential security risks. Protecting the confidentiality, integrity, and availability of EPHI becomes even more critical.

The security standards in HIPAA were developed for two primary purposes.

◆ First, and foremost, the implementation of appropriate security safeguards protects certain electronic healthcare information that may be at risk.

- Second, protecting an individual's health information, although permitting the appropriate access and use of that information, ultimately promotes the use of electronic health information in the industry.

## The Privacy Rule and Security Rule Compared

The Privacy Rule sets the standards for, among other things, who may have access to PHI, while the Security Rule sets the standards for ensuring that only those who should have access to EPHI will actually have access. The primary distinctions between the two rules follow:

- **Electronic versus oral and paper:** The Privacy Rule applies to all forms of patients' protected health information, whether electronic, written, or oral. In contrast, the Security Rule covers only protected health information that is in electronic form. This includes EPHI that is created, received, maintained, or transmitted.

- **"Safeguard" requirement in Privacy Rule:** While the Privacy Rule contains provisions that currently require covered entities to adopt certain safeguards for PHI, the Security Rule provides for far more comprehensive security requirements and includes a level of detail not provided in the Privacy Rule section.

## Critical Thinking Exercise 11D: Comparing Privacy and Security Rules

The purpose of this exercise is to evaluate your understanding of the difference between the two rules.

### Case Study

You are training a new employee on the differences between the HIPAA Privacy Rule and the HIPAA Security Rule.

### Step 1

Start a supported web browser program and follow the steps listed inside the cover of this textbook to log in to the MyHealthProfessionsLab for this course.

Locate and click on Exercise 11D.

### Step 2

Follow the onscreen directions. When you have finished, click the Submit Quiz button and close the window.

## Security Standards

The security standards are divided into the categories of administrative, physical, and technical safeguards. Each category of the safeguards comprises a number of standards, which generally contain a number of implementation specifications.

- **Administrative safeguards:** In general, these are the administrative functions that should be implemented to meet the security standards. These include assignment or delegation of security responsibility to an individual and security training requirements.

- **Physical safeguards:** In general, these are the mechanisms required to protect electronic systems, equipment, and the data they hold, from threats, environmental hazards, and unauthorized intrusion. They include restricting access to EPHI and retaining off-site computer backups.

## Security Standards Matrix

### Administrative Safeguards

| Standards | Section of Rule | Implementation Specifications | Required or Addressable |
|---|---|---|---|
| Security Management Process | § 164.308Addressable(1) | Risk Analysis | Required |
| | | Risk Management | Required |
| | | Sanction Policy | Required |
| | | Information System Activity Review | Required |
| Assigned Security Responsibility | § 164.308Addressable(2) | | Required |
| Workforce Security | § 164.308Addressable(3) | Authorization and/or Supervision | Addressable |
| | | Workforce Clearance Procedure | Addressable |
| | | Termination Procedures | Addressable |
| Information Access Management | § 164.308Addressable(4) | Isolating Health Care Clearinghouse Function | Required |
| | | Access Authorization | Addressable |
| | | Access Establishment and Modification | Addressable |
| Security Awareness and Training | § 164.308Addressable(5) | Security Reminders | Addressable |
| | | Protection from Malicious Software | Addressable |
| | | Log-In Monitoring | Addressable |
| | | Password Management | Addressable |
| Security Incident Procedures | § 164.308Addressable(6) | Response and Reporting | Required |
| Contingency Plan | § 164.308Addressable(7) | Data Backup Plan | Required |
| | | Disaster Recovery Plan | Required |
| | | Emergency Mode Operation Plan | Required |
| | | Testing and Revision Procedure | Addressable |
| | | Applications and Data Criticality Analysis | Addressable |
| Evaluation | § 164.308Addressable(8) | | Required |
| Business Associate Contracts and Other Arrangement | § 164.308(b)(1) | Written Contract or Other Arrangement | Required |

**Figure 11-5** HIPAA Security Standards Matrix.

◆ **Technical safeguards:** In general, these are primarily the automated processes used to protect data and control access to data. They include using authentication controls to verify that the person signing onto a computer is authorized to access that EPHI, or encrypting and decrypting data as it is being stored and/or transmitted.

In addition to the safeguards just listed, the Security Rule also contains several standards and implementation specifications that address organizational requirements, as well as policies and procedures and documentation requirements.[18]

---

[18]Adapted from *Security 101 for Covered Entities*, HIPAA Security Series (Baltimore, MD: Centers for Medicare and Medicaid Services, November 2004 and revised March 2007).

## Physical Safeguards

| Standards | Section of Rule | Implementation Specifications | Required or Addressable |
|---|---|---|---|
| Facility Access Controls | § 164.310Addressable(1)) | Contingency Operations | Addressable |
| | | Facility Security Plan | Addressable |
| | | Access Control and Validation Procedures | Addressable |
| | | Maintenance Records | Addressable |
| Workstation Use | § 164.310(b)Required | | Required |
| Workstation Security | § 164.310(c)Required | | Required |
| Device and Media Controls | § 164.310(d)(1) | Disposal | Required |
| | | Media Re-use | Required |
| | | Accountability | Addressable |
| | | Data Backup and Storage | Addressable |

## Technical Safeguards

| Standards | Section of Rule | Implementation Specifications | Required or Addressable |
|---|---|---|---|
| Access Control | § 164.312Addressable(1) | Unique User Identification | Required |
| | | Emergency Access Procedure | Required |
| | | Automatic Logoff | Addressable |
| | | Encryption and Decryption | Addressable |
| Audit Controls | § 164.312(b) | | Required |
| Integrity | § 164.312(c)(1) | Mechanism to Authenticate Electronic Protected Health Information | Addressable |
| Person or Entity Authentication | § 164.312(d) | | Required |
| Transmission Security | 164.312(e)(1) | Integrity Controls | Addressable |
| | | Encryption | Addressable |

## Organizational Requirements

| Standards | Section of Rule | Implementation Specifications | Required or Addressable |
|---|---|---|---|
| Business Associate Contracts or Other Arrangements | § 164.314(a)(1) | Business Associate Contracts Other Arrangements | Required |
| Requirements for Group Health Plans | §164.314(b)(1) | Implementation Specifications | Required |

**Figure 11-5** (*continued from previous page*)

## Implementation Specifications

An implementation specification is an additional detailed instruction for implementing a particular standard. Implementation requirements and features within the categories were listed in the Security Rule by alphabetical order to convey that no one item was considered to be more important than another.

Implementation specifications in the Security Rule are either "Required" or "Addressable." Addressable does not mean optional.

To help you understand the organization of safeguards, security standards, and implementation specifications, a matrix of the HIPAA Security Rule is provided in Figure 11-5. The matrix is a part of the official rule and published as an appendix to the rule.[19] You may wish to refer to Figure 11-5 as we discuss each of the following sections.

# Administrative Safeguards[20]

The name *Security Rule* sounds very technical, but the largest category of the rule is Administrative Safeguards. The Administrative Safeguards comprise over half of the HIPAA security requirements.

Administrative Safeguards are the policies, procedures, and actions to manage the implementation and maintenance of security measures to protect EPHI. The Administrative Standards are as follows:

## Security Management Process

The Security Management Process is the first step. It is used to establish the administrative processes and procedures. There are four implementation specifications in the Security Management Process standard.

1. **Risk Analysis** Identify potential security risks and determine how likely they are to occur and how serious they would be.

2. **Risk Management** Make decisions about how to address security risks and vulnerabilities. The risk analysis and risk management decisions are used to develop a strategy to protect the confidentiality, integrity, and availability of EPHI.

3. **Sanction Policy** Define for employees what the consequences of failing to comply with security policies and procedures are.

4. **Information System Activity Review** Regularly review records such as audit logs, access reports, and security incident tracking reports. The information system activity review helps to determine if any EPHI has been used or disclosed in an inappropriate manner.

## Critical Thinking Exercise 11E: How to Assess Security Risk

This exercise will help you understand how to analyze security risks for HIPAA compliance.

### Case Study

You are sent by your boss to attend a meeting on assessing security risks.

---

[19] Figure adapted from: Appendix A to Subpart C of Part 164, Health Insurance Reform: Security Standards; Final Rule.
[20] Adapted from *Security Standards: Administrative Safeguards*, HIPAA Security Series #2 (Baltimore, MD: Centers for Medicare and Medicaid Services, May 2005 and revised March 2007).

### Step 1

Start a supported web browser program and follow the steps listed inside the cover of this textbook to log in to the MyHealthProfessionsLab for this course.

Locate and click on Exercise 11E.

### Step 2

Watch a short video and answer the follow-up questions. When you have finished, click the Submit Quiz button and close the window.

## Assigned Security Responsibility

Similar to the Privacy Rule, which requires an individual be designated as the privacy official, the Security Rule requires one individual be designated the security official. The security official and privacy official can be the same person, but do not have to be. The security official has overall responsibility for security; however, specific security responsibilities may be assigned to other individuals. For example, the security official might designate the IT Director to be responsible for network security. Figure 11-6 shows a staff meeting at which security policy is being reviewed.

Courtesy Brand New Images/Iconica/ Getty Images
**Figure 11-6** Medical office staff review security policy and appoint the security officer.

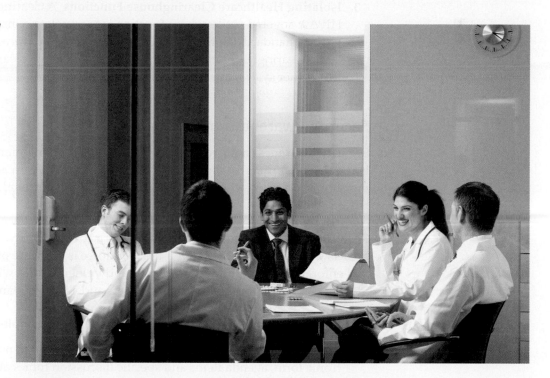

## Workforce Security

Within Workforce Security there are three addressable implementation specifications:

1. **Authorization or Supervision** Authorization is the process of determining whether a particular user (or a computer system) has the right to carry out a certain activity, such as reading a file or running a program.

2. **Workforce Clearance Procedure** Ensure members of the workforce with authorized access to EPHI receive appropriate clearances.

3. **Termination Procedures** Whether the employee leaves the organization voluntarily or involuntarily, termination procedures must be in place to remove access

privileges when an employee, contractor, or other individual previously entitled to access information no longer has these privileges.

## Information Access Management

Restricting access to only those persons and entities with a need for access is a basic tenet of security. By managing information access, the risk of inappropriate disclosure, alteration, or destruction of EPHI is minimized. This safeguard supports the "minimum necessary standard" of the HIPAA Privacy Rule.

The Information Access Management standard has three implementation specifications.

1. **Access Authorization** In the Workforce Security standard (see preceding section) the healthcare organization determines who has access. This section requires the organization to identify who has authority to grant that access and the process for doing so.

2. **Access Establishment and Modification** Once a covered entity has clearly defined who should get access to what EPHI and under what circumstances, it must consider how access is established and modified.

3. **Isolating Healthcare Clearinghouse Functions** A clearinghouse is a unique HIPAA-covered entity whose function is to translate nonstandard transactions into HIPAA standards. In the very rare case that your healthcare organization also operates a clearinghouse, the rule requires the isolation of clearinghouse computers from other systems in the organization.

## Security Awareness and Training

Security awareness and training for all new and existing members of the workforce is required. Figure 11-7 illustrates training an employee. In addition, periodic retraining should be given whenever environmental or operational changes affect the security of EPHI.

Regardless of the Administrative Safeguards a covered entity implements, those safeguards will not protect the EPHI if the workforce is unaware of its role in adhering to and enforcing them. Many security risks and vulnerabilities within covered entities are internal. This is why the Security Awareness and Training standard is so important.

The Security Awareness and Training standard has four implementation specifications.

1. **Security Reminders** Security reminders might include notices in printed or electronic form, agenda items and specific discussion topics at monthly meetings, focused reminders posted in affected areas, as well as formal retraining on security policies and procedures.

2. **Protection from Malicious Software** One important security measure that employees need to be reminded of is that malicious software is frequently brought into an organization through e-mail attachments and programs that are downloaded from the Internet. As a result of an unauthorized infiltration, EPHI and other data can be damaged or destroyed or, at a minimum, can require expensive and time-consuming repairs.

3. **Log-In Monitoring** Security awareness and training also should address how users log on to systems and how they are supposed to manage their passwords. Typically, an inappropriate or attempted login is when someone enters multiple

**Figure 11-7** Training
medical staff on security
policy and procedures.

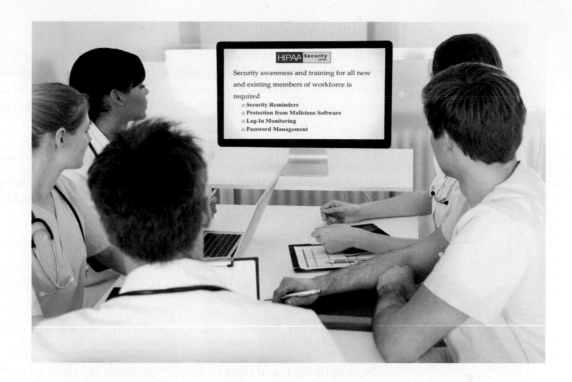

combinations of user names or passwords to attempt to access an information system. Fortunately, many information systems can be set to identify multiple unsuccessful attempts to log in. Other systems might record the attempts in a log or audit trail. Still other systems might disable a password after a specified number of unsuccessful login attempts. Once capabilities are established, the workforce must be made aware of how to use and monitor them.

4. **Password Management** In addition to providing a password for access, entities must ensure that workforce members are trained on how to safeguard the information. Train all users and establish guidelines for creating passwords and changing them during periodic change cycles.

## Security Incident Procedures

Security incident procedures must address how to identify security incidents and provide that the incident be reported to the appropriate person or persons. Examples of possible incidents include the following:

◆ Stolen or otherwise inappropriately obtained passwords that are used to access EPHI

◆ Corrupted backups that do not allow restoration of EPHI

◆ Virus attacks that interfere with the operations of information systems with EPHI

◆ Physical break-ins leading to the theft of media or mobile devices containing EPHI

◆ Failure to terminate the account of a former employee that is then used by an unauthorized user to access information systems with EPHI

◆ Providing media with EPHI, such as a PC hard drive or laptop, to another user who is not authorized to access the EPHI before removing the EPHI stored on the media

There is one required implementation specification for this standard:

1. **Response and Reporting** Establish adequate response and reporting procedures for these and other types of events

## Contingency Plan

What happens if a healthcare facility experiences a power outage, a natural disaster, or other emergency that disrupts normal access to healthcare information? A **contingency plan** consists of strategies for recovering access to EPHI should the organization experience a disruption of critical business operations. The goal is to ensure that EPHI is available when it is needed.

The Contingency Plan standard includes five implementation specifications:

1. **Data Backup Plan** Data backup plans are an important safeguard and a required implementation specification. Most covered entities already have backup procedures as part of current business practices.

2. **Disaster Recovery Plan** These are procedures to restore any loss of data.

3. **Emergency Mode Operation Plan** When operating in emergency mode because of a technical failure or power outage, security processes to protect EPHI must be maintained.

4. **Testing and Revision Procedures** Periodically test and revise contingency plans.

5. **Application and Data Criticality Analysis** Analyze software applications that store, maintain, or transmit EPHI and determine how important each is to patient care or business needs. A prioritized list of specific applications and data will help determine which applications or information systems get restored first or that must be available at all times.

## Evaluation

Ongoing evaluation of security measures is the best way to ensure all EPHI is adequately protected. Periodically evaluate strategy and systems to ensure that the security requirements continue to meet the organization's operating environments.

## Critical Thinking Exercise 11F: Developing a Contingency Plan

The purpose of this exercise is to let you see how you would apply what you have learned in this section.

### Case Study

You are part of a committee assigned the task of developing your healthcare facility's contingency plan.

### Step 1

Start a supported web browser program and follow the steps listed inside the cover of this textbook to log in to the MyHealthProfessionsLab for this course.

Locate and click on Exercise 11F.

### Step 2

Watch a short video and answer the follow-up questions. When you have finished, click the Submit Quiz button and close the window.

# Real-Life Story

## Contingency Plans Ensure Continued Ability to Deliver Care

**by Tanya Townsend**

*Chief information Officer at HSHS —Eastern Division in Green Bay, Wisconsin.*

Several years ago I had the opportunity to set up a new hospital that used all-digital health records—that is, there were no paper patient records, charts, or orders. As I talked to other hospitals and IT professionals about our accomplishments, one question I was frequently asked was, "What are your contingency plans in case of a power or system failure?"

Much of our plan was designed to avoid an outage in the first place. We had several redundancies in place to prevent that. For example, there are two WAN (wide-area network) connections—completely separate links going out different sides of the building to our core data center. The idea is that if one of those lines were to become disconnected for any reason, the other would seamlessly continue to function. In actual capacity they are balanced to make sure that can be accomplished. We also have redundancies on the LAN (local-area network) with wireless access points. As mobile as we are, we are very dependent on wireless.

For data protection we have multiple data centers. On the hospital side we have two different data centers that are redundant. On the ambulatory side there are three. In addition to these data centers, we also back up all the data in real time to another off-site location in Madison, which is a couple of hours away.

Should we lose connectivity because both links are down, we have a satellite antenna on the roof that can access the backup data in Madison. So as long as you can still power up your computer, you can get to the historical information. Electrical power can be supplied by an emergency generator that is designed to come online automatically in the event of a power loss.

Should the systems ever be completely down, we still need to take care of patients. In that event, we have downtime procedures for using paper forms that would allow us to continue to function. The necessary forms can be printed on demand but we have some preprinted copies on hand in case a power loss prevented us from printing. Once the system again becomes available, we have a policy and process for incorporating that paper documentation back into the system so we are not forced to carry that paper record forward.

The other area where we have built redundancy is our voice communications. We are using Voice-over-IP technology for our telecommunications, so a power or network outage would mean our phones would not work either. We plan for that by having cell phones and radios available. We also have certain phones that use traditional phone lines so we can continue to communicate.

We do a practice run, a mock downtime situation twice a year. One run is just simulated, but for the second one we actually take the systems down to make sure that we know how we are going to function. We also have planned outages, where we need to take the system down because we are upgrading it or doing maintenance on it. We continue to strive to keep those outages as brief as possible, but in those events we go to our downtime procedures and we continuously learn and improve on these.

## Business Associate Contracts and Other Arrangements

The Business Associate Contracts and Other Arrangements standard is comparable to the Business Associate Contract standard in the Privacy Rule, but is specific to business associates that create, receive, maintain, or transmit EPHI. The standard has one implementation specification:

1. **Written Contract or Other Arrangement** Covered entities should have a written agreement with business associates ensuring the security of EPHI. Government agencies that exchange EPHI should have a Memorandum of Understanding.

# Physical Safeguards[21]

The Security Rule defines physical safeguards as physical measures, policies, and procedures to protect a covered entity's electronic information systems and related buildings and equipment from natural and environmental hazards and unauthorized intrusion.

## Facility Access Controls

Facility Access Controls are policies and procedures to limit physical access to electronic information systems and the facility or facilities in which they are housed.

There are four implementation specifications.

1. **Access Control and Validation Procedures** Access Control and Validation are procedures to determine which persons should have access to certain locations within the facility based on their role or function.

2. **Contingency Operations** Contingency operations refer to physical security measures to be used in the event of the activation of contingency plans.

3. **Facility Security Plan** The Facility Security Plan defines and documents the safeguards used to protect the facility or facilities. Some examples include the following:

   ◆ Locked doors, signs warning of restricted areas, surveillance cameras, alarms

   ◆ Property controls such as property control tags, engraving on equipment

   ◆ Personnel controls such as identification badges, visitor badges, or escorts for large offices

   ◆ Private security service or patrol for the facility

   In addition, all staff or employees must know their roles in facility security.

4. **Maintenance Records** Document facility security repairs and modifications such as changing locks, making routine maintenance checks, or installing new security devices.

## Workstation Use

Inappropriate use of computer workstations can expose a covered entity to risks, such as virus attacks, compromise of information systems, and breaches of confidentiality. Specify the proper functions to be performed by electronic computing devices.

Workstation use also applies to workforce members using off-site workstations that can access EPHI. This includes employees who work from home, in satellite offices, or in another facility.

## Workstation Security

Although the Workstation Use standard addresses the policies and procedures for how workstations should be used and protected, the Workstation Security standard addresses how workstations are to be physically protected from unauthorized users.

## Device and Media Controls

Device and Media Controls are policies and procedures that govern the receipt and removal of hardware and electronic media that contain EPHI, into and out of a facility, and the movement of these items within the facility.

---

[21]Adapted from *Security Standards: Physical Safeguards*, HIPAA Security Series #3 (Baltimore, MD: Centers for Medicare and Medicaid Services, February 2005 and revised March 2007).

The Device and Media Controls standard has four implementation specifications, two required and two addressable.

1. **Disposal** When disposing of any electronic media that contains EPHI, make sure it is unusable or inaccessible.

2. **Media Reuse** Instead of disposing of electronic media, covered entities may want to reuse it. The EPHI must be removed before the media can be reused.

3. **Accountability** When hardware and media containing EPHI are moved from one location to another, a record should be maintained of the move. Laptop computers, tablets, smartphones, and portable media present a special challenge. Portable technology has gotten smaller, less expensive, and has an increased capacity to store large quantities of data, making accountability even more important and challenging.

4. **Data Backup and Storage** This specification protects the availability of EPHI and is similar to the Data Backup Plan for the contingency plan.

## Technical Safeguards[22]

The Security Rule defines technical safeguards as "the technology and the policy and procedures for its use that protect electronic protected health information and control access to it."

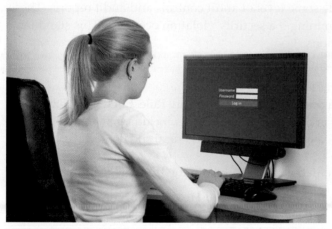

**Figure 11-8** A medical office employee logs on using a unique user ID and secure password.

Because security technologies are likely to evolve faster than legislative rules, specific technologies are not designated by the Security Rule. Where the CMS guidance documents provide examples of security measures and technical solutions to illustrate the standards and implementation specifications, these are just examples. The Security Rule is *technology neutral*; healthcare organizations have the flexibility to use any solutions that help them meet the requirements of the rule.

### Access Control

The Access Control standard outlines the procedures for limiting access to only those persons or software programs that have been granted access rights by the Information Access Management administrative standard (discussed earlier). Figure 11-8 shows a logon screen, one of the most common methods of access control.

Four implementation specifications are associated with the Access Controls standard.

1. **Unique User Identification** Unique User Identification provides a way to identify a specific user, typically by name or number. This allows an entity to track specific user activity and to hold users accountable for functions performed when logged into those systems.

2. **Emergency Access Procedure** Emergency Access procedures are documented instructions and operational practices for obtaining access to necessary EPHI during an emergency situation. Access Controls are necessary under emergency conditions, although they may be very different from those used in normal operational circumstances.

3. **Automatic Logoff** As a general practice, users should log off the system they are working on when their workstation is unattended. However, there will be times

---

[22]Adapted from *Security Standards: Technical Safeguards*, HIPAA Security Series #4 (Baltimore, MD: Centers for Medicare and Medicaid Services, May 2005 and revised March 2007).

when workers may not have the time, or will not remember, to log off a workstation. Automatic logoff is an effective way to prevent unauthorized users from accessing EPHI on a workstation when it is left unattended for a period of time.

Many applications have configuration settings for automatic logoff. After a predetermined period of inactivity, the application will automatically log off the user. Some systems that may have more limited capabilities may activate an operating system screen saver that is password protected after a period of system inactivity. In either case, the information that was displayed on the screen is no longer accessible to unauthorized users.

4. **Encryption and Decryption** Encryption is a method of converting regular text into code. The original message is encrypted by means of a mathematical formula called an *algorithm*. The receiving party uses a key to convert (decrypt) the encoded message back into plain text. Encryption is part of access control because it prevents someone without the key from viewing or using the information.

## Audit Controls

Audit Controls are "hardware, software, and/or procedural mechanisms that record and examine activity in information systems."

Most information systems provide some level of audit controls and audit reports. These are useful, especially when determining if a security violation occurred. This standard has no implementation specifications.

## Integrity

Protecting the integrity of EPHI is a primary goal of the Security Rule. EPHI that is improperly altered or destroyed can result in clinical quality problems, including patient safety issues. The integrity of data can be compromised by both technical and nontechnical sources.

There is one addressable implementation specification in the Integrity standard.

1. **Mechanism to Authenticate Electronic Protected Health Information** Once risks to the integrity of EPHI data have been identified during the risk analysis, security measures are put in place to reduce the risks.

## Person or Entity Authentication

The Person or Entity Authentication standard has no implementation specifications. This standard requires "procedures to verify that a person or entity seeking access to electronic protected health information is the one claimed."

There are several ways to provide proof of identity for authentication.

◆ Require something known only to that individual, such as a password or PIN.

◆ Require something that individuals possess, such as a smart card, a token, or a key. An example of a smart card is shown in Figure 11-9.

◆ Require something unique to the individual, such as a biometric. Examples of biometrics include fingerprints, voice patterns, facial patterns, or iris patterns.

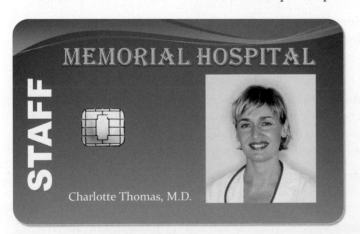

**Figure 11-9** A staff ID card that uses smart card technology.

Most covered entities use one of the first two methods of authentication. Many small provider offices rely on a password or PIN to authenticate the user. Fingerprint recognition can be used to control access to many mobile devices.

## Transmission Security

Transmission Security procedures are the "measures used to guard against unauthorized access to electronic protected health information that is being transmitted."

The Security Rule allows for EPHI to be sent over an electronic open network as long as it is adequately protected. This standard has two implementation specifications.

1. **Integrity Controls** Protecting the integrity of EPHI maintained in information systems was discussed previously in the Integrity standard. Integrity in this context is focused on making sure the EPHI is not improperly modified during transmission. A primary method for protecting the integrity of EPHI being transmitted is through the use of network communications protocols. Using these protocols, the computer verifies that the data sent is the same as the data received.

2. **Encryption** As previously described in the Access Control standard, encryption is a method of converting an original message of regular text into encoded or unreadable text that is eventually decrypted into plain comprehensible text.

   Encryption is necessary for transmitting EPHI over the Internet. There are various types of encryption technology available, but for encryption technologies to work properly both the sender and receiver must be using the same or compatible technology. Currently no single interoperable encryption solution for communicating over open networks exists.

# Organizational, Policies and Procedures, and Documentation Requirements[23]

In addition to the standards in the Administrative, Physical, and Technical Safeguards categories of the Security Rule, there also are four other standards that must be implemented. These are listed in the Security Standards Matrix (Figure 11-5), and they must not be overlooked.

## Organizational Requirements

There are two implementation specifications of this standard.

1. **Business Associate Contracts** The Business Associate Contracts are used if the business associate creates, receives, maintains, or transmits EPHI. The Business Associate must meet the Security Rule requirements.

2. **Other Arrangements** The Other Arrangements implementation specifications apply when both parties are government entities. There are two alternative arrangements:

   ◆ A memorandum of understanding (MOU), which accomplishes the objectives of the Business Associate Contracts section of the Security Rule

   ◆ A law or regulation applicable to the business associate that accomplishes the objectives of the Business Associate Contracts section of the Security Rule

---

[23]Adapted from *Security Standards: Organizational, Policies and Procedures*, HIPAA Security Series #5 (Baltimore, MD: Centers for Medicare and Medicaid Services, May 2005 and revised March 2007).

## Policies and Procedures

Although this standard requires covered entities to implement policies and procedures, the Security Rule does not define either "policy" or "procedure." Generally, policies define an organization's approach. Procedures describe how the organization carries out that approach, setting forth explicit, step-by-step instructions that implement the organization's policies. Policies and procedures may be modified as necessary.

## Documentation

The Documentation standard has three implementation specifications.

1. **Time Limit** Retain the documentation required by the rule for 6 years from the date of its creation or the date when it last was in effect, whichever is later.

2. **Availability** Make documentation available to those persons responsible for implementing the procedures to which the documentation pertains.

3. **Updates** Review documentation periodically, and update as needed, in response to environmental or operational changes affecting the security of the electronic protected health information.

The Security Rule also requires that a covered entity document the rationale for all security decisions.

# Minimizing the Risk of Mobile Devices

Healthcare professionals use smartphones, laptops, and tablets in their work. Whether it is a personal device or one supplied by the healthcare facility, you must protect and secure protected information. CMS offers the following tips:

◆ Use a password, fingerprint, or other authentication.

◆ Install or enable encryption if built into the device.

◆ Install and activate remote wiping and/or remote disabling to erase data on a lost or stolen device.

◆ Install and enable a firewall.

◆ Install and enable security software and keep security software up to date.

◆ Disable and do not install file sharing apps.

◆ Research apps before downloading. Use only known or trusted sources.

◆ Maintain physical control of the device.

◆ Use adequate security over Wi-Fi networks.

◆ Delete all stored PHI before discarding or reusing the mobile device.

Cautious healthcare organizations reduce security risk by not permitting personal devices to access PHI. Instead they provide properly secured tablets and smartphones for employees to use at work. If an organization allows providers and professionals to use mobile devices for work, the organization should have reasonable and appropriate mobile device policies and procedures. The policies and procedures should describe any configuration requirements for mobile devices used by providers and professionals for work.

## Critical Thinking Exercise 11G: Securing EHR Access

The purpose of this exercise is to let you see how you would apply what you have learned in this section.

### Case Study

A medical assistant in Dr. Anderson's office uses a laptop computer to connect to the EHR via a secure wireless network. She starts a patient encounter, documents the patient's vital signs, then leaves to get the doctor. You are challenged to find ways of ensuring only authorized users can access EPHI.

### Step 1

Start a supported web browser program and log in to the MyHealthProfessionsLab for this course.

Locate and click on Exercise 11G.

### Step 2

Watch a short video and answer the follow-up questions. When you have finished, click the Submit Quiz button and close the window.

## Breach Notification Requirements[24]

The HITECH Act also added new requirements regarding the occurrence of a breach of unsecured protected health information. A *breach* is defined as an impermissible use or disclosure under the Privacy Rule that compromises the security or privacy of the PHI such that the use or disclosure poses a significant risk of financial, reputation, or other harm to the affected individual.

There are three exceptions to the definition of "breach":

◆ Unintentional acquisition, access, or use of PHI by an employee of a covered entity or business associate

◆ Inadvertent disclosure of PHI from an authorized person to another authorized person at the covered entity or business associate

◆ If the covered entity or business associate has a good faith belief that the unauthorized individual, to whom the impermissible disclosure was made, would not have been able to retain the information

Covered entities must notify affected individuals, the Secretary of Health and Human Services, and, in certain circumstances, the media following the discovery of a breach of unsecured PHI. Business associates must notify covered entities if a breach has occurred. The OCR must post a list of breaches that affect 500 or more individuals.

### Individual Notice

Covered entities must provide affected individuals written notice by first-class mail, or alternatively, by e-mail if the affected individual has agreed to receive such notices electronically. If the covered entity has insufficient or out-of-date contact information for 10 or more individuals, the covered entity must provide substitute individual notice by

---

[24]HIPAA Breach Notification Rule, 45 CFR subsection 164.400-414.

either posting the notice on the home page of its web site or by providing the notice in major print or broadcast media where the affected individuals likely reside. If the covered entity has insufficient or out-of-date contact information for fewer than 10 individuals, the covered entity may provide substitute notice by an alternative form of written, telephone, or other means.

These individual notifications must be provided without unreasonable delay and in no case later than 60 days following the discovery of a breach and must include, to the extent possible, a description of the breach, a description of the types of information that were involved in the breach, the steps affected individuals should take to protect themselves from potential harm, a brief description of what the covered entity is doing to investigate the breach, mitigate the harm, and prevent further breaches, as well as contact information for the covered entity. Additionally, for substitute notice provided via web posting or major print or broadcast media, the notification must include a toll-free number for individuals to contact the covered entity to determine if their PHI was involved in the breach.

## Media Notice

Covered entities that experience a breach affecting more than 500 residents of a State or jurisdiction are, in addition to notifying the affected individuals, required to provide notice to prominent media outlets serving the State or jurisdiction. Covered entities will likely provide this notification in the form of a press release to appropriate media outlets serving the affected area. Like individual notice, this media notification must be provided without unreasonable delay and in no case later than 60 days following the discovery of a breach and must include the same information required for the individual notice.

## Notice to the Secretary

In addition to notifying affected individuals and the media (where appropriate), covered entities must notify the Secretary of Health and Human Services of breaches of unsecured PHI. Covered entities will notify the Secretary by visiting the HHS web site and filling out and electronically submitting a breach report form. If a breach affects 500 or more individuals, covered entities must notify the Secretary without unreasonable delay and in no case later than 60 days following a breach. If, however, a breach affects fewer than 500 individuals, the covered entity may notify the Secretary of such breaches on an annual basis. Reports of breaches affecting fewer than 500 individuals are due to the Secretary no later than 60 days after the end of the calendar year in which the breaches occurred.

## Notification by a Business Associate

If a breach of unsecured PHI occurs at or by a business associate, the business associate must notify the covered entity following the discovery of the breach. A business associate must provide notice to the covered entity without unreasonable delay and no later than 60 days from the discovery of the breach. To the extent possible, the business associate should provide the covered entity with the identification of each individual affected by the breach as well as any information required to be provided by the covered entity in its notification to affected individuals.

# Electronic Signatures for Health Records

The HIPAA Security Rule was originally titled "Security and Electronic Signature Standards." The original Security Rule also proposed a standard for electronic signatures. The final rule covered only security standards.

The Electronic Signatures in Global and National Commerce Act[25] made digital signatures as binding as their paper-based counterparts for commerce. However, HIPAA does not yet require the use of electronic signatures, because HIPAA does not yet have a Rule for Electronic Signature standards.

Today, shopping web sites, banking and credit card web sites, and even Medicare provider enrollment sites accept the user's entry of an ID and pin or password as an Electronic Signature for purposes of accepting the terms of an official policy or even a contract.

Most EHR systems allow a clinician using an authenticated login to "sign" his or her encounter notes, by clicking a button or checkbox that finalizes the note. Once "signed" the document is "sealed," and the software will permit no further edits or changes to it, except by adding an amendment document, which leaves the original intact.

## HIPAA Privacy, Security, and You

As someone who will work with patients' health records, it is especially important for you to understand the regulations regarding privacy and security. Follow the privacy policy and security rules at your place of work. Know who the privacy and security officials are. Ask them if you have any questions regarding policies at your practice or if you feel that you need additional training.

It is especially important not to give others your password and to always log out of a medical records computer when you are not using it. Remember to treat every medical record (paper or electronic) in a confidential manner. You are only permitted to access a patient's PHI for work-related purposes and within the limitations prescribed by law.

## Chapter Eleven Summary

The Health Insurance Portability and Accountability Act, or HIPAA, was passed in 1996. The Administrative Simplification Subsection (Title 2, f) (hereafter just called HIPAA) has four distinct components:

1. Transactions and code sets

2. Uniform identifiers

3. Privacy

4. Security

HIPAA regulates health plans, clearinghouses, and healthcare providers as "covered entities" or a "covered entity" with regard to these four areas.

HIPAA standardized formats for EDI or Electronic Data Interchange by requiring specific Transaction Standards. These currently are used for nine types of transactions between covered entities. This was the first of the Administrative Simplification Subsections to be implemented. This section also requires standardized code sets such as HCPCS, CPT-4, ICD10-CM, and others to be used.

---

[25]Electronic Signatures in Global and National Commerce Act (ESIGN), Pub.L. 106–229, 14 Stat. 464, enacted June 30, 2000, 15 U.S.C. ch. 96.

HIPAA also established uniform identifier standards, to be used on all claims and other data transmissions. These include the following:

◆ National provider identifier for doctors, nurses, and other healthcare providers

◆ Federal employer identification number used to identify employer-sponsored health insurance

◆ National health plan identifier, a unique identification number that will be assigned to each insurance plan, but is not yet implemented

The privacy and security rules use two acronyms: PHI, which stands for Protected Health Information, and EPHI, which stands for Protected Health Information in an Electronic Format.

The HIPAA privacy standards are designed to protect a patient's identifiable health information from unauthorized disclosure or use in any form, while permitting the practice to deliver the best healthcare possible. To comply with the law, privacy activities in the average medical office might include the following:

◆ Providing a copy of the office privacy policy informing patients about their privacy rights and how their information can be used

◆ Asking the patient to acknowledge receiving a copy of the policy or signing a consent form

◆ Obtaining signed authorization forms and in some cases tracking the disclosures of patient health information when it is to be given to a person or organization outside the practice for purposes other than treatment, billing, or payment

◆ Adopting clear privacy procedures for its practice

◆ Training employees so that they understand the privacy procedures

◆ Designating an individual to be responsible for seeing that the privacy procedures are adopted and followed

◆ Securing patient records containing individually identifiable health information so that they are not readily available to those who do not need them

The Privacy Rule does not require providers to obtain patient "consent" to use and disclose PHI for the purposes of treatment, payment, and healthcare operations. In general, the practice can use PHI for almost anything related to treating the patient, running the medical practice, and getting paid for services. This means doctors, nurses, and other staff can share the patient's chart within the practice.

Authorization differs from consent in that it does require the patient's permission to disclose PHI. Some examples of instances that would require an authorization would include sending the results of an employment physical to an employer, immunization records, or the results of an athletic physical to the school.

The authorization form must include a date signed, an expiration date, to whom the information may be disclosed, what is permitted to be disclosed, and for what purpose the information may be used. The authorization must be signed by the patient or a representative appointed by the patient. Unlike the open concept of consent, authorizations are not global. A new authorization is signed each time there is a different purpose or need for the patient's information to be disclosed.

Practices are permitted to disclose PHI without a patient's authorization or consent when it is requested by an authorized government agency. Generally, such requests are for legal (law enforcement, subpoena, court orders, and so on) public health purposes, or for enforcement of the Privacy Rule itself. Providers also are permitted to disclose PHI concerning on-the-job injuries to workers' compensation insurers, state administrators, and other entities to the extent required by state law.

Whether the practice has disclosed PHI based on a signed authorization or to comply with a government agency, the patient is entitled to know about it. The Privacy Rule gives the individuals the right to receive a report of all disclosures made for purposes other than treatment, payment, or operations. Therefore, in most cases the medical office must track the disclosure and keep the records for at least six years.

Most healthcare providers and health plans use the services of a variety of other persons or businesses. The Privacy Rule allows covered providers and health plans to disclose protected health information to these "business associates." The Privacy Rule requires that a covered entity obtain a written agreement from its business associate, which states the business associate will appropriately safeguard the protected health information it receives or creates on behalf of the covered entity.

Congress provided civil and criminal penalties for covered entities that misuse personal health information. The privacy rule is enforced by the HHS Office for Civil Rights (OCR).

The Privacy Rule sets the standards for, among other things, who may have access to PHI, whereas the Security Rule sets the standards for ensuring that only those who should have access to EPHI actually will have access. The Privacy Rule applies to all forms of patients' protected health information, whether electronic, written, or oral. In contrast, the Security Rule covers only protected health information that is in electronic form.

HIPAA and the Omnibus HIPAA rule give patients the right to copies of their own health records in paper or electronic form.

Security standards were designed to provide guidelines to all types of covered entities, while affording them flexibility regarding how to implement the standards. Covered entities may use appropriate security measures that enable them to reasonably implement a standard.

Security standards were designed to be "technology neutral." The rule does not prescribe the use of specific technologies, so that the healthcare community will not be bound by specific systems or software that may become obsolete.

The security standards are divided into the categories of administrative, physical, and technical safeguards.

**Administrative safeguards.** In general, these are the administrative functions that should be implemented to meet the security standards. These include assignment or delegation of security responsibility to an individual and security training requirements.

**Physical safeguards.** In general, these are the mechanisms required to protect electronic systems, equipment, and the data they hold from threats, environmental hazards, and unauthorized intrusion. They include restricting access to EPHI and retaining off-site computer backups.

**Technical safeguards.** In general, these are primarily the automated processes used to protect data and control access to data. They include using authentication controls to verify that the person signing onto a computer is authorized to access that EPHI, or encrypting and decrypting data as it is being stored or transmitted.

Breach Notification Requirements require covered entities to notify affected individuals, the Secretary of Health and Human Services, and, in certain circumstances, the media of the occurrence of a breach of unsecured PHI. Business associates must notify covered entities if a breach has occurred. The OCR must post a list of breaches that affect 500 or more individuals.

The original Security Rule also proposed a standard for electronic signatures. The final rule covered only security standards.

The Electronic Signatures in Global and National Commerce Act made digital signatures as binding as their paper-based counterparts.

## Testing Your Knowledge of Chapter 11

### Step 1

Start a supported web browser program and follow the steps listed inside the cover of this textbook to log in to the MyHealthProfessionsLab for this course.

Locate and click on Chapter 11 Test.

### Step 2

Answer the test questions. When you have finished, click the Submit Test button to close the window.

# 12

# EHR Coding and Reimbursement

## Learning Outcomes

*After completing this chapter, you should be able to:*

◆ Explain why billing codes are important in an EHR system

◆ Understand the relationship between the encounter diagnoses and the ICD-10-CM code set

◆ Identify and assign more specific levels of ICD-10-CM codes

◆ Use E&M calculator software

◆ Show how Evaluation and Management (E&M) codes are determined

◆ Name and describe key components of E&M codes

◆ Read and understand the tables used in CMS E&M guidelines

◆ Explain how the level of key components determines the level of the E&M code

◆ Correctly use and document the time factor to change the level of an E&M code

## The EHR and Reimbursement

There is no question that healthcare providers must be paid for their services, but the vast majority of those payments are from insurance plans, which require the use of standard codes. Some clinical workers ignore or resist a discussion of the relationship of the EHR to reimbursement, considering it the responsibility of the HIM or billing departments. Unfortunately, that is not the case.

Whether the clinician is a doctor, nurse, or medical assistant, how and what that person documents in the patient chart has everything to do with what the medical facility is going to be paid for treating the patient.

Insurance plan audits follow this dictum: *If it isn't documented, it wasn't done.* This means no matter how long the medical assistant and patient discussed the patient's history and symptoms; no matter how thoroughly the nurse assessed the patient; no matter how brilliant the doctor's diagnosis; if those findings aren't documented with sufficient detail in the chart, the auditor will assume that those portions of the encounter were never performed.

Knowing there is a direct relationship between the completeness of your clinical documentation and the financial well-being of your medical facility can help you understand the necessity of this chapter. If your interest is primarily clinical and not administrative, have no fear of this chapter. It is not intended to train you as a medical coder or billing specialist. A complete medical coding course could not be taught in one chapter anyway.

The U.S. government, Medicare, and insurance regulations financially affect all healthcare facilities. Adoption of an EHR system can not only improve patient care, as described in earlier chapters, but can also ensure reimbursement for services provided. The purpose of this chapter is to help you understand the guidelines used for calculating reimbursement for outpatient services by analyzing a patient's encounter note recorded in an EHR. We are going to focus on two key areas:

1. Proper coding of diagnoses

2. Factors of Evaluation and Management

## HIPAA-Required Code Sets

HIPAA[1] law regulates many things, including the privacy and security of health records. It also standardized healthcare transactions and required the use of the ICD-10-CM, CPT-4, and HCPCS code sets.

### Diagnoses Codes Justify Billing

Chapter 2 briefly introduced ICD-10-CM codes and discussed their use for mortality and morbidity studies. Since the topic of this chapter is EHR coding and reimbursement you may get the impression that ICD-10-CM codes are "billing" codes because reimbursement is tied to the diagnoses codes and they are required by HIPAA for claims and other transactions. Also, because there is a similarly named, but unrelated set of codes used for hospital billing called ICD-10PCS. ICD-10-CM codes are important for other reasons beyond billing, including statistical studies of causes of death, disease, and injury. ICD-10-CM provides an internationally recognized system of codifying the patient's condition. That said, in this chapter we are discussing ICD-10-CM primarily as it is used for outpatient billing, which requires that one or more ICD-10-CM codes be assigned to every procedure. Also reimbursement for most inpatient hospitals is based entirely on the Medical Severity Diagnostic Related Group (MS-DRG) determined from the primary and secondary diagnoses assigned by the attending physician. However, we will not be discussing inpatient billing.

First, the diagnosis must correspond to the procedure. For example, you cannot bill for an eye exam using the diagnosis for a broken toe.

Second, the ICD-10-CM code should be as specific as possible. ICD-10-CM codes are alphanumeric, from three to seven characters long. The first three characters identifying

---

[1]Health Insurance Portability and Accountability Act, Administrative Simplification Subsection, Title 2, subsection f.

a category are followed by a decimal point and up to four additional characters, which subdivide the category to further specify or refine the description of the condition. Insurance billing rules require clinicians to code to the most specific level. Not all codes have a sixth or seventh character, but a code that has an applicable seventh character is considered invalid without the seventh character.[2] The level of specificity is best understood by example, as you will see in Exercise 12A.

Each of the encounters you have documented in previous chapter exercises included an Assessment finding that was from the Medcin domain of Diagnoses, Syndromes and Conditions. Medcin and other EHR nomenclatures contain a "cross-walk" or internal reference table that can automatically produce ICD-10-CM codes at the specificity level of the diagnosis the clinician selected. Furthermore, Quippe has a code review feature the clinician can use to see the ICD-10-CM code and, when necessary, find a more specific level diagnosis.

## Primary and Secondary Diagnoses

The concept of the primary diagnosis is also important. The **primary diagnosis** is the reason why the patient came to the office or hospital. Other conditions that are addressed during the visit are listed as **secondary diagnoses** (also called **comorbidity**). In a hospital, secondary diagnoses are classified as POA, present on admission, or HAC, hospital acquired condition.

Any conditions that exist concurrently with the primary diagnosis should be reviewed, examined, or treated and documented in the exam note. These are usually on the problem list, which you learned about in Chapter 7.

## Multiple Diagnoses

Multiple diagnoses occur mainly in patients with ongoing or chronic conditions requiring regular visits. It is correct and appropriate to continue to use diagnosis codes from past visits for as long as the patient continues to have the illness or condition and that condition is clearly documented in the record. For example, a patient with diabetes mellitus—well controlled might be seen regularly. With this disease, on some visits the patient will likely have other problems as well. However, the diagnosis "Diabetes Mellitus—well controlled" should be included in every visit note and on insurance claims for those visits.

## Guided Exercise 12A: Using Code Review

In this exercise you will use Code Review to see the ICD-10-CM codes corresponding to the assessment findings and to select more specific codes where available. Because we are focusing on only the assessment, the encounter note you create will be medically incomplete.

### Case Study

Unfortunate Sally Sutherland, who has been your patient for many previous exercises, presents today with bronchitis-like symptoms. For the purpose of this exercise you are only going to document her diagnoses and a lab test.

---

[2]ICD-10-CM Official Guidelines for Coding and Reporting FY 2016, CMS.gov, January 2016.

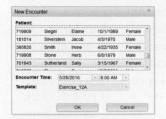

**Figure 12-1** New Encounter window with Sally Sutherland selected.

**Figure 12-2** Selecting Code Review on the View drop-down menu opens Code Review in the bottom of the pane.

## Step 1

Start a supported web browser program and log in to the MyHealthProfessionsLab for this course.

Locate and click on the link **Exercise 12A**. This will open the Quippe software window with the New Encounter window displayed in the center.

## Step 2

In the New Encounter window patient list, locate and click on **Sutherland, Sally** as shown in Figure 12-1, and then click the OK button. You do not need to set the date and time of the encounter for this exercise.

## Step 3

Sally has two active problems. Remember, Active Problems are reviewed every visit, even when they are not the primary reason for the visit. Proceed to the Assessment section, locate and click on **hyperlipidemia** until it turns red.

Click the View button on the toolbar and select Code Review from the drop-down menu (shown at the top of Figure 12-2. The Code Review grid (shown at the bottom of the figure) will be displayed.

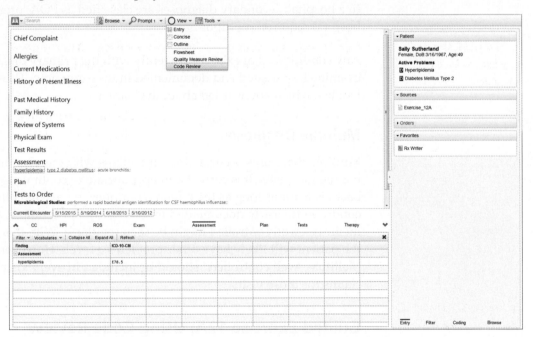

The first column lists the findings in the note, which have crosswalks to other standard code sets. The column labeled ICD-10-CM contains the diagnosis code. For hyperlipidemia it is E78.5.

Code Review can also display codes from additional vocabularies and code sets such as CPT-4, LOINC, SNOMED, RxNorm, and others.

## Step 4

The other problem on Sally's active problems list is **type 2 diabetes mellitus**. Locate it in the Assessment section and click on it until it turns red.

For type 2 diabetes the Code Review shows the ICD-10-CM code E11. This three-character code identifies an ICD-10 category, but it is not coded as specific as it should be.

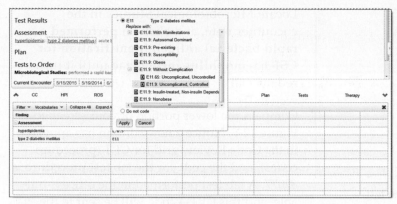

**Figure 12-3** Pop-up to select more specific ICD-10-CM code for diabetes.

Locate and click on the cell in the grid containing the ICD-10-CM code **E11**. A pop-up window listing more specific diagnosis codes will open as shown in Figure 12-3.

*Tip*: If the pop-opens too low on your screen, click any white space in the pop-up window to reposition it at the top of the Code Review grid.

The ICD-10-CM pop-up uses a tree structure similar to the Browse button, with which you are familiar.

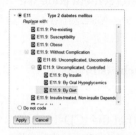

**Figure 12-4** ICD-10-CM pop-up scrolled, Uncomplicated, Controlled expanded to By Diet (highlighted).

Sally's diabetes is without complication, controlled by diet. Locate **Without Complication** in the pop-up, and click the plus symbol to expand the tree.

Click the plus symbol next to "Uncomplicated, Controlled" to further expand the tree. Scroll the list, as shown in Figure 12-4, to locate **E11.9 By Diet**, and then *double-click* on it. The pop-up window will close.

### Step 5

Locate the Assessment section and notice that selecting a new diagnosis in the ICD-10-CM pop-up window added a corresponding finding to the encounter note: "type 2 diabetes mellitus – uncomplicated, controlled by diet."

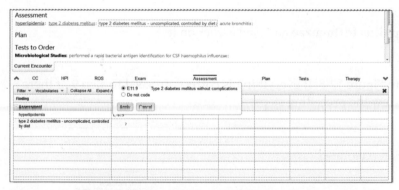

**Figure 12-5** Pop-up to apply ICD-10-CM code E11.9 for type 2 diabetes without complications.

Locate the row for type 2 diabetes in the Code Review and notice a '?' in the ICD-10-CM column. Code Review displays a question mark to tell the clinician to open the pop-up window. A question mark appears either when the finding is too general and there are more than one possible code choices, or, as in this case, when the diagnosis code doesn't match the finding.

In this case, we have changed the finding to a more specific diagnosis, but have not yet applied the more specific level of ICD-10-CM. Locate and click on the Code Review cell with the question mark to invoke the pop-up window shown in Figure 12-5.

Click in the circle next to **E11.9 Type 2 diabetes mellitus without complications**, and click the Apply button. The pop-up will close and the code E11.9 will replace the question mark in the grid.

### Step 6

As mentioned earlier, Medcin also contains crosswalks to additional code sets and clinical vocabularies.

The clinician tests Sally for the flu by taking a swab of her throat and nostrils and performing an in-office test.

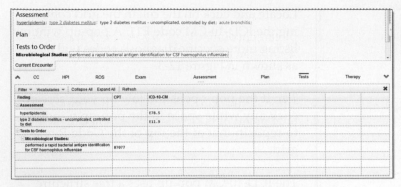

**Figure 12-6** Code Review shows the CPT-4 code for the lab test.

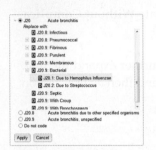

**Figure 12-7** Changing Acute bronchitis to a more specific diagnosis via the ICD-10-CM pop-up window.

Locate Microbiological Studies in the encounter note, and click on **performed a rapid bacterial antigen identification for CSF haemophilus influenzae** until it turns red.

Compare the lower portion of your screen to Figure 12-6. Notice a new column has appeared in the Code Review grid for CPT (procedure codes), and the code for the lab test procedure is 87077. A lab test performed in the office is billable, and this CPT-4 code will be sent to the practice management system billing module along with the ICD-10-CM codes, and the CPT-4 evaluation and management code we will learn about in the next section.

### Step 7

The test results confirm the clinician's diagnosis. Locate **acute bronchitis** in the Assessment section and click on it until it turns red.

Locate the row for acute bronchitis in the Code Review and notice that the ICD-10-CM code J20 is not specific enough. Using what you have learned in step 4, click on the cell in the grid containing the ICD-10-CM code **J20** to open the pop-up window. Scroll the list downward.

Locate and click on the plus symbol next to "Bacterial" to expand the tree as shown in Figure 12-7.

Locate **Due to Haemophilus Influenzae** and *double-click* on it.

### Step 8

Compare your screen to Figure 12-8. If everything is correct, proceed to step 9. If there are any differences, review the preceding steps, and correct your errors.

**Figure 12-8** Correctly completed encounter note; Code Review shows ICD-10-CM and CPT-4 codes.

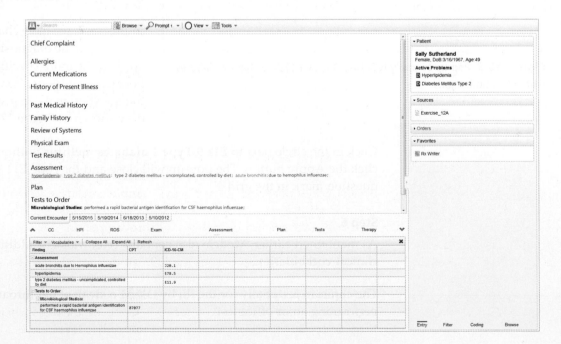

**Step 9**

If you wish to print a copy of your completed encounter notes for yourself or because your instructor requires you to turn them in, then print or download the PDF at this time.

Locate and click the blue Quippe icon button on the toolbar to display the drop-down menu, and then select the Submit for Grade menu option. This will complete Exercise 12A.

Although in previous chapters we used general diagnoses for upper respiratory infections, with the advent of ICD-10-CM clinicians have had to learn to use more specific levels of diagnoses. The advantage of using an EHR with a codified nomenclature is that software like Code Review can alert the clinician when the level of ICD-10-CM code is not as specific as it should be. It also makes it easy to select not only the code, but the finding as well so the ICD-10-CM code sent to the billing system will always be in sync with the encounter note in the event the claim is audited.

## CPT-4 and HCPCS Codes

In addition to standard codes for diagnoses, HIPAA requires the use of CPT-4 and HCPCS codes for procedures. CPT-4 stands for Current Procedural Terminology, fourth edition. It was developed and is maintained by the American Medical Association (AMA). HCPCS stands for Healthcare Common Procedure Coding System. It was developed by the CMS to code for supplies, injectable medications, and blood products. CPT-4 is incorporated into the HCPCS standard even though it is separately maintained by the AMA.

## Evaluation and Management (E&M) Codes

Although the majority of CPT-4 codes represent a specific medical procedure, such as the lab test performed in the previous exercise, the portion of the CPT-4 code set most frequently used is the Evaluation and Management (E&M) codes. This is because E&M CPT-4 codes are used to bill for nearly every kind of patient encounter, including medical office visits, inpatient hospital exams, nursing home visits, consults, emergency room (ER) doctors, and scores of other services. E&M codes are used by virtually all specialties.

At one time E&M billing was based on the provider's judgment of how complex the visit was. However, Medicare developed strict guidelines for determining how the level of exam justified the level of E&M code. These guidelines were adopted by virtually all payers.

The E&M guidelines were published in 1995. Specialists, however, found fault with the 1995 guidelines. For example, an ophthalmologist performs an in-depth exam of the eyes but does not typically perform a complete head-to-toe review of systems. Under the 1995 guidelines, the ophthalmologist would never meet the criteria for higher level codes. In response, the guidelines were revamped in 1997. Today physicians are allowed to use either the 1995 or 1997 guideline, whichever best suits their practice, but not both. This chapter uses the 1997 guideline, because it is the most recent.

E&M guidelines determine the CPT-4 E&M code based almost exclusively on the findings documented in the encounter note. Gone are the days when a clinician might perform a very adequate physical but scribble only a few lines in the chart. With exception of psychiatric services, the length of time spent with the patient is no longer the controlling factor, although it can be an overriding factor as we will see in a later exercise.

## Four Levels of E&M Codes

There are four levels of E&M codes for each type of visit. The levels represent the least complicated exam (level 1) to the most complex exam (level 4). The level is important because a provider's "allowed payment" amount is proportionate to the level of the exam (with level 1 paying the least and level 4 paying the most).

Where the service is rendered is an important consideration as well. There are separate categories of E&M codes for different locations such as office visits, inpatient exams, ER exams, and so on. Each category of E&M codes has at least four codes representing the four levels of service. Some categories have more than four E&M codes because there are subcategories—for example, new patient versus established patient. Most exercises in this chapter use the E&M codes for outpatient office visits.

## How the Level of an E&M Code Is Determined

Seven components are evaluated to determine the level of E&M services:

◆ History

◆ Examination

◆ Medical decision making

◆ Counseling

◆ Coordination of care

◆ Nature of presenting problem

◆ Time

Three components—history, examination, and medical decision making—are the key components in determining the level of E&M services. The level of each key component is determined separately. The level of E&M code is derived from the highest level of two or three key components. There is one exception. For services such as psychiatry, which consist predominantly of counseling or coordination of care, time is the key or controlling factor determining the level of E&M service.

This chapter explains each of the components, the levels within the key components, and how they are combined to calculate the E&M code. A later exercise will also show how time can become an overriding factor, justifying a higher level code for visits that require more time for counseling the patient.

## Undercoding

Even with an EHR, some providers still use a paper "encounter" form such as the one shown in Figure 12-9 to communicate CPT-4 and ICD-10-CM codes to the billing department. In such an office the clinician checks or circles the procedure and writes the diagnosis codes on a paper form, which is routed to administrative personnel to be posted into the practice management system for billing. These clinicians are at risk. If they select a code that is at a higher level than the encounter note supports, they can be fined. To avoid risk, many practices undercode (choosing a code one level below what they believe to be correct), taking the attitude "better safe than sorry." This is bad for

# Family Practice Management Superbill Template

From the American Academy of Family Practice (AAFP) Family Practice Management Toolkit
(http://www.aafp.org/fpm/20060900/43inse.html)

| Date of service: | Waiver? ☐ | |
|---|---|---|
| Patient name: | Insurance: | |
| | Subscriber name: | |
| Address: | Group #: | Previous balance: |
| | Copay: | Today's charges: |
| Phone: | Account #: | Today's payment: check# |
| DOB:          Age:          Sex: | Physician name: | Balance due: |

| RANK | Office visit | New | Est | RANK | Office procedures | | RANK | Laboratory | |
|---|---|---|---|---|---|---|---|---|---|
| | Minimal | | 99211 | | Anoscopy | 46600 | | Venipuncture | 36415 |
| | Problem focused | 99201 | 99212 | | Audiometry | 92551 | | Blood glucose, monitoring device | 82962 |
| | Expanded problem focused | 99202 | 99213 | | Cerumen removal | 69210 | | Blood glucose, visual dipstick | 82948 |
| | Detailed | 99203 | 99214 | | Colposcopy | 57452 | | CBC, w/ auto differential | 85025 |
| | Comprehensive | 99204 | 99215 | | Colposcopy w/biopsy | 57455 | | CBC, w/o auto differential | 85027 |
| | Comprehensive (new patient) | 99205 | | | ECG, w/interpretation | 93000 | | Cholesterol | 82465 |
| | Significant, separate service | -25 | -25 | | ECG, rhythm strip | 93040 | | Hemoccult, guaiac | 82270 |
| | **Well visit** | **New** | **Est** | | Endometrial biopsy | 58100 | | Hemoccult, immunoassay | 82274 |
| | < 1 y | 99381 | 99391 | | Flexible sigmoidoscopy | 45330 | | Hemoglobin A1C | 85018 |
| | 1-4 y | 99382 | 99392 | | Flexible sigmoidoscopy w/biopsy | 45331 | | Lipid panel | 80061 |
| | 5-11 y | 99383 | 99393 | | Fracture care, cast/splint | 29____ | | Liver panel | 80076 |
| | 12-17 y | 99384 | 99394 | | Site: | | | KOH prep (skin, hair, nails) | 87220 |
| | 18-39 y | 99385 | 99395 | | Nebulizer | 94640 | | Metabolic panel, basic | 80048 |
| | 40-64 y | 99386 | 99396 | | Nebulizer demo | 94664 | | Metabolic panel, comprehensive | 80053 |
| | 65 y + | 99387 | 99397 | | Spirometry | 94010 | | Mononucleosis | 86308 |
| | **Medicare preventive services** | | | | Spirometry, pre and post | 94060 | | Pregnancy, blood | 84703 |
| | Pap | | Q0091 | | Tympanometry | 92567 | | Pregnancy, urine | 81025 |
| | Pelvic & breast | | G0101 | | Vasectomy | 55250 | | Renal panel | 80069 |
| | Prostate/PSA | | G0103 | | **Skin procedures** | **Units** | | Sedimentation rate | 85651 |
| | Tobacco counseling/3-10 min | | 99406 | | Burn care, initial | 16000 | | Strep, rapid | 86403 |
| | Tobacco counseling/>10 min | | 99407 | | Foreign body, skin, simple | 10120 | | Strep culture | 87081 |
| | Welcome to Medicare exam | | G0344 | | Foreign body, skin, complex | 10121 | | Strep A | 87880 |
| | ECG w/Welcome to Medicare exam | | G0366 | | I&D, abscess | 10060 | | TB | 86580 |
| | Flexible sigmoidoscopy | | G0104 | | I&D, hematoma/seroma | 10140 | | UA, complete, non-automated | 81000 |
| | Hemoccult, guaiac | | G0107 | | Laceration repair, simple | 120____ | | UA, w/o micro, non-automated | 81002 |
| | Flu shot | | G0008 | | Site: _____ Size: _____ | | | UA, w/ micro, non-automated | 81003 |
| | Pneumonia shot | | G0009 | | Laceration repair, layered | 120____ | | Urine colony count | 87086 |
| | **Consultation/preop clearance** | | | | Site: _____ Size: _____ | | | Urine culture, presumptive | 87088 |
| | Expanded problem focused | | 99242 | | Lesion, biopsy, one | 11100 | | Wet mount/KOH | 87210 |
| | Detailed | | 99243 | | Lesion, biopsy, each add'l | 11101 | | **Vaccines** | |
| | Comprehensive/mod complexity | | 99244 | | Lesion, destruct., benign, 1-14 | 17110 | | DT, <7 y | 90702 |
| | Comprehensive/high complexity | | 99245 | | Lesion, destruct., premal., single | 17000 | | DTP | 90701 |
| | **Other services** | | | | Lesion, destruct., premal., ea. add'l | 17003 | | DtaP, <7 y | 90700 |
| | After posted hours | | 99050 | | Lesion, excision, benign | 114____ | | Flu, 6-35 months | 90657 |
| | Evening/weekend appointment | | 99051 | | Site: _____ Size: _____ | | | Flu, 3 y + | 90658 |
| | Home health certification | | G0180 | | Lesion, excision, malignant | 116____ | | Hep A, adult | 90632 |
| | Home health recertification | | G0179 | | Site: _____ Size: _____ | | | Hep A, ped/adol, 2 dose | 90633 |
| | Post-op follow-up | | 99024 | | Lesion, paring/cutting, one | 11055 | | Hep B, adult | 90746 |
| | Prolonged/30-74 min | | 99354 | | Lesion, paring/cutting, 2-4 | 11056 | | Hep B, ped/adol 3 dose | 90744 |
| | Special reports/forms | | 99080 | | Lesion, shave | 113____ | | Hep B-Hib | 90748 |
| | Disability/Workers comp | | 99455 | | Site: _____ Size: _____ | | | Hib, 4 dose | 90645 |
| | **Radiology** | | | | Nail removal, partial | 11730 | | HPV | 90649 |
| | | | | | Nail removal, w/matrix | 11750 | | IPV | 90713 |
| | | | | | Skin tag, 1-15 | 11200 | | MMR | 90707 |
| | **Diagnoses** | | | | **Medications** | **Units** | | Pneumonia, >2 y | 90732 |
| 1 | | | | | Ampicillin, up to 500mg | J0290 | | Pneumonia conjugate, <5 y | 90669 |
| 2 | | | | | B-12, up to 1,000 mcg | J3420 | | Td, >7 y | 90718 |
| 3 | | | | | Epinephrine, up to 1ml | J0170 | | Varicella | 90716 |
| 4 | | | | | Kenalog, 10mg | J3301 | | **Immunizations & Injections** | **Units** |
| **Next office visit** | | | | | Lidocaine, 10mg | J2001 | | Allergen, one | 95115 |
| Recheck | Prev | PRN | _____ D W M Y | | Normal saline, 1000cc | J7030 | | Allergen, multiple | 95117 |
| Instructions: | | | | | Phenergan, up to 50mg | J2550 | | Imm admin, one | 90471 |
| | | | | | Progesterone, 150mg | J1055 | | Imm admin, each add'l | 90472 |
| | | | | | Rocephin, 250mg | J0696 | | Imm admin, intranasal, one | 90473 |
| | | | | | Testosterone, 200mg | J1080 | | Imm admin, intranasal, each add'l | 90474 |
| **Referral** | | | | | Tigan, up to 200 mg | J3250 | | Injection, joint, small | 20600 |
| To: | | | | | Toradol, 15mg | J1885 | | Injection, joint, intermediate | 20605 |
| | | | | | **Miscellaneous services** | | | Injection, joint, major | 20610 |
| Instructions: | | | | | | | | Injection, ther/proph/diag | 90772 |
| | | | | | | | | Injection, trigger point | 20552 |
| **Physician signature** | | | | | | | | **Supplies** | |
| X _____ | | | | | | | | | |

**Figure 12-9** Encounter form (also known as a superbill, routing slip, or charge ticket).

the practice financially; they are losing payment for their work. When clinicians under-code by one level, it is the same as seeing 80 patients and getting paid for seeing 60.

## Accurate Coding

The clinician using an EHR does not worry about the mandate "If it isn't documented, it wasn't done" because it is always documented. EHR systems that use standardized nomenclatures have a codified record of the encounter. This enables the software to use data in the encounter note to calculate the correct E&M code for billing.

EHR systems analyze the amount and type of data and accurately determine the correct E&M code at the correct level. Many EHR systems can show the provider how the calculation was determined, thus giving the provider confidence that the code can be substantiated. In addition to E&M codes, the EHR can identify CPT-4 codes for other procedures performed during the encounter as you saw in the previous exercise.

When the EHR is an integrated component of practice management software, or when it is interfaced to a practice management system, the ICD-10-CM, CPT-4, and HCPCS codes can transfer directly to the billing or charge posting module. Most practice management systems do not post the charges automatically, but transfer them as "pending" charges. The charges are reviewed by a billing or coding specialist before being "posted" to the patient's account or billed to insurance.

# Using EHR Software to Understand E&M Codes

In the remaining exercises, we are going to focus on understanding E&M codes. The Student Edition software contains an E&M code calculator. You are going to use the E&M calculator window to help you understand the CMS Documentation Guidelines for Evaluation and Management Services.

One difference from previous chapters is that the Guided Exercises using the E&M calculator start with a significant portion of the findings already recorded so you can concentrate on understanding the E&M guidelines. The next four Guided Exercises incorporate quite a bit of reading material within the steps, but require very little data entry. If you cannot finish an exercise in the allotted time, you can quit the exercise and redo it later without affecting your grade by using the Quit Encounter option (explained in Chapter 3, Exercise 3B, step 2). When you use the Quit option, any findings you have added during the exercise will *not* be saved, and you *will* have to re-add them when you start over. However, in the next four exercises you usually will only need to select the patient and click a few findings to get back to the step where you left off.

## Guided Exercise 12B: Calculating the E&M Code from an Encounter

In this exercise, you are going to learn how to use the E&M calculator by using a partially completed encounter that is already in your system. Using an encounter with some of the findings already recorded will allow you to focus on understanding the E&M codes themselves without worrying about creating the note.

### Case Study

Mary Williams is the 26-year-old mother who brought her infant Tyrell to the pediatri-cianin a previous chapter. She is being seen at the family care clinic for stuffy sinus. The healthcare provider who entered the encounter data has not yet recorded the history or vital signs.

### Step 1

Start a supported web browser program and follow the steps listed inside the cover of this textbook to log in to the MyHealthProfessionsLab for this course.

Locate and click on the link **Exercise 12B**. This will open the Quippe software window with the New Encounter window displayed in the center.

### Step 2

In the New Encounter window patient list, locate and click on **Williams, Mary** as shown in Figure 12-10, and then click the OK button. You do not need to set the date and time of the encounter for this exercise.

### Step 3

Compare your screen to Figure 12-11. The encounter note was created using the Adult URI List and therefore some of the findings should look familiar to you.

Because we are going to be using the information from the encounter note to calculate the E&M code, take a few minutes to look at the encounter note on your screen. It contains a Review of Systems, but nothing in the History sections.

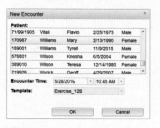

**Figure 12-10** Select patient Mary Williams.

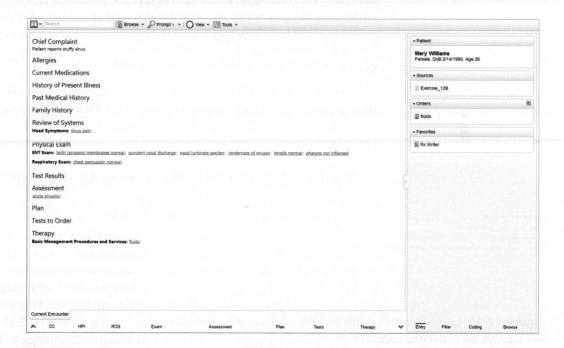

**Figure 12-11** Mary Williams' initial encounter note for Exercise 12B.

### Step 4

Compare the number of body systems in the Physical Findings section of the note with the number of body systems in the Review of Systems section.

When you are sufficiently familiar with the encounter note, locate and click the Tools button in the toolbar at the top of your screen. Select E&M calculator from the drop-down menu shown at the top of Figure 12-12.

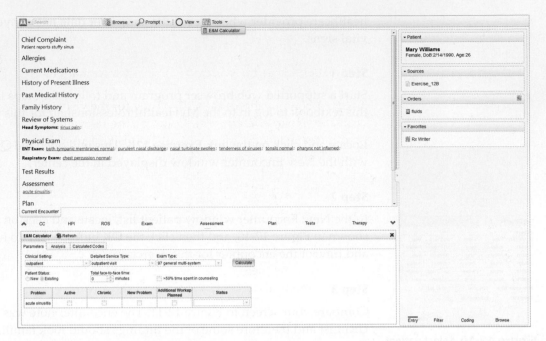

**Figure 12-12** The Tools button menu option (above) invokes the E&M Calculator in the pane below the encounter note.

The E&M Calculator will be displayed below the encounter note in the bottom portion of the workspace pane. The E&M Calculator has three tabs. The first tab has four fields that determine the type of E&M codes applicable to the encounter (outpatient or inpatient, service and exam type, and whether the patient is new or an existing patient). Two additional fields concern the time the clinician spent with the patient. These will be explained in a later exercise. Leave the fields set to their default values.

### Step 5

At the bottom of the tab is a grid of problems documented in the Assessment section of the encounter note. This encounter has one problem, acute sinusitis. We will learn more about this section in Exercise 12D. For the next few exercises do not check any of the boxes in the grid.

Click on the Calculate button located to the right of Exam Type.

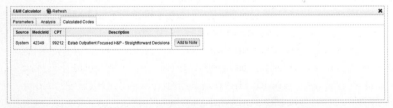

**Figure 12-13** Calculate button on the first tab calculates the CPT-4 code and displays the Calculated Codes tab.

### Step 6

Clicking the Calculate button will analyze the findings in the note and, in the context of the information selected on the first tab, will determine the E&M code whose level is supported by the amount and type of data in the encounter note. The E&M Calculator will automatically change to the third tab, labeled "Calculated Codes," as shown in Figure 12-13.

The grid on the Calculated Codes tab contains 5 columns, Source, MedcinId, CPT, Description, and a button to add a finding, for the procedure code and description in the note.

The Source column indicates whether the code was derived purely by the system or was overridden by the clinician. The clinician does not have to accept the calculated code and can choose to override it if, for example, the encounter note contained extensive amounts of free-text or annotated drawings for which the clinician felt the calculator was not giving enough credit.

The MedcinId can be ignored; it is purely informational.

The CPT column shows the CPT-4 code for the visit, in this case 99212. The Description is an abbreviated description, summarizing relevant factors the code represents, in this case, an established patient, outpatient visit, focused history and physical, with straight-forward medical decision making.

## Key Components

You will recall from an earlier discussion that history, examination, and medical decision making are the key components that determine the level of E&M services. The CPT-4 E&M code description lists the three key components and their levels. The levels of the key components listed in the description for code 99212 are focused history and physical, medical decision making straightforward.

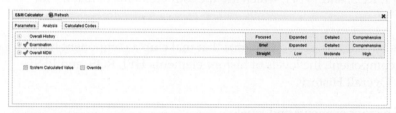

**Figure 12-14** The E&M calculator Analysis tab displays levels of the three key components.

### Step 7

Locate the E&M calculator tab labeled Analysis and click on it. The analysis tab allows the clinician to see how findings in the encounter note meet the E&M guideline. The tab (as shown in Figure 12-14) displays three rows. The rows are the three key components: History, (physical) Examination, and Medical Decision Making (MDM). Plus symbols preceding the component names expand the rows to show their elements, similar to the behavior of other tree structures in Quippe.

## Levels of Key Components

The key components each have levels of their own, which are determined separately by methods we will explain later. Components levels have a name, such as brief, extended, low, high, simple, or complex, which equate to numerical levels 1 to 4. In the E&M analysis grid these are shown in the four columns on the right, which sequence from the lowest level (1) to the rightmost column, which represents the highest level (4). The cell level for which the number of findings is sufficient to meet the guidelines is identified by changing the color of the cell and displaying the level name in bold type. For example, in Figure 12-14 the level 1 cells are peach colored for Examination and Overall MDM and the level names Brief and Straight are in bold type, whereas none of the levels for Overall History are peach and none of the level names are bold. This means there are insufficient history findings to meet even level 1. (Note: The colors on your computer screen may be different.)

The level of an E&M code is derived from the highest level of two or three key components. Over the course of the next few exercises we will discuss each of the key components, the levels within the key components, and how they are combined to calculate the E&M code.

## Key Component: History

### Step 8

We will begin with the key component History. Locate and click the plus symbol next to Overall History. The component will expand the rows to show elements which make up the history component as shown in Figure 12-15.

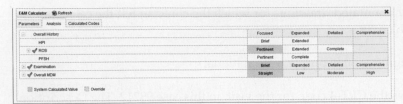

**Figure 12-15** Expanded Overall History displays levels of History elements.

The E&M History component includes the following elements:

◆ **CC**, which is an acronym for Chief Complaint. A Chief Complaint is required for all levels of History, thus it is not shown in the grid.

◆ **HPI**, which is an acronym for History of Present Illness.

◆ **ROS**, which is an acronym for Review of Systems.

◆ **PFSH**, which is an acronym for Past History, Family History, and Social History.

As you can see from the list, the key component History comprises the many sections of the encounter note with the word history in the label, but also includes the sections Allergies, Current Medications, and Review of Systems.

The expanded rows of history on the E&M calculator analysis tab shown in Figure 12-15 are Overall History, HPI, ROS, and PFSH, which are the four elements of history for E&M calculation.

Just as key components have levels, so too elements that make up a component have levels. For the History component, the levels of history elements HPI, ROS, and PFSH determine the level for Overall History.

Let us now discuss the history elements and levels.

**History of Present Illness (HPI)** The HPI is a chronological description of the development of the patient's present illness from the first sign and/or symptom or from the previous encounter to the present. HPI includes the following characteristics:

◆ Location

◆ Quality

◆ Severity

◆ Duration

◆ Timing

◆ Context

◆ Modifying factors

◆ Associated signs and symptoms

HPI has two named levels, brief and extended. The levels are determined by the quantity of findings:

**Brief** (consists of one to three items in the HPI)

**Extended** (consists of at least four items in the HPI or the status of at least three chronic or inactive conditions)

Locate the History of Present Illness section of the encounter note. There are no findings; therefore, neither of the levels in the HPI row was met.

**Step 9**

Locate the row labeled ROS. The word "Pertinent" in the first level column is bold, meaning ROS has enough findings for level 1 but not enough for level 2. A plus symbol in the ROS row indicates that we could expand the row to see the findings which were counted in this level, but in this case it isn't necessary, as you can see there is only one finding in the Review of Systems section of the encounter note.

**Review of Systems (ROS)** The ROS level is determined by the number of systems reviewed. You are familiar with ROS from previous exercises. ROS has three levels:

Problem **Pertinent** (ROS inquires about the system directly related to the problems identified in the HPI.)

**Extended** (ROS inquires about the system directly related to the problems identified in the HPI and a number of additional systems. Extended level requires two to nine systems be documented.)

**Complete** (ROS inquires about the systems directly related to the problems identified in the HPI plus all additional body systems. At least ten organ systems must be reviewed to meet the requirement for Complete.)

## Step 10

**Past, Family, and/or Social History (PFSH)** The PFSH consists of a review of three areas:

◆ Past history (the patient's past experiences with illnesses, operations, injuries, and treatments)

◆ Family history (a review of medical events in the patient's family, including diseases that may be hereditary or place the patient at risk)

◆ Social history (an age-appropriate review of past and current activities)

PFSH level is determined by the number of findings in these three history types. PFSH has two levels:

**Pertinent** (at least one item in any of PFSH area directly related to the problems identified in the HPI)

**Complete** (a review of two or all three of the PFSH history areas, depending on the category of the E&M service. Complete requires all three history areas for services that include a comprehensive assessment of a new patient or reassessment of an existing patient. A review of two of the three history areas is sufficient for other services.)

Look at the column under PFSH on your screen. In this encounter, no PFSH was recorded.

## Step 11

The level for the key component History is shown on the tab in the row Overall History. The key component History has four possible levels:

1. Problem Focused

2. Expanded Problem Focused

3. Detailed

4. Comprehensive

The component level is derived from the levels of the HPI, ROS, and PSFH elements. Figure 12-16 shows the elements required to reach each level of overall history.[3]

---

[3]Figure adapted from *1997 Documentation Guidelines for Evaluation and Management Services* (Washington, DC: U.S. Department of Health and Human Services, 1997).

**Figure 12-16** Table of elements required for each level of History.

**Table of Elements Required for Each Level of History**

| | Level of History | CC | History of Present Illness (HPI) | Review of Systems (ROS) | Past, Family, and/or Social History (PFSH) |
|---|---|---|---|---|---|
| | | | **History Elements** | | |
| 1 | *Problem Focused* | * | Brief (1–3 elements) | (No elements required) | (No elements required) |
| 2 | *Expanded Problem Focused* | * | Brief (1–3 elements) | Problem Pertinent (related to HPI) | (No elements required) |
| 3 | *Detailed* | * | Extended (4 or more) | Extended (2–9 body systems) | Pertinent (1 or more) |
| 4 | *Comprehensive* | * | Extended (4 or more) | Complete (10 or more body systems) | Complete (2 areas Past, Family, or Social) |

* Chief Complaint is expected for all Types of History.

The levels of the key component History are listed in the first column of Figure 12-16. The row for each History level lists the minimum number of elements (findings) required in HPI, ROS, and PFSH columns to meet that level. For example, locate the row for History level 2 in Figure 12-16. Notice that one finding in HPI and one finding in ROS would meet the requirements for overall history level 2.

Compare the HPI, ROS, and PFSH rows on your screen to the chart in Figure 12-16. Do you see why the overall history does not have any level? It is because only the ROS has a level, and HPI is required for level 1.

The extent of history of present illness, review of systems, and past, family, or social history that is obtained and documented is dependent on clinical judgment and the **nature of the presenting problems**. However, for purposes of understanding the overall history matrix, let us add some findings.

**Step 12**

Drag the symptom sinus pain from the Review of Systems section and drop it on the heading History of Present Illness. (Click and hold the left mouse button as you drag the finding upwards. Release the mouse button when the finding is on the heading. Make certain the finding is still red after it is moved.)

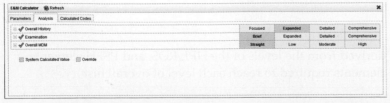

**Figure 12-17** History level changed by moving a symptom to the HPI section of encounter note.

Locate and click the Refresh button on the E&M Calculator. This will cause the note to be reanalyzed and the E&M Calculator to change to the Calculated Codes tab. Notice that moving the symptom did not change the code. It is still 99212. However, click on the analysis tab (shown in Figure 12-17) and notice that overall history now has a level.

## Step 13

Click back on the Calculated Codes tab. Locate and click the Add to Note button. This will add the E&M code to the encounter note.

Close the E&M Calculator by clicking the X in the right corner of the calculator.

Compare your screen to Figure 12-18. If everything is correct, proceed to step 14. If there are any differences, review the preceding steps, and correct your errors.

**Figure 12-18** Correctly completed encounter note for Exercise 12B with CPT-4 code.

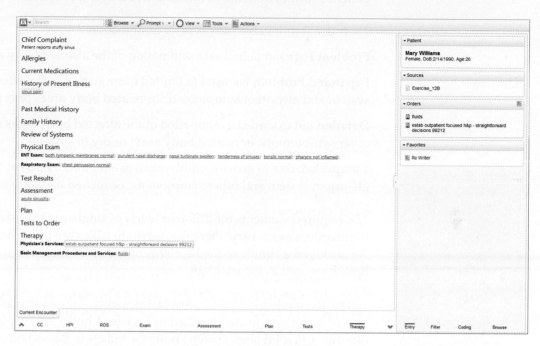

## Step 14

If you wish to print a copy of your completed encounter notes for yourself or because your instructor requires you to turn them in, then print or download the PDF at this time.

Locate and click the blue Quippe icon button on the toolbar to display the drop-down menu, and then select the Submit for Grade menu option. This will complete Exercise 12B.

# Key Component: Examination

The second key component is the **Physical Examination component**. Examination guidelines have been defined for a general multisystem exam and the following 10 single-organ systems:

◆ Cardiovascular

◆ Ears, Nose, and Throat

◆ Eyes

◆ Genitourinary (Female or Male)

◆ Hematologic/Lymphatic/Immunologic

◆ Musculoskeletal

◆ Neurological

◆ Psychiatric

◆ Respiratory

◆ Skin

A general multisystem examination or a single-organ system examination may be performed by any physician, regardless of specialty. The type and content of examination are selected by the examining physician and are based on clinical judgment, the patient's history, and the nature of the presenting problems.

There are four levels of any type of examination:

**Problem Focused** (a limited examination of the affected body area or organ system)

**Expanded Problem Focused** (a limited examination of the affected body area or organ system and any other symptomatic or related body areas or organ systems)

**Detailed** (an extended examination of the affected body areas or organ systems and any other symptomatic or related body areas or organ systems)

**Comprehensive** (a general multisystem examination, or complete examination of a single-organ system and other symptomatic or related body areas or organ systems)

The required elements for different levels of single-organ system exams and the general multisystem exam vary; therefore, separate tables are published for each type of system. An abridged example of the Elements of General Multisystem Examination table[4] has been reprinted in Figure 12-19.

Within the guideline tables, individual elements of the examination pertaining to a body area or organ system are identified by bullets. A bullet is a typographic character that looks like this: • (a solid black circle). Locate the bullets in the second column of Figure 12-19.

If you have taken a class in medical coding or read the CPT-4 book, you may be familiar with the concept of "the number of bullets required to meet a level of E&M coding." This simply means how many findings in the encounter note correspond to elements in the guideline table with bullet characters printed next to them.

## Guided Exercise 12C: Understanding the Examination Component

In this exercise, continue using the E&M calculator as you read about the E&M key component: Examination.

### Step 1

Start a supported web browser program and log in to the MyHealthProfessionsLab for this course.

Locate and click on the link **Exercise 12C**. This will open the Quippe software window with the New Encounter window displayed in the center.

### Step 2

In the New Encounter window patient list, locate and click on **Williams, Mary** as shown previously in Figure 12-10, and then click the OK button. You do not need to set the date and time of the encounter for this exercise.

---

[4]Ibid.

| Elements of General Multisystem Examination | |
| --- | --- |
| **System/Body Area** | **Exam Elements** |
| Constitutional | • Measurement of any three of the following seven vital signs: (1) sitting or standing blood pressure, (2) supine blood pressure, (3) pulse rate and regularity, (4) respiration, (5) temperature, (6) height, (7) weight (may be measured and recorded by ancillary staff) <br> • General appearance of patient (e.g., development, nutrition, body habitus, deformities, attention to grooming) |
| Eyes | • Inspection of conjunctivae and lids <br> • Examination of pupils and irises (e.g., reaction to light and accommodation, size and symmetry) <br> • Ophthalmoscopic examination of optic discs (e.g., size, C/D ratio, appearance) and posterior segments (e.g., vessel changes, exudates, hemorrhages) |
| Ears, Nose, Mouth, and Throat | • External inspection of ears and nose (e.g., overall appearance, scars, lesions, masses) <br> • Otoscopic examination of external auditory canals and tympanic membranes <br> • Assessment of hearing (e.g., whispered voice, finger rub, tuning fork) <br> • Inspection of nasal mucosa, septum, and turbinates <br> • Inspection of lips, teeth, and gums <br> • Examination of oropharynx: oral mucosa, salivary glands, hard and soft palates, tongue, tonsils, and posterior pharynx |
| Neck | • Examination of neck (e.g., masses, overall appearance, symmetry, tracheal position, crepitus) <br> • Examination of thyroid (e.g., enlargement, tenderness, mass) |
| Respiratory | • Assessment of respiratory effort (e.g., intercostal retractions, use of accessory muscles, diaphragmatic movement) <br> • Percussion of chest (e.g., dullness, flatness, hyperresonance) <br> • Palpation of chest (e.g., tactile fremitus) <br> • Auscultation of lungs (e.g., breath sounds, adventitious sounds, rubs) |
| Cardiovascular | |
| Chest (Breasts) | • Inspection of breasts (e.g., symmetry, nipple discharge) <br> • Palpation of breasts and axillae (e.g., masses or lumps, tenderness) |
| Gastrointestinal (Abdomen) | • Examination of abdomen with notation of presence of masses or tenderness <br> • Examination of liver and spleen <br> • Examination for presence or absence of hernia <br> • Examination (when indicated) of anus, perineum and rectum, including sphincter tone, presence of hemorrhoids, rectal masses <br> • Obtain stool sample for occult blood test when indicated |

**Figure 12-19** Table of Elements of General Multisystem Examination (abridged sample).

## Step 3

Practice what you have learned in the previous exercise. Invoke the E&M Calculator by clicking the Tools button on the toolbar and selecting E&M Calculator from the drop-down menu.

Notice that the drop-down field for Exam Type is set to "97 general multi-system." This is the guideline that will be used for calculating the level of the Examination component. Although there are guidelines for single-organ systems, the 97 general multi-system guideline may be used by any specialty.

Click on the Calculate button.

When the code 99212 is displayed, click on the Analysis tab and click the plus symbol next to Examination to expand the row.

Because the expanded Examination row has so many entries it will be easier for you to perform subsequent steps if you increase the proportion of the workspace pane allocated to the E&M Calculator. This is accomplished by the same process you used to resize flow sheets in a previous chapter. Position your mouse pointer on the small line at the bottom of the navigation bar (circled in red in Figure 12-20). When the mouse pointer changes to two arrows, click and hold the left mouse button while dragging the line upward until the E&M calculator portion of your screen resembles Figure 12-20.

**Figure 12-20** Encounter pane with HPI positioned at the top, E&M pane expanded to show the Examination section.

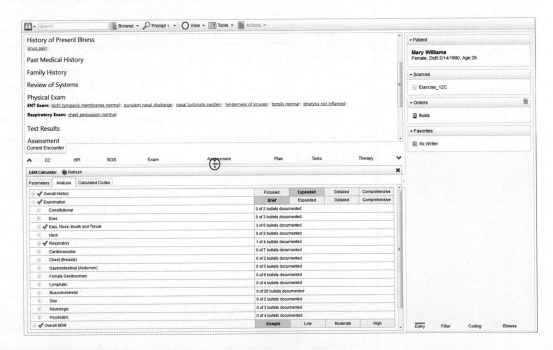

## Step 4

The E&M calculator and encounter note portions of the workspace can be scrolled separately. It will be useful for you to scroll the encounter note portion until History of Present Illness is positioned at the top of the pane, as shown in Figure 12-20.

Locate the Examination component in the Analysis tab. As with the other key components the four columns on the right of the Examination row list the four possible levels. For this encounter note the Examination component level is Brief.

The expanded rows beneath Examination list the body/system areas of the General Multipurpose Examination. For each body/system, the column on the right has a pair of numbers and the words "bullets documented." For example, locate the row for Ears, Nose, Mouth, and Throat; you will see "3 of 6 bullets documented." This means the clinician examined three of six elements in that body/system.

The number of bullets possible for each body/system correlates to the table in Figure 12-19.

### Step 5

Unlike the key component History where the number of findings equated to number of history elements, the Examination component is not determined by the number of findings, but by the number of bullets satisfied within a body/system (the bullets in Figure 12-19).

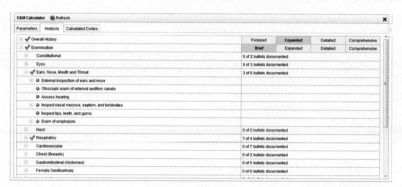

**Figure 12-21** E&M calculator showing bullets for Ears, Nose, Mouth, and Throat.

Locate the row Ears, Nose, Mouth, and Throat, and click the plus symbol to expand it, as shown in Figure 12-21. Here you can see bullets next to six exam elements. Turn to Figure 12-19 in your text, and locate the section of the table for Ears, Nose, Mouth, and Throat. Compare the list of exam elements in Figure 12-19 with the descriptions in the expanded rows below Ears, Nose, Mouth, and Throat on your screen.

In Figure 12-21, blue bullets indicate exam elements with findings, while grayish-black bullets indicate bulleted exam elements that do not have a finding.

### Step 6

Look at the Physical Exam section of the encounter note and count the number of findings in the ENT exam.

Why, if there are six findings documented, are only three bullets met?

If you suppose it is because half the findings are normal (blue), you are mistaken. Findings do not have to be abnormal; normal findings count as well. The guidelines state: "A brief statement or notation indicating 'negative' or 'normal' is sufficient to document normal findings related to unaffected areas or asymptomatic organ systems."[5]

To find the correct answer to the question compare the bulleted descriptions in the expanded rows below Ears, Nose, Mouth, and Throat with the findings in the encounter note. Of the six findings, most were about the nasal, sinus, and throat. Findings about auditory canals, hearing, lips, and gums were not recorded, so those bullets were not met.

Before proceeding to the next step, locate the minus symbol next to Ears, Nose, Mouth, and Throat and click it to collapse the expanded ENT rows. Your screen should again resemble Figure 12-20.

---

[5]*1997 Documentation Guidelines for Evaluation and Management Services* (Washington, DC: U.S. Department of Health and Human Services, 1997).

## Levels of Key Component: Examination

From the previous discussion we see that the level of the examination component is not based on quantity of findings alone, but on the number of bullets in an examination guideline that are satisfied per body/system section.

Of course, the number of bullets required to be satisfied varies by the type of Exam guideline applied. In this exercise we are using the "97 General multi-system guideline." If the clinician were to select the ENT guideline, the E&M Calculator would give more weight to the ENT elements and require more bullets.

The Table of Elements Required for Each Level of Examination[6] in Figure 12-22 defines the level of Examination by the number of bullets met in the number of body systems examined.

**Figure 12-22** Table of Elements Required for Each Level of Examination.

### Table of Elements Required for Each Level of Examination

| | Level of Examination | Examination Elements by Type of Exam | |
| --- | --- | --- | --- |
| | | General Multisystem Examinations | Single Organ System Examinations |
| 1 | Problem Focused (Brief) | 1 to 5 elements identified by a bullet (•) in one or more organ systems or body areas. | 1 to 5 elements identified by a bullet (•), whether in a box with a shaded or unshaded border.* |
| 2 | Expanded Problem Focused | At least 6 elements identified by a bullet (•) in one or more organ systems or body areas. | At least 6 elements identified by a bullet (•), whether in a box with a shaded or unshaded border.* |
| 3 | Detailed Examination | At least 6 organ systems or body areas; for each system/area selected at least 2 elements identified by a bullet (•). Alternatively, at least 12 elements identified by a bullet (•) in 2 or more organ systems or body areas. | At least 12 elements identified by a bullet (•), whether in a box with a shaded or unshaded border.* Exception: requirement reduced to 9 elements for Eye and psychiatric examinations. |
| 4 | Comprehensive Examination | At least 9 organ systems or body areas; for each system/area selected all elements identified by a bullet (•). | Every element in each box with a shaded border and at least 1 element in each box with an unshaded border; Plus all elements identified by a bullet (•) whether in a box with a shaded or unshaded border.* |

\* This refers to sections of the printed tables for Single Organ System Exams, which are outlined with a shaded border.

## Step 7

Look at your E&M calculator. Green check marks appear in two rows of body areas of the Examination section, Ear, Nose, Mouth and Throat, and Respiratory. Follow the rows to the right to locate the number of bullets met: Ear, Nose, Mouth and Throat—3 of 6 bullets documented; Respiratory—1 of 4 bullets documented.

Refer to the table in Figure 12-22. Level 1 (Brief) is defined as a "Problem Focused Exam," when there are one to five elements identified by a bullet (in Figure 12-19). Although this encounter has seven physical exam findings, they satisfied only four bullets.

---

[6]Ibid.

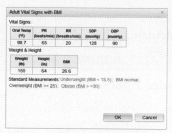

**Figure 12-23** Adult Vital Signs with BMI form for Mary Williams.

## Step 8

Since this encounter is missing vital signs, which are physical exam findings, let us add some.

Click the Browse button on the toolbar, and expand Sample Custom Content, Shared Content, Student Edition Forms. Click on "Adult BMI + Vitals" to highlight it, and click the Add to Note button. The form pop-up window shown in Figure 12-23 will be displayed.

Enter the following vital signs for Mary in the corresponding fields of the form:

| | |
|---|---|
| Temperature: | **98.7** |
| Pulse: | **65** |
| Respiration: | **20** |
| SBP: | **128** |
| DBP: | **90** |
| Weight: | **155** |
| Height: | **64** |

When you have entered all of the vital signs, compare your screen to Figure 12-23 and then click the OK button to close the form and add the findings.

## Step 9

Locate and click the Refresh button at the top of the E&M Calculator. The Calculated Codes tab will redisplay. Notice that the E&M code did not change. It is still 99212.

Click the Analysis tab. Notice that the Examination level did not change. It is still Brief.

Click the plus symbol in the Examination row to expand the section. Notice that Constitutional now has a green checkmark. Follow the row to the right and notice that it says "1 of 2 bullets documented."

Sum the number of bullets in the examination section now listed as documented. There are five. Refer to the table in Figure 12-22 and notice that level 1 is one to five bullets.

Locate the Constitutional row of the E&M calculator and click on the plus symbol to expand it. The bullet that has been satisfied is "Three of seven vital signs." The bullet that was not met was "general appearance of the patient."

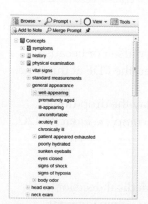

**Figure 12-24** Browse Concepts drop-down list showing well-appearing highlighted.

## Step 10

Click on any whitespace in the encounter note that does not cause a finding or heading to have focus.

Click the Browse button, and the plus symbols to expand Concepts, physical examination, and general appearance. Click on well-appearing to highlight it (as shown in Figure 12-24) and then click the Add to Note button.

Locate the added finding in the encounter note and click it until it turns red:

- not well-appearing

## Step 11

Locate and click the Refresh button at the top of the E&M Calculator. The Calculated Codes tab will redisplay. This time the E&M code changed to 99213.

Locate and click the Add to Note button. The E&M code and description will be added to the encounter note.

Click the Analysis tab. Notice that the Examination level now reads Expanded.

Click the plus symbol in the Examination row to expand the section. Sum the number of bullets in the examination section that are listed as documented. There are six. Refer to the table in Figure 12-22 and notice that level 2 is "At least 6 elements identified by a bullet."

## Step 12

Close the E&M Calculator by clicking the X in the right corner of the calculator.

Compare your screen to Figure 12-25. If everything is correct, proceed to step 13. If there are any differences, review the preceding steps, and correct your errors.

**Figure 12-25** Correctly completed encounter note for Exercise 12C.

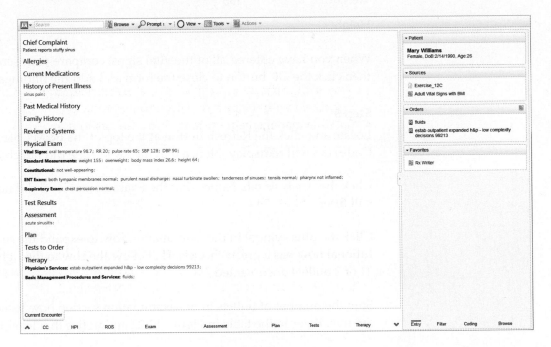

## Step 13

If you wish to print a copy of your completed encounter notes for yourself or because your instructor requires you to turn them in, then print or download the PDF at this time.

Locate and click the blue Quippe icon button on the toolbar to display the drop-down menu, and then select the Submit for Grade menu option. This will complete Exercise 12C.

## Key Component: Medical Decision Making

The third key component is Medical Decision Making (MDM). Medical decision making refers to the complexity of establishing a diagnosis or selecting a management option as measured by the following elements:

◆ **Number of possible diagnoses or management options** that must be considered. This element has four levels. The level is determined by the number and types of problems addressed during the encounter, the complexity of establishing a diagnosis, and the management decisions that are made by the clinician. The levels are:

Level 1: Minimal

Level 2: Limited

Level 3: Multiple

Level 4: Extensive

In addition to the actual number of diagnoses findings recorded, the number and type of diagnostic tests employed may be an indicator of the number of possible diagnoses. Problems that were reviewed also are counted. Consulting or seeking advice from others is another indicator of complexity of diagnostic or management problems.

Amount or complexity of medical records, diagnostic tests, or other information that must be obtained, reviewed, and analyzed. There are four levels for this element as well:

Level 1: Minimal or None

Level 2: Limited

Level 3: Moderate

Level 4: Extensive

**Risk of significant complications, morbidity or mortality, as well as comorbidities,** associated with the patient's presenting problems, the diagnostic procedures, or the possible management options. Risk also has four levels:

Level 1: Minimal

Level 2: Low

Level 3: Moderate

Level 4: High

As you can see, each of the elements of medical decision making has four levels. The overall level of the MDM component is derived from the highest level of two of the three elements. Let us look at how it is determined.

## Guided Exercise 12D: Understanding the MDM Component

In this exercise, continue using the E&M calculator as you read about the E&M key component Medical Decision Making.

### Step 1

Start a supported web browser program and follow the steps listed inside the cover of this textbook to log in to the MyHealthProfessionsLab for this course.

Locate and click on the link **Exercise 12D**. This will open the Quippe software window with the New Encounter window displayed in the center.

### Step 2

In the New Encounter window patient list, locate and click on **Williams, Mary** as shown previously in Figure 12-10, and then click the OK button. You do not need to set the date and time of the encounter for this exercise.

## Step 3

Practice what you have learned in the previous exercise. Invoke the E&M Calculator by clicking the Tools button on the toolbar and selecting E&M Calculator from the drop-down menu.

Click the Calculate button. Because we are continuing from the previous exercise, the Calculated Codes tab will display CPT-4 code 99213 since there are now six elements with bullets in the Examination component.

Click on the Analysis tab. Locate and click the plus symbol for the row Overall MDM to expand the section.

Dx/Mgt stands for Diagnosis and/or Management Options. Click the plus symbol next to Dx/Mgt to expand the row as shown in Figure 12-26.

**Figure 12-26** Encounter note with the E&M Analysis tab showing expanded rows of Overall MDM.

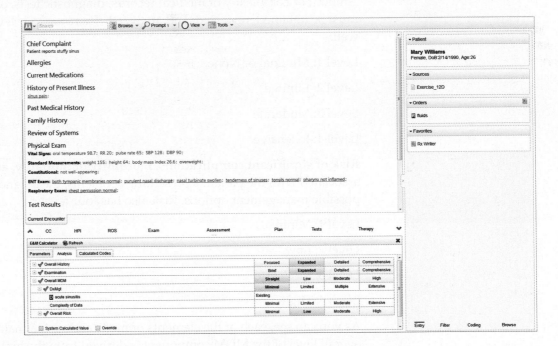

Notice the Overall MDM level is "Straight," Dx Mgt is "Minimal," and Overall Risk is "Low." Complexity of Data does not have any level set.

## Step 4

In the previous exercises we have ignored four questions at the bottom of the first tab of the E&M Calculator because they only apply to MDM and were not, at that point, relevant.

MDM element levels can be affected by factors of the problem assessment that may not be explicitly documented in the encounter note such as the following:

- ◆ Is the problem active or inactive?
- ◆ Is the problem chronic or not?
- ◆ Is the problem new to the examiner?
- ◆ Is additional workup planned for the problem?
- ◆ Is the problem stable or worsening?

Click on the E&M Calculator tab labeled "Parameters." Locate the problem grid at the bottom.

The Problem grid allows clinician to add information for the E&M calculator about each problem by checking boxes for active, chronic, new, or additional workup. A drop-down list lets the provider inform the E&M calculator of the problem status, but unlike the ICD-10-CM Code Review in the previous exercise, which actually changed the diagnosis finding, setting problem status in the E&M Calculator does not alter a problem status that has been recorded in the Detail pop-up window Status field. This encounter has only one diagnosis. If there were additional diagnoses, there would be a row in the grid for each.

Ms. Williams has a new problem. She is coming today because it is getting worse.

Click the following checkboxes:

✓ Active

✓ New Problem

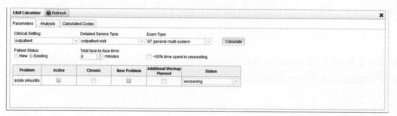

**Figure 12-27** E&M Parameter tab with Problem grid checkboxes checked and Status set.

In the Status field click the down-arrow and select **worsening** from the drop-down list. Compare your problem grid to Figure 12-27.

Locate the Refresh button at the top of the E&M Calculator and click it. This will recalculate the code and redisplay 99213 in the Calculated Codes tab. Adding diagnosis information did not change the E&M code, but it did change the MDM level.

### Step 5

Click on the Analysis tab and then the plus symbols to expand the Overall MDM and Dx/Mgt rows as shown in Figure 12-28. Notice that because the problem is active, new to the clinician, and worsening, it changed the level of Dx/Mgt from level 1, minimal, to level 3, multiple.

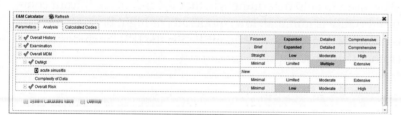

**Figure 12-28** Dx/Mgt level changed by adding problem information.

### Step 6

The next element of MDM is the complexity of medical records, diagnostic tests and other information that must be obtained and reviewed. This encounter doesn't have any orders.

The clinician orders a test for the flu. Click in the Search box on the toolbar at the top of the screen, type **rapid bacterial antigen**, and press the Enter key on your keyboard.

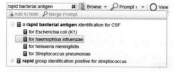

**Figure 12-29** Search results for rapid bacterial antigen identification for CSF, for haemophilus influenzae selected

In the search results list, click the plus symbol next to "rapid bacterial antigen identification for CSF" to expand the tree. Click on **for haemophilus influenzae** to highlight it, as shown in Figure 12-29, and then click the Add to Note button.

Locate the added finding in the encounter note Tests to Order section and click on it until it turns red.

● rapid bacterial antigen identification for CSF for haemophilus influenzae

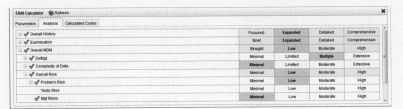

**Figure 12-30** Level of Overall MDM determined by the highest two of three elements.

**Step 7**

Locate the Refresh button at the top of the E&M Calculator and click it. Click on the Analysis tab and then the plus symbols to expand the Overall MDM and Dx/Mgt rows. Notice that complexity of level now has a minimal level where previously there was no level.

The level of Overall Risk is low. Click the plus symbol for Overall Risk to expand the rows below it, as shown in Figure 12-30. The level of Problem Risk is low, and the Test does not present a risk, so it has no level.

**Step 8**

Look at the encounter note Therapy section (scrolling the encounter pane portion of the workspace if necessary). The clinician ordered the patient to drink plenty of fluids.

Look at the last row of the E&M Calculator Analysis tab, Mgt Risks. The risk level for this row is "minimal" because there is little risk involved when drinking fluids.

The E&M guidelines use a special table for calculating the overall level of risk[7] (shown in Figure 12-31). However, risk differs from the other two MDM elements in that risk level is the highest level of any *one* column in the table.

The table in Figure 12-31 is used to help determine whether the risk of significant complications, morbidity, or mortality is minimal, low, moderate, or high. Because the determination of risk is complex and not readily quantifiable, the table includes common clinical examples rather than absolute measures of risk.

Locate the Overall Risk row in the E&M calculator window. Notice that the level of the overall risk column is "low," because that was the level of the highest of the three risk elements, Problem Risk. You will see another example of this aspect of risk in Guided Exercise 12E.

## Determining the Level of Medical Decision Making

There are four levels of Medical Decision Making:

Level 1: **Straight**forward

Level 2: **Low** Complexity

Level 3: **Moderate** Complexity

Level 4: **High** Complexity

The individual levels from each of the elements we have discussed, number of diagnoses, amount or complexity of data, and the level of risk are used to determine the level for Medical Decision Making.

---

[7]Figure adapted from *1997 Documentation Guidelines for Evaluation and Management Services* (Washington, DC: U.S. Department of Health and Human Services, 1997).

## Table of Risk

| Level of Risk | Presenting Problem(s) | Diagnostic Procedure(s) Ordered | Management Options Selected |
|---|---|---|---|
| 1 Minimal | • One self-limited or minor problem, e.g., cold, insect bite, tinea corporis | • Laboratory tests requiring venipuncture<br>• Chest x-rays<br>• EKG/EEG<br>• Urinalysis<br>• Ultrasound, e.g., echocardiography<br>• KOH prep | • Rest<br>• Gargles<br>• Elastic bandages<br>• Superficial dressings |
| 2 Low | • Two or more self-limited or minor problems<br>• One stable chronic illness, e.g., well-controlled hypertension, non–insulin dependent diabetes, cataract, BPH<br>• Acute uncomplicated illness or injury, e.g., cystitis, allergic rhinitis, simple sprain | • Physiologic tests not under stress, e.g., pulmonary function tests<br>• Non-cardiovascular imaging studies with contrast, e.g., barium enema<br>• Superficial needle biopsies<br>• Clinical laboratory tests requiring arterial puncture<br>• Skin biopsies | • Over-the-counter drugs<br>• Minor surgery with no identified risk factors<br>• Physical therapy<br>• Occupational therapy<br>• IV fluids without additives |
| 3 Moderate | • One or more chronic illnesses with mild exacerbation, progression, or side effects of treatment<br>• Two or more stable chronic illnesses<br>• Undiagnosed new problem with uncertain prognosis, e.g., lump in breast<br>• Acute illness with systemic symptoms, e.g., pyelonephritis, pneumonitis, colitis<br>• Acute complicated injury, e.g., head injury with brief loss of consciousness | • Physiologic tests under stress, e.g., cardiac stress test, fetal contraction stress test<br>• Diagnostic endoscopies with no identified risk factors<br>• Deep needle or incisional biopsy<br>• Cardiovascular imaging studies with contrast and no identified risk factors, e.g., arteriogram, cardiac catheterization<br>• Obtain fluid from body cavity, e.g., lumbar puncture, thoracentesis, culdocentesis | • Minor surgery with identified risk factors<br>• Elective major surgery (open, percutaneous, or endoscopic) with no identified risk factors<br>• Prescription drug management<br>• Therapeutic nuclear medicine<br>• IV fluids with additives<br>• Closed treatment of fracture or dislocation without manipulation |
| 4 High | • One or more chronic illnesses with severe exacerbation, progression, or side effects of treatment<br>• Acute or chronic illnesses or injuries that pose a threat to life or bodily function, e.g., multiple trauma, acute MI, pulmonary embolus, severe respiratory distress, progressive severe rheumatoid arthritis, psychiatric illness with potential threat to self or others, peritonitis, acute renal failure<br>• An abrupt change in neurologic status, e.g., seizure, TIA, weakness, sensory loss | • Cardiovascular imaging studies with contrast with identified risk factors<br>• Cardiac electrophysiological tests<br>• Diagnostic endoscopies with identified risk factors<br>• Discography | • Elective major surgery (open, percutaneous, or endoscopic) with identified risk factors<br>• Emergency major surgery (open, percutaneous, or endoscopic)<br>• Parenteral controlled substances<br>• Drug therapy requiring intensive monitoring for toxicity<br>• Decision not to resuscitate or to de-escalate care because of poor prognosis |

**Figure 12-31** Table for determining level of risk.

The chart in Figure 12-32 shows the level of elements required for each level of medical decision making.[8] The level of MDM (shown in the first column of Figure 12-32) is determined by the highest levels of any two of the three elements.

**Table of Levels of Medical Decision Making**

| Level of MDM | Medical Decision Making | Number of diagnoses or management options | Amount and/or complexity of data to be reviewed | Risk of complications and/or morbidity or mortality |
|---|---|---|---|---|
| 1 | *Straightforward* | Minimal | Minimal or None | Minimal |
| 2 | *Low Complexity* | Limited | Limited | Low |
| 3 | *Moderate Complexity* | Multiple | Moderate | Moderate |
| 4 | *High Complexity* | Extensive | Extensive | High |

### Step 9

Compare the chart in Figure 12-32 to the E&M calculator window.

Locate the row labeled "Overall MDM," which is level 2, **low**.

Looking at the rows for the individual elements, notice that Dx/Mgt is level 3, **multiple**, but Overall Risk is level 2, **low**. Even though Dx/Mgt is level 3, the rule states that the MDM level is set to the highest of two out of three elements. Since there are not two level 3 elements, the MDM is set to level 2.

## Other Components: Counseling, Coordination of Care, and Time

The **Time component** is considered the key or controlling factor to qualify for a particular level of E&M services *only* when **counseling** or **coordination of care** dominates more than 50 percent of the encounter (face-to-face time in the office or other outpatient setting, floor/unit time in the hospital or nursing facility).

**Face-to-face time** incorporates the total time both before and after the visit, such as taking patient history, performing the exam, reviewing lab results, planning for follow-up care, and communicating with other providers about the patient's case.

### Step 10

Click on the E&M Calculator Parameters tab.

In the center of the E&M calculator window, above the problem grid, are two fields related to time (circled in Figure 12-33). The first field is used to enter the total face-to-face time. The second field is a check box used to indicate that counseling (or coordination of care) exceeded 50 percent of the face-to-face time for the visit.

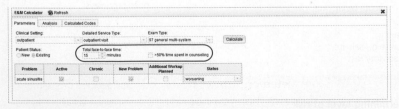

**Figure 12-33** Parameters tab, Total face-to-face time and Counseling fields circled.

---

[8]Ibid.

The E&M calculator allows you to record the amount of face-to-face time even when you are not using counseling time as a factor. It is a good practice to record the face-to-face time for each encounter.

The clinician spent 15 minutes face-to-face time with Ms. Williams. Locate "Total face-to-face time" and enter **15** in the field. You can type minutes in the field or use the arrow buttons. Each click of the up-arrow button increments the field in 5-minute intervals. The down-arrow button de-increments in 5-minute intervals. Do *not* check the >50% checkbox.

Click on the Calculate button. The tab will change to the Calculated Codes tab This will not change the E&M code because time does not become a factor until it is more than half of the face-to-face time. In Guided Exercise 12F you will learn to use both of these time-related fields to change the E&M code and to document the results in your encounter note.

Click on the Add to Note button. The CPT-4 code and description will be added to the note.

### Step 11

Close the E&M Calculator by clicking the X in the right corner of the calculator.

Compare your screen to Figure 12-34. If everything is correct, proceed to step 12. If there are any differences, review the preceding steps, and correct your errors.

**Figure 12-34 Completed encounter note with the CPT-4 code for Exercise 12D.**

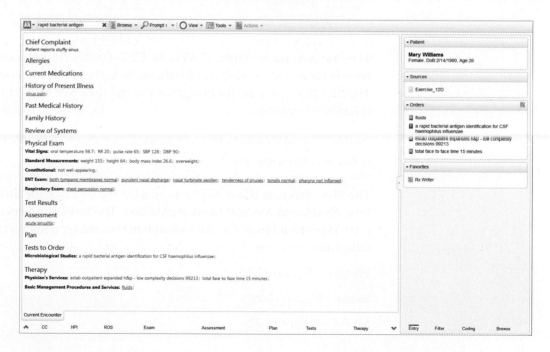

### Step 12

If you wish to print a copy of your completed encounter notes for yourself or because your instructor requires you to turn them in, then print or download the PDF at this time.

Locate and click the blue Quippe icon button on the toolbar to display the drop-down menu, and then select the Submit for Grade menu option This will complete Exercise 12D.

# Putting It All Together

Momentarily leaving the element of time aside, you will see that the levels of each of the three *key components* combine to determine the level of the E&M code.

The chart in Figure 12-35 shows the E&M codes used for the category of outpatient office visits. It will help you to visualize how the relationship of the key components determines the E&M code. You will also notice that there are different code sets for new versus established patients.

**Figure 12-35** Relationship of key component levels determines the E&M code.

### Relationship of Key Elements to E&M Codes for Outpatient Visits

| E&M Code | Type of Patient | # of Key Elements Met | History Level | Exam Level | Medical Decision Making | Face-to-face Time |
|---|---|---|---|---|---|---|
| 99201 | New | All 3 | 1 | 1 | 1 | 10 min |
| 99202 | New | All 3 | 2 | 2 | 1 | 20 min |
| 99203 | New | All 3 | 3 | 3 | 2 | 30 min |
| 99204 | New | All 3 | 4 | 4 | 3 | 45 min |
| 99205 | New | All 3 | 4 | 4 | 4 | 60 min |
| 99211 | Established | 2 of 3 | Presentation of Problem Minimal Documentation Req. | | | 5 min |
| 99212 | Established | 2 of 3 | 1 | 1 | 1 | 10 min |
| 99213 | Established | 2 of 3 | 2 | 2 | 2 | 15 min |
| 99214 | Established | 2 of 3 | 3 | 3 | 3 | 25 min |
| 99215 | Established | 2 of 3 | 4 | 4 | 4 | 40 min |

The first column in Figure 12-35 is the CPT-4 code. The second column indicates if the code is for a new or established patient. Note that there are two groups of codes listed. The first five codes are for new patients, and then five different codes are listed for established patients.

The third column, labeled "# of Key Elements Met," indicates how many key components determine the E&M code.

The blue, green, and lavender columns list the levels of the three key components: History, Exam, and Medical Decision Making. The level numbers under each key component are derived from the individual tables in the sections you have just completed. The tables are:

History—Figure 12-16

Exam—Figure 12-19

MDM—Figure 12-32

The final column lists the number of minutes per type of visit used by the E&M calculator. Time will be discussed further in Guided Exercise 12F.

## Evaluating Key Components

Once the level of each of the key components has been determined, calculating the level of the E&M code is fairly straightforward. The E&M code level is determined by the lowest level of the key components considered. However, different requirements apply when determining the E&M code for new versus established patients.

Scan down the third column of Figure 12-35. Note that the number of key components for a new patient is "All 3." Notice that for established patients it is "2 of 3." This does not mean that an encounter will not have findings for all three components—in most cases it will. It means that, for an established patient, the two key components with the highest levels are considered and the lowest level of the two determines the E&M code.

For example, consider an encounter that has:

History Level 1 (Problem Focused)

Exam Level 2 (Expanded Problem Focused)

MDM Level 3 (Moderate Complexity)

The E&M code for an established patient will be level 2 because the elements with the highest levels (Exam and MDM) are the relevant elements and Exam has the lower level of the two.

Now compare the E&M codes for a new patient. Locate the section of the table in Figure 12-35 for new patients. What E&M code would be used when History is level 1 (Problem Focused), Exam is level 2 (Expanded Problem Focused), and MDM is level 2 (Low Complexity)?

If you answered 99201, you are correct. The E&M code for new patients is determined by all three elements. Even though the Exam and MDM components are level 2, if the History level is not 2, then the lower code must be used.

Having tried to determine a code manually, you can appreciate the value that an E&M calculator brings to an EHR system. Remember that the level of each of the key components is a combination of elements:

◆ To qualify for a given level of history, the quantity and types of HPI, ROS, and PFSH must be met.

◆ To qualify for a given level of exam, the number of "bulleted" items in the appropriate number of body systems must be met.

◆ To qualify for a given level of medical decision making, two of the three elements (the number of diagnosis, the amount of data, and the risk assessment) must be either met or exceeded.

If you can imagine trying to count bullets from your encounter notes, calculate the amount of and types of history, and determine the level of decision making in your head—all while you are seeing the patient—you can understand why so many doctors code at the wrong level, just to be safe. You also can appreciate the skill required of medical coders who do this manually.

## How Changes in Key Components Affect the E&M Code

At this point, you should have a good understanding on how an E&M code is determined from the key components of the encounter. However, what raises the E&M code for an encounter to the next level is not always apparent.

The level of E&M code for an established patient is dependent on two of three of the key components. Merely adding more findings to any one component may bring that component to a higher level, but that does not necessarily mean that the visit as a whole will qualify for the higher level E&M code.

For example, in Guided Exercise 12B (Figure 12-17) an established patient had:

History Level 2 Problem Focused (Expanded)

Exam Level 1 Problem Focused (Brief)

MDM Level 1 Straight Forward (Straight)

The E&M code was level 1 (99212) because one of the two highest key components was a level 1. Even if the level of History was raised to three, the E&M code would still be level 1 because the exam component was only level 1.

Work must be performed and documented in the appropriate areas to result in a higher E&M code. The next exercise demonstrates how changes to key components affect an increase to the level of an E&M code.

In the next exercise, you are going to add findings to an existing encounter to study the effects on E&M coding.

---

### Fraud and Abuse

The goal of these exercises is to provide an experiential understanding of concepts discussed in this chapter. They should not be construed as having any other purpose.

It is unethical and illegal to maximize payment by means that contradict regulatory guidelines. The HHS Office of Inspector General (OIG) investigates allegations of medical billing fraud and abuse. It does not matter if coding errors are made deliberately or inadvertently; OIG still treats it as fraud and abuse.

The student should not get the impression that it is okay to up-code to maximize reimbursement unless legally entitled by documentation and service provided. Similarly, a clinician cannot adjust the time factor unless it is substantiated in the documentation. Diagnoses or procedures should not be inappropriately included or excluded to affect or alter payment or insurance policy coverage requirements.

EHR systems support accurate, complete, and consistent coding practices by documenting the encounter with codified nomenclature that can be analyzed and used to determine the levels of billing justified. Medical coders must adhere to the coding conventions, official coding guidelines, and official rules, and assign codes that are clearly and consistently supported by clinical documentation in the health record.

---

## Guided Exercise 12E: Calculating E&M for a More Complex Visit

In this exercise, you are going to add findings to an existing encounter to study the effects on E&M coding.

### Step 1

Start a supported web browser program and log in to the MyHealthProfessionsLab for this course.

Locate and click on the link **Exercise 12E**. This will open the Quippe software window with the New Encounter window displayed in the center.

### Step 2

In the New Encounter window patient list, locate and click on **Williams, Mary** as shown previously in Figure 12-10, and then click the OK button. You do not need to set the date and time of the encounter for this exercise.

### Step 3

When the encounter note is displayed, study it a moment. You will recall from Guided Exercise 12C that, even with the vital signs added, this patient encounter note produced a calculated E&M code of 99212. You do not need to run the E&M calculator yet. In the following steps, you are going to add findings and study their effect on the levels of E&M key components.

**History**   There is one history finding, sinus pain, located in HPI. Although the E&M Calculator will count a HPI finding as a body system, History level is determined by the relationship between HPI, ROS, and PFSH.

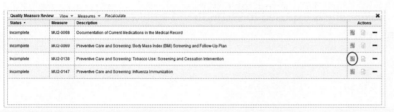

**Figure 12-36** Quality Measures Review for Mary Williams.

### Step 4

Perhaps you noticed the CQM Tobacco Status had not been documented. This is a Personal History finding.

Click the View button and select Quality Measure Review from the drop-down menu. The CQM grid will open in the pane below the encounter note as shown in Figure 12-36.

When Ms. Williams brought her infant son Tyrell for his well-baby checkup she stated that she is not smoking or drinking because she is nursing, but her husband smokes cigarettes and drinks moderately.

Locate the CQM Preventive Care and Screening Tobacco Use, Actions column, and click the wizard button (circled in Figure 12-36).

### Step 5

When the Tobacco CQM pop-up opens, click the following checkbox:

✓ Never Smoked

Compare your screen to Figure 12-37 and then click the Finish button.

### Step 6

Ms. Williams is not taking any medications. Locate the CQM Documentation of Current medication, and click the wizard button in the Actions column. When the pop-up opens, click the following checkbox:

✓ Medication list is documented

Compare your screen to Figure 12-38 and then click the Finish button.

Her BMI is already documented in the note, and giving a flu shot while someone is ill is contraindicated. Click the minus symbol in the Actions column for the two remaining CQMs (Body Mass Index Screening and Influenza Immunization).

Close the Quality Measures Review by clicking the X in the right corner of the view.

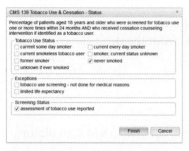

**Figure 12-37** CQM wizard for Tobacco Use & Cessation – Status.

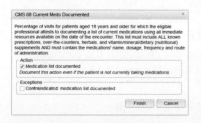

**Figure 12-38** CQM wizard for Current Meds Documented.

**Step 7**

Because this encounter note was for an URI, load the Adult URI list.

Click any white space in the encounter pane that does not give focus to a heading or finding.

Click the Browse button on the toolbar and the plus symbols to expand Sample Custom Content, Shared Content, and Student Edition Lists. Locate and click on Adult URI to highlight it, and then click on the Add to Note button.

Ms. Williams has no allergies and did not have an URI prior to this. As stated earlier she is not taking medication. Locate and click the following findings until they turn blue and their descriptions change:

- allergy
- taking medication
- recent upper respiratory infection

Because her husband smokes, she is exposed to secondhand smoke. Click on the following finding until it turns red.

- to smoke

**Step 8**

Proceed to the Review of Systems section. Ms. Williams is not feeling well, and her nasal passages feel blocked, but she is having nasal discharge. Click on the findings until they turn red.

- not feeling well
- headache
- nasal discharge
- nasal passage blockage

She does not have a fever, chills, swollen glands, earache, cough, difficulty breathing, or muscle aches. Click on the Review of Systems heading to highlight the section. Click the Actions button on the toolbar and select Otherwise normal from the drop-down menu.

Compare your screen to Figure 12-39.

**Step 9**

Click the Tools button on the toolbar and select E&M Calculator. The E&M Calculator will open in the pane below the encounter note.

Click on the Calculate button. Notice the calculated code is still 99212 even though we added numerous history findings.

Click on the Analysis, tab and then click the plus symbol to expand Overall History as shown in Figure 12-40. While the Overall History level has not changed, the elements ROS and PFSH have increased to level 2 when compared with Figure 12-15.

If you refer back to the table in Figure 12-16, you will see the following:

◆ An increase in the number of findings for HPI will only affect the level of history if ROS and PFSH contain data as well.

**Figure 12-39** Upper portion of the encounter note with the History and Review of Systems sections completed.

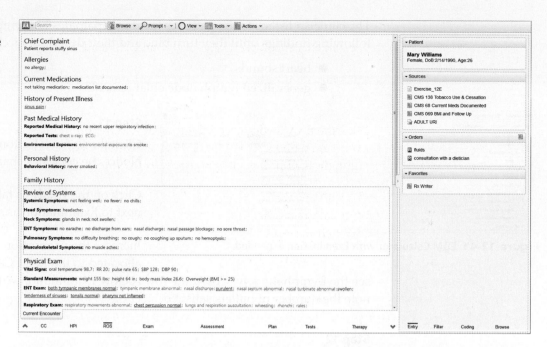

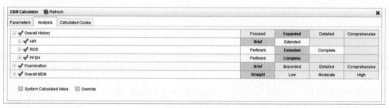

**Figure 12-40** E&M Calculator with Overall History expanded.

◆ An increase in the number of body systems in ROS will only affect the level of history if HPI contains at least four findings and PFSH contains at least one.

◆ Adding even one finding for PFSH will only affect the level of history if HPI contains at least four findings and ROS contains at least two body systems.

◆ A "Complete" level of PFSH will only affect the overall history level when HPI contains at least four findings and ROS has at least 10 systems.

Click on the minus symbol next to Overall History to collapse the rows below it, and then click the plus symbol next to Examination to prepare for the next step.

### Step 10

**Examination**   Exams provide the most direct, but not the easiest, means to reach a higher level code. More systems examined, and more bullet points that are met, mean that more work has been done and therefore a higher level of E&M code is justified. However, consider the following:

◆ In a general multisystem examination, six or more elements with a bullet are required to reach the second level.

◆ The third level is reached when you have at least two elements in six or more systems/body areas.

◆ The fourth level requires all of the bulleted items in at least nine systems/body areas.

With the vital signs the encounter has five bullets documented. Six are required for the next level.

Scroll the upper pane so that the Physical Exam section is at the top.

The clinician listens to the patient's heart and palpates her lymph nodes. Click on the following findings until they turn blue and their descriptions change.

- heart sounds
- generalized lymph node enlargement

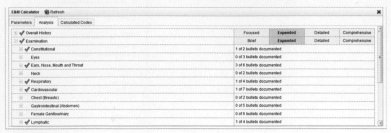

**Figure 12-41** E&M Calculator with Examination expanded.

### Step 11

Click the Refresh button on the E&M Calculator. Notice the code has changed to 99213.

Click on the Analysis tab and the plus symbol next to Examination as shown in Figure 12-41.

Increase the proportion of the workspace pane allocated to the E&M Calculator until you can see the Lymphatic row. Count the rows below Examination with green checkmarks and note the number of bullets satisfied.

### Step 12

**Medical Decision Making**   Click on the E&M Parameters tab and then click the following checkboxes:

✓ Active

✓ New Problem

In the Status field click the down-arrow and select **worsening** from the drop-down list. Your screen should resemble Figure 12-27, shown previously.

Locate the Refresh button at the top of the E&M Calculator and click it. Click on the Analysis tab and then the plus symbols to expand the Overall MDM and Dx/Mgt rows. Your screen should resemble Figure 12-28, shown previously.

### Step 13

The clinician orders inhaled nasal steroids and a blood analysis test: complete blood count with differential. Locate and click the following findings until they turn red:

- inhaled / nasal steroids
- complete blood count with differential

Locate and click the Refresh button at the top of the E&M Calculator. Click on the Analysis tab and then the plus symbols to expand the Overall MDM and Dx/Mgt rows. Compare the Plan and Tests to Order sections of your screen to Figure 12-42. In the E&M Calculator portion notice that the Overall MDM and Overall Risk levels have increased to level 3. The Complexity of data row, which previously did not have a level, is now level 1.

The level of MDM is determined by two out of three elements in the table shown in Figure 12-32. However, the risk table in Figure 12-31 indicates that managing prescribed medications raises the risk to Level 3. Therefore, ordering the inhaled nasal steroids increased the Risk level.

Click on the Calculated Codes tab, and then click the Add to Note button. The CPT-4 code and description will be added to the note.

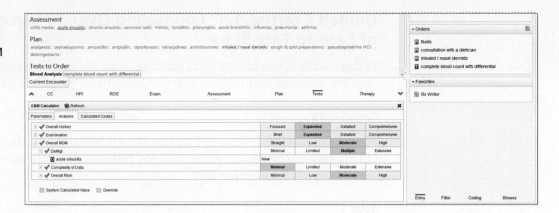

**Figure 12-42** Encounter Plan and Test findings; E&M Calculator with Overall MDM and Dx/Mgt expanded.

## Step 14

Close the E&M Calculator by clicking the X in the right corner of the calculator.

Click the View button on the toolbar and select Concise from the drop-down menu. Compare your screen to Figure 12-43. If everything is correct, proceed to step 15. If there are any differences, review the preceding steps, and correct your errors.

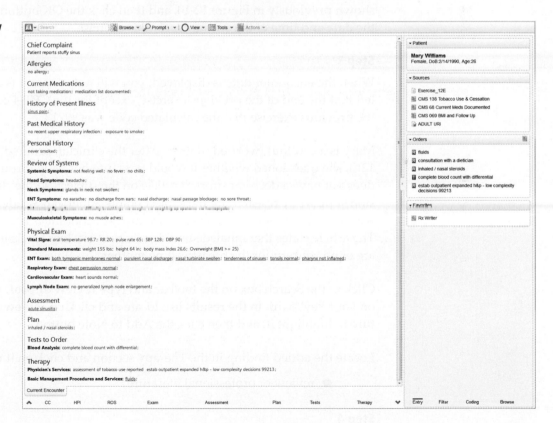

**Figure 12-43** Concise view of the correctly completed encounter note for Exercise 12E.

## Step 15

If you wish to print a copy of your completed encounter notes for yourself or because your instructor requires you to turn them in, then print or download the PDF at this time.

Locate and click the blue Quippe icon button on the toolbar to display the drop-down menu, and then select the Submit for Grade menu option. This will complete Exercise 12E.

## Guided Exercise 12F: Counseling Over 50 Percent of Face-to-Face Time

In this exercise, you are going to continue with the previous encounter, documenting time the clinician spent counseling the patient and providing patient education.

**Case Study**

Mary Williams is a 26-year-old mother who is breastfeeding her infant son, Tyrell. Not only is she concerned about her sinusitis, but also about the steroids or her illness passing into Tyrell through her milk.

**Step 1**

Start a supported web browser program and log in to the MyHealthProfessionsLab for this course.

Locate and click on the link **Exercise 12F**. This will open the Quippe software window with the New Encounter window displayed in the center.

**Step 2**

In the New Encounter window patient list, locate and click on **Williams, Mary** as shown previously in Figure 12-10, and then click the OK button. You do not need to set the date and time of the encounter for this exercise.

**Step 3**

When the encounter note is displayed, you will notice that it is essentially where you left it at the end of the previous exercise, except for the CPT-4 code. You will recall from the previous exercise that the calculated code was 99213.

Mary is a cautious, worried mother. After the clinician ordered medication (in Exercise 12E), she questioned whether it would pass into her baby through her milk. The clinic does not have a decision support article on the subject, so the clinician performs decision support by researching the subject on the American Academy of Family Physicians web site and locates an evidence-based article, *Medications in the Breast-Feeding Mother*. The article states that inhaled steroids achieve very low levels in maternal plasma and are of no concern for the breastfeeding mother.

Click in the Search box on the toolbar and type **review of prof**, then press the Enter key on your keyboard. In the results list, locate and click on **review of professional literature** to highlight it, and then click the Add to Note button.

Locate the added finding in the Therapy section and click on it until it turns red.

- review of professional literature

**Step 4**

Mary is also afraid that Tyrell could catch what she has by nursing and asks if she should quit. The clinician reassures her that her sinus infection will not transfer through milk and encourages her to continue breastfeeding. However, noting her high BMI, the clinician is concerned that she lose weight through a safe diet that maintains adequate nutritional levels for her and her milk.

Since child safety is an issue, the clinician suggests a cool mist vaporizer, and that she ask her husband not to smoke in the house.

Document the additional orders and the extra counseling. Locate and click on the following findings until they turn red:

- cool mist vaporizer
- avoid second hand tobacco smoke
- patient education about a specific disorder
- breast feeding encouraged
- education, guidance and counseling
- dietary education
- patient education about weight control

*Right-click* on **breast feeding encouraged** and select Details from the Actions drop-down menu. In the Details pop-up window click the down-arrow in the prefix field and select **continue** from the drop-down list. Click the OK button to close the Details window. The description should read "continue breast feeding encouraged."

Compare the Therapy and Counseling and Education sections of your screen to those in Figure 12-44.

**Figure 12-44** Upper pane showing sections of the encounter note; E&M Calculator showing the 99213 code.

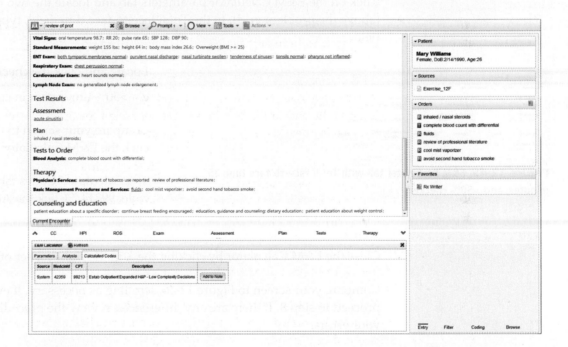

**Step 5**

Click the Tools button on the toolbar and select E&M Calculator. In the parameters tab, click the following checkboxes.

✓ Active

✓ New Problem

In the Status field, click the down-arrow and select **worsening** from the drop-down list. Your problem grid should resemble Figure 12-27 shown previously.

Click the Calculate button. Compare the E&M calculator portion of Figure 12-44 to your results.

Notice that, even with the extra therapy and counseling findings, the level of the E&M code is still 99213.

### Step 6

The clinician spent quite a long time answering Mary's questions and counseling and educating her. What the clinician failed to do was document the extra time spent counseling.

**Time**   As you learned earlier, time can be a factor when more than 50 percent of the face-to-face time is spent counseling the patient. Both the face-to-face time and the counseling time must be documented.

When counseling or coordination of care represent over 50 percent of the face-to-face time of the visit, time becomes a key or controlling factor to the level of E&M services. The guideline states, "If the physician elects to report the level of service based on counseling and/or coordination of care, the total length of time of the encounter (face-to-face or floor time, as appropriate) should be documented and the record should describe the counseling and/or activities to coordinate care."[9]

Click on the E&M Calculator parameters tab and locate the two fields related to time (above the problem grid). In the Total face-to-face time field, type **25** in the minutes field.

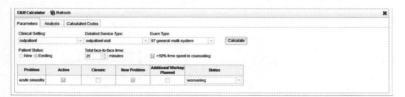

**Figure 12-45** E&M Parameter tab with Total face-to-face time 25 minutes, and >50% checked.

Locate and click the checkbox:

✓   >50% time spent in counseling

Compare your screen to Figure 12-45, and then click the E&M Calculator Refresh button.

The Calculated Codes tab should display "CPT-4 code: 99214." Click the Add to Note button.

### Step 7

Close the E&M Calculator by clicking the X in the right corner of the calculator.

Compare your screen to Figure 12-46, scrolling as necessary. If everything is correct, proceed to step 8. If there are any differences, review the preceding steps, and correct your errors.

### Step 8

If you wish to print a copy of your completed encounter notes for yourself or because your instructor requires you to turn them in, then print or download the PDF at this time.

Locate and click the blue Quippe icon button on the toolbar to display the drop-down menu, and then select the Submit for Grade menu option. This will complete Exercise 12F.

---

[9]*1997 Documentation Guidelines for Evaluation and Management Services* (Washington, DC: U.S. Department of Health and Human Services, 1997).

**Figure 12-46** Completed Encounter with E&M code, time, and counseling.

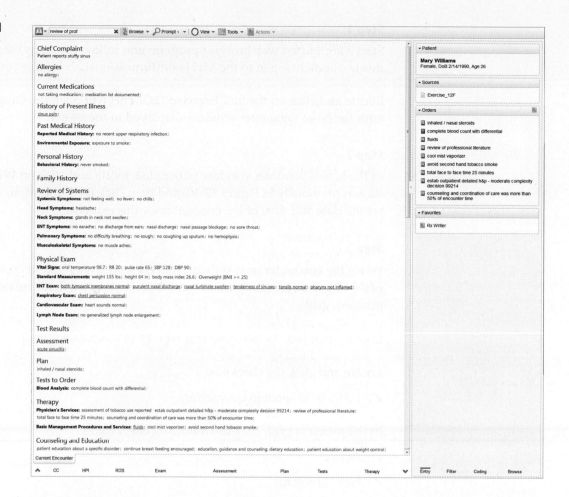

## Critical Thinking Exercise 12G: Understanding How Procedures Are Posted to the Billing System

EHR systems that are integrated with practice management or billing software can transfer the Procedure and Diagnosis (CPT-4, HCPCS, and ICD-10-CM) codes from the EHR directly into the practice management billing system.

In most healthcare facilities the codes that are transferred from the EHR do not post automatically to the billing system. Most systems hold these as "pending" charges until they are reviewed by a billing or coding expert, who may make modifications to the codes before posting them as charges. Here are a few examples of why this is necessary:

◆ Certain procedures are considered part of another procedure (bundled).

◆ Under certain conditions a coding specialist may need to add procedure modifier codes.

◆ Certain codes may represent a supply or sample for which the doctor does not wish to charge the patient.

In this exercise, you are going to complete the previous encounter, documenting time the clinician spent counseling the patient, posting the CPT-4 code, and reviewing the codes.

### Case Study

Mary Williams' encounter is completed. In this exercise, you are going to calculate the E&M code again and view the ICD-10-CM code for her diagnosis.

### Step 1

Start a supported web browser program and follow the steps listed inside the cover of this textbook to log in to the MyHealthProfessionsLab for this course.

Locate and click on the link **Exercise 12G**. This will open the Quippe software window with the New Encounter window displayed in the center.

### Step 2

In the New Encounter window patient list, locate and click on **Williams, Mary** as shown previously in Figure 12-10, and then click the OK button. You do not need to set the date and time of the encounter for this exercise.

### Step 3

When the encounter note is displayed, click the Tools button on the toolbar and select E&M Calculator. In the parameters tab locate the two fields related to time (above the problem grid).

Locate Total face-to-face time and type **25** in the minutes field.

Locate and click the checkbox:

✓ >50% time spent in counseling

In the problem grid, click the following checkboxes:

✓ Active

✓ New Problem

In the Status field, click the down-arrow and select **worsening** from the drop-down list. Your problem grid should resemble Figure 12-45 shown previously.

Click the Calculate button. When the Calculated Codes tab displays the CPT-4 code, click the Add to Note button.

Close the E&M Calculator by clicking the X in the right corner of the calculator.

### Step 4

Your version of the Student Edition is not interfaced to a billing system and therefore does not have a system to transfer the codes into. However, it does post codes to the patient encounter. You can view the codes that would be transferred to a practice management system in Code Review.

Click the View button on the toolbar and select Code Review from the drop-down menu.

When the Code Review pane opens, scroll it all the way to the bottom as shown in Figure 12-47. Next, scroll the encounter note portion of the workspace pane all the way to the bottom of the encounter note.

Compare your screen to Figure 12-47.

Not all of the codes displayed in Code Review will be sent to the practice management system. For example, CPT-4 code 85025 for the complete blood count with differential lab test will not be posted because the test was not performed, but simply ordered.

**Figure 12-47** Upper pane – encounter note with E&M code, time, and counseling; lower pane – Code Review.

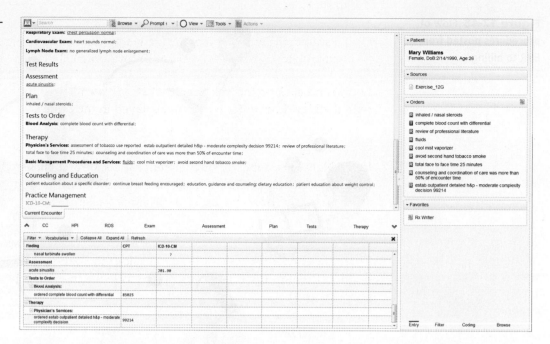

### Step 5

The ICD-10-CM codes for all diagnoses in the Assessment section will transfer automatically to the practice management system billing module. However, because the Student Edition is not interfaced to a billing system, you are going to look up the code and type it in the encounter note. In a medical practice this is unnecessary as the software already knows the ICD-10-CM code and will transfer it. You are entering it here only so your instructor will know you identified the correct code.

Locate the diagnosis in the Assessment section of the Code Review grid. Follow the row across and locate the code displayed in the ICD-10-CM column.

### Step 6

In the encounter note pane, locate the Practice Management section and click on the line next to the label ICD-10-CM code. Type in the code you found in step 5 and press the Enter key on your keyboard.

### Step 7

If you wish to print a copy of your completed encounter notes for yourself or because your instructor requires you to turn them in, then print or download the PDF at this time.

Locate and click the blue Quippe icon button on the toolbar to display the drop-down menu, and then select the Submit for Grade menu option.

Proceed to step 8.

### Step 8

Figure 12-48 illustrates the typical method of posting charges from an EHR to a practice management billing module. Review the figure as you read the following steps:

**1** Clinician documents encounter at point of care.

**2** The EHR calculates E&M code. Clinician clicks the Add To Note button.

**3** The clinician reviews diagnosis and procedure codes and electronically "signs" or otherwise indicates the encounter is complete.

**Figure 12-48** Flow of procedures posted from EHR to billing.

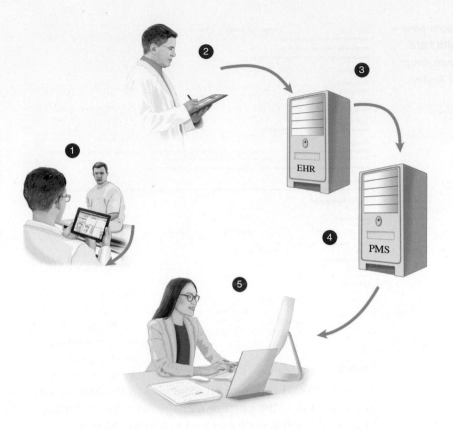

④ The EHR transfers CPT-4 and ICD-10-CM codes to the practice management system.

⑤ A billing or coding specialist reviews the "pending" charges, adds modifiers or other information, and posts them.

**Step 9**

Figure 12-49 shows a practice management billing screen used to post charges transferred from the EHR after being reviewed by a billing or coding specialist.

This completes Exercise 12G.

**Figure 12-49** Practice management system posting E&M and ICD-10-CM codes from the EHR.

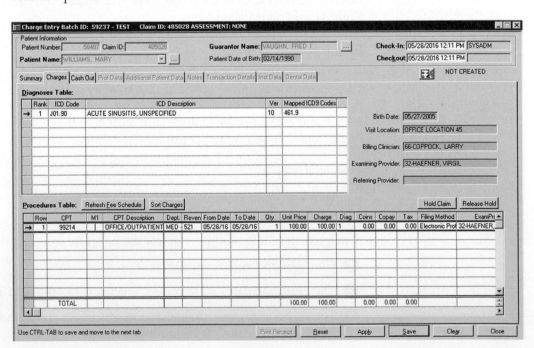

# Real-Life Story

## A New Level of Efficiency in Addition to Improved E&M Coding

**Philip C. Yount, MD**

*Ashe Medical Associates*

Every medical doctor in America reviews the patient's past medical problems, medication list, social history, and so on, but does each one always document that? I think it is safe to say that doctors, who dictate after the visit, actually get more information, examine more of the patient, and say things to the patient that they do not recall when they dictate later. Certainly when I was dictating or writing notes I did not always remember to document all that I did. To be safe, I tended to undercode; I am sure most everybody else does, too.

Our practice has been using an electronic medical record for almost three years. I would never go back to a paper-based system again. But back when I was dictating, the workflow with the paper system was to finish the visit, mark the charge and the E&M code on a paper encounter form [similar to Figure 12-9], and then dictate it later. This was really hard because during dictation I was trying both to remember the visit accurately and to make sure I dictated enough to support the level of the E&M code already selected. Now that we use an EMR, both things are done simultaneously.

These days I finish the documentation before the patient leaves. I review it, verify my documentation, and then E&M code it. I am much more accurate and I think I code higher. I think the tendency on a paper system is to always downcode rather than risk getting yourself in trouble.

I practice family medicine with two other physicians and a physician assistant. One thing we do in our quarterly meetings is to review each other's charts to see if we agree with the level of E&M coding that the other provider has charged. Our office manager randomly selects three patients' charges for each of us and prints out the exam notes for peer review. Since we have been on the electronic system, we have had very few discrepancies. Not only is the coding very accurate with the EMR, but the quarterly review itself is facilitated by the electronic records. If you had to dig up charges and pull records from a paper file system . . . well, with electronic medical records it is a lot simpler.

Did switching to electronic records increase our level of coding? I think we are all doing a much better job of coding than we were in the past and we have definitely stopped downcoding, but it is difficult to compare the coding of visits before the EMR because you would have to analyze all those old charts. I have a sense that our documentation went up 15 to 20 percent in terms of

levels, but we actually chose to measure something else. We wanted something easy to track, so we tracked the number of patient encounters instead of the coding levels.

In the first year of using the EMR, compared to the previous year, we went up 15 percent in number of visits, so it really improved our efficiency to that extent. The second year we were up 17 percent and this year we are up 5 percent above that—with no additional providers, no longer hours open, or anything else. In addition, we get done on time. I am rarely at the office after 5:00 P.M. anymore. I finish the patient's chart while the patient is still there. So there is a lot of efficiency in addition to the improved E&M coding.

The system we use does have an E&M coder that will count the points of history, review of systems, exam, and so on, and then suggest a code. Like most other EMR systems, it calculates and suggests the E&M code but the software developer does not want the responsibility for actually posting it. It is up to the doctor to decide to use the code.

Most EMR systems have templates, but there are two types. One type uses checklists of problems: "You're here for a cold; you have an earache, a cough, and a sore throat." The other type of template fills blanks in a narrative: "30-year-old male presents to the office with a history of cough, cold, fever." The ability of the system to calculate the E&M code depends on whether the template uses discrete items or sentences, because it can't count the status in those narrative sentences. However, even without using the E&M coder, the coding becomes more accurate because the electronic record is capturing the exam more accurately. A doctor can look at a finished EMR note and see the data points.

Our software uses templates and I designed the history items right into them. We don't miss documenting them now and that lends significant points to the E&M coding. But there is something else our templates do that is perhaps more toward the issue of quality of care than just coding, and that is in the plan. By building templates for certain diagnoses we include all the things we might choose in the plan. This not only helps document simple things that might have been overlooked in the old dictation method, like telling the patient to take Tylenol, but it also gives us a complete checklist of things to consider when concluding the visit.

During the first year, we built templates and customized the software to suit our practice's needs. We worked evenings at the office to overcome a steep learning curve and technological obstacles. With the system finally in place and reaching comfortable levels of proficiency, we have now come to realize a new level of efficiency in our practice.

Our workflow has improved markedly since the implementation of an electronic medical record system, allowing us to do more work in less time with the same sized staff. We are now able to accommodate more patients in a day; able to access our system from home; send prescriptions to pharmacies from our computers; scan and add outside reports to our records; and we have reduced paperwork and increased staff efficiency. Our medical recordkeeping has improved exponentially and we have added at least 20 percent to our bottom line.

## Factors That Affect the E&M Code Set

Thus far you have seen the effects of key components and time on determining the E&M code. However, you will recall that earlier in this chapter it was mentioned that there are different sets of E&M codes. E&M codes extend from 99201 through 99499. These include different codes for new versus established patients, as well as for clinical setting (location of service). It was also mentioned that a provider may choose to use the 1995 or 1997 E&M guidelines (or a single-organ guideline).

## Guided Exercise 12H: Exploring Other Factors of E&M Codes

In this exercise you are going to use the E&M calculator window to see an example of a different set of E&M codes, by changing the settings of several fields that you have not yet worked with. To maintain the focus of this exercise on exploring how E&M calculation works in alternative situations and to keep the exercise short, we will not enter all of the findings that would be documented for this type of visit.

### Case Study

Eleanore Nash is a 41-year-old female admitted to the hospital for bacterial pneumonia. She reported that she has had a "cold" for the past 2 weeks, but now she is experiencing shortness of breath with exertion, dyspnea when lying down, fever, and pain in her right chest when she coughs. She has a harsh, nonproductive cough and is experiencing extreme fatigue, and seems anxious. She has been admitted with an admission diagnosis of bacterial pneumonia. A physician from her family medical practice has come to the hospital to examine her.

### Step 1

Start a supported web browser program and follow the steps listed inside the cover of this textbook to log in to the MyHealthProfessionsLab for this course.

Locate and click on the link **Exercise 12H**. This will open the Quippe software window with the New Encounter window displayed in the center.

### Step 2

In the New Encounter window patient list, locate and click on **Nash, Eleanore** as shown in Figure 12-50. You do not need to set the date and time of the encounter for this exercise.

### Step 3

Locate and click in the blank space below the Chief Complaint label and type: **Pneumonia hospital consult**.

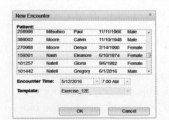

**Figure 12-50** New Encounter window with Eleanore Nash selected.

### Step 4

Click any white space in the encounter pane that does not highlight a heading or finding to restore the date tabs at the bottom of the encounter pane.

Locate and click the **5/11/2016** tab.

When the previous note is displayed, copy the following sections into the current note by clicking on the heading to outline the section, and then selecting **Copy into current note** from the drop-down menu, as indicated by the arrows in Figure 12-51. The sections to copy are:

**Allergies**

**History of Present Illness**

**Past Medical History**

**Personal History**

**Family History**

**Figure 12-51** Copy into current note the sections indicated by arrows.

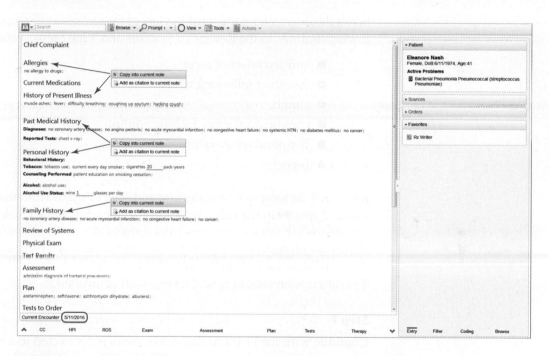

### Step 5

Scroll the encounter pane to the bottom of the note. Click on the **Therapy** section heading and select **Copy into current note** as shown in Figure 12-52.

The doctor also reviews the nursing notes and wants to cite them, but not merge them as part of the current note.

Locate and click on the section heading **Nursing Care**, but this time select **Add as citation to current note**.

Locate and click the tab at the bottom labeled **Current Encounter**.

### Step 6

Ms. Nash reports having a terrible cough with reddish sputum and then a sudden onset fever and sweating. The nursing staff has been documenting vital signs regularly in

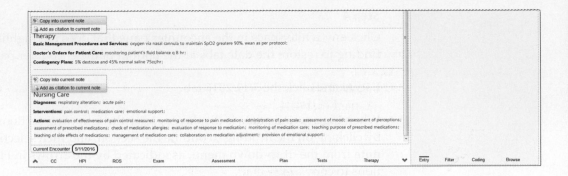

**Figure 12-52** Copy into current note the Therapy section. Add as citation to current note the Nursing Care section.

another part of the chart. The clinician checks Eleanore's most recent reading, and notices it is not that high and her fever has come down, but makes note of it.

Locate Active Problems in the right content pane under the patient's name and *double-click* Bacterial Pneumonia Pneumococcal (streptococcus pneumonia).

Scroll the encounter pane until Review of Systems is at the top. Locate and click the following findings in the Review of Systems and Vital Signs sections until they turn red:

- sudden onset of fever
- sweating following a fever
- cough
- coughing up rusty looking sputum
- temporal temperature
- fever

*Right-click* on temporal temperature and select Details from the Actions drop-down menu. Type: **99** in the value field and **F** in the units field. Click the OK button.

*Right-click* on **fever** and select Details from the Actions drop-down menu. Click in the Status field and select **well-controlled** from the drop-down list. Click the OK button. The description should read: "fever – well-controlled."

### Step 7

Continue with the Physical Exam. Ms. Nash is connected to a vital signs monitor, which reports, gathers, and displays her BP, HR, RR, and O₂ Sat. The physician notes her heart rate is high even though she is currently on oxygen and her breath rate is normal.

Locate and click the following Vital Signs until they turn red:

- RR
- pulse rate
- tachycardia

*Right-click* on **RR** and select Details from the Actions drop-down menu. Type **20** in the value field, click the Units field and select **breaths/min** from the drop-down list. Click the OK button.

*Right-click* on **pulse rate** and select Details from the Actions drop-down menu. Type **101** in the value field, click the Units field, and select **bpm** from the drop-down list. Click the OK button.

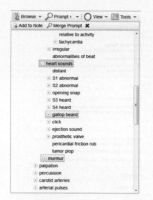

**Figure 12-53** List of clinical concepts. Add to note: heart sounds, gallop heard, and murmur.

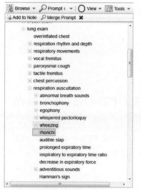

**Figure 12-54** List of clinical concepts. Add to note: wheezing and rhonchi.

### Step 8

The doctor listens to her chest. Locate Cardiovascular Exam and click on tachycardia.

● tachycardia

Click the Browse button on the toolbar and the clinical concept list should open to tachycardia, as shown in Figure 12-53.

Click the red pushpin at the top of the Browse list to hold it open.

Locate and click on **heart sounds** to highlight it, and then click the Add to Note button. Click the plus symbol next to it to expand the tree.

Locate and click on **gallop heard** to highlight it, and then click the Add to Note button.

Locate and click on **murmur** to highlight it, and then click the Add to Note button.

Click the Browse button to close the drop-down list.

The added findings are likely red. Click on each of the following until they turn blue and their descriptions change:

● heart sounds
● gallop heard
● murmur

### Step 9

Document the Respiratory Exam. Locate and click on lung exam until it turns red.

● lung exam

Click the Browse button on the toolbar and the clinical concept list should open to lung exam, as shown in Figure 12-54. Click the plus symbol to expand respiration auscultation.

Locate and click on **wheezing** to highlight it, and then click the Add to Note button.

Locate and click on **rhonchi** to highlight it, and then click the Add to Note button.

Scroll the list slightly downward to locate and click on **examination of sputum** to highlight it, and then click the Add to Note button.

Click the Browse button to close the drop-down list.

The three added findings should all be red. If any of them are not, click on them. Locate the following unentered finding and click it until it turns red:

● wet rales

Compare your Review of Systems and Physical Exam findings to the upper portion of Figure 12-55. If everything is correct, proceed to step 10. If there are any differences, review the preceding steps, and correct your errors.

### Step 10

Click the Tools button on the toolbar and select E&M Calculator. The parameters tab will display. The first row has three fields with drop-down lists that we have not previously explored.

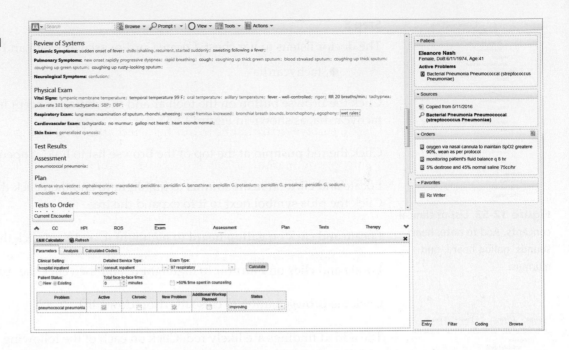

**Figure 12-55** Encounter pane shows correctly added findings. E&M Calculator fields are correctly set.

**Clinical Setting**  As you may recall from the table in Figure 12-35, CPT-4 has different sets of codes for new patients versus existing patients. Similarly, there are different CPT-4 code sets for clinical setting in which the visit takes place and the type of service the clinician is providing. The settings of the first two fields are used by the E&M Calculator to select from the proper category of CPT-4 codes.

Click the down-arrow for the Clinical Setting field and select **hospital inpatient**. As you can see from the drop-down list there are different CPT-4 codes for emergency departments, long-term care facilities, home visits, and more.

**Detailed Service Type**  Within categories of E&M codes for different locations there are also subcategories of the types of services that might be rendered. The Detailed Service Type field is used to indicate the type of service that was performed in a given setting.

Click the down-arrow for the Detailed Service Type field and select **Consult inpatient** from the drop-down list.

Note, the Detailed Service Type is related to the Clinical Setting selected—that is, the drop-down list of Detailed Service choices changes based on the type of facility selected in the Clinical Setting field.

**Exam Type**  You will recall that, in our discussion of the key component Examination, there are guidelines for 10 different single organ system exams in addition to the general multisystem exam. Also, clinicians are permitted to use either the 1995 or 1997 guideline, whichever best suits their practice. The Exam Type field allows the clinician to select the appropriate guideline for the E&M calculator to use.

Click the down-arrow for the Exam Type field and select **97 respiratory** from the drop-down list.

### Step 11

Locate the Problem grid and click the boxes for the following:

✓ Active

✓ New Problem

Click the down-arrow in the Status field and select **improving** from the drop-down list.

Compare your parameter tab to the E&M Calculator portion of Figure 12-55. If everything is correct, click the Calculate button.

### Step 12

When the Calculated Codes tab displays the CPT-4 code, notice that inpatient services use an entirely different set of E&M codes than you have seen in previous exercises for outpatient services (99212, 99213, and 99214).

Click the Add to Note button. The CPT-4 code and description will be added to the note.

Close the E&M Calculator by clicking the X in the right corner of the calculator.

### Step 13

Click the View button on the toolbar and select Concise from the drop-down menu. Compare your screen to Figure 12-56. If everything is correct, proceed to step 14. If there are any differences, review the preceding steps, and correct your errors.

**Figure 12-56** Concise view of correctly completed encounter for Exercise 12H.

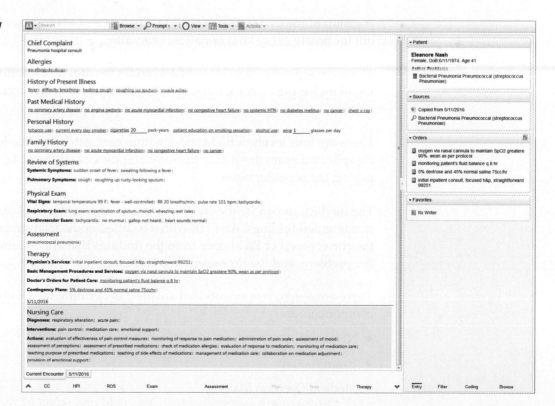

**Step 14**

If you wish to print a copy of your completed encounter notes for yourself or because your instructor requires you to turn them in, then print or download the PDF at this time.

Locate and click the blue Quippe icon button on the toolbar to display the drop-down menu, and then select the Submit for Grade menu option. This will complete Exercise 12H.

## Chapter Twelve Summary

CPT-4 and ICD-10-CM codes are national standards that are required on insurance claims for outpatient and other services.

ICD-10-CM is the latest revision to the International Classification of Diseases. It was adopted for use in the United States in 2015. In addition to the statistical uses discussed in Chapter 2 ICD-10-CM codes are also required for insurance claims. For both inpatient and outpatient facilities, the use of the correct ICD-10-CM code on a claim serves to explain or justify the medical reason for the services being billed.

Reimbursement for most inpatient hospitals is based entirely on the Diagnostic Related Group (DRG) determined from the primary and secondary diagnoses assigned by the attending physician.

Outpatient billing requires one or more ICD-10-CM codes be assigned to every procedure and the diagnosis must be appropriate to the procedure.

The use of HCPCS and CPT-4 codes for procedures is also required. CPT stands for Current Procedural Terminology. It was developed and is maintained by the AMA.

A group of the CPT-4 codes called Evaluation and Management (E&M) codes is used to bill for nearly every kind of patient encounter.

There are separate categories of E&M codes for different locations such as outpatient, inpatient hospital exams, nursing home visits, consults, emergency room doctors, and so on.

There are four levels of E&M codes within each category. The levels represent the least complicated exam (level 1) to the most complex exam (level 4), with higher levels paying the provider more.

The medical record for the encounter must support the level of E&M code billed with documented findings. An EHR with a codified nomenclature can accurately calculate the correct level of E&M code from the findings that are documented, information about the problem, and the time spent in counseling.

There are seven components that are used in defining the level of E&M services. These components are:

◆ History

◆ Examination

◆ Medical Decision Making

- Counseling
- Coordination of Care
- Nature of Presenting Problem
- Time

The first three of these components, History, Examination, and Medical Decision Making, are called key components. Each of the key components has subcomponents called elements that determine the level of the component. Once the level of each of the key components is determined, the results are evaluated to calculate the correct level of E&M code.

Time is used to adjust the level of the E&M code only when counseling/coordination of care exceeds 50 percent of the face-to-face time.

Because the level of E&M code is dependent on the levels of multiple key components, merely adding more findings to only one key component may bring that component to a higher level, but that does not necessarily mean that the visit as a whole will qualify for the higher level E&M code.

## Testing Your Knowledge of Chapter 12

### Step 1

Log in to MyHealthProfessionsLab following the directions printed inside the cover of this textbook.

Locate and click on Chapter 12 Test.

### Step 2

Answer the test questions. When you have finished, click the Submit Test button to close the window.

## Testing Your Skill Exercise 12J: Counseling an Established Patient

Now that you have performed all the exercises in Chapter 12, this exercise will help you and your instructor evaluate your acquired skills. Use the information in the case study and the features of the software you already know to document the patient's encounter. You will then calculate the E&M code and post it to the encounter.

### Case Study

Lisa Marie Juarez is a 50-year-old established patient with Type 2 diabetes and benign hypertension who complained of a lump in the right breast during her last checkup. A mammogram was ordered and performed. The chief reason for this visit is to review mammogram results.

The clinician has received the report and digitized images and is going to refer her to an oncologist. The patient is anxious and apprehensive. The clinician will access and review with her a decision support document on cancer survivorship. After spending 30 minutes face-to-face time, more than half of it counseling her, the clinician invokes the E&M Calculator, notes the time, active problems, and the new problem, calculates the code, and adds it to the note.

Here are Lisa Marie's vital signs:

| | |
|---|---|
| Temperature: | **98.6** |
| Pulse: | **96** |
| Respiration: | **30** |
| SBP: | **148** |
| DBP: | **96** |
| Weight: | **150** |
| Height: | **62** |

### Step 1

Start a supported web browser program and follow the steps listed inside the cover of this textbook to log in to the MyHealthProfessionsLab for this course.

Locate and click on the link **Exercise 12J**. This will open the Quippe software window with the New Encounter window displayed in the center.

### Step 2

Locate and click on the patient name, and click the OK button. In this exercise, you do not need to set the date or time of the encounter.

### Step 3

Read the case study *carefully*.

Hint: What is her present illness? Drag the finding from Review of Systems and drop it on HPI. Next, save time by copying her Current Medication, Personal History, and Family History into the note from her 5/18/2016 visit.

### Step 4

After recording the test results, primary diagnosis, and therapy findings, the clinician will create a problem section based on the diagnosis.

Clinicians always document active problems every visit, even when they are not the primary reason for the visit. Hint: *Double-click* on each diagnosis in her Active Problems list, and create a Problem section for it.

After creating the problem sections the clinician documents the Review of Systems and Physical Exam as "Otherwise Normal."

### Step 5

Once you have calculated the E&M code and added it to the note, click the View button, and select Code Review. Scroll the Code View downward until you locate the problem section.

For each problem click the question mark in the ICD-10-CM column and select a more specific ICD-10-CM code, and then click the apply button.

### Step 6

If you wish to print a copy of your completed encounter notes for yourself or because your instructor requires you to turn them in, use the Create PDF option, and then print or download the PDF at this time.

Submit your completed work for a grade. This will complete Exercise 12J.

# Comprehensive Evaluation of Chapters 7–12

This comprehensive evaluation will enable you and your instructor to determine your understanding of the material covered in the second half of this book. Complete both the written test and the hands-on exercises provided below. Depending on the time provided, it may be necessary to do this in two separate sessions. Your instructor will advise you. Do not begin Part II if there will not be enough class time to complete it.

## Part I—Testing Your Knowledge of Chapters 7–12

### Step 1

Log in to MyHealthProfessionsLab following the directions printed inside the cover of this textbook.

Locate and click on Comprehensive Evaluation Test 2.

### Step 2

Answer the test questions. When you have finished, click the Submit Test button to close the window.

<table>
<tr><td>ALERT</td></tr>
<tr><td>Make certain you set the date and time correctly for this exercise.</td></tr>
</table>

## Part II—Critical Thinking Exercise CE3: Examination of a Patient with Arterial Disease

In this exercise, you will use the skills you have acquired to document this patient encounter. Complete each step in sequential order using the instructions and other information provided.

### Case Study

Brenda Green is a 54-year-old flight attendant with a history of hypertension and possible peripheral arterial disease of the legs. During her last visit, she complained of pain in the legs and cold feet following exercise. After performing an ankle-brachial index test in the office, the clinician ordered an angiogram. Brenda is coming today for the results of her test and a follow-up exam.

### Step 1

Start a supported web browser program and follow the steps listed inside the cover of this textbook to log in to the MyHealthProfessionsLab for this course.

Locate and click on the link **Exercise CE3**. This will open the Quippe software window with the New Encounter window displayed in the center.

### Step 2

In the New Encounter window patient list, locate and click on **Green, Brenda**.

Set the date to **May 31, 2016**, and the time to **10:15 AM** before clicking on the OK button.

### Step 3

Enter the Chief complaint: **Patient reports leg pain after exercise**.

### Step 4

Begin the visit by copying the Past Medical History, Assessment, and Tests to Order sections from her 5/18/2016 visit.

Return to the Current Encounter tab and drag **angiography of bilateral extremities** from Tests to Order and drop it on Test Results.

*Right-click* on angiography of bilateral extremities, and select Details from the drop-down menu. Change the Prefix to "**report for**."

### Step 5

Click on the tab for her 5/17/2016 visit. Copy the Current Medications and Plan sections into the current note.

Return to the Current Encounter tab and drag the prescription drug **atenolol** from Plan and drop it on Current Medications.

*Right-click* on atenolol, and select Details from the drop-down menu. Clear the Prefix by changing it from "ordered" to blank.

### Step 6

The clinician is going to treat her atherosclerosis by prescribing a blood thinner to prevent blood clots.

Locate Rx Writer in the right content pane under Favorites and click it.

Write a prescription for warfarin sodium, 1 milligram tablet

1 tab twice a day for 30 days, 3 refills, generic.

### Step 7

Patients on warfarin must have a blood test regularly. Search for **INR**. In the search results list, click the plus symbol next to INR and select **in blood or platelet poor plasma** and Add to Note. Locate the INR finding and click it until it turns red.

### Step 8

*Right-click* on the diagnosis in the Assessment section and create a problem group.

*Right-click* on the diagnosis and select **Prompt** from the drop-down menu.

### Step 9

Locate Past Medical History and drag the four findings in the Other group upward and drop them on the HPI section. Be certain they are still red.

Proceed to Personal History. Ms. Green has never smoked, but she has two martinis every night at cocktail hour.

- never smoked
- alcohol use
- hard liquor

Type **2** in the quantity field and select **glasses per day** from the drop-down list.

Proceed to Review of Systems, Cardiovascular symptoms and click all three findings until they turn red.

### Step 10

Document Brenda's vital signs and information about her active problem by using the **Hypertension** Wizard form.

When the form pop-up opens, enter Brenda's vital signs in the corresponding fields on the form as follows:

| | |
|---|---|
| Temperature: | **98.6** |
| Pulse: | **78** |
| Respiration: | **22** |
| SBP: | **130** |
| DBP: | **90** |
| Weight: | **210** |
| Height: | **68.5** |

### Step 11

Locate and click on the checkbox for the diagnosis:

✓ Y Systemic HTN

The clinician performs the Quick Screening Exam and finds everything normal. Click the Otherwise Normal button, and then the Next button to order medications. The clinician renews her atenolol and hydrochlorothiazide.

Click the Finish button.

### Step 12

*Right-click* on the assessment **systemic HTN** and create problem 2.

Click the View button on the toolbar and select Flowsheet view from the drop-down menu.

Scroll the flow sheet to the bottom, locate the row for ordered **pulse oximetry with ankle/brachial index**, and Copy Forward the result. Close the flow sheet view.

### Step 13

Locate Laboratory Studies and drag the finding you have just copied upward and drop it on Test Results.

*Right-click* on **pulse oximetry with ankle/brachial index**, select Details from the drop-down menu, and change the Prefix from "ordered" to **reviewed**.

### Step 14

The clinician advises her that, to avoid further blood clots, she must walk every day and exercise at home. Proceed to the Therapy section and click the following findings until they turn red.

- exercises as prescribed
- home exercises

### Step 15

The clinician reviews Decision support information on Deep Vein Thrombosis (DVT), and also prints and discusses DVT patient education materials with her, explaining the risk of blood clots from high-altitude flight. Ms. Green appears to understand.

### Step 16

The clinician also annotated a drawing to further explain the problem, and reviewed preventive measures. You will do these activities in the next exercise. For now, use what you have learned in Chapter 12 to invoke the E&M Calculator, calculate the E&M code, and add it to the note.

The clinician spent 35 minutes with Ms. Green, with more than half spent counseling. Also, both problems are active. Be certain to check the one that is new before you click the Calculate button.

### Step 17

If you wish to print a copy of your completed encounter notes for yourself or because your instructor requires you to turn them in, use the Create PDF option, and then print or download the PDF at this time.

Submit your completed work for a grade. This will complete Exercise CE3.

If time permits, proceed to Part III. Do not start the next exercise unless there will be enough time to complete it.

## Part III—Critical Thinking Exercise CE4: Counseling and Education for a Patient with Arterial Disease

In this exercise, you will continue with Brenda Green's visit, performing Clinical Quality Review and annotating a drawing to supplement the patient education materials you reviewed with her in the previous exercise.

### Step 1

Start a supported web browser program and follow the steps listed inside the cover of this textbook to log in to the MyHealthProfessionsLab for this course.

Locate and click on the link **Exercise CE4**. This will open the Quippe software window with the New Encounter window displayed in the center.

### Step 2

In the New Encounter window patient list, locate and click on **Green, Brenda**.

Set the date to **May 31, 2016**, and the time to **10:15 AM** before clicking on the OK button.

**Step 3**

When the encounter note is displayed, you will notice some but not all of the findings from the previous exercise are displayed. Have no concern. You have already been graded on the previous exercise. The number of findings displayed has been reduced only for convenience in this exercise.

In the Chief complaint type **CQM and Drawing** followed by *your name*.

**Step 4**

Continuing with Ms. Green's visit, the clinician clicks the View button and selects Quality Measures Review. Using wizards, document the CQMs as follows:

Current Medications have been reconciled.

The BMI and Follow Up – Plan is Dietary education, guidance, and counseling.

Tobacco use screening: Brenda has never smoked.

Breast Cancer screening, the clinician orders a mammogram.

Skip the influenza immunization screening.

Controlling High Blood Pressure is adequately controlled.

**Step 5**

Create an annotated drawing to explain the angiography results to the patient.

*Hint:* Click on a white space in the encounter pane, so no heading or finding has focus. Click the Browse button on the toolbar, and expand the trees "Sample Custom Content," "Shared Content," "Images," and "Full Body."

Add the anatomical image **Full Body Cardiovascular Front** to the encounter note.

An anatomical drawing similar to Figure C-1 will be inserted into the Physical Exam section of the encounter note.

Click on the image. The Drawing Editor tools will be invoked in the right pane.

Drag the lower right corner of the drawing canvas until it is a comfortable size for you to annotate.

**Step 6**

As closely as possible, replicate the drawing in Figure C-1.

Draw a blue circle over the femoral artery midway between the groin and the knee (as shown in Figure C-1).

Draw a horizontal line from the circle to the blank area of the drawing on the right.

Next, change the color to red by selecting the Color pallet button.

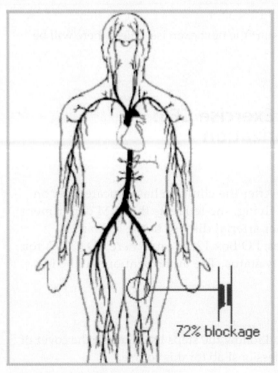

Anatomical Figure © Medicomp Systems, Inc.

**Figure C-1**  Drawing of annotations to be performed in Exercise CE-4.

72% blockage

In the blank area of the drawing, draw two vertical, parallel lines to represent an enlarged view of the artery.

Using the Pen, make a thick line on the interior of each of the parallel lines to represent the blockage in the artery (similar to Figure C-1).

Annotate the drawing. Change to the abc Text tool.

Click your mouse in the image to the right of the knee and a text field will open. Type **72% blockage**.

Compare your drawing to Figure C-1. If you need to correct the line or circle, change the tool button to "Select" and click on the object. Use the Delete button in the Toolbar and then redraw the correct element.

### Step 7

Click the Quippe icon button and select Create PDF from the drop-down menu.

Your instructor will direct you to either print the PDF and hand in your printout, or download the PDF and send it electronically.

### Step 8

Click the Quippe icon button and select Submit for Grade. This will complete Exercise CE4.

If time permits, proceed to Part IV. Do not start the next exercise unless there will be enough time to complete it.

## Part IV—Testing Your Skill Exercise CE5: Patient Signs HIPAA Authorization

### Case Study

Brenda Green is employed by an airline. After the clinician has educated her on the risks of DVT and suggested she stop flying, she requests the HIM department send her medical records pertaining to her arterial disease to the human resources department at On Time Airlines, PO Box 1234, Anywhere, ID 83207, for the purposes of determining her disability status. The authorization will be in effect for 1 year.

### Step 1

Start a supported web browser program and follow the steps listed inside the cover of this textbook to log in to the MyHealthProfessionsLab for this course.

Locate and click on the link **Exercise CE5**. This will open the Quippe software window with the New Encounter window displayed in the center.

### Step 2

In the New Encounter window patient list, locate and click on **Green, Brenda**.

You may use the current date for this exercise. Click on the OK button and the HIPAA Authorization screen will be displayed.

### Step 3

Using the information from the case study, complete the fields on the screen.

### Step 4

When you have filled in all the fields, imagine you have printed the document and Brenda has signed it. You do not need to create a PDF for this exercise unless you want to have a copy for yourself or because your instructor requires you to turn it in; in which case use the Create PDF option, and then print or download the PDF at this time.

Submit your completed work for a grade. This will complete Exercise CE5.

# Glossary

**A1C** glycosylated hemoglobin (blood glucose test also called HbA1c). A test that measures the average amount of sugar in the patient's blood over the past three months.

**ABG** A medical abbreviation for arterial blood gas.

**ABN** An acronym for Advance Beneficiary Notice—information presented to the patient in advance that the test or procedure will not be covered by Medicare or insurance. The same acronym is sometimes uses as the abbreviation for Abnormal.

**Access Control (HIPAA)** Technical policies and procedures to allow access only to those persons or software programs that have been granted rights to access EPHI.

**Accession Number** A unique number assigned to a lab test, radiology study, or a case in a cancer registry.

**Acetaminophen** A medicine used as an alternative to aspirin to relieve pain and fever. The active ingredient in Tylenol.

**Actions (button)** A Quippe toolbar button that displays a drop-down menu of actions that may be done on the finding or heading that currently has focus; for example, invoke detail entry pop-up, delete the finding, or set a section of findings otherwise normal. The options in the Actions menu change by the type of encounter note element that has focus. The Actions menu can also be invoked by right-clicking the mouse.

**Acute** Severe, but of short duration.

**Acute Self-Limiting** Problems that normally resolve themselves over a short period of time.

**Administrative Safeguards (HIPAA)** These are the administrative functions that should be implemented to meet the standards of the HIPAA Security Rule. These include assigning security responsibility to an individual and security training requirements.

**Administrative Simplification (HIPAA)** The Administrative Simplification Subsection of HIPAA covers providers, health plans, and clearinghouses. It has four distinct components: Transactions and Code Sets, Uniform Identifiers, Privacy, and Security.

**Agonal Breathing** An abnormal pattern of breathing and brainstem reflex characterized by gasping, labored breathing. It is the last respiratory pattern prior to terminal apnea.

**AHIMA** An acronym for American Health Information Management Association, the leading organization of health information professionals.

**AHRQ** An acronym for Agency for Healthcare Research and Quality, a Public Health Service agency in the Department of Health and Human Services to support research designed to improve the quality, safety, efficiency, and effectiveness of healthcare for all Americans.

**Alert** A warning, message, or reminder automatically generated by EHR systems based on logical rules.

**AMA** An acronym for American Medical Association; also an acronym for Against Medical Advice.

**Ambulatory Setting** Outpatient setting.

**Amoxicillin** An oral antibiotic; a synthetic penicillin derived from ampicillin.

**Angina Pectoris** A disease marked by brief, recurrent pain, usually in the chest and left arm, caused by a sudden decrease of the blood supply to the heart muscle.

**Angiogram** An x-ray (roentgenogram) of the flow of blood after injecting a contrast material.

**Angiography** *See* Angiogram.

**Annotated Drawing** Anatomical drawings of the body and body systems on which the clinician has marked observations and text notes.

**ANSI** An acronym for American National Standards Institute, a private, nonprofit organization that administers and creates product and communication standards in the United States. ANSI uses a voluntary consensus process to arrive at and maintain standards not only in healthcare but also in many diverse areas of industry and manufacturing.

**ARRA** an acronym for American Recovery and Reinvestment Act, federal legislation that included the HITECH Act. *See* HITECH Act.

**Assessment (chart)** The diagnosis or determination arrived at by the clinician from the medical examination, subjective and objective findings, and test results.

**Assignment of Benefits** A patient's authorization for a payer to send remittance directly to the provider.

**Asthma** A generally chronic disorder often caused by an allergic origin, characterized by wheezing, coughing, labored breathing, and a suffocating feeling.

**Asynchronous telemedicine** Independent sessions not occurring at the same time also called store-and-forward telemedicine.

**Auscultation** Listening (in this text, listening with a stethoscope).

**Authorization (HIPAA)** Authorization differs from consent in that it does require the patient's permission to disclose PHI. Under the HIPAA Privacy Rule, authorization is required for most disclosures of PHI other than for treatment of the patient, seeking payment, or operation of the healthcare facility.

**Beneficiary** The individual member covered by the health insurance policy.

**BID** A medical abbreviation for "twice daily."

**Biomedical Devices** Monitoring devices and instruments that attach to the patient or are intended for the patient to touch. Examples include telemetry devices for measuring vital signs, cardiac function, or arterial blood gas.

**BIPAP** A medical abbreviation for Bilevel Positive Airway Pressure.

**Blood Glucose Level** The amount of glucose (a type of sugar) in the blood at the time the specimen is taken. A random blood glucose test is done without regard to when the patient last ate. A fasting blood glucose test is done after a patient has not had food or drink (except water) for 12 hours.

**BMI** An acronym for Body Mass Index, a number that shows body weight adjusted for height.

**BMP** A medical abbreviation for basic metabolic panel.

**Bradycardia** Abnormally slow heart rate (less than 60 beats per minute).

**Bronchitis** A disease marked by inflammation of the bronchial tubes.

**Browse (button)** Displays the Medcin nomenclature hierarchy. Also accesses Sample Custom Content such as lists, forms, and images.

**Bullets (for E&M)** A bullet is a typographic character that looks like this: • (a solid black circle). Bullets are printed in the E&M guideline tables next to certain individual elements of the examination pertaining to a body area or organ system. The level of the examination component when calculating E&M code is determined by the number of findings in the exam that corresponded to elements in the guideline table with bullet characters printed next to them.

**Business Associate Agreement** The HIPAA Privacy Rule requires covered entities that use the services of other persons or businesses to obtain a written agreement that the business associate will comply with the protection of PHI under the Privacy Rule.

**Button (software)** A raised or indented object in the software used to invoke an action or change of state when clicked on with a mouse. Found in most Windows software programs, buttons usually contain a word or icon representing their function.

**Bypass Surgery** *See* Cardiac Bypass.

**Cardiac Bypass** A surgical shunt to divert blood supply from one circulatory path to another.

**Cardiac Catheterization** A test to evaluate the heart and arteries. A thin flexible tube is threaded through a blood vessel into the heart, then a contrast material is injected to trace the movement of blood through the coronary arteries.

**Cardiovascular** The heart and the system of blood vessels.

**CAT Scan** Computerized Axial Tomography uses multiple x-rays and a computer to generate images of cross sections of the body.

**CBC** An acronym for Complete Blood Count, which is a lab test that includes separate counts for both white and red blood cells.

**CC** *See* Chief Complaint.

**CCC** An acronym for Clinical Care Classification system used by nurses to codify documentation of patient care in any setting.

**CDA** An acronym for Clinical Document Architecture, an HL7 standard for incorporating clinical text reports or other information in a Claim Attachment.

**CDC** An acronym for the Centers for Disease Control, an agency of the U.S. Department of Health and Human Services.

**CDISC** An acronym for Clinical Data Interchange Standards Consortium, an organization that has created standards that enable sponsors, vendors, and clinicians to acquire and exchange data used in clinical drug trials. CDISC has become part of HL7.

**CDR** An acronym for Clinical Data Repository, a database used to aggregate EHR data from several disparate systems.

**Certified EHR** EHR software that has been certified by an ONC Authorized Certification Body to be capable of meeting provisions of the HITECH Act.

**CHCS II** An acronym for Composite Health Care System II, the U.S. Department of Defense Electronic Health Record System.

**CHF** A medical abbreviation for Congestive Heart Failure.

**Chief Complaint** A concise statement describing the symptom, problem, condition, diagnosis, physician-recommended return, or other factor that is the reason for the encounter, usually stated in the patient's words.

**Chronic** Disease or problem that lasts a long time or recurs often.

**Cite/Citation (software)** A feature of the software that allows findings from previous exams to be copied to the bottom of the current encounter without counting as new findings in the current encounter. Cited findings cannot be updated or changed.

**Clearinghouse** *See* Healthcare Clearinghouse.

**Clinical Concepts** Pre-correlated findings in the Medcin nomenclature.

**Clinical Terminology** An organized list of medical phrases and codes. *See* Nomenclature.

**Clinical Vocabulary** An organized list of medical phrases and codes. *See* Nomenclature.

**CME** An acronym for Continuing Medical Education, courses required to maintain licenses for licensed healthcare professionals.

**CMS** An acronym for the Centers for Medicare and Medicaid Services, an agency of the U.S. Department of Health and Human Services (formerly HCFA).

**COB** Coordination of Benefits; when a patient is covered by more than one health insurance plan, the plans involved determine how much each plan is to pay. A HIPAA transaction permits the plans to do this electronically.

**Codified Data (chart)** EHR data with each finding assigned a standard code assures uniformity of the medical records, eliminates ambiguities about the clinician's meaning, and facilitates communication between multiple systems.

**Comorbidity** A diagnosed condition that coexists with the principal reason for hospitalization and will affect the treatment or length of stay.

**Comprehensive Metabolic Chem Panel** A blood test to determine blood sugar level, electrolytes, fluid balance, kidney function, and liver function. The panel measures (in blood) the sodium, potassium, calcium, chloride, carbon dioxide, glucose, blood urea nitrogen (BUN), creatinine, total protein, albumin, bilirubin, alkaline phosphatase transferase (ALP), aspartate amino transferase (AST), and alamine amino transferase (ALT).

**Consent (HIPAA)** Under the revised HIPAA Privacy Rule, a patient gives consent to the use of their PHI for purposes of treatment, payment, and operation of the healthcare practice by acknowledging that they have received a copy of the office's privacy policy. HIPAA privacy consent should not be confused with *informed* consent to perform a medical procedure.

**Content Pane** Right pane of Quippe software displays patient information, active problems, sources and orders in current encounter, and Rx Writer.

**Contingency Plan** Strategies for recovering access to EPHI should a medical office experience an emergency, such as a power outage or disruption of critical business operations. The goal is to ensure that EPHI is available when it is needed.

**Coordination of Care** Consultation or follow-up by two or more healthcare providers or facilities on a patient's care plan.

**Counseling** Therapeutic or educational services that are primarily rendered verbally to the patient.

**Covered Entity (HIPAA)** HIPAA refers to healthcare providers, plans, and clearinghouses as Covered Entities. In the context of this book, think of covered entity as the medical practice and all of its employees.

**CPOE** An acronym for Computerized Physician Order Entry; also for Computerized Provider Order Entry.

**CPR** A medical abbreviation for cardio-pulmonary resuscitation.

**CPRI** An acronym for Computer-Based Patient Record Institute, formed to promote the universal and effective use of electronic healthcare information systems to improve health and the delivery of healthcare was merged into HIMSS in 2002.

**CPT-4** An acronym for Current Procedural Terminology, fourth edition. CPT-4 are standardized codes for reporting medical services, procedures, and treatments performed for patients by the medical staff. CPT-4 is owned by the American Medical Association.

**CQM** An acronym for Clinical Quality Measures, data reported to CMS by a provider which indicates the quality of care provided by measuring the quantity of patients assessed or successfully treated according to evidence-based best practices.

**Cross-walk (codes)** A reference table for translating a code from one set to a code with the same meaning in another code set. For example, the Medcin and SNOMED-CT nomenclatures each have tables for translating a finding code to an ICD-10CM code.

**Cruciate Ligament (of the knee)** Two ligaments in the knee joint that cross each other from the femur to the tibia. The anterior one limits extension and rotation.

**CT (codes)** An acronym for Clinical Terms that were added to SNOMED.

**CT Scan** Computerized Tomography (*see* CAT Scan).

**CVP** A medical abbreviation for cerebral vascular pressure.

**DAW** The acronym for Dispensed As Written is used on a prescription as an instruction to dispense the exact brand of medication specified. Do not substitute a generic equivalent drug.

**Decision Support** Computer- or Internet-based systems used to improve the process and outcome of medical decisions by delivering evidence-based information to the clinician who is determining the diagnosis or treatment orders.

**Decryption** A method of converting an encrypted message back into regular text using a mathematical algorithm and a string of characters called a "key." *See also* Encryption.

**Detail Window** A pop-up window used to enter additional information about, or modify the meaning of, the finding that is selected at that time. *See* Prefix, Modifier, Results, Status, Episode, Onset, Duration, Value, Units, and Note.

**Diabetes Mellitus** A chronic form of diabetes; characterized by an insulin deficiency, an excess of sugar in the blood and urine, and by hunger, thirst, and gradual loss of weight.

**Diagnosis** A disease or condition; or the process of identifying the diseased condition. Generally codified using ICD-10CM.

**Diastolic Pressure** The measure of pressure in the arteries between heart beats.

**DICOM** An acronym for Digital Imaging and Communication. It is a standard for communication and file structure for transfer of digital images between equipment and computer systems.

**Digital Images (chart)** EHR data in image format. This includes diagnostic images, digital x-rays, as well as documents scanned into the EHR. *See also* Scanned Images. Image data usually requires specific software to view the image.

**Discrete Data (chart)** Information stored in a computer record as distinct segments. EHR data in computer format. Discrete data is typically either Fielded or Codified. Fielded data identifies the type of information by its position in the EHR record. Codified data pairs each piece of information with a code that identifies the information in a uniform way.

**Drop-down List** A standard feature in most Windows software, which displays a list of items the user may select when a mouse is clicked in the field or on a down-arrow button next to the field.

**Drug Formulary** Drug formularies are used to look up drugs by names or therapeutic class, provide an updated list of the drugs that are available in the inventory, provide information on costs, indications for use, treatment recommendations, dosage, guidelines, and prescribing information. Health insurance programs use the term *formulary* for plan-specific drug lists.

**DTaP** An acronym for Diphtheria, Tetanus, acellular Pertussis (whooping cough); a combination vaccine.

**DUR** An acronym for Drug Utilization Review, which is the process of comparing a prescription drug to a patient's history and recent medications for contraindications, overdosing, underdosing, allergic reactions, drug-to-drug interactions, and drug/food interactions.

**Duration (detail window)** The Duration field is used to enter a number and a unit of time related to the duration of the currently selected finding. The time unit can be "second," "minute," "hour," "day," "week," "month," "year," or their plurals.

**Dx/Mgt Options** An abbreviation used in the E&M calculator for Diagnosis and/or Management Options. The number of possible diagnoses and management options are factors in the Medical Decision Making component when determining the E&M code.

**Dysplasic Polyp** Abnormal growth, a tumor.

**E&M (codes)** An acronym for Evaluation and Management codes, which are a subset of CPT-4 codes used to bill for nearly every kind of patient encounter, such as physician office visits, inpatient hospital exams, nursing home visits, consults, emergency room doctors, and scores of other services. *See also* Key Components.

**E&M Calculator** A pop-up window in EHR software, which calculates then displays Evaluation and Management codes by analyzing the findings in the current encounter note.

**ECG** An acronym for Electrocardiogram.

**EDI** An acronym for Electronic Data Interchange. Information exchanged electronically as data in codified transactions.

**EHR** An acronym for Electronic Health Records—the portions of a patient's medical records that are stored in a computer system as well as the functional benefits derived from having an electronic health record.

**Electrolyte Panel** A blood test that measures the levels of the minerals sodium, potassium, and chloride in the blood. The test also measures the level of carbon dioxide, which takes the form bicarbonate when dissolved in the blood. Certain medications can create an electrolyte imbalance, which is often the reason an Electrolyte Panel is ordered for patients on those medications.

**Electronic Signature** A method of marking an electronic record as "signed" having the same legal authority as a written signature. The electronic signature process involves the successful identification and authentication of the signer at the time of the signature, binding of the signature to the document, and nonalterability of the document after the signature has been affixed. .

**Eligible Professionals** Providers designated as eligible to receive incentive payments under the HITECH Act.

**EMR** An acronym for Electronic Medical Record.

**Encounter** The medical record of an interaction between a patient and a healthcare provider.

**Encryption** A method of converting an original message of regular text into encoded text, which is unreadable in its encrypted form. The text is encrypted by means of an algorithm using a private "key." *See also* Decryption.

**Endoscopy** Examination of the digestive tract using a flexible tube with a light and camera.

**ENT** An acronym for Ears, Nose, and Throat.

**EPHI (HIPAA)** Protected Health Information in electronic form.

**Episode (detail window)** The record data regarding the frequency or interval of occurrence of a finding.

**ER** An abbreviation for Emergency Room or emergency department.

**Evidence-based** Developed by analyzing scientific evidence from current research and studies to determine the effectiveness.

**E-Visit** An E-visit is a patient encounter conducted over the Internet, without an office visit. The patient enters symptom, history, and HPI information, which is then reviewed by a clinician, who communicates via the Internet to ask additional questions, and provides a diagnosis, treatment orders, and patient education. E-visits are used only for nonurgent visits and are reimbursed by a growing number of insurance plans.

**Exacerbate** To cause a disease or its symptoms to become more severe; to aggravate the condition.

**Face-to-Face Time** The total time both before and after a patient visit (in the office or other or outpatient setting) such as taking patient history, performing the exam, reviewing lab results, planning for follow-up care, and communicating with other providers about the patient's case.

**Family History** Diseases, conditions, or syndromes that close members of the patient's family have had, that may be predictors of the same or a similar condition developing in the patient.

**FDA** An acronym for Food and Drug Administration, an agency of the U.S. Department of Health and Human Services. This federal agency regulates prescription and nonprescription drugs.

**FEIN** Federal Employer Identification Number—a number assigned by the U.S. Internal Revenue Service, also known as a business tax ID.

**FEV**1 Forced Expired Volume in one second; the volume of air expired in the first second of maximal exhalation after a full inhalation. This can be used to measure how quickly full lungs can be emptied.

**Fielded Data** Information packets identified by their position in a computer record.

**Findings** Clinical concepts that have a positive or negative (abnormal or normal) result.

**Floor/Unit Time** The total time both before and after a patient visit (in the hospital or nursing facility) such as taking patient history, performing the exam, reviewing lab results, planning for follow-up care, and communicating with other providers about the patient's case.

**Flow Sheet (software)** A feature of the software that presents data from multiple encounters in column format resembling a spreadsheet. Flow sheets allow findings from any previous encounter to be copied forward into the current note.

**Forms (software)** Forms are used to consistently display a desired group of findings in a presentation that allows for quick entry of not only the selected findings but of any detail fields as well. Forms are selected from the Browse button on the toolbar. Multiple forms may be used to document an encounter.

**Formulary** *See* Drug Formulary.

**Formulary Compliance Checking** A function of electronic prescription systems to verify that a drug about to be prescribed will be covered by the patient's insurance.

**Fraud and Abuse** As pertains to insurance billing, fraud and abuse is to maximize reimbursement by means that contradict regulatory guidelines. Examples include coding for services that were not justified or not performed, or unbundling a single complex procedure into multiple procedure codes instead of posting the correct code that represents the procedure as a whole.

**Free Text** EHR data that is not codified; may be attached to a codified finding as

supplemental notes. For example, Chief Complaint is a free-text field.

**FVC** An acronym for Forced Vital Capacity.

**Gallop** An abnormal heartbeat marked by three distinct sounds, like the gallop of a horse.

**Gastrointestinal** The stomach and the intestines.

**Generalized Pallor** An unusual paleness or lack of color, especially in the face.

**Genitourinary** The genital and urinary organs.

**GI/GU** An acronym for Gastrointestinal/Genitourinary body systems.

**Glucose Monitor** Home device used by diabetes patients to monitor glucose levels.

**GMDN** An acronym for Global Medical Device Nomenclature, used to identify the medical devices for ordering, inventory, or regulatory purposes, but does not provide for the codification of data from the devices.

**Google™** An Internet web site that provides a free, high-speed index of nearly every piece of information on the World Wide Web. The name is derived from Googol, the mathematical term for the number 1 followed by 100 zeros. Access Google by typing the address http://www.google.com in an Internet browser.

**Granularity** The degree or level of detail represented by a code in a nomenclature or medical coding system.

**Group Number** A number assigned by the insurance company to an employer-sponsored health plan.

**Growth Charts** A graph of growth measurements gathered from statistical studies of the growth rate of well-babies in a reference population.

**Guarantor** The person or entity financially responsible for any copay or patient due portion of a charge.

**H&P** An acronym for History and Physical.

**HAC** An acronym for Hospital Acquired Condition, an infection or other medical problem occurring after admission.

**HCAHPS** An acronym for Hospital Consumer Assessment Healthcare Providers and Systems, a standardized survey instrument and data collection methodology developed by NCQA for measuring patients' perspectives on care.

**HCFA** An acronym for the Health Care Financing Administration, which has since been renamed CMS. *See* CMS.

**HCPCS** An acronym for Healthcare Common Procedure Coding System. HCPCS is an extended set of billing codes for reporting

medical services, procedures, and treatments including codes not listed in CPT-4 codes.

**HDL** High Density Lipoprotein cholesterol in blood plasma, sometimes referred to as good cholesterol because of its tendency to pull LDL cholesterol out of the artery wall.

**Healthcare Clearinghouse** A computer system or covered entity that performs the specific function of translating nonstandard EDI transactions into HIPAA-compliant transactions.

**Health Level 7 (HL7)** A nonprofit organization and the leading messaging standard used by healthcare computer systems to exchange information.

**Health Plan or Payor** A for-profit or non-profit company, government entity, or employer self-sponsored plan providing health insurance coverage to patients.

**HEENT** An acronym for Head, Eyes, Ears, Nose, Mouth, Throat (body system).

**Hematocrit** A blood test to determine the ratio of packed red blood cells to the volume of whole blood; also the result of the test.

**Hematologic** Blood and blood-forming organs (discussed in the text as a component of a physical exam).

**Hemoglobin A1c** See A1c.

**Hepatic Function Panel** A blood test used to determine liver function and liver disease. The panel measures total protein, albumin, bilirubin, alkaline phosphatase transferase (ALP), aspartate amino transferase (AST), and alamine amino transferase (ALT).

**HepB** An acronym for Hepatitis B (vaccine).

**HHCC** An acronym for Home Health Care Classification nursing codes developed to codify documentation by home care nurses; the code set has evolved for use in all clinical settings and is now referred to as CCC.

**HHS** An acronym for U.S. Department of Health and Human Services.

**Hib** An acronym for Haemophilus Influenza Type B (vaccine).

**HIMSS** An acronym for Healthcare Information and Management Systems Society, which is an organization that provides leadership in healthcare for the management of technology, information, and change through member services, education and networking opportunities, and publications. Members include healthcare professionals, hospitals, corporate healthcare systems, clinical practice groups, HIT supplier organizations, healthcare consulting firms, and government agencies.

**HIPAA** An acronym for Health Insurance Portability and Accountability Act (of 1996). HIPAA law regulates many things; however, medical offices often use the term

**HIPAA** when they actually mean only the Administrative Simplification Subsection of HIPAA. *See* Administrative Simplification (HIPAA).

**History (Key Component)** The E&M component of an encounter document consisting of chief complaint, history of present illness, past medical history, family history, social history, and review of systems.

**HIT** An acronym for Health Information Technology; also Healthcare Information Technology.

**HITECH Act** An acronym for the Health Information Technology for Economic and Clinical Health Act, federal legislation that promoted the widespread adoption of EHR systems by authorizing incentive payments for providers that use EHR.

**HIV** An acronym for Human Immunodeficiency Virus (disease).

**HL7** An acronym for Health Level Seven, the leading messaging standard used to exchange clinical and administrative data between different healthcare computer systems.

**Holter Monitor** A device worn by the patient to record the heart rhythm continuously for 24 hours. This provides a record that can be analyzed by a cardiologist to determine any irregular or abnormal activity of the heart. Named for Dr. Norman Holter, its inventor.

**HPI** An acronym for History of Present Illness, which is a chronological description of the development of the patient's present illness from the first sign or symptom or from the previous encounter to the present.

**Hyperlipidemia** High levels of fat in the blood, such as cholesterol and triglycerides.

**Hypertension** A disease of abnormally high blood pressure.

**Hypotension** Abnormally low blood pressure.

**ICD-10CM** An acronym for International Classification of Diseases, Tenth Revision. In the United States ICD-10-CM is the standard for diagnosis codes.

**ICD-10-PCS** International Classification of Diseases, Tenth Revision, Procedure Coding System (but not derived from the ICD-10 codes). PCS stands for Procedure Coding System, and is the standard for inpatient procedure codes.

**Icon (software)** In computer software, a small image usually used on a button to represent the purpose of the button—for example, a picture of a printer on the Print button.

**ICU** An acronym for Intensive Care Unit, a special section of the hospital with monitoring equipment and staff for seriously ill patients.

**IHS** An acronym for Indian Health Service, an agency of the U.S. Department of Health and Human Services responsible for providing federal health services to American Indians and Alaska natives.

**Immunologic** The immune system; discussed as a component of evaluation during a physical exam.

**Implementation Specifications** An additional detailed instruction for implementing a specific security standard under the HIPAA Security Rule.

**Incidental Disclosures (HIPAA)** HIPAA Privacy Rule permits incidental uses and disclosures of protected health information when the covered entity has in place reasonable safeguards and minimum necessary policies and procedures to protect an individual's privacy.

**Information System Activity Review (HIPAA)** A regular review of records such as audit logs, access reports, and security incident tracking reports. The information system activity review helps to determine if any EPHI is used or disclosed in an inappropriate manner.

**Informed Consent** The patient's agreement to receive medical treatment after having been provided sufficient information to make an informed decision.

**Inpatient** A hospital patient who stays overnight.

**Interoperability** The ability for a computer system to exchange data with a different system or software.

**IOM** An acronym for Institute of Medicine of the National Academies, a nonprofit organization created to provide unbiased, evidence-based, and authoritative information and advice concerning health and science policy.

**IPV** Inactivated Polio Virus (Salk vaccine).

**JCAHO** Joint Commission on Accreditation of Healthcare Organizations.

**Key Component** There are seven components that are evaluated to calculate the CPT-4 code for E&M services. Three of the components—history, examination, and medical decision making—are called the key components because they are used to determine the level of E&M services. *See also* E&M Codes.

**Kiosk** An unattended computer terminal for use by the patients in the waiting area.

**LAN** An acronym for Local Area Network, a network of computers that share data and programs located on a central computer called a server.

**Laparoscopy** Examination of the abdominal cavity through a small incision using a fiber optic instrument.

**LDL** Low Density Lipoprotein cholesterol in blood plasma; sometimes referred to as bad cholesterol, it is often associated with clogged arteries.

**Leapfrog Group** A coalition of 150 of the largest employers who created a strategy that tied purchase of group health insurance benefits to quality care standards, promoted Computerized Physician Order Entry, and the use of an EHR.

**Lipids Test Panel** A blood test that measures the levels of lipids (fats) in the bloodstream. A lipids profile measures total cholesterol, triglycerides, HDL (high-density lipoprotein), and LDL (low-density lipoprotein).

**LIS** An acronym for Laboratory Information System, a computer system that connects to and collects data from lab test instruments.

**List** A subset of the nomenclature (typically) used for a particular condition or type of exam, making it easier to locate frequently used clinical concepts.

**Login** A computer screen requiring the user to enter their name or ID (and password) before gaining access to the programs; or the action of entering a program through such a screen. EHR software typically requires the user to "log in." Note that some systems use the term "log on" for this function.

**LOINC** An acronym for Logical Observation Identifier Names and Codes. LOINC was created and is maintained by the Regenstrief Institute, affiliated with the Indiana University School of Medicine, and is an important clinical terminology for laboratory test orders and results.

**Lymphatic System** A network of lymph nodes and small vessels that collects lymph and returns it to the bloodstream.

**Macular Degeneration** A disease marked by the loss of central vision in both eyes.

**Malicious Software** Software such as viruses, Trojans, and worms create an unauthorized infiltration to computer networks that can damage or destroy data or create the need for expensive and time-consuming repairs. Malicious software is frequently brought into an organization through e-mail attachments and programs that are downloaded from the Internet. One requirement of the HIPAA Security Rule is to protect against malicious software.

**Mammogram** An x-ray of the breast that can be used to detect tumors before they can be seen or felt.

**Mammography** *See* Mammogram.

**MDM** An acronym for Medical Decision Making (a key component).

**Meaningful Use** Criteria that providers must meet to qualify for incentive payments under the HITECH Act.

**MEDCIN** A medical nomenclature and knowledge base developed by Medicomp Systems, Inc. Recognized as a national standard, it is incorporated in many commercial EHR systems as well as the U.S. Department of Defense CHCS II system.

**Medical Decision Making (MDM)** A key component in calculating the level of E&M code; the level of complexity in Medical Decision Making is determined by the number of diagnoses and management options, the amount or complexity of data to be reviewed, and the risk of complications or morbidity or mortality.

**Medical Decision Support** *See* Decision Support.

**Member Number** A unique number assigned by the insurance plan to a covered individual. Sometimes called an insurance id number.

**Menu Bar** The Menu Bar consists of a row of words across the top of the Document/Image System screen: File, Select, View, Setup, and Help. Clicking the mouse on any of the words on the Menu Bar will display a drop-down list of related software functions. Clicking the mouse on an item in the drop-down list will invoke that function.

**Metformin** An oral medication used along with a diet and exercise program to control high blood sugar in diabetic patients.

**Microscopy** Studies or images of studies performed using a microscope.

**Minimum Necessary Standard (HIPAA)** A standard in the HIPAA Privacy Rule intended to limit unnecessary or inappropriate access to and disclosure of PHI beyond what is necessary. The minimum necessary standard does not apply to disclosures to or requests for information used by a healthcare provider for treatment of the patient.

**MMR** An acronym for a combination of vaccines to immunize against Measles, Mumps, Rubella (German measles).

**Modifier (detail window)** The Modifier field is used to modify a selected finding. For example, the finding "Pain" may be qualified as mild, severe, and such.

**Morbidity** A diseased state or symptom.

**MOU** An acronym for Memorandum of Understanding (between government entities). It can be used between government agencies to meet the HIPAA Security Rule requirement in lieu of Business Associate agreements.

**Mouse (computer)** A computer device for moving the pointer or cursor on the screen, selecting items, and invoking actions in operating system and application software.

**Mouse Button** A button on the mouse that when pressed causes a software program to invoke some action. The following applies only to the Student Edition software. A single click of the left button is used to record, highlight, or select a finding, heading, button, or other object. Active Problems require a double-click of the left mouse button to invoke a merge prompt of related findings. (Double-click is to press the left button twice in quick succession.) Clicking and holding the left button while moving the mouse will drag a finding, resize a flow sheet, or make a mark when annotating a drawing. Clicking the right button on a finding or heading invokes the Actions drop-down menu for the type of item clicked.

**Mouse Pointer** Typically an arrow shape that moves over the Window program in relationship to the movements of the mouse by the user. It also is sometimes referred to as a "cursor." When flow sheets, Clinical Quality Measures, or drawing images are used in the Student Edition software, the shape of the mouse pointer will change to a double-ended arrow at points where the pane or drawing object may be resized by dragging.

**MPI** An acronym for Master Person Index, a central database of demographic information for persons registered in a healthcare facility or organization.

**MRI** An acronym for Magnetic Resonance Imaging, which uses magnetic fields and pulses of energy to create images of organs and structures inside the body that cannot be seen by x-ray or CAT scan.

**Musculoskeletal** Components of the physical exam involving both the musculature and the skeleton.

**MVV** An acronym for Maximal Voluntary Ventilation, which is a measurement of the total volume of air that a person can breathe in and out of the lungs in 1 minute.

**NASA** An acronym for National Aeronautics and Space Administration.

**Nasal Turbinate** Spongy, spiral-shaped bones in the nose passages.

**Nature of the Presenting Problem** The degree or severity of the problem for which the patient is being seen or treated.

**Navigation Bar** A strip at the bottom of the Quippe workspace pane listing the principal headings in the encounter template. Clicking on a link in the Navigation bar highlights the corresponding section and if necessary scrolls the encounter pane to the highlighted section.

**NCQA** An acronym for the National Committee for Quality Assurance, a not-for-profit organization dedicated to improving healthcare quality by measuring the performance of providers and health plans. NCQA is the developer of the HEDIS and PCMH standards.

**NCVHS** An acronym for National Committee on Vital and Health Statistics, an advisory panel within the U.S. Department of Health and Human Services, which selects national standards for HIPAA and recommends standards for the federal government initiatives on Electronic Health Records.

**NDC** An acronym for National Drug Code. The NDC is the standard identifier for human drugs. It is assigned and used by the pharmaceutical industry.

**NEC** An acronym for Not Elsewhere Classified (diagnosis codes).

**Neurological Disorders** Disorders of the nervous system.

**Nevi** Moles on the skin; plural of nevus.

**NHII** An acronym for National Health Information Infrastructure, a plan to make EHR records available wherever the patient is treated.

**NHS** An acronym for National Health Service, the national medical system in the United Kingdom.

**NLM** An acronym for the United States National Library of Medicine; a unit of the National Institute of Health, it is the world's largest medical library.

**Nomenclature** A system of names created by a recognized group or authority and used in a field of science. An EHR nomenclature is an organized list of medical phrases and codes that helps to standardize the way clinicians record information. These are also referred to as clinical vocabularies or clinical terminologies.

**NOS** An acronym for Not Otherwise Specified (diagnosis codes).

**Note (detail window)** The Note field (in detail windows) is used to enter a free-text note attached to the currently selected finding. (*See also* Free Text.)

**NPI** An acronym for National Provider Identifier for doctors, nurses, and other healthcare providers.

**OB** Obstetrics is the field of specialty concerned with pregnancy, childbirth, and the period following.

**Objective (chart)** The clinician's observations and findings from the physical exam.

**OCR (computer)** An acronym for Optical Character Recognition, which is software that can analyze scanned document images, identify typed characters, and convert them into computer text.

**OCR (HIPAA)** An acronym for Office for Civil Rights, an agency of the Department of Health and Human Services that enforces the HIPAA Privacy Rule, in addition to other federal laws.

**OIG** An acronym for Office of Inspector General (Department of Health and Human Services).

**ONC** An acronym for the Office of National Coordinator for Health Information Technology, an agency of the U.S. Department of Health and Human Services responsible for creating a national health information network and encouraging the use of EHR systems.

**ONC-ATCB** An acronym for organizations designated by the Office of the National Coordinator as Authorized Testing and Certification Body for purposes of certifying EHR systems.

**Onset (detail window)** The Onset field is used to enter a number and a unit of time related to the onset of the currently selected finding. The time unit can be "second," "minute," "hour," "day" "week," "month," "year," or their plurals. Alternatively, a date can be typed in mm/dd/yyyy format.

**Otitus Media** Inflammation of the middle ear, often accompanied by pain, fever, dizziness, or hearing abnormalities.

**Otolaryngeal** Ears, Nose, and Throat.

**Outpatient** A patient who is examined or treated at a healthcare facility but is not hospitalized overnight. In this textbook, outpatient applies to all medical offices and clinics without overnight accommodation.

**PAC(S)** An acronym for Picture Archive and Communication System, a computer system that stores diagnostic images such as x-rays and CAT scans.

**Pane (software)** Two windows within the Student Edition software, each capable of displaying and updating information. The left pane displays the encounter note, flow sheet, drawing canvas, and Clinical Quality Measures Review. The right pane, generally referred to as the content pane, displays patient information, active problems, orders, drawing tools, and sources of clinical concepts currently displayed in the encounter pane such as forms, lists, merge prompts, and items copied from previous encounters.

**Patient Account** A unique number assigned at patient registration to an individual or family to which charges and payments are applied.

**Patient-Centered Medical Home** An approach to providing comprehensive primary care in a healthcare setting that facilitates partnerships between individual patients, their personal physicians, and when appropriate, the patient's family.

**PDF** An acronym for Portable Document Format, a file format that retains the layout and fonts of the original document.

**PEA** A medical abbreviation for Pulseless Electrical Activity.

**PEFR** An acronym for Peak Expiratory Flow Rate of air exhaled from the lungs.

**Pending Order** A lab test or diagnostic procedure that has been ordered but for which no results have been received.

**Percent Effort** The portion of a scheduled appointment that will require the scheduled provider's presence in the room.

**Percentiles** Lines on a pediatric growth chart representing the growth rate of well-babies in a reference population.

**Personal Representative (HIPAA)** The HIPAA Privacy Rule allows a patient to appoint a personal representative and requires covered entities to treat an individual's personal representative as the individual with respect to uses and disclosures of the individual's protected health information and the individual's rights under the Privacy Rule.

**Pertinent Negatives** Findings that are negative or within normal limits, the absence or normality of which help to rule out conditions the patient does not have.

**Pertussis** Whooping cough (vaccine).

**PET** Positron Emission Tomography combines CT (Computer Tomography) and nuclear scanning using a radioactive substance called a tracer, which is injected into a vein. A computer records the tracer as it collects in certain organs, then converts the data into a three-dimensional image of the organ, which can be used to detect or evaluate cancer.

**PFSH** An acronym for Past History, Family History, and Social History, obtained from patient or other family member.

**Pharmacy Benefit Manager** A company that serves as a middleman between the health insurance plan and pharmacy to identify if a drug is covered and what the patient copay will be.

**Pharynx** The muscular and membranous cavity leading from the mouth and nasal passages to the larynx and esophagus.

**PHI (HIPAA)** An acronym for Protected Health Information; a patient's personally identifiable health information (in any form) is protected by the HIPAA Privacy Rule.

**Phlebotomist** A medical technician who draws blood specimens.

**PHR** An acronym for Personal Health Record, an electronic health record owned and maintained by the patient.

**Physical Examination (Key Component)** The E&M component of an encounter document consisting of vital signs, measurements, findings of direct examination, or observation of the patient.

**Physical Safeguards (HIPAA)** The HIPAA Security Rule requirements to implement physical mechanisms to protect electronic systems, equipment, and EPHI from threats, environmental hazards, and unauthorized intrusion. They include restricting access to EPHI and retaining off-site computer backups.

**PIN** An acronym for Personal Identification Number, a secret number used like a password.

**PKI** An acronym for Public Key Infrastructure, which is used to secure messages or electronically sign documents.

**Plan of Treatment** Prescribed therapy, medication, orders, and patient instructions for treatment or management of the diagnosed condition.

**PMS** A medical abbreviation for Premenstrual Syndrome.

**POA** Acronym for "present on admission," which is an indicator that a condition was present at the time of the order for inpatient admission. The POA indicator is required for each primary and secondary diagnosis on an inpatient claim.

**Point-of-care Documentation** The ability to completely document the encounter while both the patient and provider are present.

**Point-of-care Testing** Laboratory tests that can be performed in the office or at a bedside in a hospital without requiring a specimen to be sent to a reference laboratory or pathology department.

**Policy Holder** The employee or individual in whose name a health insurance policy is obtained.

**Policy Number** A unique id assigned to a healthcare policy by the insurance plan.

**Polydipsia** Excessive, abnormal thirst.

**Posting** A term used for the act of entering data into the practice management or hospital system—for example, entering charges and payments into the patient accounting system.

**Prefix (detail window)** The Prefix field (in detail windows) is used to qualify a selected finding. The prefix will change the meaning of a finding and sometimes the section in which it would normally appear. For example, asthma without a prefix is a diagnosis. With the prefix "History of," it is past medical history. With the prefix "Family," it is about someone other than the patient.

**Primary Diagnosis** The principal reason for the patient's visit, or the most important of several conditions present.

**Privacy Official (HIPAA)** One individual designated by the medical practice as having overall responsibility for the HIPAA Privacy Rule.

**Privacy Policy** Covered entities are required to adopt a privacy policy, which meets the requirements of the HIPAA Privacy Rule, and to provide a copy of it to patients.

**Privacy Rule (HIPAA)** Federal privacy protections for individually identifiable health information.

**PRN** A medical abbreviation for "as needed."

**Problem List** Acute conditions for which the patient was recently seen as well as chronic conditions such as high blood pressure, diabetes, and so on, which are monitored at nearly every visit, and can affect decisions about medications and treatments for even unrelated illness.

**Problem-Oriented Chart** A method of documenting or viewing a patient's chart by grouping each problem or condition with the correlating treatment plan findings related to that condition.

**Proctosigmoidoscopy** *See* Sigmoidoscopy.

**Prompt (button)** A button on the toolbar with a numeral indicating how many findings are merged when using the Intelligent Prompting feature. Prompt 1 displays the least number of findings; Prompt 3 displays the most.

**Protocol** Standard plans of therapy used to treat a disease or condition.

**PSA** An acronym for Prostate-Specific Antigen, a test used to detect possible cancer of the prostate gland in men.

**Psittacosis** An infection acquired from raising birds.

**Pulmonary Embolism** Obstruction of the pulmonary artery or one of its branches by an abnormal particle such as a blood clot.

**Purulent Discharge** Pus or puslike discharge.

**PVC** An acronym for Pneumococcal Conjugate (vaccine).

**Quippe** A clinical documentation tool used as the basis of commercial EHR applications to incorporate the Medcin knowledge base and utilize the rich intelligence and functionality of Medcin. Quippe is the basis for the Student Edition software for this book.

**Radiologists** Specialists who interpret x-rays, CAT scans, and other diagnostic images.

**Radiology Information System** Software used to schedule, bill, and track diagnostic tests that are interpreted by radiologists.

**RAM** An acronym for Random Access Memory, a measure of the quantity of computer memory.

**Reference Laboratory** A pathology laboratory that tests medical specimens, usually located outside the medical facility.

**RELMA** A free software program provided by Regenstrief Institute to assist with LOINC coding. *See also* LOINC.

**Remote Access** The ability to access the EHR from outside the medical facility network by using a direct-dial connection or a secure connection through the Internet.

**Requisition Number** *See* Accession Number.

**Resectable** Surgically removable.

**Review of Systems** An inventory of body systems starting from the head down, often referred to as ROS. The body systems in a standard ROS are Constitutional symptoms, HEENT (Head, Eyes, Ears, Nose, Mouth, Throat), Cardiovascular, Respiratory, Gastrointestinal, Genitourinary, Musculoskeletal, Integumentary (skin and/or breast), Neurological, Psychiatric, Endocrine, Hematologic/Lymphatic, and Allergic/Immunologic.

**Rhinitis** Inflammation of the mucus membrane of the nose.

**RHIO** An acronym for Regional Health Information Organizations, entities formed to facilitate data exchange of patient medical information in a region or state.

**Rhonchi** Rattling or snoring sounds heard in the chest when there is a partial bronchial obstruction.

**RIS** An acronym for Radiology Information System.

**Risk Analysis (HIPAA)** Identify potential security risks, and determine the probability of occurrence and magnitude of risks.

**Risk Management (HIPAA)** Making decisions about how to address security risks and vulnerabilities.

**ROS** An acronym for Review of Systems. *See* Review of Systems.

**RT** An acronym for Respiratory Therapist.

**Rx** An abbreviation for therapy orders including, but not limited to drug prescriptions.

**Rx Writer (button)** Located in the content pane, favorites group; invokes the prescription writer.

**Rx Norm** A nonproprietary vocabulary developed by the NLM to codify drugs at the level of granularity needed in clinical practice.

**Sanction Policy (HIPAA)** An office policy to deter noncompliance so that workforce members understand the consequences of failing to comply with security policies and procedures.

**Scanned Data (chart)** Exam Notes, Letters, Reports, and other documents that have been converted to an image by use of a scanner, then stored in the EHR. The data is accessible by a person viewing the chart, but the image contents cannot be used as data by the system for trend analysis, health maintenance, or similar purposes.

**Scroll Bar (software)** A scroll bar is a feature of most Windows software that automatically appears on the right of a list or text that is too long to fit in the window. The scroll bar has a button that can be moved by pressing the mouse button when dragging the mouse. The information in the window (or window pane) scrolls respective to the movement of the mouse.

**Search (toolbar textbox)** A word search used to quickly locate all findings in the nomenclature containing either matching words or synonyms of the search word.

**Secondary Diagnosis** A condition present in the patient that is not the principal reason for the visit or hospitalization.

**Secure Messaging** A recommended alternative to sending PHI in e-mail messages; secure messaging uses a secure Web page to read and write messages. The only message sent as e-mail is an alert to the receiving party that the actual message is waiting on the secure site. The contents of secure messages are stored in a secure server not in an e-mail system.

**Security Official (HIPAA)** One individual designated by the medical practice as having overall responsibility for the HIPAA Security Rule; however, specific security responsibilities may be assigned to other individuals.

**Security Reminders (HIPAA)** One of the implementation requirements in the HIPAA Security Rule, it includes notices, agenda items, and specific discussion topics at monthly meetings, as well as formal retraining about office security policies and procedures.

**Security Rule (HIPAA)** HIPAA security standards requiring implementation of appropriate security safeguards to protect health information stored in electronic form.

**Sig** Instructions for labeling a prescription (from Latin *signa*).

**Sigmoidoscopy** Examination of the rectum, colon, and sigmoid flexure using an illuminated, tubular instrument.

**Sinusitis** Inflammation of the sinus of the skull.

**SNOMED-CT** A medical nomenclature developed by the College of American Pathologists and United Kingdom's National Health Service. It is now owned, maintained, and distributed by the International Health Terminology Standards Development Organisation, a not-for-profit association in Denmark.

**SOAP** A defined structure for documenting a patient encounter by organizing the information into four sections. The acronym SOAP represents the first letter of each of the section titles: subjective, objective, assessment, and plan.

**Specimen** Blood, tissue, urine, stool, or other physiological sample to be analyzed or cultured in laboratory test.

**Spirometer** An instrument that measures how much and how quickly air can enter and leave the lungs. Measurements may include VC (Vital Capacity), FVC (Forced Vital Capacity), PEFR (Peak Expiratory Flow Rate), MVV (Maximal Voluntary Ventilation), and FEV (Forced Expired Volume).

**Spirometry** An objective measurement useful in the diagnosis and management of asthma and other lung conditions. (*See* Spirometer.)

**SSL** An acronym for Secure Socket Layer that transparently encrypts and decrypts Web pages over the Internet.

**Status (detail window)** The Status field (in detail windows) is used to add the status of the currently selected finding. Examples include worsening, improving, resolved, and similar designations.

**Store-and-forward Telemedicine** *See* Asynchronous Telemedicine.

**Stress Test** An electrocardiogram performed before, during, and after strenuous exercise, to measure heart function.

**Subjective (chart)** The patient describes in his or her own words what the problem is, what the symptoms are, and what he or she is experiencing.

**Systolic Pressure** The measure of pressure exerted on the walls of the arteries when the muscle contracts.

**Tablet (computer)** A self-contained battery-operated computer thinner than a laptop computer but using a finger or special stylus to replace the mouse, thus allowing the computer to be used as though the user was writing on a tablet.

**Tachypnea** Fast breathing.

**Td** An abbreviation for Tetanus and Diphtheria toxoids vaccine.

**Technical Safeguards (HIPAA)** Primarily automated processes used to protect EPHI data and control access to data. They include using authentication controls to verify that the person signing onto a computer is authorized to access that EPHI, or encrypting and decrypting data as it is being stored or transmitted.

**Telemedicine** Uses communication technology to deliver medical care to a patient in another location, usually through online consultation with that person's physician.

**Telemonitors** Biomedical devices worn by the patient to capture vital signs or other data during the course of normal activity. The data is then downloaded or transmitted to the EHR.

**Teleradiology** Uses communication technology to enable a radiologist in another location to interpret diagnostic images remotely.

**Template** A Quippe template is the starting point for an encounter note and defines the layout, visual style, and placement rules for the note.

**Text Data (chart)** Information stored in the EHR as word processing, blocks of text, or text reports. The data is searchable but neither codified nor standardized and is generally not indexed.

**Text Files** EHR data consisting of alphanumeric characters arranged in paragraphs and not in a fielded structure.

**Time Component** The portion of the encounter in which the clinician spent face-to-face time with the patient, but which also includes reviewing lab results, planning for follow-up care, and communicating with other providers about the patient's case.

**Toolbar** A "Toolbar" is a row of icon buttons, the purpose of which is to allow quick access to commonly used functions.

**Total Cholesterol** A blood test that measures the total of all cholesterol in the blood, including both HDL (high-density lipoprotein) and LDL (low-density lipoprotein).

**Transactions and Code Sets (HIPAA)** HIPAA regulations requiring all covered entities to use standard EDI transaction formats and standard codes within those transactions for claims, remittance advice and payments, claim status, eligibility, referrals, enrollment, premium payments, claim attachments, report of injury, and retail drug claims.

**Tree (software)** A standard Windows software method of displaying hierarchical lists using small plus and minus symbols to indicate where additional hierarchical levels are hidden from view. The tree structure is used in the Student Edition nomenclature and search lists to navigate the domains of clinical concepts. Clicking the mouse on the plus sign next to an item will "expand the tree" to display additional related findings in an indented list. Clicking on the minus sign next to an item will "collapse the tree," hiding all items in the indented list within the collapsed item. The purpose of the tree structure is to allow the user to quickly navigate extremely long lists by viewing only the level of hierarchy necessary.

**Trend Analysis** Comparing data from different dates, tests, or events to correlate the changes in the results with changes in the patient's health.

**Trending** Comparing a patient's results or measurements from several tests or visits.

**Triage** The screening of patients for allocation of treatment based on the urgency of their need for care. ER triage is often a sim-

plified, organ-specific review of systems conducted by the triage nurse, based on the presenting complaint.

**UMDNS** An acronym for Universal Medical Device Nomenclature System, which is used to identify the medical devices for ordering, inventory, or regulatory purposes, but does not provide for the codification of data from the devices.

**UMLS** An acronym for Unified Medical Language System from the National Library of Medicine. UMLS is not itself a medical terminology but, rather, a resource of software tools and data created from many medical nomenclatures to facilitate the development of EHR.

**Undercode** Intentionally selecting an E&M code one level below that to which the provider is entitled.

**Uniform Identifiers (HIPAA)** HIPAA regulations require all covered entities to adopt and use standard identification numbers for plans, providers, and employers in all HIPAA EDI transactions.

**Unit (detail window)** The Unit field (in detail windows) shows the currently selected unit for the currently selected finding, provided a standard unit exists. If more than one unit is available for selection, a drop-down list will be available.

**URI** An acronym for Upper Respiratory Infection. An infection affecting the nose, nasal passages, or upper part of the pharynx.

**URL** An acronym for Universal Resource Locator, the address of a web site—for example, www.pearson.com.

**U.S. Preventive Services Task Force** An independent panel of experts in primary care and prevention sponsored by AHRQ that systematically reviews the evidence of effectiveness and develops recommendations for clinical preventive services based on the patient's age, sex, and risk factors for disease. These recommendations are published by the AHRQ and also are incorporated in EHR systems from several vendors.

**UTI** A medical abbreviation for Urinary Tract Infection.

**VA** A common abbreviation for U.S. Department of Veteran Affairs.

**Value (detail window)** The Value field (in detail windows) is used to enter a numerical value for those findings that have a numeric value (for example, blood pressure, weight, test results, and similar designations).

**Varicella** Chicken pox (vaccine).

**Vasoconstrictor** An agent or drug that initiates or induces narrowing of the lumen (cavity) of blood vessels.

**VC** An acronym for Vital Capacity, a measure of the amount of air that can be forcibly exhaled after a full inhalation. An indicator of the breathing capacity of the lungs.

**Vital Signs** Functional measurements recorded at nearly every visit—temperature, respiration rate, pulse rate, and blood pressure; most clinics measure height and weight as well.

**Vital Statistics** Statistics of birth, death, disease, and health of a population.

**VPN** An acronym for Virtual Private Network. Data sent over a public network is encrypted and decrypted without user intervention to attain a level of security similar to a private network.

**WEP** An acronym for Wired Equivalent Privacy, a protocol for securing the content of signals sent over a wireless network.

**WHO** An acronym for World Health Organization.

**Wi-Fi** An abbreviation for Wireless Fidelity, a type of fast wireless computer networking. *See also* Wireless Network.

**Wireless Network** A local area computer network using radio signals in place of wired network cables.

**WNL (chart)** An acronym for Within Normal Limits in medical charts.

**Workspace** The left pane of Quippe, which displays the encounter note, flow sheet, clinical measures review, and code review.

**Workstation** A personal computer, usually connected to a main computer (server) via a network.

**XML** An acronym for eXtensible Mark-up Language, a file format similar to the hypertext mark-up language files, which contain fielded data with "tags" or names for the fields.

**X-Ray** Traditionally an image made by the passage of short wave radiation through the body onto photographic film. Digital receptors have now replaced film, allowing the image to be captured and stored in a computer form without photo processing.

# Index

## Acronyms Used in This Book

| | | | | |
|---|---|---|---|---|
| ABG | Arterial Blood Gas | | EDI | Electronic Data Interchange |
| ABN | Advance Beneficiary Notice | | EFT | Electronic Funds Transfer |
| ABN | Abnormal | | EHR | Electronic Health Record |
| ACA | Affordable Care Act | | EMR | Electronic Medical Record |
| ACE | angiotensin-converting-enzyme | | ENT | Ears, Nose, Throat |
| AHIMA | American Health Information Management Association | | EPHI | Protected Health Information in Electronic form |
| AHRQ | Agency for Healthcare Research and Quality | | EPs | Eligible Professionals |
| AMA | Against Medical Advice | | ER | Emergency Department or Emergency Room |
| ARRA | American Recovery and Reinvestment Act | | FDA | Food and Drug Administration |
| BID | Twice Daily | | FEIN | Federal Employer Identification Number |
| BIPAP | Bilevel Positive Airway Pressure | | GI | Gastrointestinal |
| BMI | Body Mass Index | | H&P | History and Physical |
| BMP | Basic Metabolic Panel | | HAC | Hospital Acquired Condition |
| CAT | Computerized Axial Tomography | | HCAHPS | Hospital Consumer Assessment Healthcare Providers and Systems |
| CBC | Complete Blood Count | | HCPCS | Healthcare Common Procedure Coding System |
| CC | Chief Complaint | | | |
| CCC | Clinical Care Classification system | | HDL-C | High-Density Lipoprotein (cholesterol test) |
| CCU | Critical Care Unit | | HEENT | Head, Eyes, Ears, Nose, (Mouth), and Throat |
| CDC | Centers for Disease Control and Prevention | | HepB | Hepatitis B (vaccine) |
| CDISC | Clinical Data Interchange Standards Consortium | | HHS | U.S. Department of Health and Human Services |
| CDR | Clinical Data Repository | | Hib | Haemophilus influenzae type B (vaccine) |
| CHF | Congestive Heart Failure | | HIE | Health Information Exchange |
| CIR | Citywide Immunization Registry (New York City) | | HIM | Health Information Management |
| | | | HIMSS | Health Information Management Systems Society |
| CME | Continuing Medical Education | | HIPAA | Health Insurance Portability and Accountability Act |
| CMS | Centers for Medicare and Medicaid Services | | | |
| COB | Coordination of Benefits | | HITECH | Health Information Technology for Economic and Clinical Health |
| CPOE | Computerized Provider Order Entry | | | |
| CPR | Cardio-Pulmonary Resuscitation | | HIV | Human Immunodeficiency Virus |
| CPRI | Computer-Based Patient Record Institute | | HL7 | Health Level 7 |
| CPT-4 | Current Procedural Terminology, 4th Revision | | HPI | History of Present Illness |
| | | | ICD-9-CM | International Classification of Diseases, ninth revision, with clinical modifications |
| CRNA | Certified Registered Nurse Anesthesiologist | | | |
| CT | Computed Tomography | | ICD-10CM | International Classification of Diseases, tenth revision, with clinical modifications |
| CVP | Cerebral Vascular Pressure | | | |
| DAW | Dispense As Written | | IMH | Instant Medical History |
| DICOM | Digital Imaging and Communications in Medicine | | IOM | Institute of Medicine |
| | | | IPV | Inactivated Polio Virus (vaccine) |
| DTaP | Diphtheria, Tetanus, Pertussis (vaccine) | | IT | Information Technology |
| DUR | Drug Utilization Review | | JCAHO | The Joint Commission on Accreditation of Healthcare Organizations |
| DVT | Deep Vein Thrombosis | | | |
| E&M | Evaluation and Management codes | | LAN | Local Area Networks |
| ECG or EKG | Electrocardiogram | | LIS | Laboratory Information System |